TECHNIQUES • IN *Therapeutic* ARTHROSCOPY

TECHNIQUES • IN

Therapeutic ARTHROSCOPY

Edited by J. Serge Parisien, MD, FACS

With illustrations by Gary Welch

Raven Press • New York

Distributed in the USA and Canada by:
Raven Press
1185 Avenue of the Americas
New York, NY 10036
USA

ISBN: 0-7817-0054-X

Library of Congress Cataloging-in-Publication Data
Techniques in therapeutic arthroscopy / edited by
J. Serge Parisien.
p. cm.
Includes bibliographical references and index.
ISBN 0-7817-0054-X
1. Joints—Endoscopic surgery. 2. Arthroscopy. I.
Parisien, J. Serge.
[DNLM: 1. Arthroscopy—methods. 2. Joints—surgery.
WE 312 T2556]
RD686.T36 1993
617.4'72059—dc20
92-49803

British Library Cataloguing-in-Publication Data
A catalogue record for this book is available
from the British Library.

Printed in Hong Kong by Imago

10 9 8 7 6 5 4 3 2 1

Editor/Project Manager: Elizabeth Greenspan
Illustration Director: Laura Pardi Duprey
Illustrators: Interior and Cover, Gary Welch;
Chapter 7, Steven J. Harrison
Line Drawings: Patricia Gast
Art Director/Cover Design: Kathryn Greenslade
Design and Layout: Paul Fennessy,
Thomas Tedesco
Typesetting Supervisor: Erick Rizzotto
Editorial Assistant: David Yoon

To my parents, to my wife, May,
and to my children, Christine and Alex

Preface

Major technological advances in fiberoptics and microsurgical instruments have contributed hugely to the present state of arthroscopic surgery. The usefulness of many of the techniques developed in the past decade has been demonstrated.

My purpose in editing *Techniques in Therapeutic Arthroscopy* is to present readers with a textbook that focuses on the various arthroscopic techniques most commonly used today. The intended readers (orthopedic residents, fellows, general orthopedic surgeons, arthroscopic surgeons, and sports medicine specialists) are already familiar with the basic principles of diagnostic arthroscopy and have an excellent knowledge of the indications and contraindications of arthroscopic surgery, so the contributors have emphasized the principles and fine points of the various techniques. Thus, pitfalls can be avoided and complications minimized.

Procedures for meniscal resection and repair and synovial and articular pathology are presented, using a wealth of color illustrations that make the written explanation simpler and clearer. When the indications for surgery exist in a patient who presents with anterior cruciate ligament injury, various arthroscopic methods, using either autogenous tissue, allograft, or synthetic materials, are presented. Particular attention is paid to critical details.

Shoulder arthroscopic techniques are still evolving. Procedures such as acromioclavicular joint debridement and subacromial decompression have been refined. Some of the relatively new procedures that deal with shoulder instability will probably withstand the test of time, since they are based on sound principles.

Other chapters are devoted to specific surgical arthroscopic techniques for the carpal tunnel, the elbow, the wrist, the hip, the ankle, and the subtalar and temporomandibular joints.

With great indebtedness to my co-authors, who have authoritatively and skillfully covered various aspects of arthroscopic surgery, I am dedicating this book to the pioneering works of the many orthopedic surgeons from all over the world.

J. Serge Parisien, M.D., F.A.C.S.

Acknowledgments

I take this opportunity to pay special tribute to a few important people in my professional life:

To my father, Vastey Parisien, who was a superb orthopedic surgeon and who taught me so many things; to our "Chief," Dr. Henry Mankin, who, when I was a resident, set a lasting example in teaching, research, and patient care and who is still an inspiration to all of his "boys"; and to Dr. Herman Robbins for his teaching and encouragement.

I owe much to the many wonderful orthopedic residents of the Hospital for Joint Diseases, my devoted scrub nurse Cecilia Sarmiento, and Dr. David Present, a good friend and one of my brilliant pupils, for making it exciting to work at the same place for the past 20 years. I also wish to thank Elizabeth Greenspan and the editing staff of Gower for their professionalism. I extend my gratitude to Gary Welch for the superb quality of his illustrations and to the photography department of the Hospital for Joint Diseases.

Finally, I am indebted to my daughter, Christine, for her diligent help and understanding during the preparation of this book.

J. Serge Parisien, M.D., F.A.C.S.

Contributors

LOUIS U. BIGLIANI, MD
Associate Professor of Clinical Orthopaedic Surgery
Chief, Shoulder Service
The New York Orthopaedic Hospital
Columbia-Presbyterian Medical Center
New York, New York

EDWARD S. BITTAR, MD, PHD
Associate Clinical Professor
Department of Orthopaedics
University of Florida
Gainesville, Florida

EUGENE J. CHANDLER, MD
Director, Arthroscopic Surgery Center
Scottsdale, Arizona

JAMES C.Y. CHOW, MD
Orthopaedic Research of Southern Illinois
Orthopaedic Clinic of Mt. Vernon
Mt. Vernon, Illinois
Clinical Assistant Professor
Southern Illinois University School of Medicine
Springfield, Illinois

JAMES C. ESCH, MD
Tri-City Medical Center and North Coast Surgery Center
Oceanside, California
Clinical Instructor
Division of Orthopaedics and Rehabilitation
University of San Diego
San Diego, California

GREGORY C. FANELLI, MD
Sports Injury Clinic
Department of Orthopaedic Surgery
Geisinger Medical Center
Danville, Pennsylvania

EVAN L. FLATOW, MD
Assistant Professor of Orthopaedic Surgery
Shoulder Service
The New York Orthopaedic Hospital
Columbia-Presbyterian Medical Center
New York, New York

FREDDIE H. FU, MD
Blue Cross of Western Pennsylvania Professor of Orthopaedic Surgery
Vice Chairman, Clinical Department of Orthopaedic Surgery
University of Pittsburgh
Pittsburgh, Pennsylvania

JAMES M. GLICK, MD
Senior Attending Orthopaedic Surgeon
Mount Zion Hospital Campus
University of California
San Francisco, California
Associate Clinical Professor, Orthopaedic Surgery
University of California
San Francisco, California

JAMES F. GUHL, MD
Arthroscopy & Sports Medicine Center of Southeastern Wisconsin
St. Francis Hospital Sports Performance Center
Clinical Instructor
Department of Orthopaedics
Medical College of Wisconsin
Milwaukee, Wisconsin

JAMES A. HILL, MD
Associate Professor of Clinical Orthopaedic Surgery
Northwestern University Medical School
Chicago, Illinois

MEHRDAD M. MALEK, MD
Director, Washington Orthopaedic and Knee Clinic
Associate Professor
Department of Orthopaedics
Howard University
Washington, DC

DAVID S. MENCHE, MD
Associate Director, Sports Medicine Center
Medical Director, Physical/Occupational Therapy
Hospital for Joint Diseases Orthopaedic Institute
New York, New York

JAMES S. MULHOLLAN, MD
Arkansas Knee Clinic
Little Rock, Arkansas

ERIC J. OLSON, MD
Staff Orthopaedic Surgeon
Walter Reed Army Medical Center
Washington, DC
Assistant Professor of Surgery
Uniformed Services University of the Health Sciences
Bethesda, Maryland

J. SERGE PARISIEN, MD, FACS
Chief, Arthroscopic Surgery Service
Attending Physician, Sports Medicine Service
Hospital for Joint Diseases Orthopaedic Institute
Associate Professor of Clinical Orthopaedic Surgery
New York University Medical School
New York, New York
Founding Member, International Arthroscopy Association

MARK I. PITMAN, MD
Director, Sports Medicine Center
Hospital For Joint Diseases Orthopaedic Institute
New York, New York

DONALD J. ROSE, MD
Assistant Attending Orthopaedic Surgeon
Director, Harkness Center for Dance Injuries
Hospital for Joint Diseases Orthopaedic Institute
New York, New York

STUART I. SPRINGER, MD
Affiliated with the Hospital for Joint Diseases Orthopaedic Institute
Chairman, International Arthroscopy Center
Hospital for Joint Diseases Orthopaedic Institute
New York, New York

JAMES W. STONE, MD
Arthroscopy & Sports Medicine Center of Southeastern Wisconsin
St. Francis Hospital Sports Performance Center
Milwaukee, Wisconsin

MOHAN THOMAS, DDS, FACD, FICD
Chairman, Division of Oral/Maxillofacial Surgery
Director, Center for Corrective Jaw Surgery and Temporomandibular Disorders
Hospital for Joint Diseases Orthopaedic Institute
Clinical Assistant Professor
Mt. Sinai School of Medicine
New York, New York

EUGENE M. WOLF, MD
Department of Orthopaedic Surgery
California Pacific Medical Center
San Francisco, California

Contents

Section One

The Knee

chapter One

Arthroscopic Meniscectomy

J. Serge Parisien

Arthroscopic meniscal procedures are the most common operations performed on the knee. Depending on the patient's age, the location, and the nature of the tear, partial meniscectomy or meniscal repair is indicated. The menisci are important structures of the knee, and their well-known functions include load distribution, shock absorption, lubrication, nutrition, and joint stability.[1–10] It has also been shown that the vascularity of the meniscus is much greater in the young. The medial and lateral geniculate arteries form a perimeniscal capillary plexus that supplies the peripheral border of the meniscus as well as 10% to 30% of the width of the medial border and 10% to 25% of the width of the lateral border, with the exception of the popliteal corner.[11] Because of this rich vascular network, tears of the peripheral area of the meniscus usually respond very well to primary or even delayed repair. In many instances, however, owing to the patient's age and to the location and type of tears, a partial meniscectomy is the only alternative for a torn symptomatic meniscus. As emphasized by O'Connor,[12] American pioneer of arthroscopic meniscal surgery, a successful outcome is dependent on the following factors: accurate recognition of the tear pattern, excision of the offending meniscal fragment or fragments, and careful trimming of the remaining meniscal rim after its stability has been confirmed by probing.

INSTRUMENTATION

The procedure is done in an outpatient facility under general, spinal, or epidural anesthesia. Local anesthesia, in cooperative patients, can also be used. A unit containing the TV monitor and VCR is usually placed on the opposite side of the leg being operated on (Fig. 1.1). The following instruments are necessary for partial resection of the meniscus: a 4 or 5 mm arthroscope with 25° or 30° inclination that will fit a hand-held video camera; a probe; hand-held instruments such as knives (rosette, retrograde, meniscotome), scissors, basket punches of various sizes and angles, rotary 90° basket punches, grasping forceps, and power equipment (shaver and meniscus cutter); and a magnetic retriever. A leg-holding device is another important piece of equipment, useful to control the varus and valgus stresses on the knee that are essential for maximal exposure of the menisci (Fig. 1.2). A tourniquet is always applied on the thigh, above or underneath the leg holder. Although some arthroscopists advocate its use in all meniscal surgery, there is little need to inflate the tourniquet during the procedure, if a pump that can pressurize the irrigation fluid is available. While the operated knee is flexed with the lower part of the operating table bent at 90°, the other lower extremity is kept in slight flexion at the hip, well padded, with a bolster under the thigh. Some surgeons advocate the use of a lithotomy leg support to position the nonoperated leg away from the operated knee.

Since Ringer's lactate has been shown to support chondrocyte metabolism better than normal saline, it is used more frequently in some centers as a fluid medium during arthroscopic procedures.

PORTALS

Although most arthroscopic partial meniscectomies can be performed through the anteromedial and anterolateral

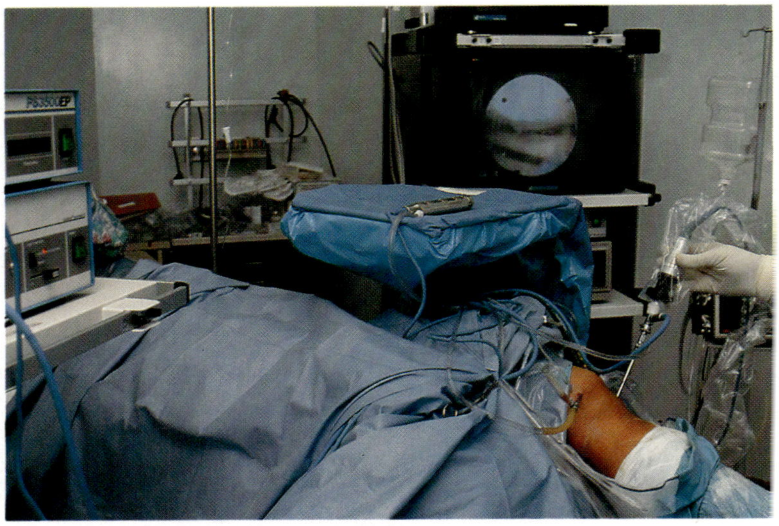

Figure 1.1
Operating room set up with TV camera and infusion pump.

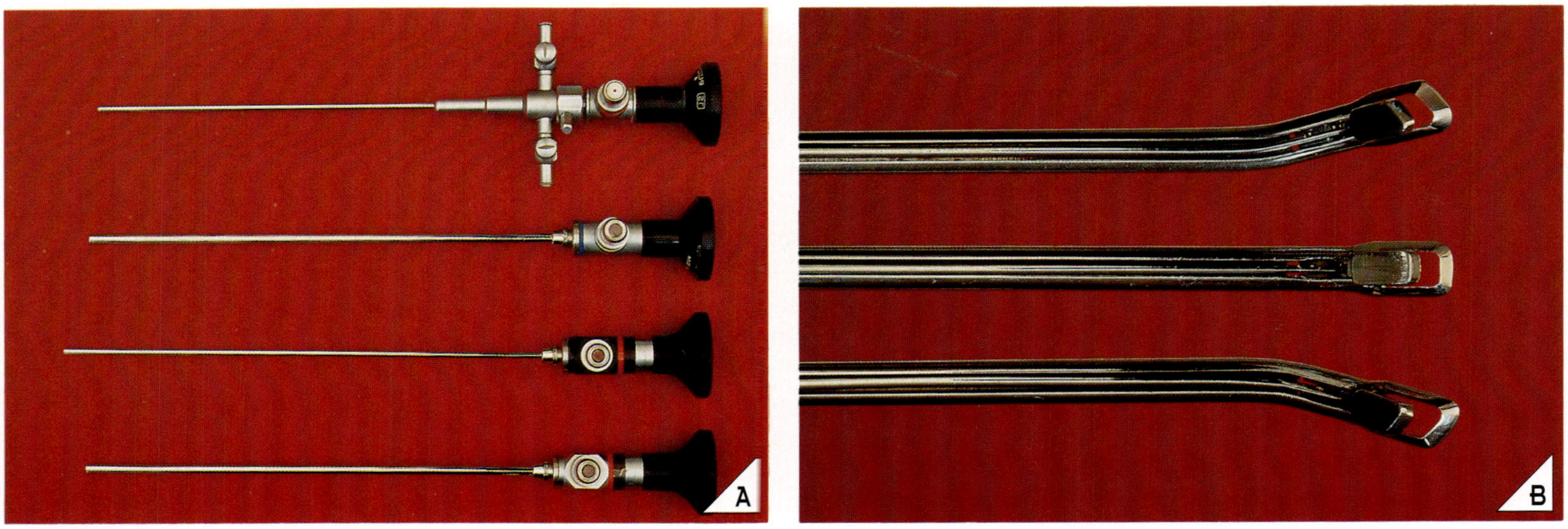

Figure 1.2
(A) Scopes of various sizes and angulations. (B) Duckbill baskets (Acufex). (continued on next page)

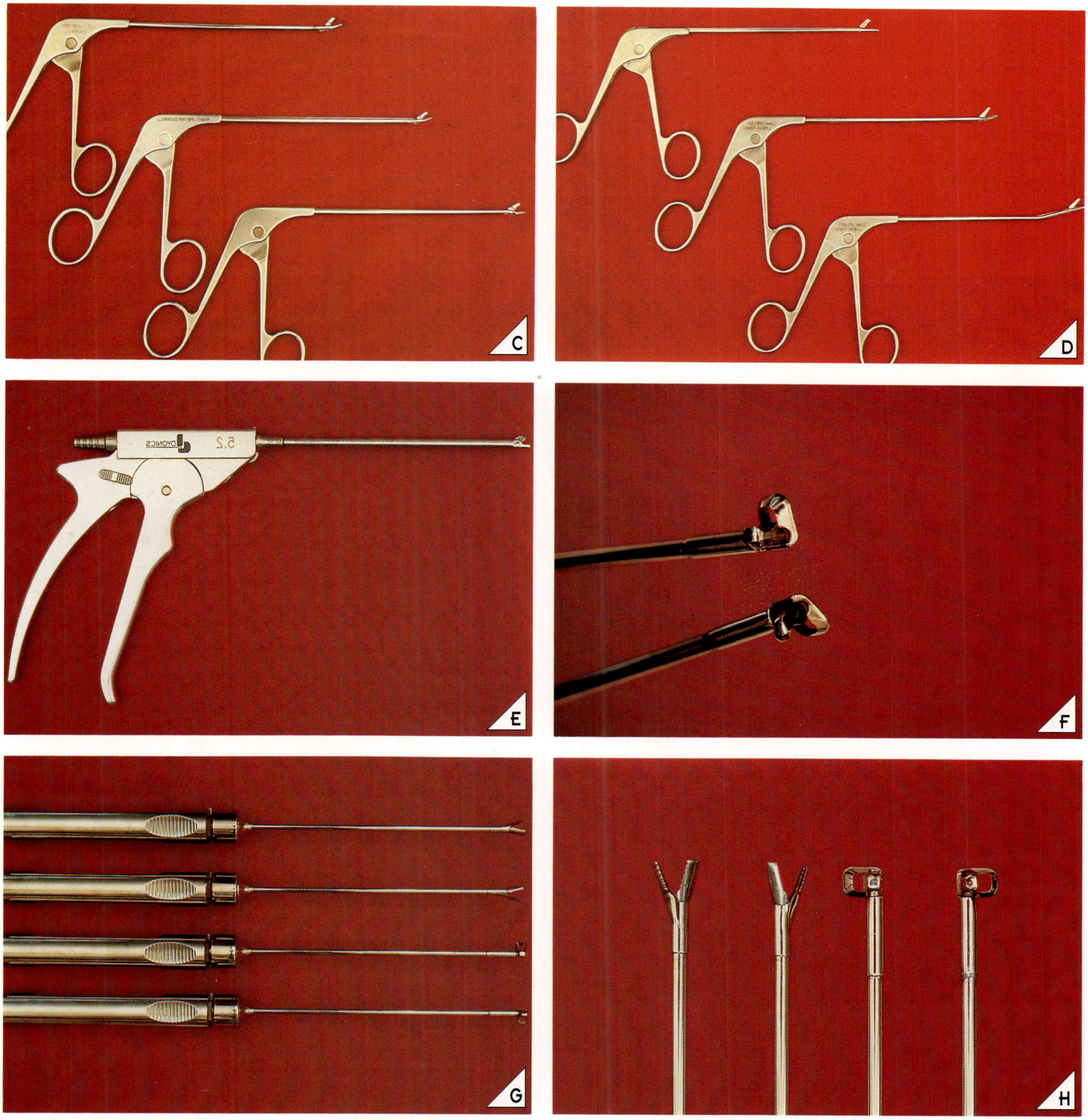

Figure 1.2 (continued)

(C) Basket forceps. (D) Various shapes of basket punches. (E) Suction basket (Dyonics). (F) Rotary baskets. (G) Rotary basket and scissors (Acufex). (H) Close up of rotary baskets and scissors.

portals, familiarity with the other portals is necessary in the case of difficult tears that may require a combination of portals (Fig. 1.3).

For a complete examination of the knee, the anterolateral portal is the most commonly used. It is located 1 cm lateral to the patellar tendon, below the inferior pole of the patella.

The anteromedial portal is medial to the patellar tendon, above the tibial plateau. This approach provides excellent visualization of the anterior half of the lateral meniscus and of the posteromedial aspect of the knee. The anteromedial portal is best developed after introducing a percutaneous spinal needle while viewing from the anterolateral portal. An accessory anteromedial portal may have to be developed higher for probing and instrumentation of the lateral compartment.

The central portal is placed through a midline incision approximately 1 cm below the patella. It gives good visualization of the posterior compartment as well as the posterior cruciate ligament.

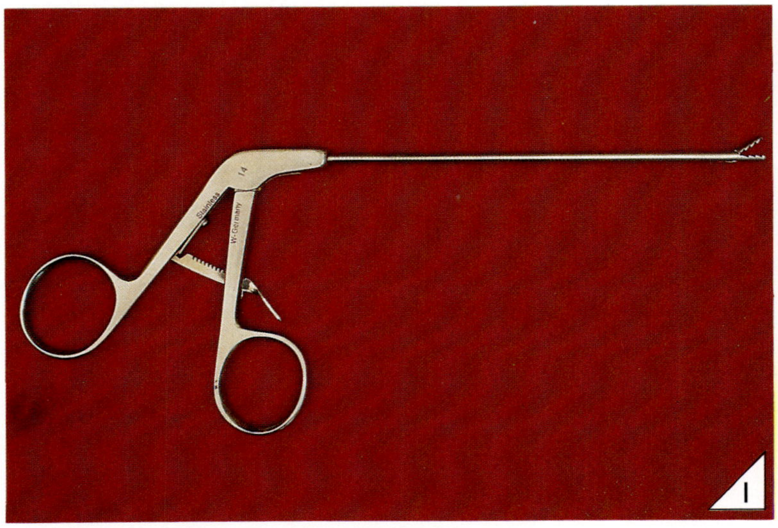

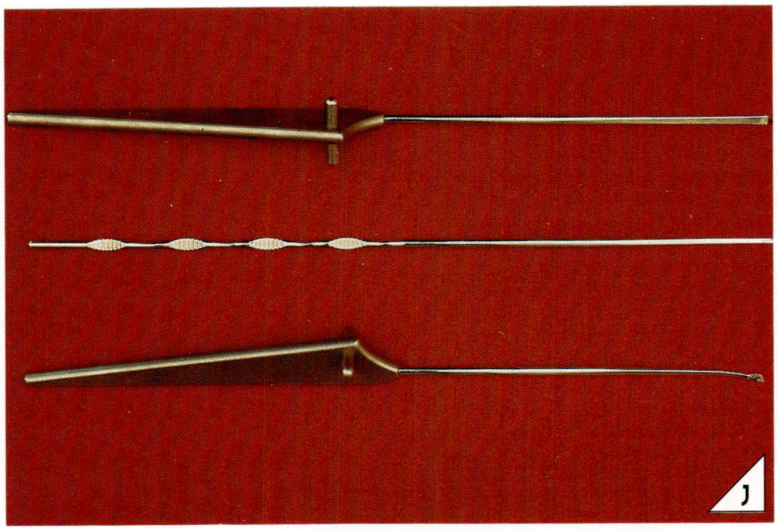

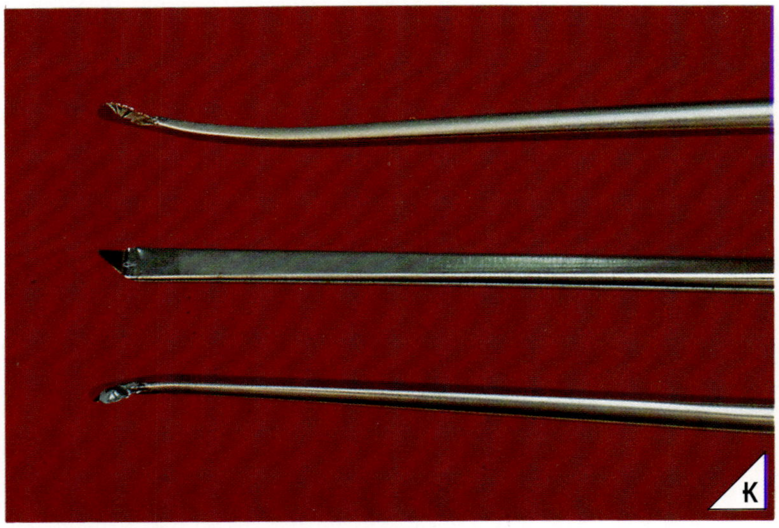

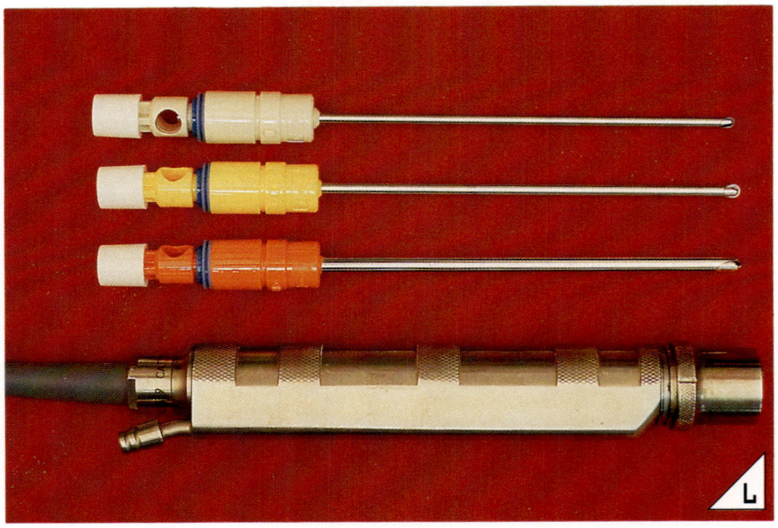

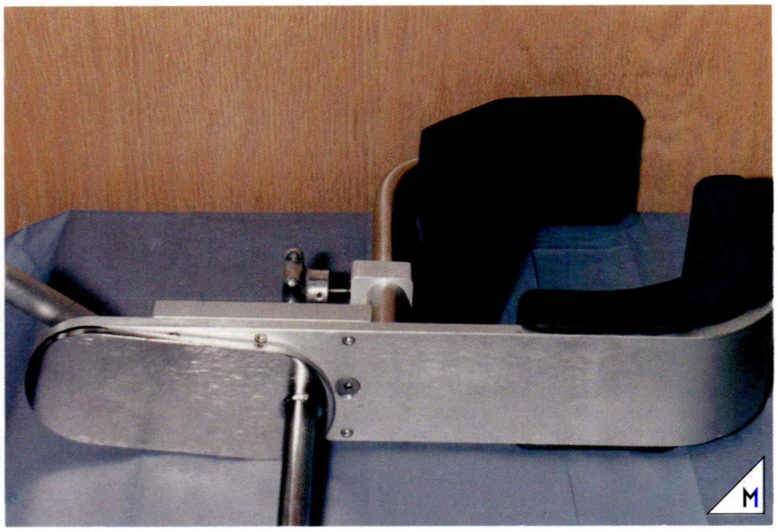

Figure 1.2 (continued)
(I) Grasping forceps. (J) Various knives. (K) Close up of knives. (L) High speed power instrumentation. (M) Leg holder.

The posteromedial portal is posterior to the medial collateral ligament, slightly above the joint line. The site for this portal can be determined using a spinal needle with the knee flexed at 90° while visualizing the distended posteromedial corner of the knee through the anterolateral portal.

The posterolateral portal is proximal to the head of the fibula and anterior to the biceps femoris tendon.

The suprapatellar approaches, lateral and medial, are located approximately 1 cm above the superior pole of the patella.

The midpatellar approaches are placed on the medial and lateral aspects of the patella, at the middle border. They provide excellent visualization of the anterior horns of the menisci. The use of a 70° arthroscope will improve the visualization of the posterior aspect of the knee.

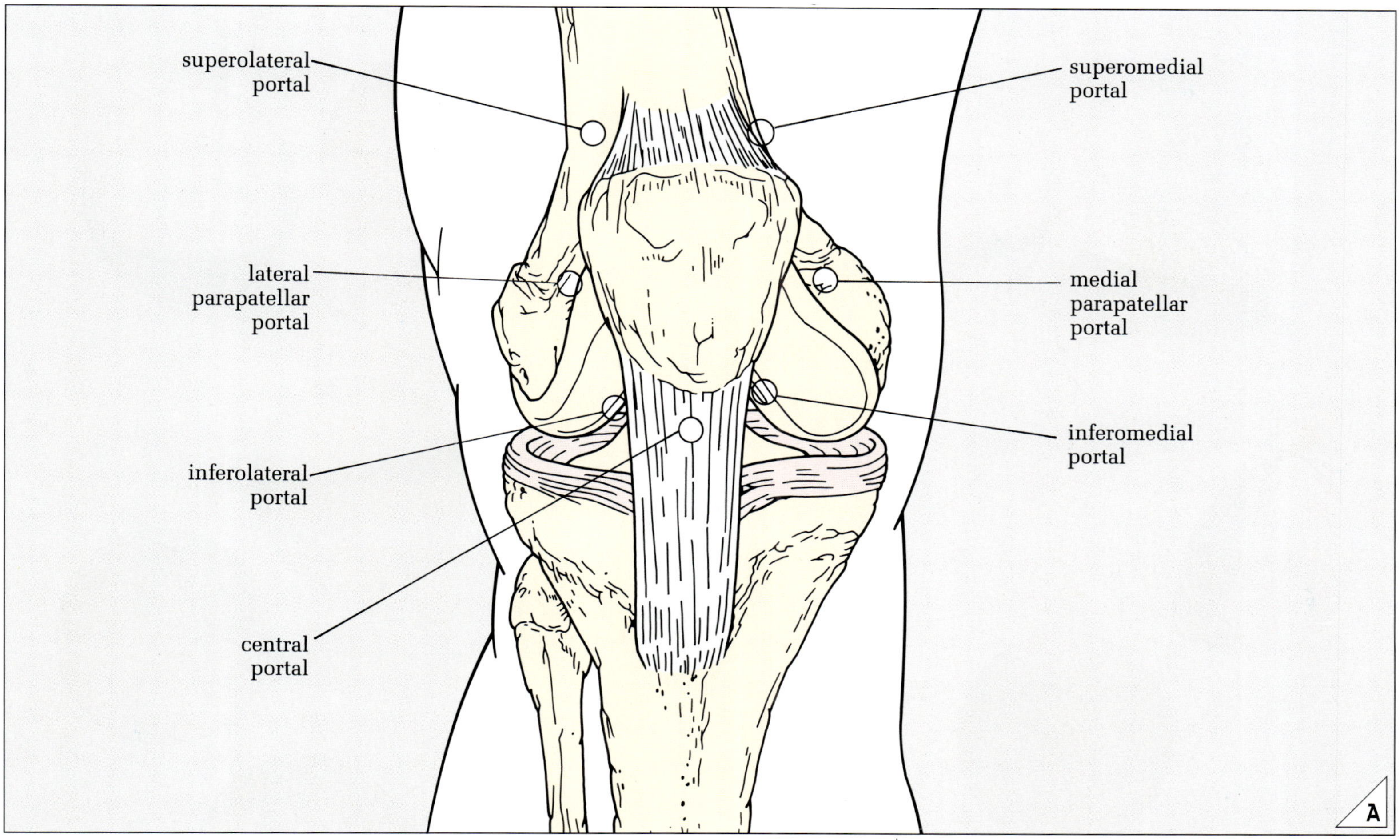

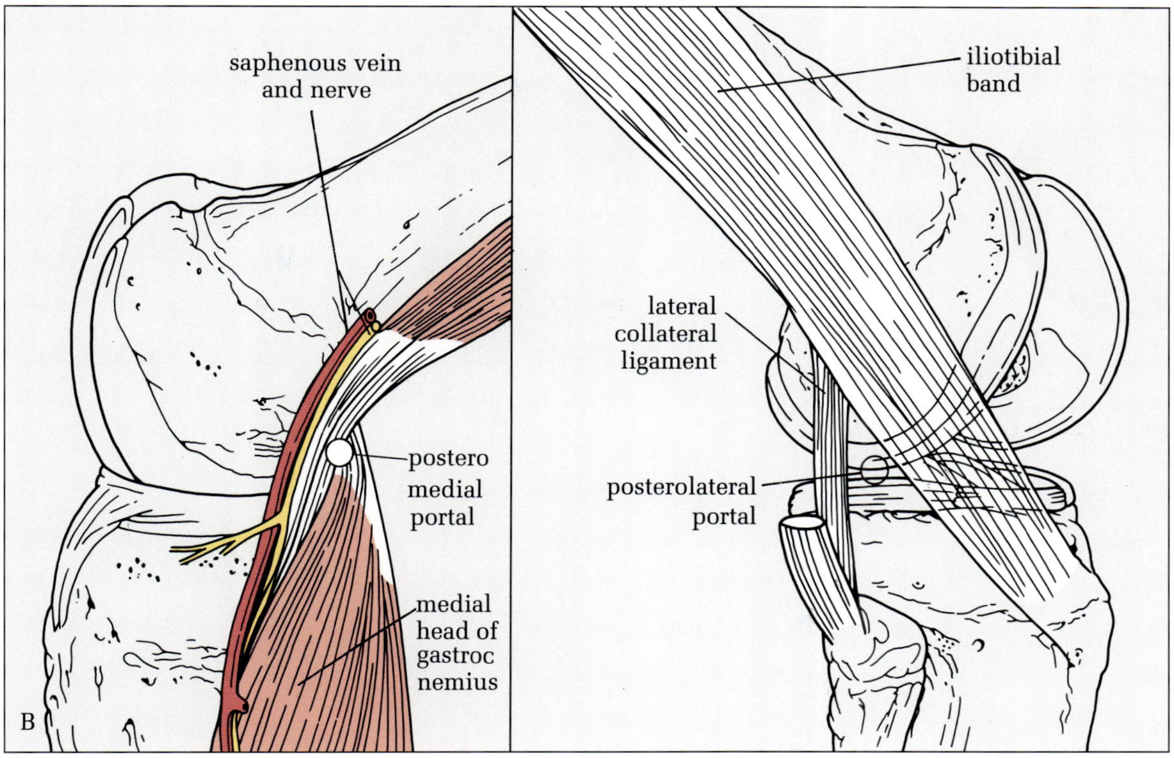

Figure 1.3
Anterior (A), posteromedial (B), and posterolateral (C) portals. **(continued on next page)**

MEDIAL MENISCUS

The medial meniscus has a C-shaped configuration, with the anterior half much narrower than the posterior half. The medial meniscus, unlike the lateral meniscus, is firmly attached to the joint capsule along its periphery (Fig. 1.4).

Patterns of Tears

Tears can be vertical longitudinal, vertical transverse (radial), oblique, horizontal, or degenerative. They are described as complex when many components exist in combination (Fig. 1.5).

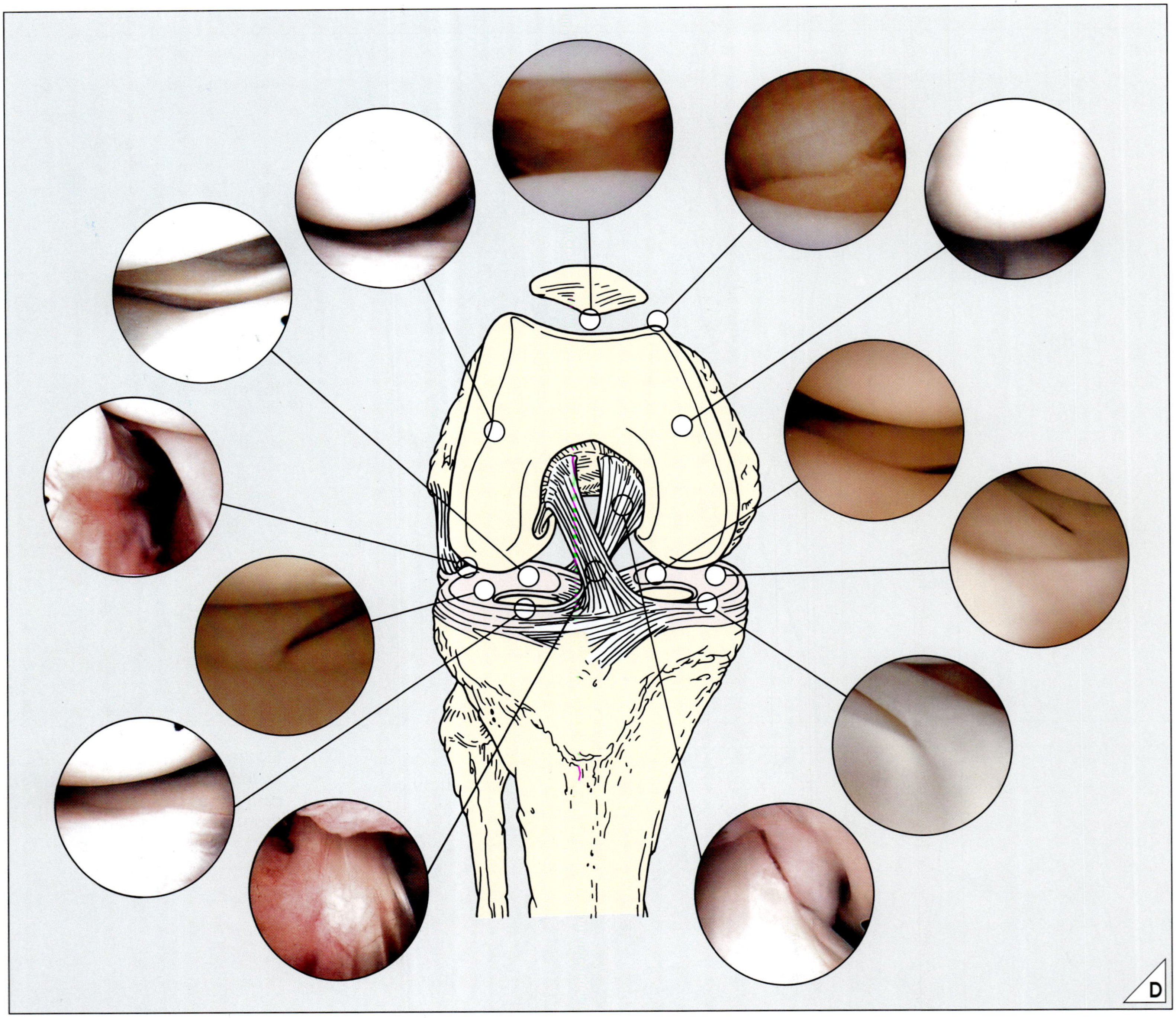

Figure 1.3 (continued)
(D) Arthroscopic visualization of various areas of a normal knee.

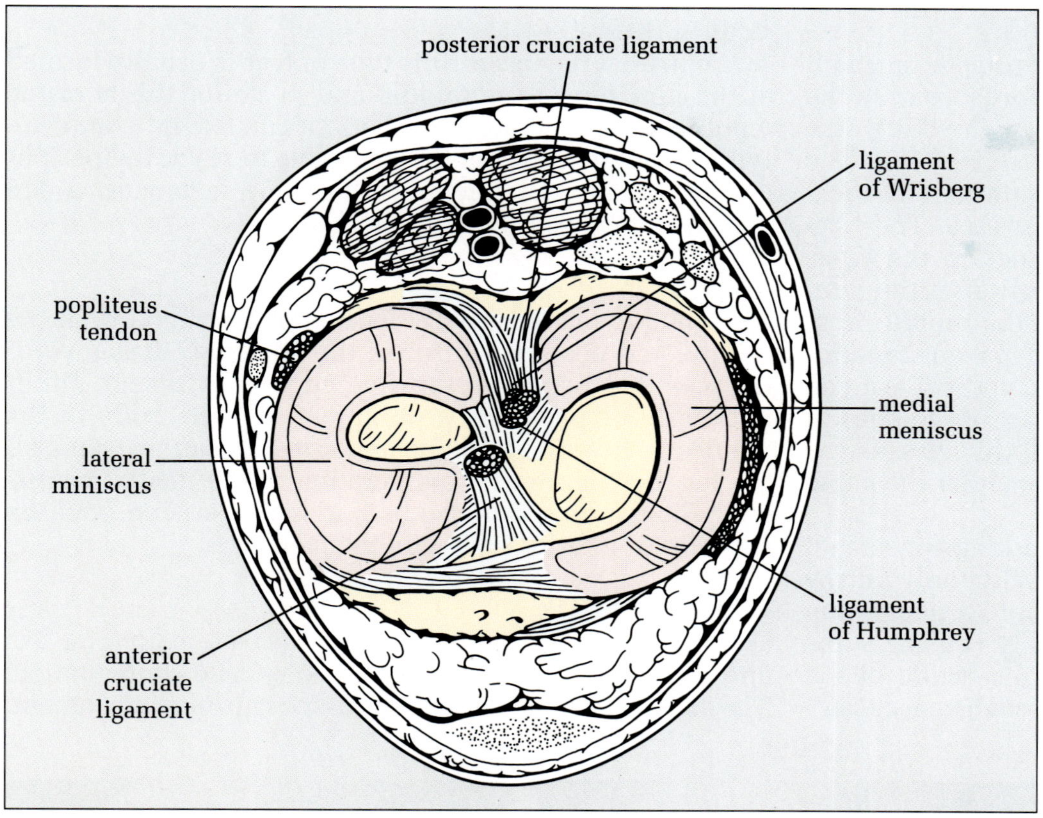

Figure 1.4
Transverse section of the knee joint.

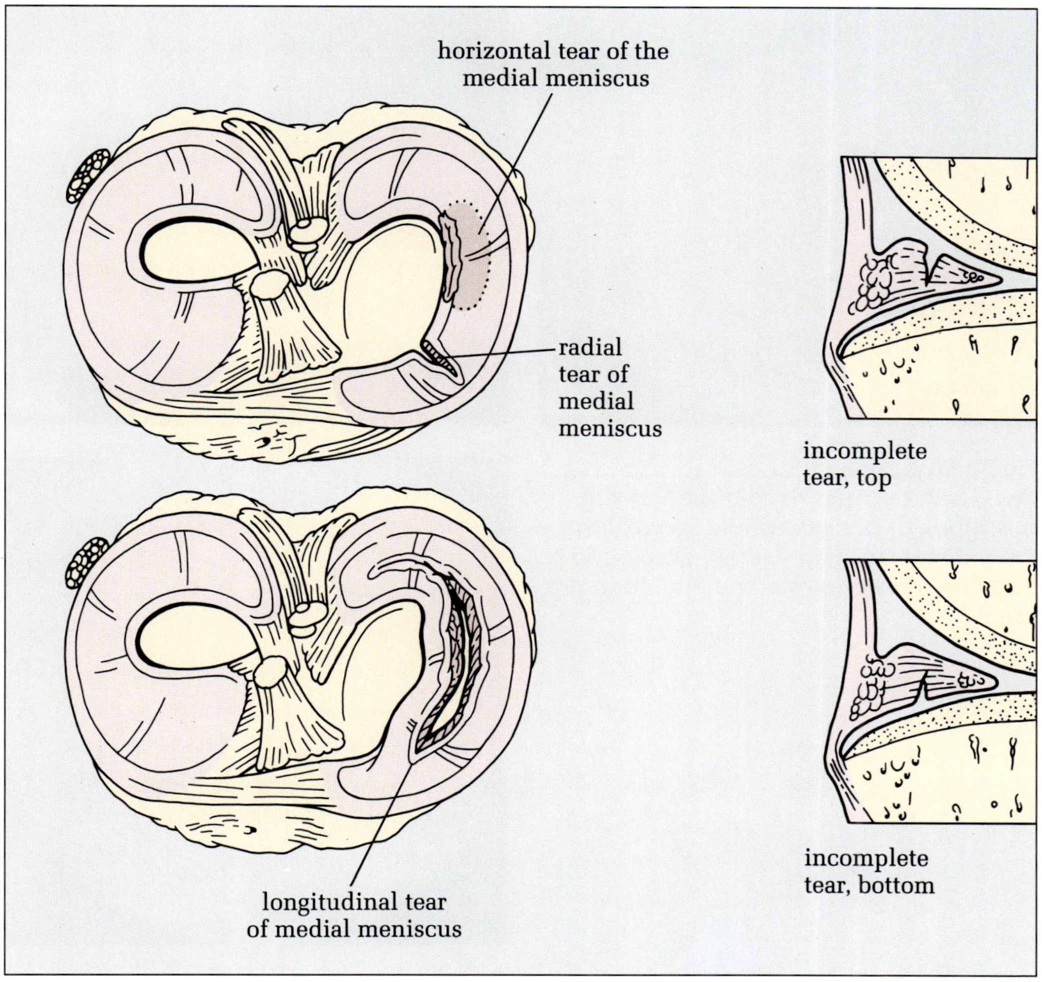

Figure 1.5
Various types of tears of the medial meniscus.

Vertical longitudinal tear

These tears are common with anterior cruciate ligament instability. A tear can involve half, two thirds, or even the full circumference of the medial meniscus, in which case it is termed the classic bucket-handle tear (Fig. 1.6). The mobile fragment can be responsible for intermittent locking when it moves into the intercondylar area. The fragment can also, in some situations, be stuck in the intercondylar notch, with a lack of full extension of the joint present on examination. A division of the mobile fragment will create two separate meniscal flaps, one anterior and one posterior, of various lengths. The vertical tear can be short and located at the posterior aspect of the knee. It can be complete when it involves the full thickness of the meniscus or incomplete when it involves either the superior or inferior surface (Fig. 1.7).

At times the meniscus will appear normal on visual examination and will show some abnormality only during probing. The examiner's probe will fall into a depression in the substance of the meniscus, possibly causing some displacement of the meniscus towards the center of the joint. This is the classic interstitial or intrasubstance tear.

Radial tear

In the medial meniscus, this type of tear is usually located at the junction of the middle and posterior thirds of the meniscus or at the posterior horn. It can extend completely into the full width of the meniscus to reach the peripheral meniscal attachments or, in some instances, it can have a vertical component (Fig. 1.8).

Oblique and flap tears

The oblique tear is usually located at the junction of the middle and posterior thirds of the meniscus. It is a vertical tear that begins at the free edge and travels, either anteriorly or posteriorly, obliquely into the body of the meniscus. It varies in shape and size and can be responsible for the "flap tear" configuration of the medial meniscus. The flap tear can also be horizontal, arising from the superior or inferior surface of the meniscus.

Horizontal tear

This tear gives rise to two meniscal leaves, a superior leaf and an inferior leaf, of variable thickness and configuration. The cleft can extend completely to the capsular attachment.

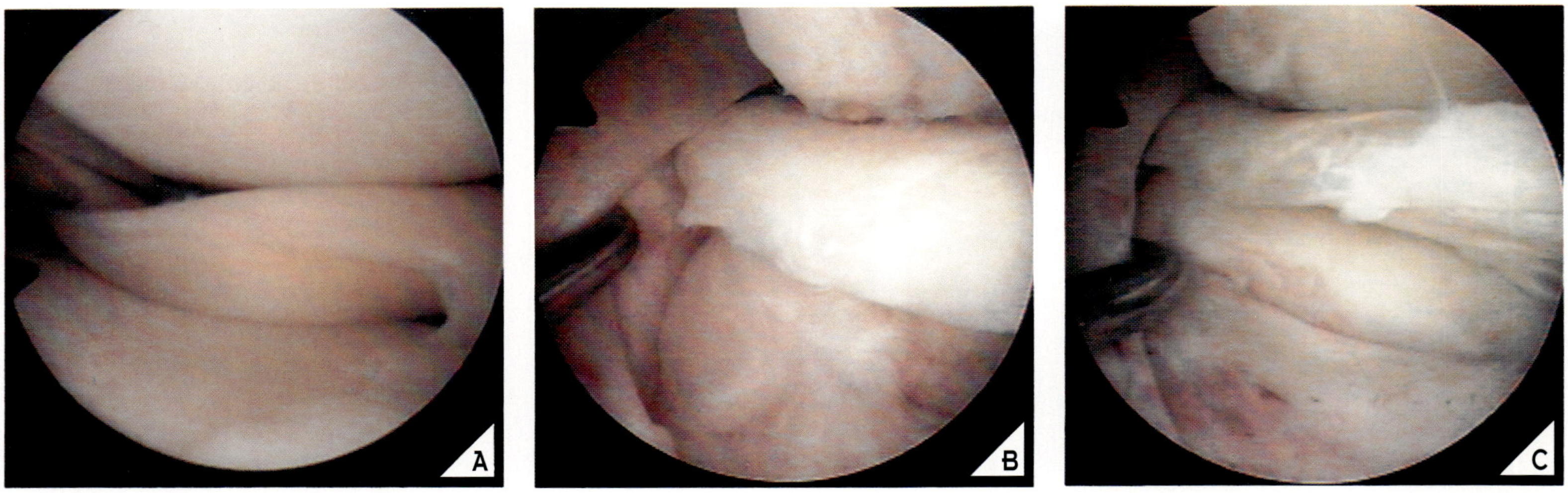

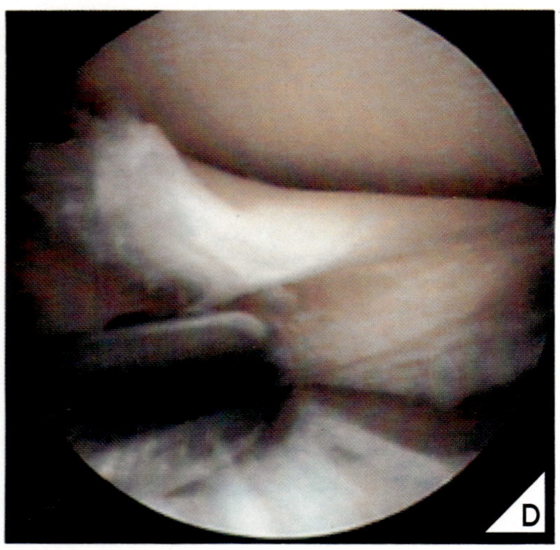

Figure 1.6
(A–D) Arthroscopic visualization of various types of bucket-handle tears of the medial meniscus right knee. Displaced fragments are shown in the intercondylar area.

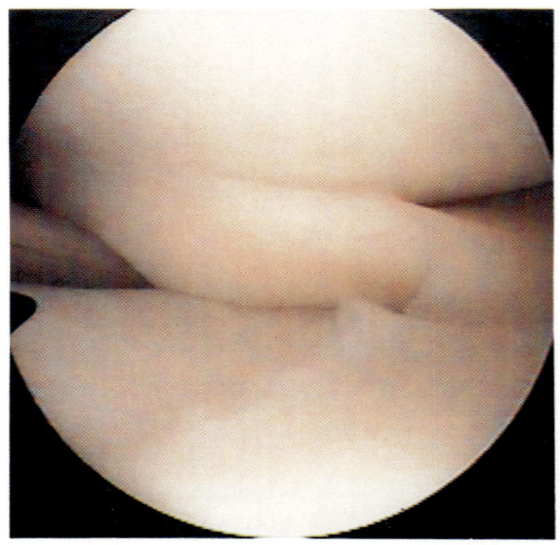

Figure 1.7
Vertical tear of the posterior horn of the medial meniscus right knee.

Degenerative tear

These tears are common in older patients and represent one component of a degenerative joint process. The meniscus is usually fibrillated, and various flaps are present. Chondromalacic areas of the articular cartilage of the tibial plateau or femoral condyles are also present.

Surgical Technique

Vertical longitudinal (bucket-handle) tear

The arthroscope is placed in the anterolateral portal for a complete arthroscopic evaluation of the knee. A probe is used in the anteromedial portal to assess the nature and extent of the tear. This anteromedial portal, developed after a spinal needle is placed through the skin to choose the location of the skin incision, is used for instrumentation. Once it is determined that the bucket-handle tear needs excision, the displaced fragment is reduced, to improve visualization of the posterior horn and to facilitate its division. Basket scissors are used to partially divide the posterior axilla of the mobile meniscal fragment, leaving only a few fibers of attachment. Then the anterior attachment is cut with the same scissors very close to the axilla of the tear so that there will be no remaining anterior flap that may be very difficult to remove later. The anterior attachment can also be divided with a curved rosette knife. When the attachment is at the very anterior horn of the meniscus, a 45° angled knife will make the job easier, or scissors can be placed through the anterolateral portal with the arthroscope switched to the anteromedial portal. Grasping forceps are then placed through the anteromedial portal to grasp the fragment by its very anterior end, thus allowing its smooth removal from the joint. After removal of the mobile fragment, the probe is used to check the stability of the remaining rim and to look for any other vertical or cleavage tears. Basket forceps or a motorized shaver are used to gently trim the remaining rim, excising any irregularities of the free border (Fig. 1.9). If the displaced bucket-handle cannot be relocated, a three-portal technique is needed.

Through the anteromedial portal, grasping forceps are used to grip the divided anterior attachment of the meniscus and to place it under tension. A third portal through the patellar tendon, or very close to it, is made after the exact location has been confirmed by means of a spinal needle, allowing introduction of a meniscotome or basket forceps to cut the posterior attachment (Fig. 1.10).

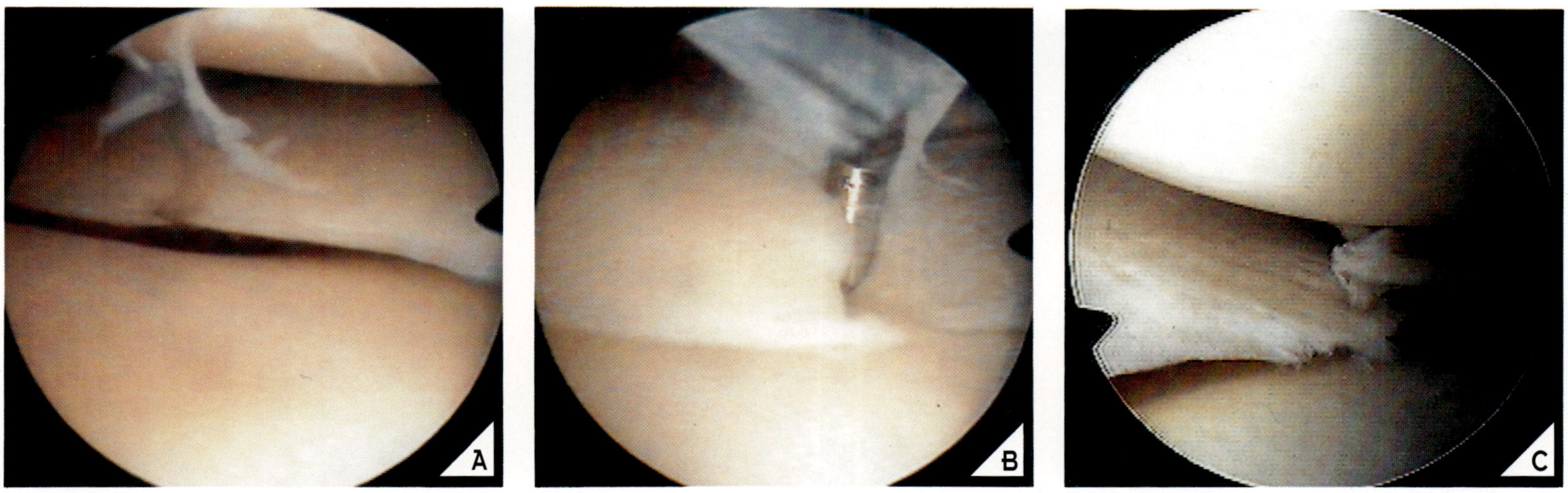

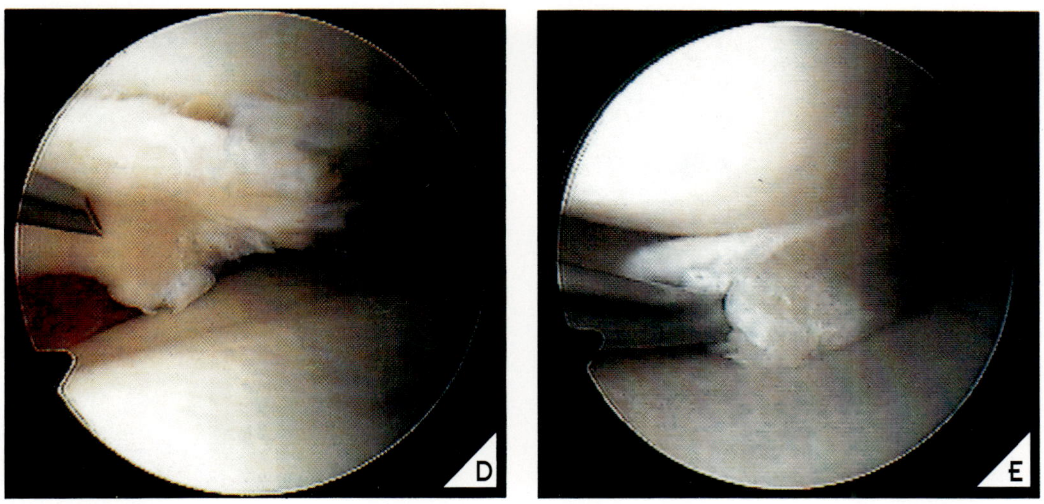

Figure 1.8
(A–E) Various types of radial tears in the medial meniscus left knee.

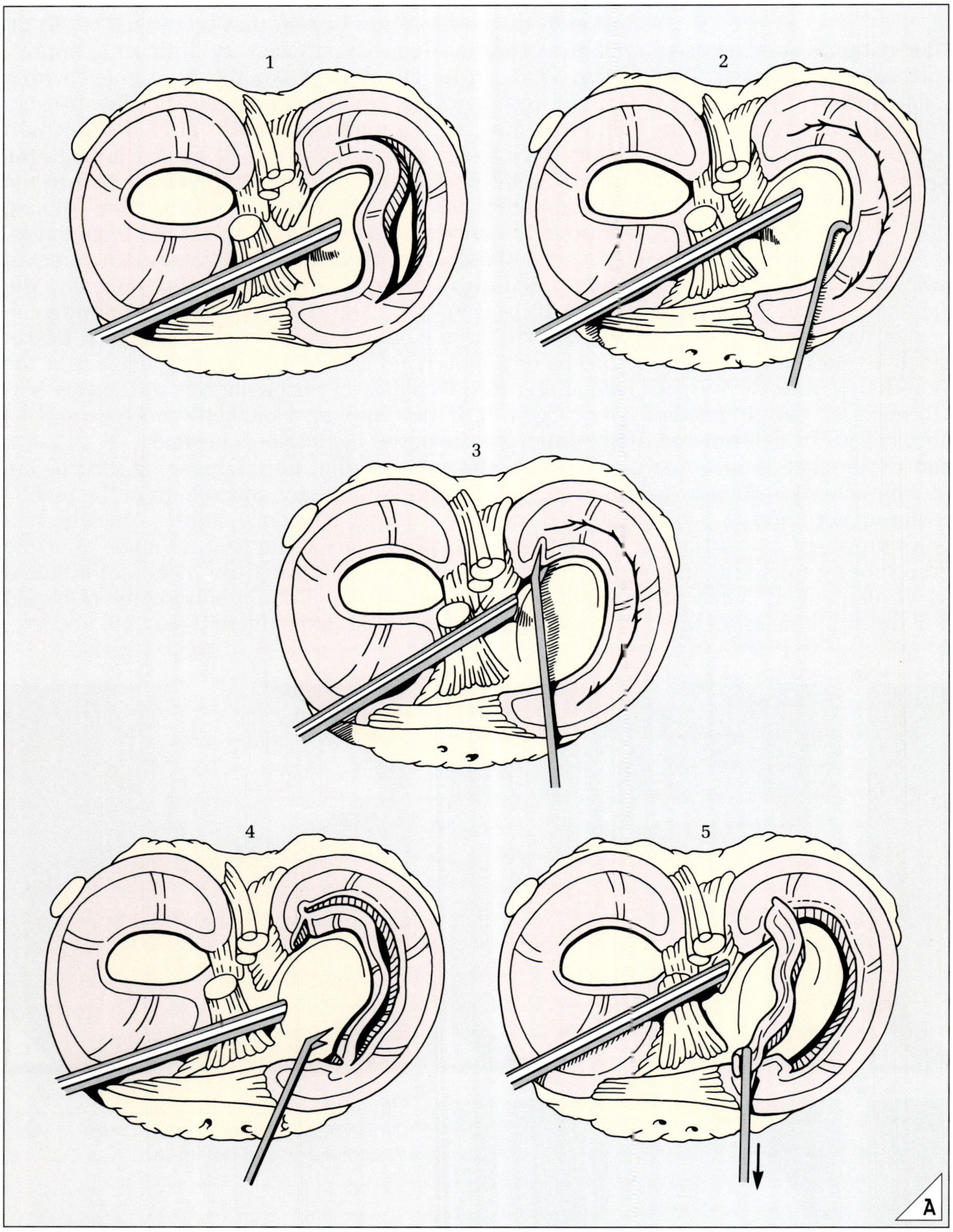

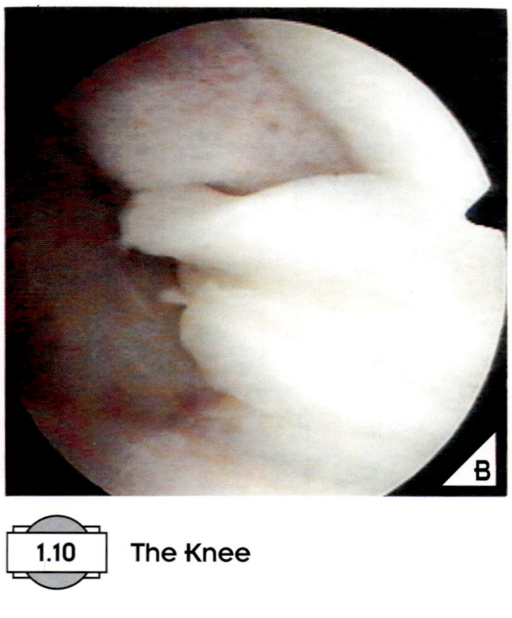

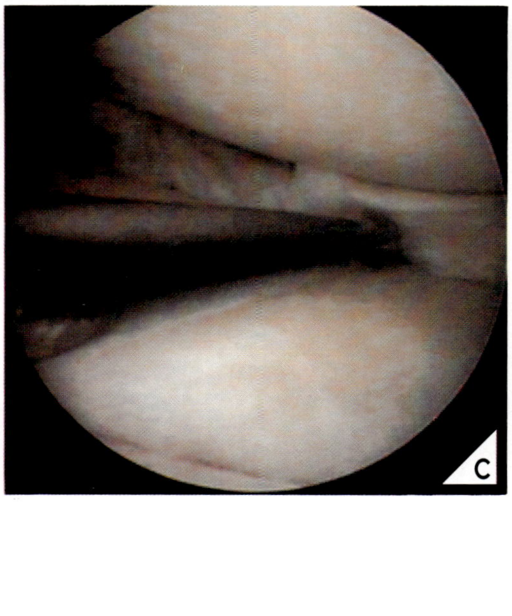

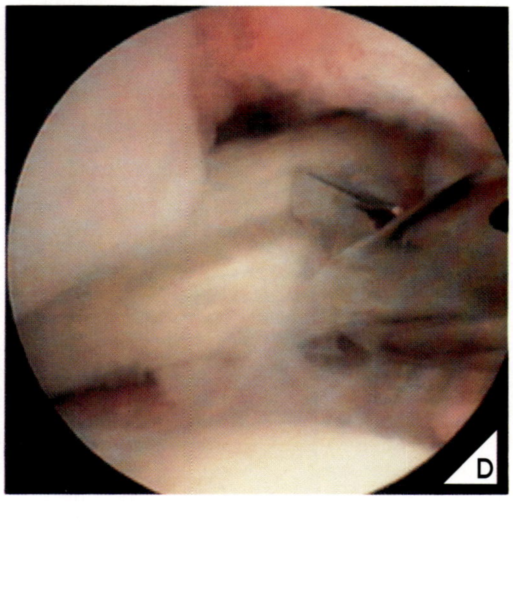

Figure 1.9
(A) Schematic illustration of excision of a bucket-handle tear in the medial meniscus right knee. This is a two-portal approach. (B–F) Arthroscopic visualization of the steps of excision of a bucket-handle tear of the medial meniscus right knee.

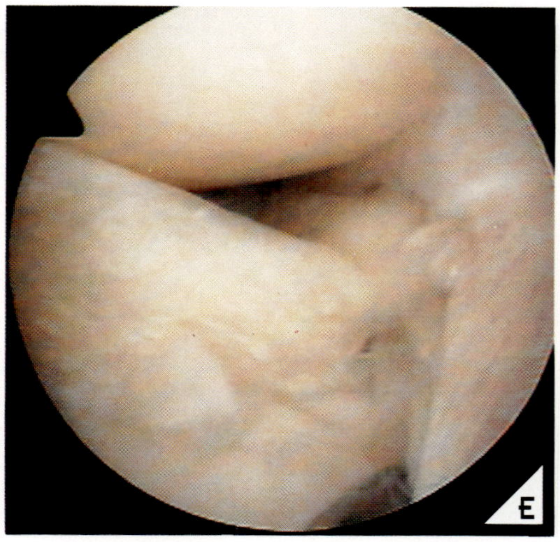

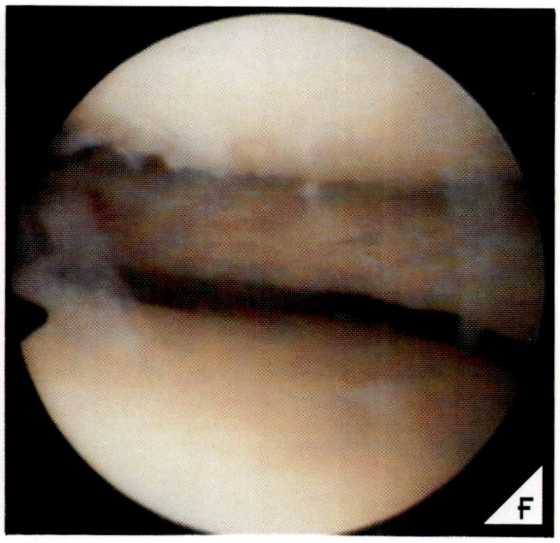

Figure 1.9 (continued)

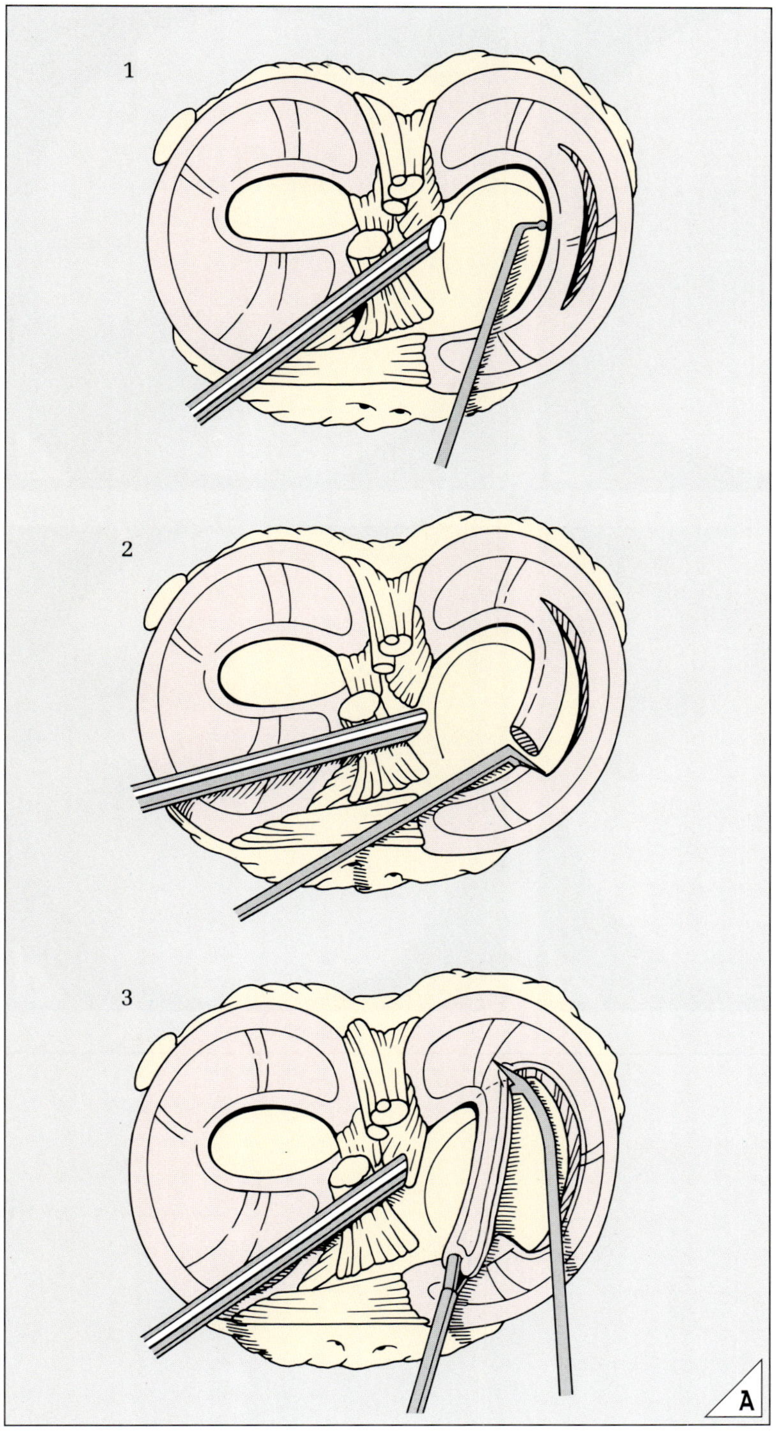

Figure 1.10
Schematic illustration (A) and arthroscopic visualizations (B–J) of the steps of excision of a bucket-handle tear of the medial meniscus right knee. This is a three-portal approach.

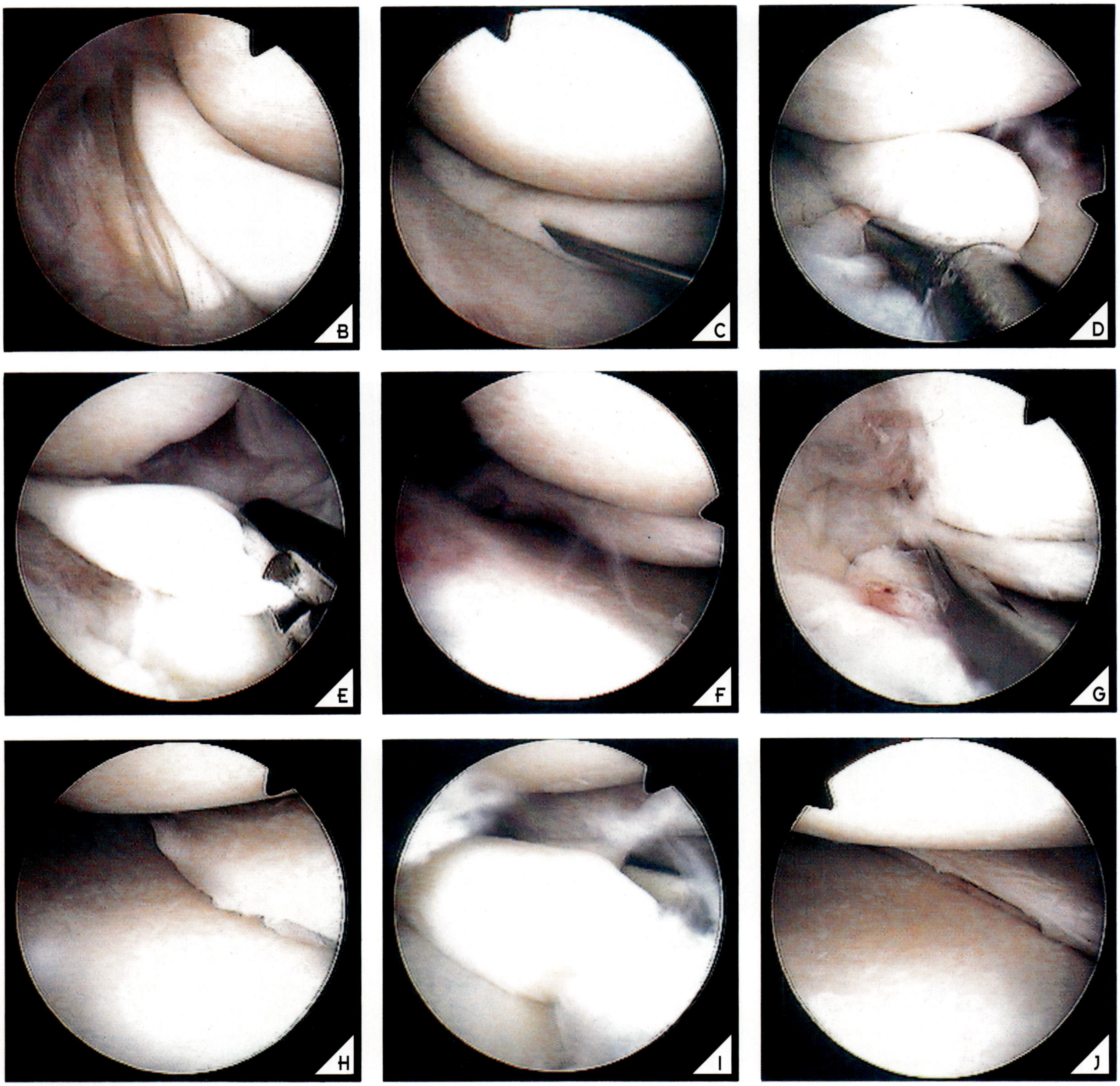

Figure 1.10 (continued)

Short vertical tears occur very commonly in the posterior horn of the medial meniscus. If one is located in the vascular area of a young individual, it should be repaired by use of the techniques described in Chapter 2. If the tear is not repairable, the mobile unstable fragment should be excised. The posterior attachment is cut, leaving a small bridge of meniscus, and the anterior horn is completely divided using the same surgical instrumentation, followed by extraction of the fragment. Probing and trimming of the remaining meniscal rim complete the procedure (Fig. 1.11).

An incomplete vertical tear larger than 1.5 cm and involving the superior or inferior surface should be resected or salvaged, depending on whether or not it meets the

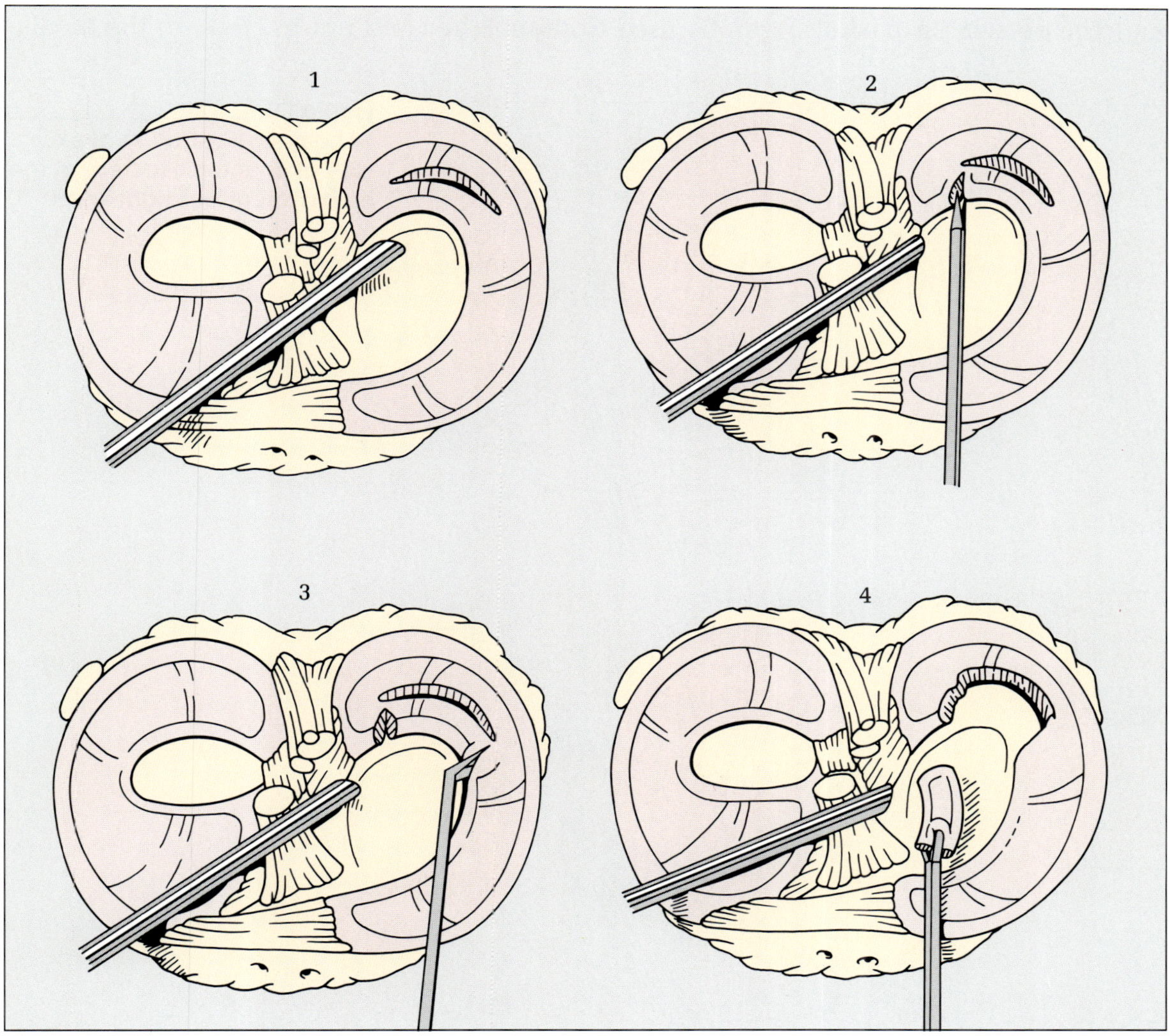

Figure 1.11 Schematic illustration of excision of a short vertical tear of the posterior horn of the medial meniscus right knee.

criteria for meniscal repair. A symptomatic interstitial tear can be resected using a combination of retrograde knife and basket punch (Fig. 1.12).

Radial tear

Careful probing of this type of tear is necessary to ascertain its true extent into the substance of the meniscus and its association with a vertical longitudinal component. Small radial tears are rare in the medial meniscus, and can be trimmed back to normal tissue with a basket. Larger radial tears sometimes involve the full width of the meniscus and may be resected with basket forceps. The adjacent areas of such a tear should also be excised, to contour the remaining meniscus evenly (Fig. 1.13).

Oblique and flap tears

Small oblique tears are usually resected with basket forceps or a motorized instrument. The large oblique tear can be removed in one piece. A percutaneous spinal needle can be used to immobilize and put traction on the menis-

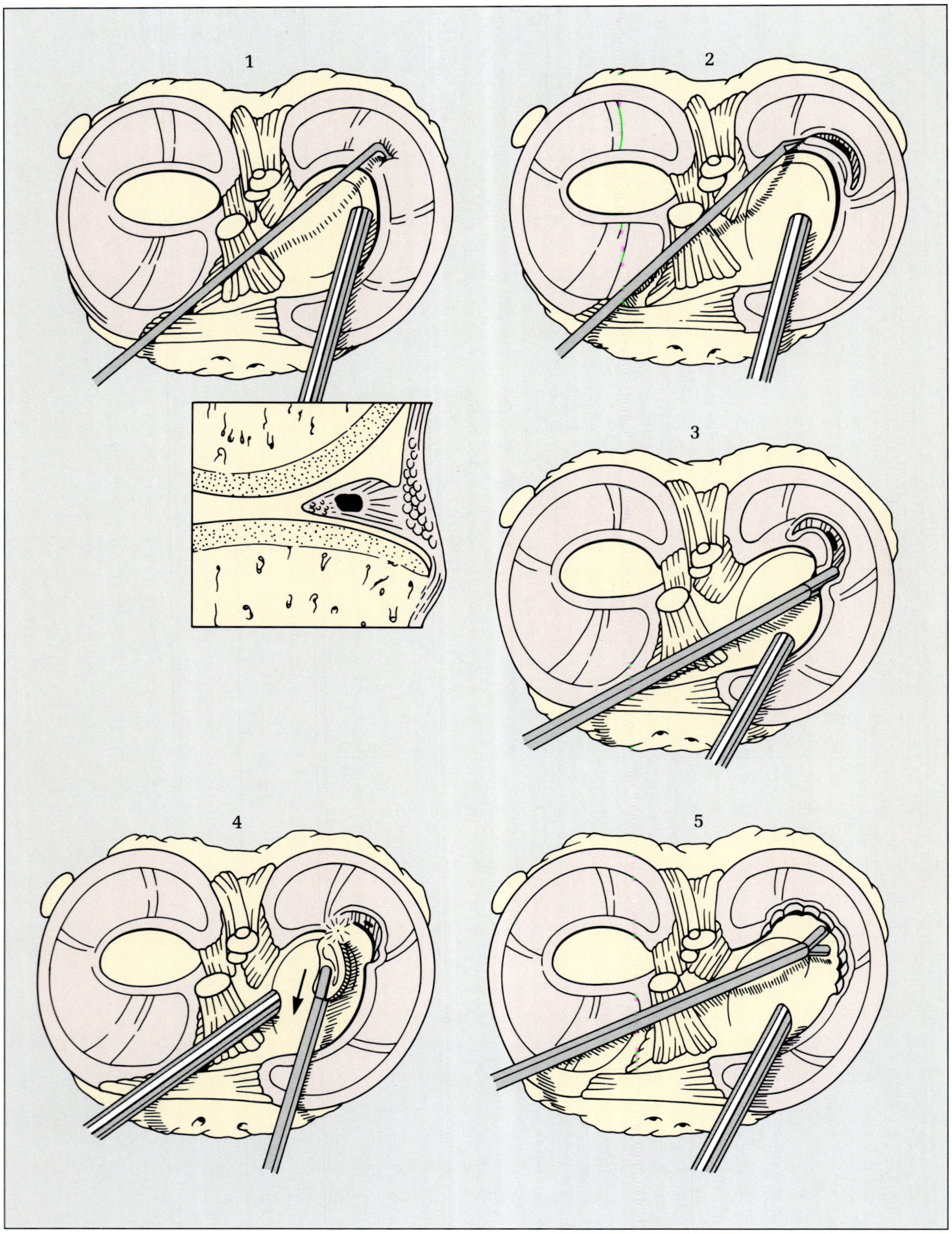

Figure 1.12 Schematic illustration of excision of an interstitial tear of the medial meniscus right knee.

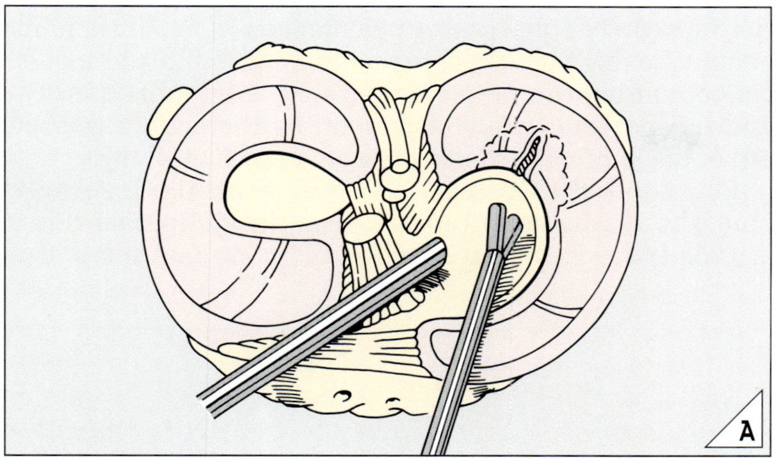

Figure 1.13

(A) Schematic illustration of excision of a radial tear in the medial meniscus right knee. (B–G) Excision of radial tear of a medial meniscus right knee using a basket forceps. At the same time chondroplasty of the medial femoral condyle is performed with a banana knife and a rasp.

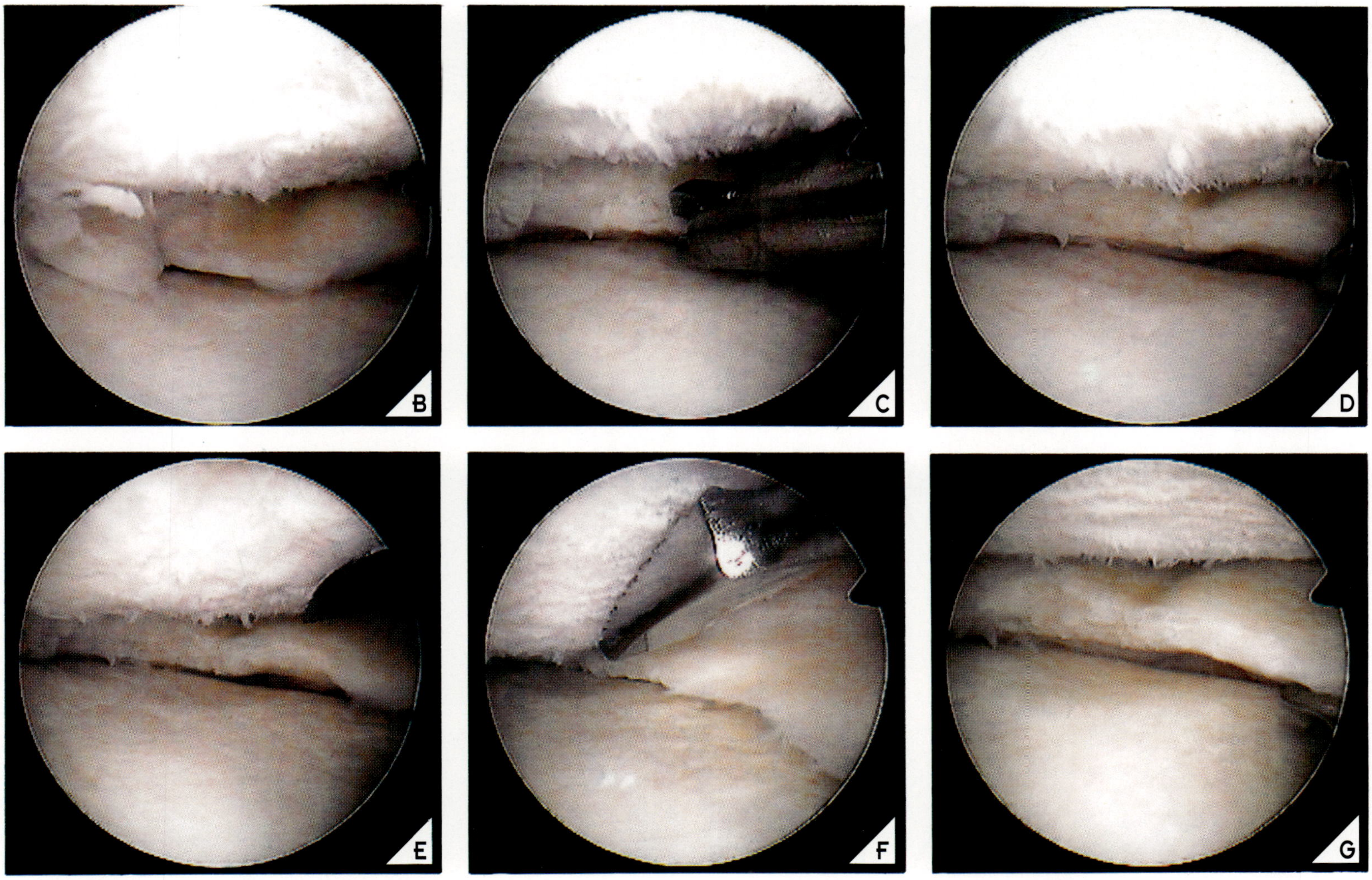

cal fragment while arthroscopic scissors amputate the base. The rim should be probed and gently trimmed with a basket or motorized cutter.

Excision of a small superior flap tear can be accomplished with basket forceps. A large flap can be avulsed after the base is divided incompletely with scissors, leaving a tenuous attachment to the meniscus. The remaining rim of the meniscus should be probed and contoured. The inferior flap can be lifted with a percutaneous spinal needle for better visualization of the base. Final trimming and meniscal contouring can be performed with a motorized instrument. Any meniscal debris should be thoroughly washed out of the joint with copious lavage (Figs. 1.14, 1.15).

Flaps can also be inverted underneath the meniscus. One should be suspicious when the meniscus has a rounded edge in one area instead of the normal sharp, free

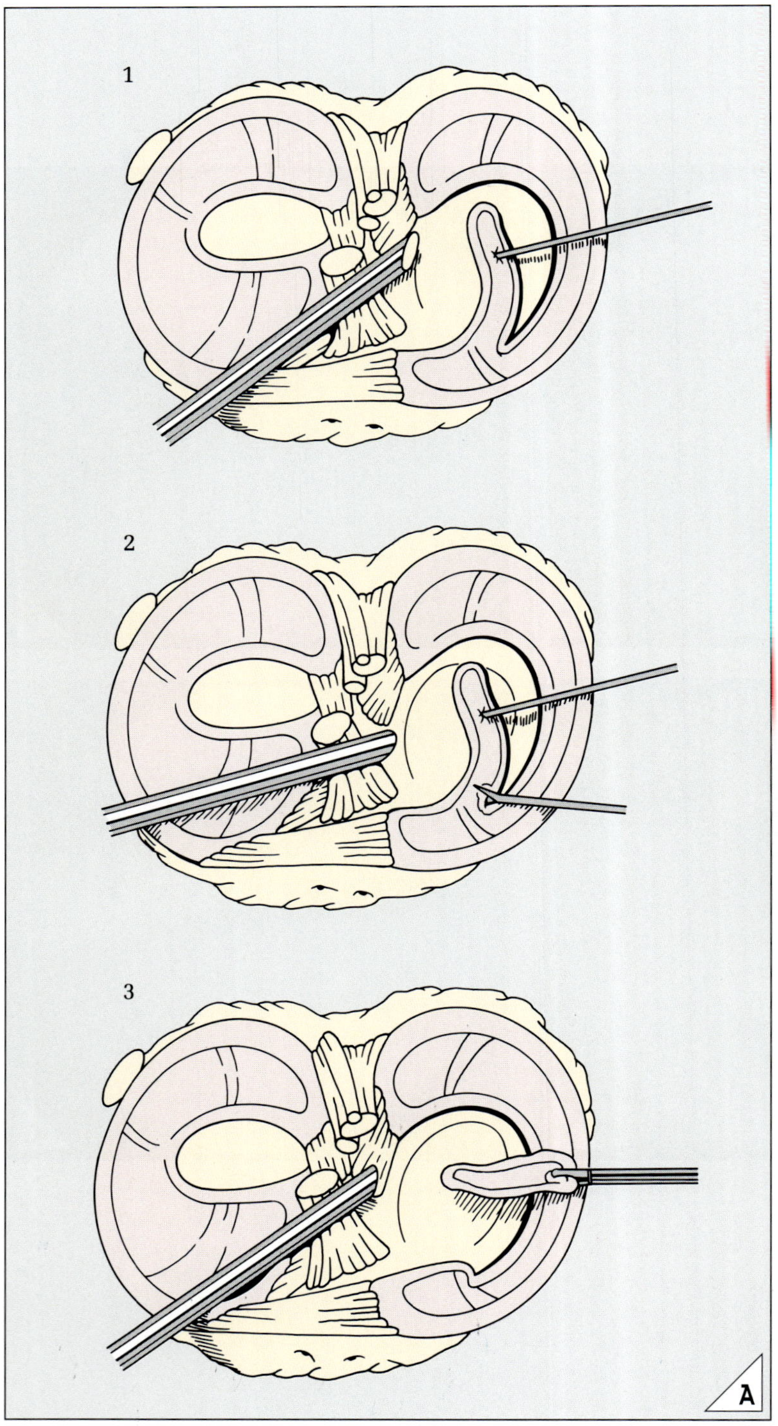

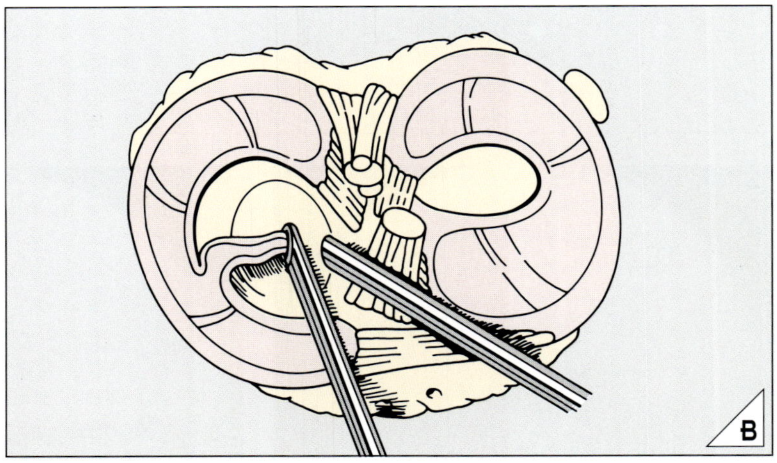

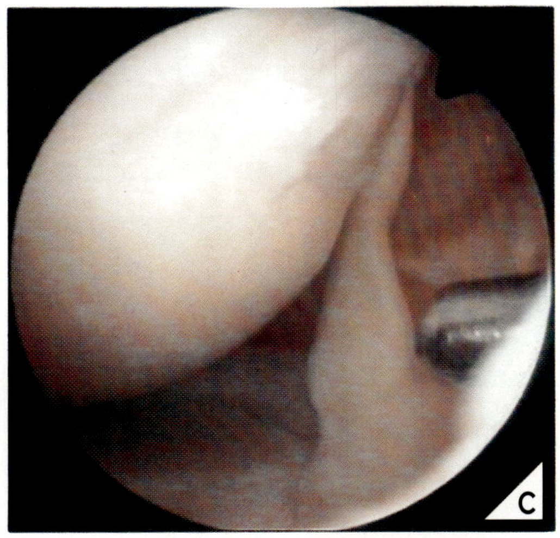

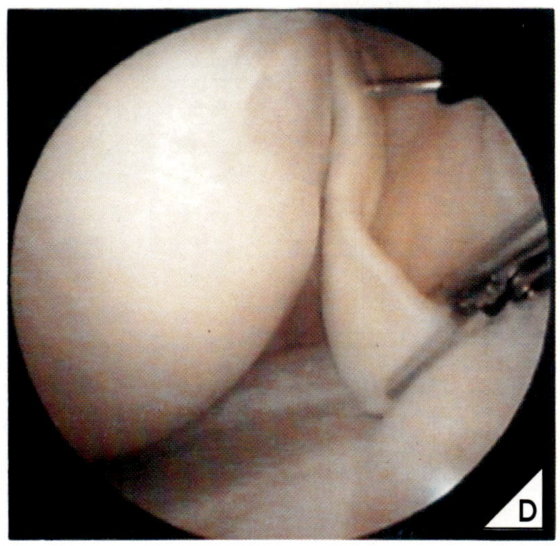

Figure 1.14
(A) Schematic illustration of excision of a flap tear in the anterior horn of the medial meniscus right knee using hand instruments. (B) Excision of a flap tear left knee using motorized instruments. (C–E) Arthroscopic visualization of the steps of excision of a flap tear in the anterior horn of the medial meniscus right knee. (F) Excision of flap tear of the medial meniscus left knee using a shaver.

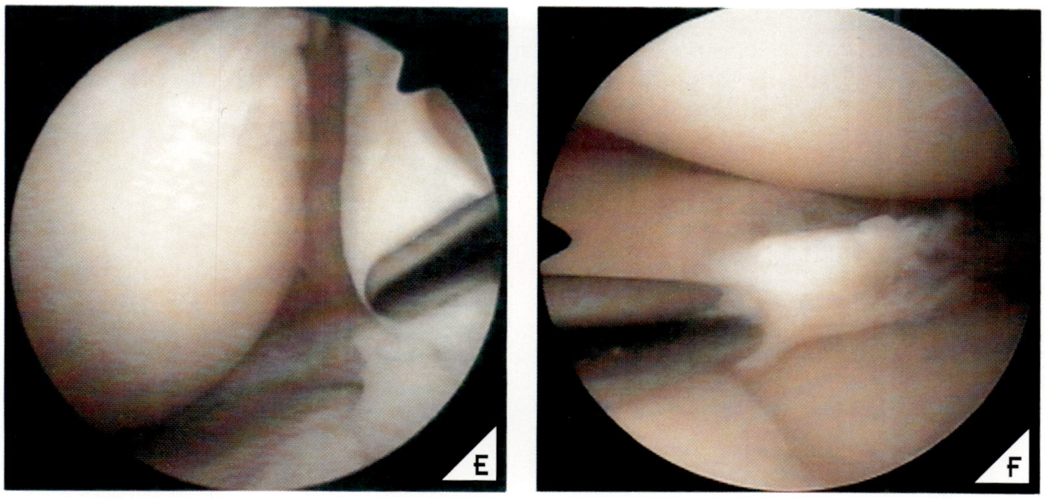

Figure 1.14 (continued)

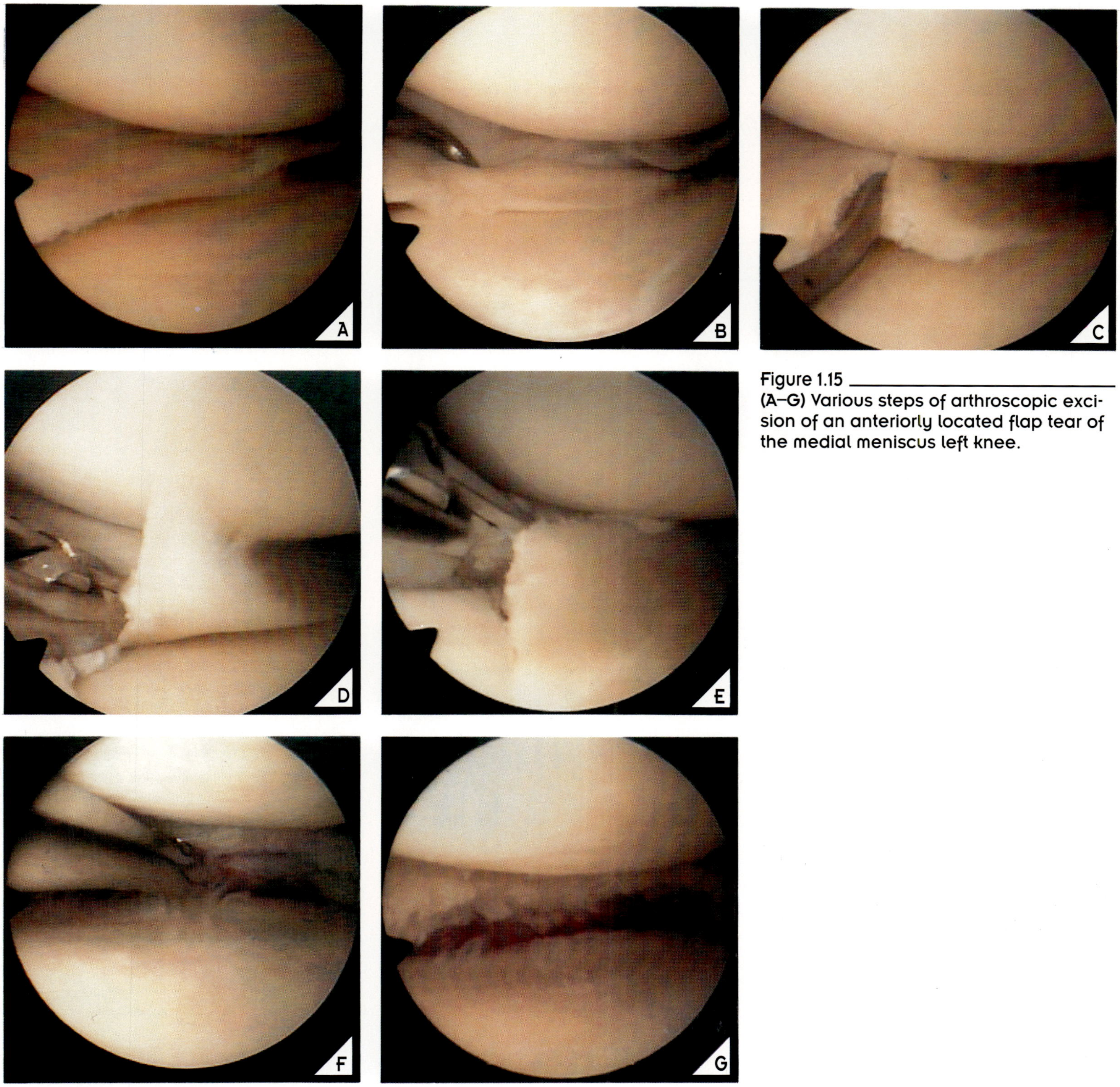

Figure 1.15
(A–G) Various steps of arthroscopic excision of an anteriorly located flap tear of the medial meniscus left knee.

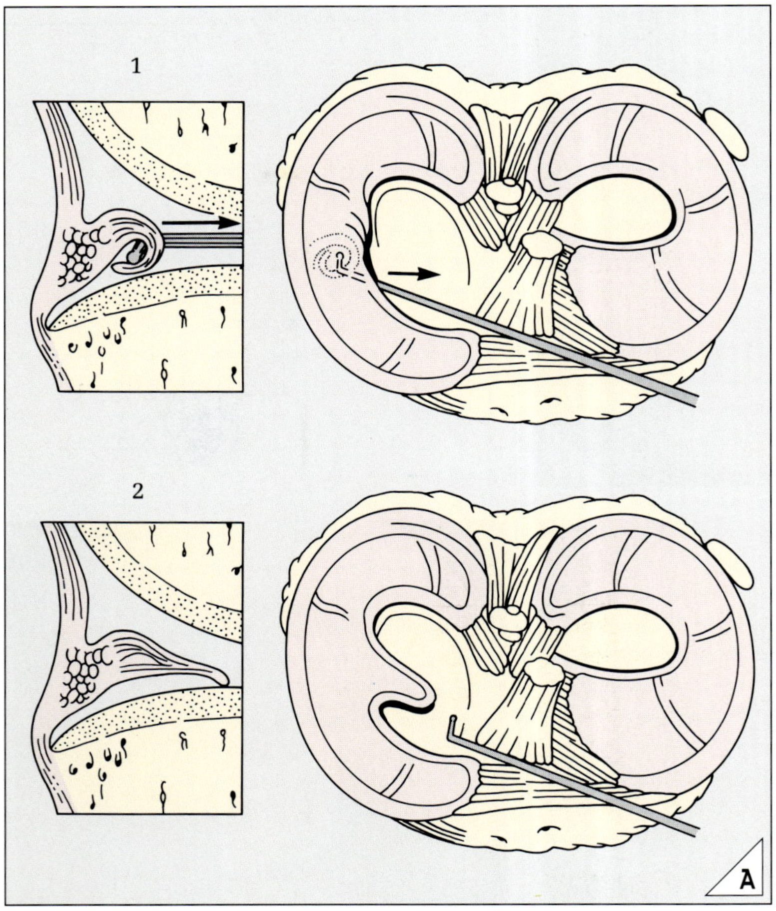

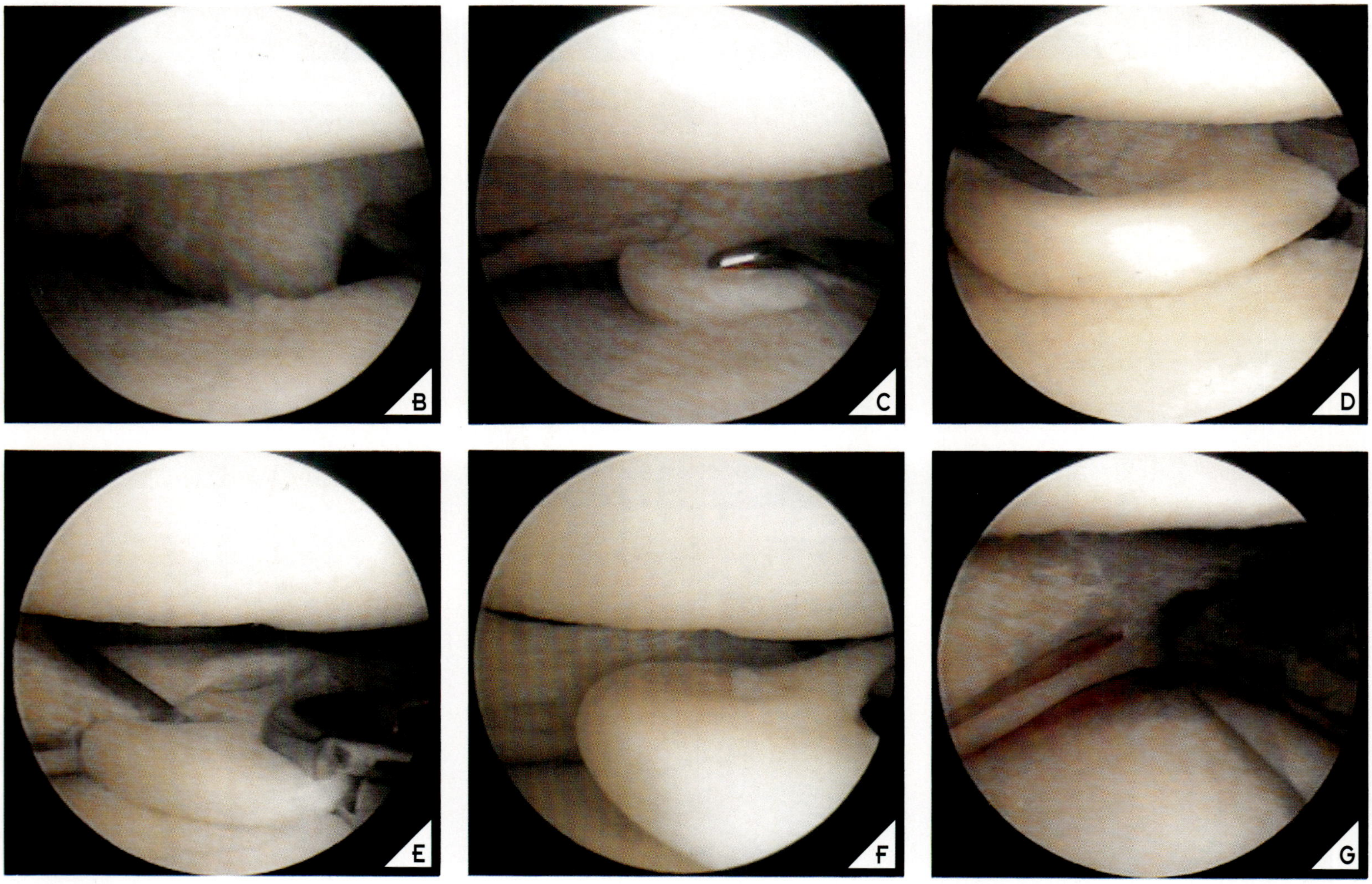

Figure 1.16

Schematic illustration (A) and arthroscopic visualization (B–G) of various steps of the excision of a posteriorly located inverted flap tear in the medial meniscus left knee.

edge. Probing will usually deliver a meniscal fragment of variable size. Complete resection can be done as previously described (Fig. 1.16).

Horizontal tear

This tear exhibits two leaves, one superior and one inferior. It is important to probe a horizontal tear carefully to judge its limits and rule out the existence of a vertical tear at the periphery of one of the leaves. When both leaves are of equal thickness, the unstable one should be excised. When both are stable, it is preferable to remove the inferior leaf. If the superior leaf is thicker but unstable at the periphery because of a tear, the inferior leaf can be excised and the superior one repaired. It is always advisable to gently trim the free border of the remaining leaf, which is usually degenerated and friable. Arthroscopic excision of the horizontal tear can be performed by use of a combination of instruments, such as basket forceps and a meniscal cutter. The inner edge of the leaf to be resected is trimmed towards the periphery. Once the well vascularized peripheral area is reached, it is not necessary to be too aggressive with the resection. This more peripheral aspect of the cleavage component of the tear will heal and will smooth out with the passage of time. Thorough lavage and suction of the joint, to remove loose meniscal fragments, complete the procedure (Figs. 1.17, 1.18).

Degenerative tear

A degenerative meniscal tear can be isolated, but more often is a component of a larger picture, the degenerative knee of an older patient (Figs. 1.19–1.24).

When the degenerative tear is isolated, arthroscopic

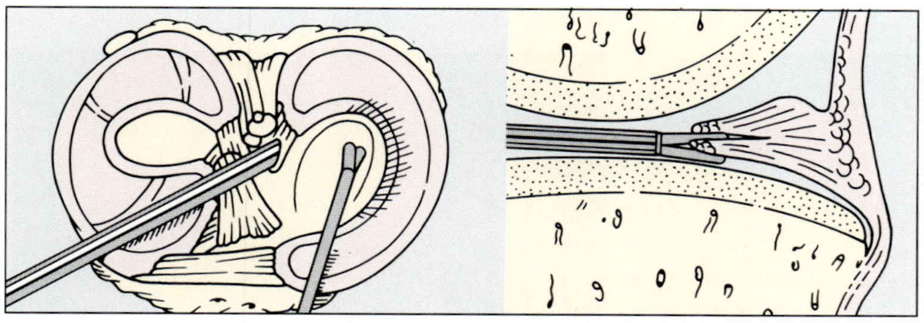

Figure 1.17
Schematic illustration of excision of a horizontal tear in the medial meniscus right knee.

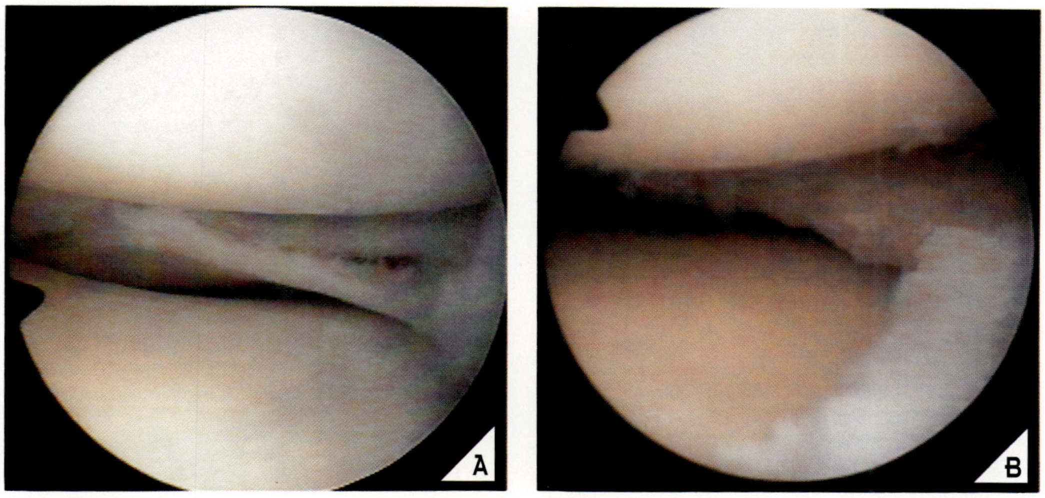

Figure 1.18
Arthroscopic visualization of a horizontal tear in the medial meniscus right knee before (A) and after (B) excision.

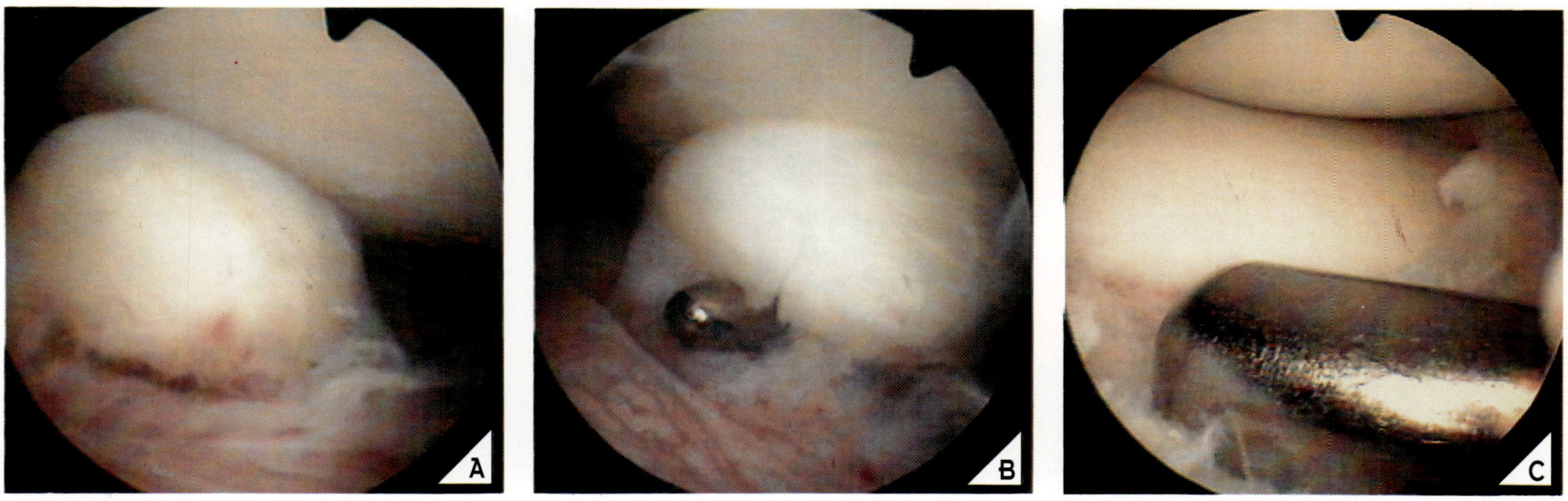

Figure 1.19
(A–C) Arthroscopic visualization of the excision of an anterior horn flap tear in the medial meniscus right knee.

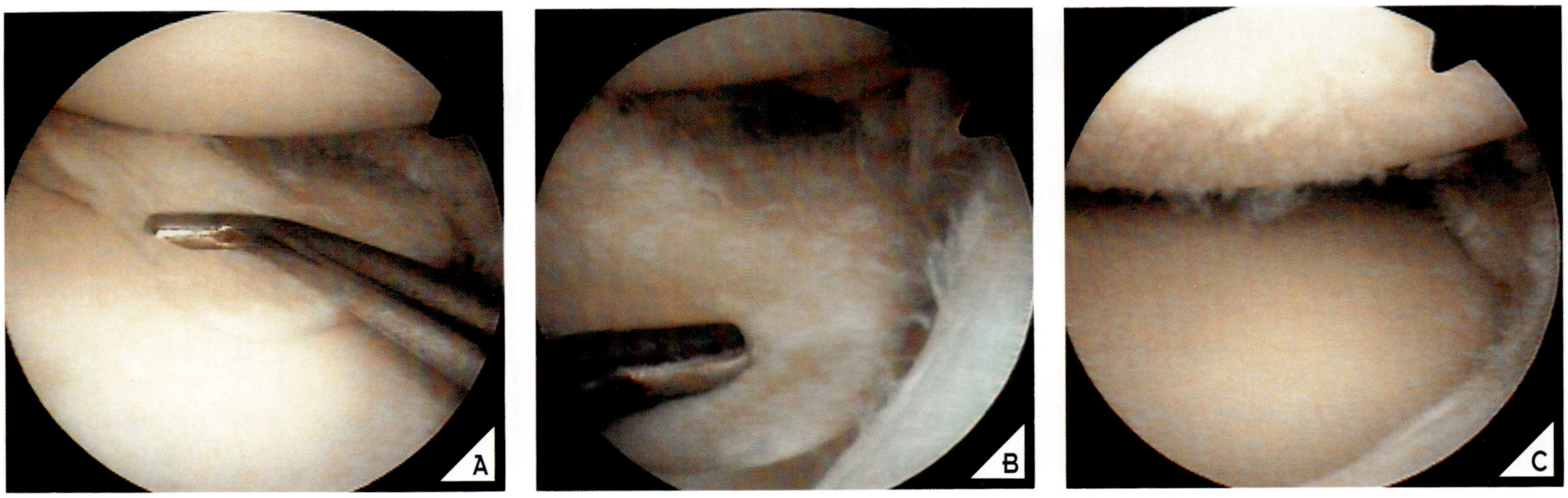

Figure 1.20
(A–C) Posteriorly-based degenerative flap tear in the medial meniscus right knee before and after excision.

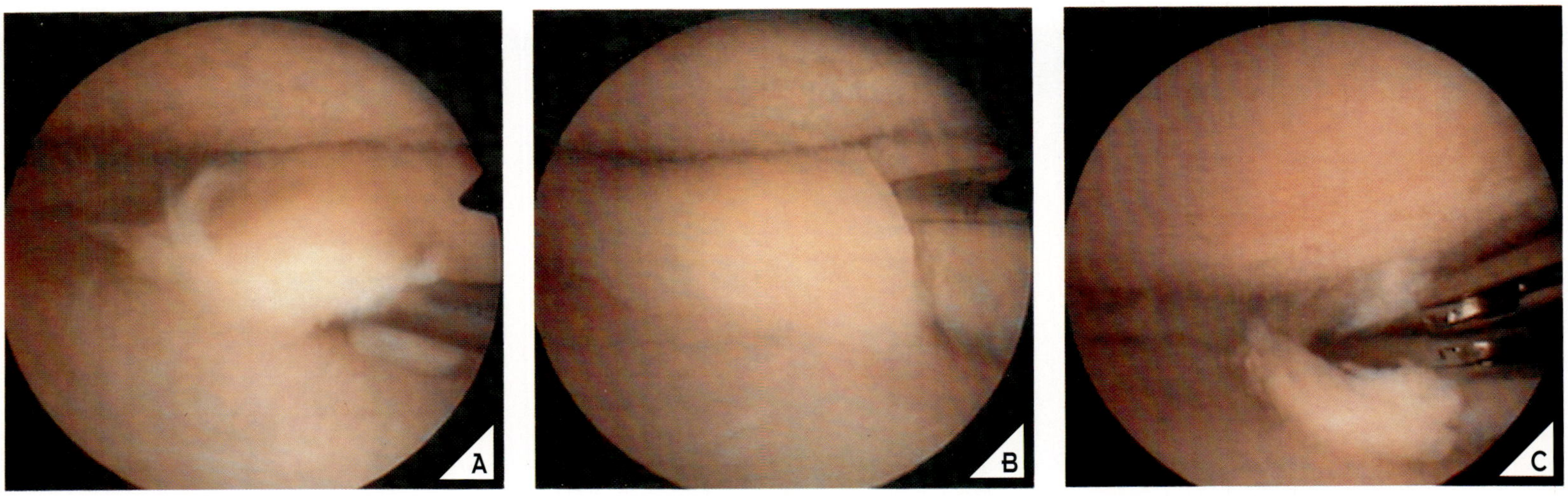

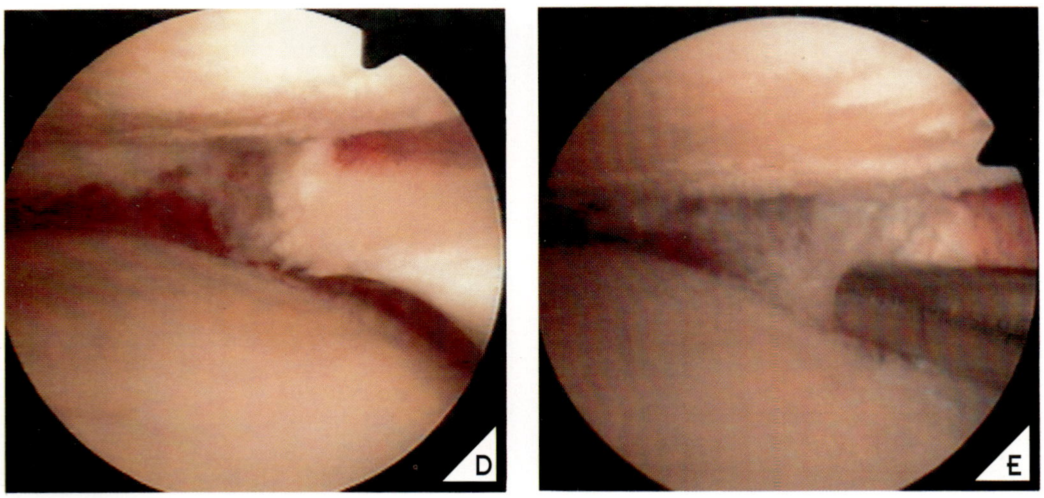

Figure 1.21
(A–E) Steps of excision of an anteriorly-based degenerative flap tear in the medial meniscus right knee.

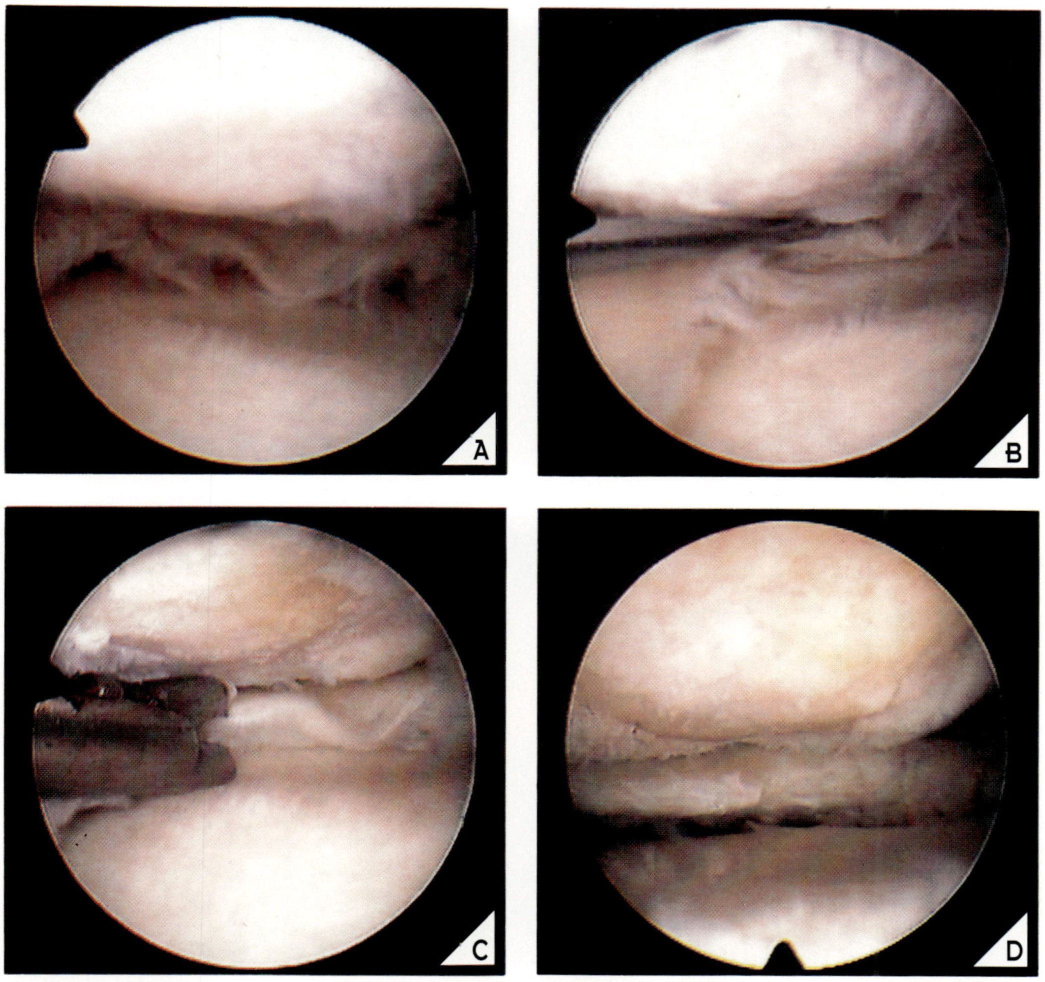

Figure 1.22
(A–D) Steps of excision of a degenerative tear in the medial meniscus left knee using a suction-punch basket.

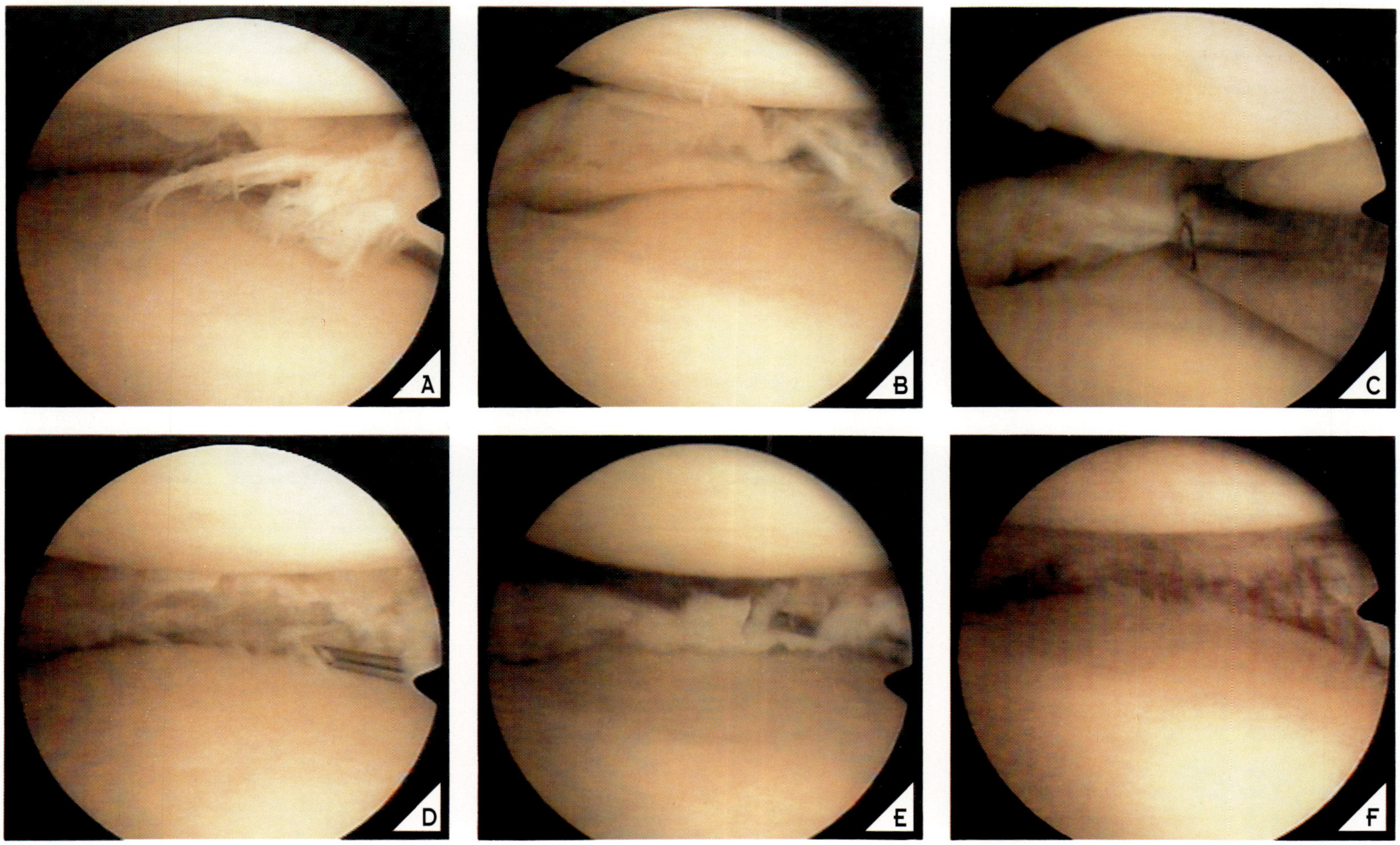

Figure 1.23
(A–F) Steps of excision of a degenerative tear in the medial meniscus right knee using a suction-punch basket. In steps D and E a percutaneous spinal needle is used to bring the superior leaf into view for proper debridement.

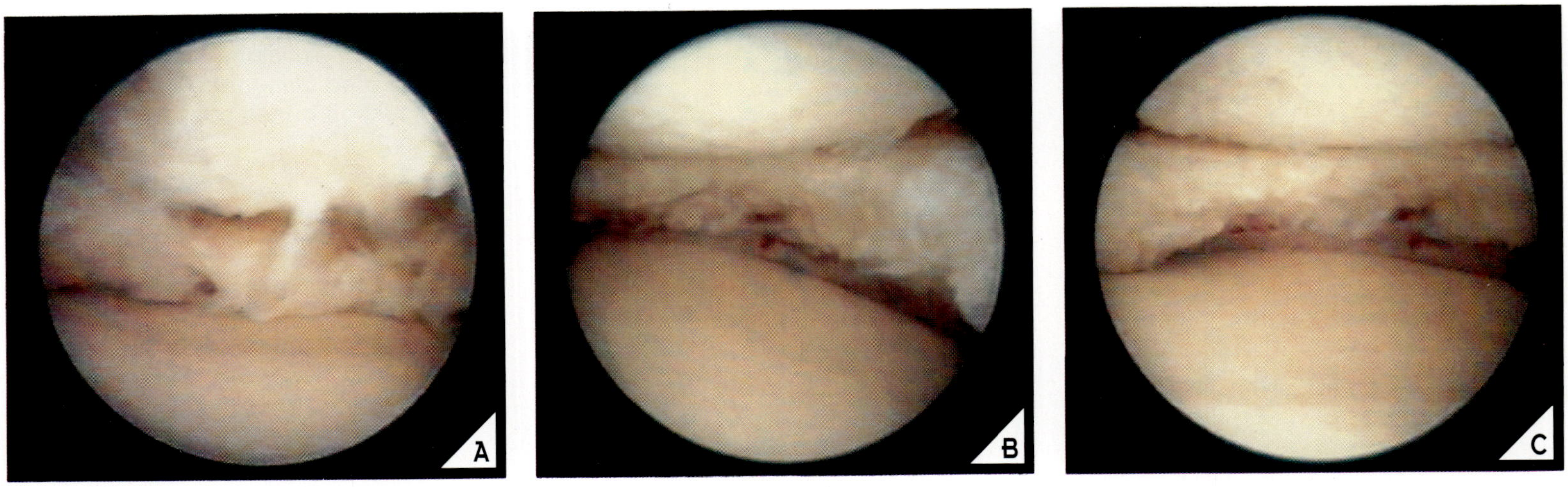

Figure 1.24
(A–C) Degenerative tear in the medial meniscus right knee before and after partial medial meniscectomy and chondroplasty of the medial femoral condyle. Basket forceps and motorized instruments were used for the arthroscopic debridement.

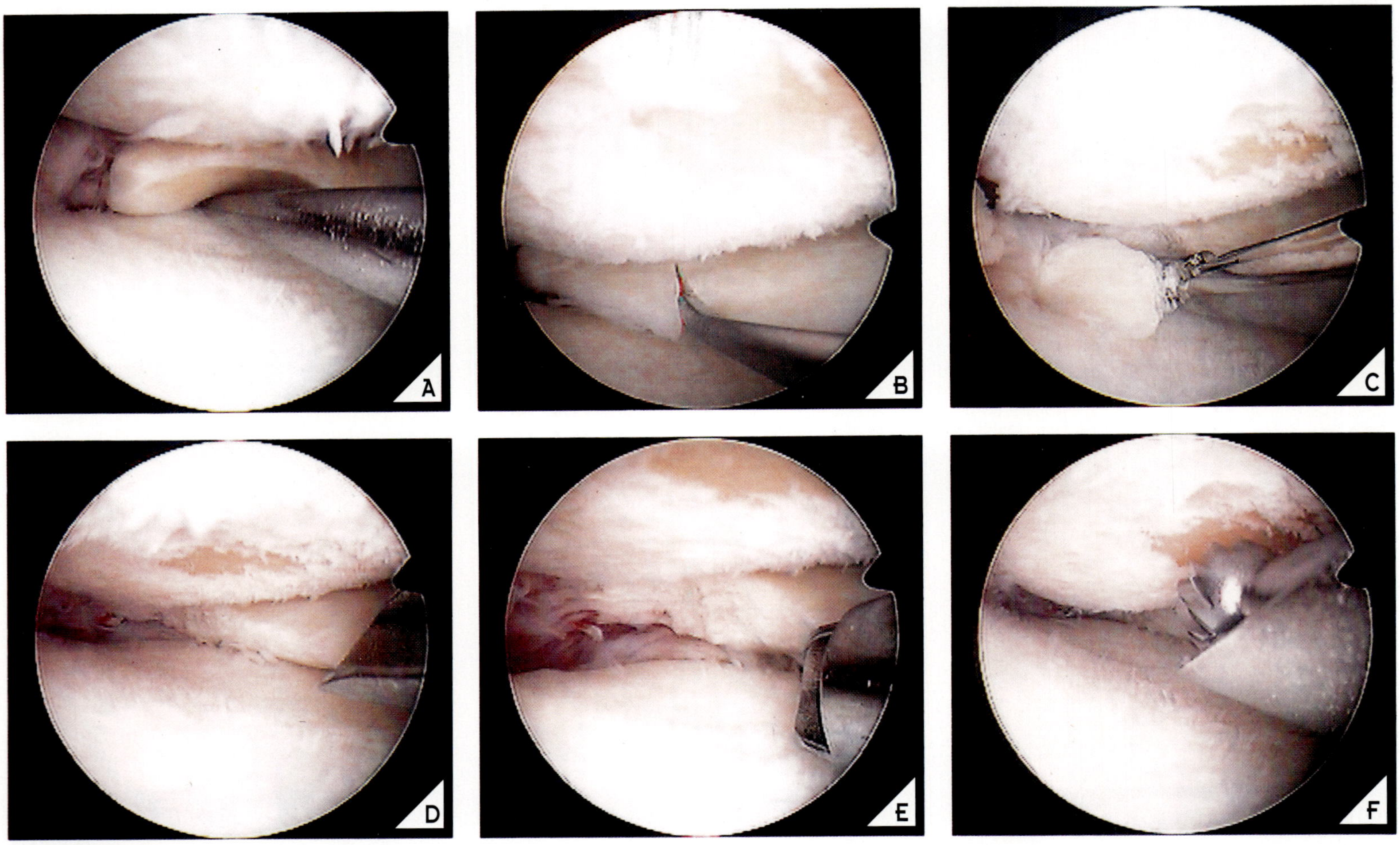

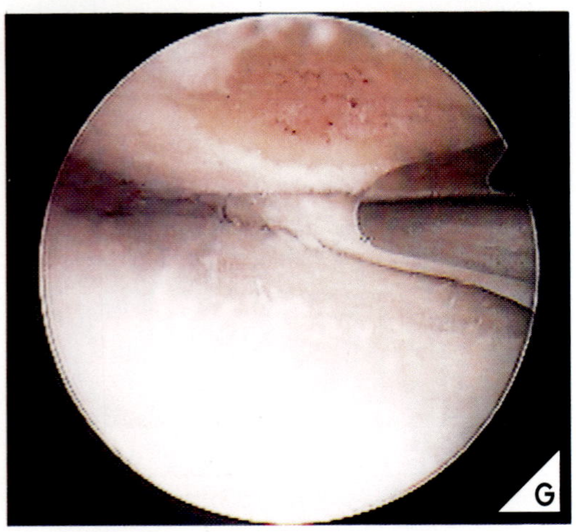

Figure 1.25
(A–G) Steps of partial medial meniscectomy and abrasion arthroplasty for a degenerative complex tear of the posterior horn of the medial meniscus right knee. A curved rosette knife, basket forceps, and an abrader were used during the arthroscopic procedure.

surgery is beneficial if these patients present with mechanical symptoms. A careful examination and assessment of the tear should be performed, and only the major flaps and unstable fragments should be excised. Basket forceps can be used, although motorized cutters are very effective for this type of degenerated tissue. When chondromalacic areas are present, shaving is done with a motorized shaver. It is not necessary to perform an abrasion arthroplasty for a partial-thickness lesion of the articular cartilage, but this procedure may be of benefit to a localized, full-thickness lesion.

When arthroscopic partial meniscectomy is done in patients with degenerative arthritis, appropriate procedures such as excision of osteophytes, partial synovectomy, and excision of loose articular cartilage fragments should complete the joint debridement. It is important to remember that the meniscus, even when degenerated, is still useful and has important functions providing it is stable. It is not unusual for patients to complain of further symptoms after arthroscopic partial meniscectomy has been performed for a degenerative meniscus.

Complex Tears

When the meniscal tear involves many planes it is referred to as a complex tear. All the components of the tear should be removed in a systematic way (Figs. 1.25–1.27). When present, flaps should be resected first, followed by excision of the larger unstable fragments. A subtotal meniscectomy, including excision of the peripheral rim of the posterior aspect of the meniscus, and salvage of the anterior horn and part of the body, is sometimes required for this type of tear.

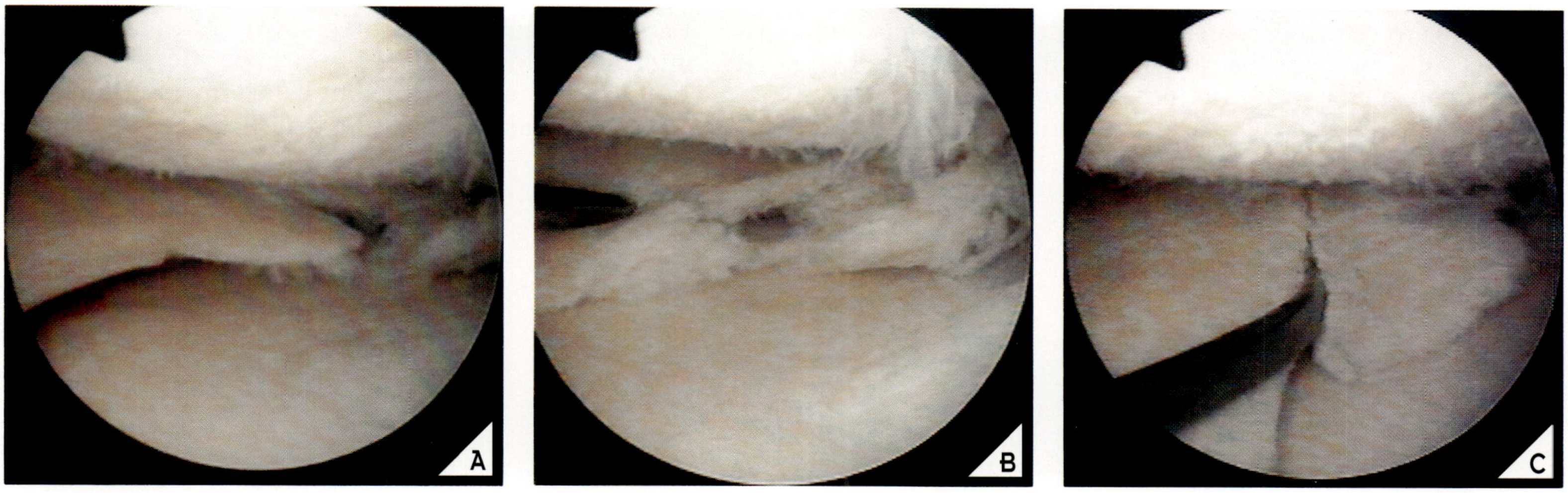

Figure 1.26
(A–C) Some steps in excision of a complex tear in the medial meniscus left knee. A curved rosette knife and motorized shaver were used.

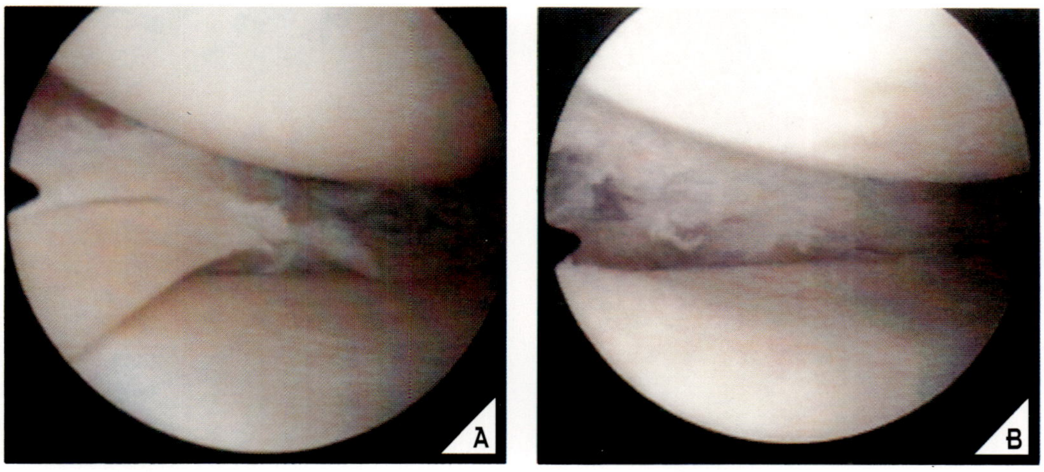

Figure 1.27
(A, B) Complex tear in the medial meniscus left knee before and after partial medial meniscectomy using a curved rosette knife and motorized shaver.

LATERAL MENISCUS

Some anatomic characteristics of the lateral compartment of the knee are worth emphasizing when arthroscopic surgery on the lateral meniscus is planned. The lateral meniscus, unlike its medial counterpart, has the appearance of a closed ring, with its anterior and posterior attachments lying between those of the medial meniscus. Its average width of 12 to 13 mm is greater than that of the medial meniscus. Fibers from the posterior horn attach to the medial femoral condyle, to form the Humphrey and Wrisberg meniscofemoral ligaments, respectively located anterior and posterior to the posterior cruciate ligament. The lateral meniscus is loosely connected to the joint capsule and has a unique relationship with the popliteus tendon posteriorly (Fig. 1.28).[13–15] This tendon passes through a hiatus in the peripheral attachment that is slightly anterior to the midcoronal plane of the meniscus. Two distinct attachments, the superior and inferior fascicles, arising respectively from the superior and inferior surfaces of the lateral meniscus, form the roof and floor of the popliteal tunnel. This normal hiatus in the lateral aspect of the lateral meniscus should not be confused with a peripheral detachment of the meniscus. The degree of integrity of the fascicles influences the arthroscopic management of a tear located in this area. The lateral inferior geniculate artery is at the meniscal level and is susceptible to injury during surgery. The lateral tibial plateau is lower than the medial and has a dome-shaped appearance in the center. Therefore, to reach the posterior horn of the lateral meniscus from the medial side, the portal should be placed close to the patellar tendon and way above the meniscus.

Patterns of Tears

Tears of the lateral meniscus also can be classified into radial (vertical transverse), vertical longitudinal, horizontal, degenerative, and complex (Fig. 1.29). Flap tears can develop from any of the three planes previously mentioned and from any of the three segments of the meniscus (anterior, middle, and posterior). In addition, cystic degeneration of the meniscus and discoid meniscus are more commonly seen on the lateral side of the knee.

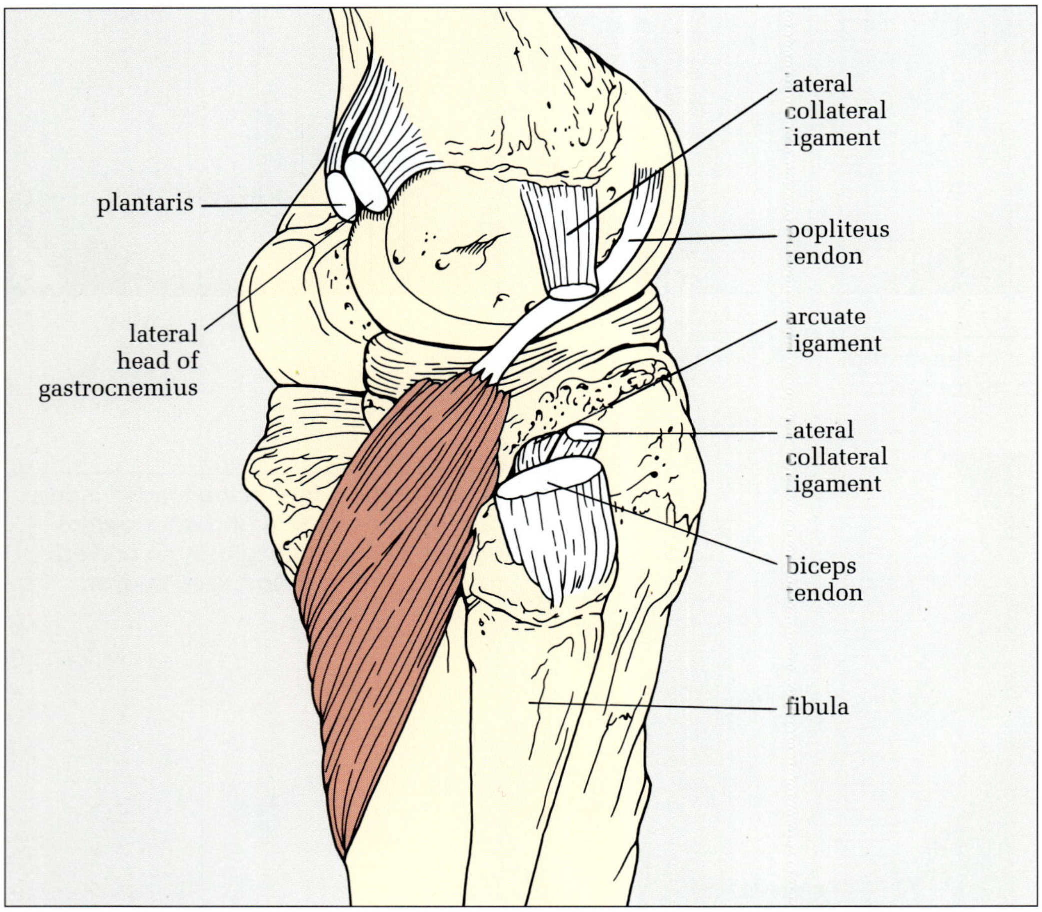

Figure 1.28 The posterolateral aspect of the left knee.

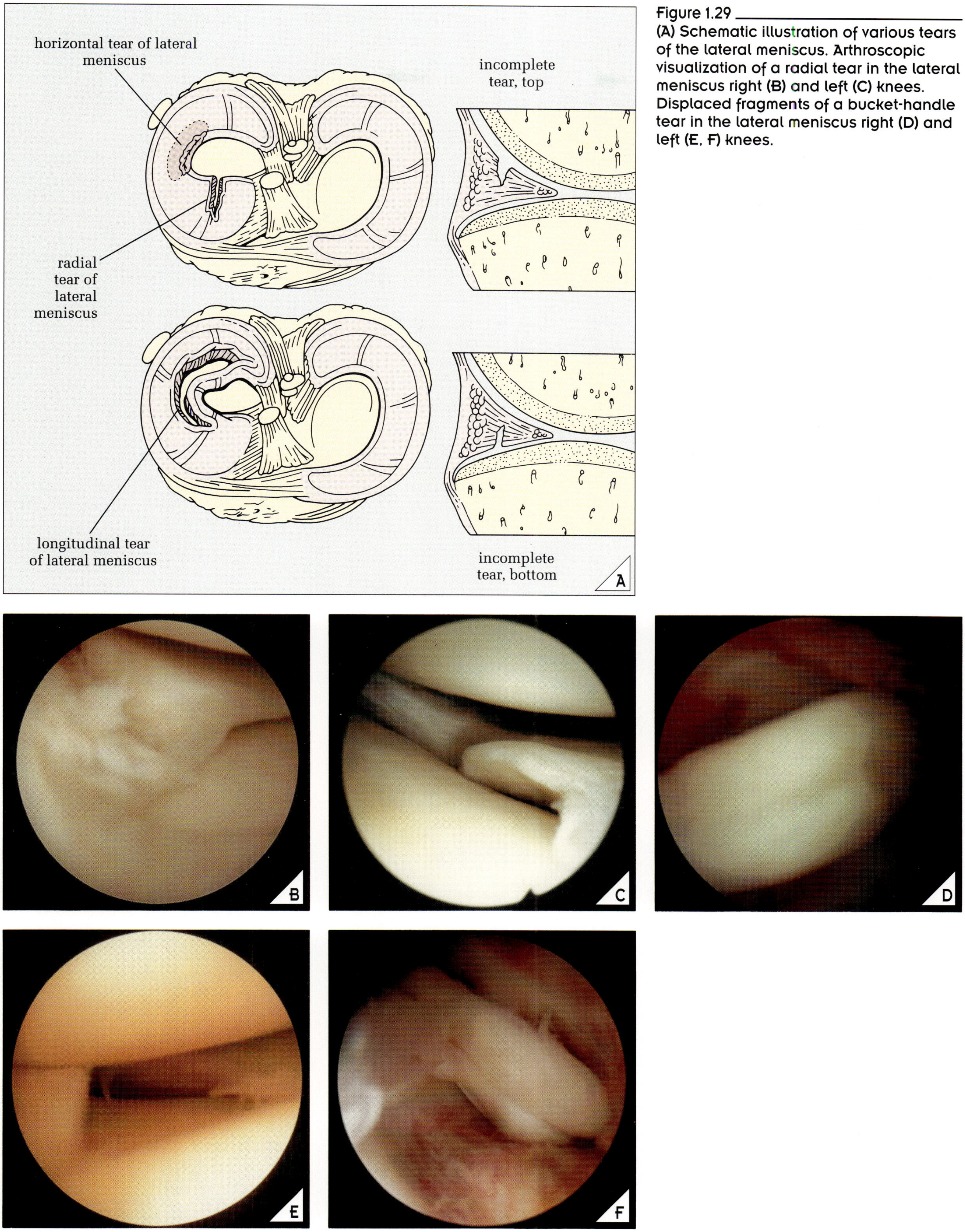

Figure 1.29

(A) Schematic illustration of various tears of the lateral meniscus. Arthroscopic visualization of a radial tear in the lateral meniscus right (B) and left (C) knees. Displaced fragments of a bucket-handle tear in the lateral meniscus right (D) and left (E, F) knees.

Surgical Technique

Radial Tear

When the radial tear involves the midsegment of the meniscus, a complete arthroscopic examination of all the compartments of the knee is performed. First, the arthroscope is placed through the anterolateral portal with the knee in varus stress. The anterior part of the tear can then be excised with a 90° rotary basket punch. The torn posterior aspect can be resected, preferably with a straight basket punch. A suction device can be introduced into the joint to remove all the loose meniscal fragments. An alternative method is to use suction basket forceps if they are available. Final probing should check the stability of the lateral meniscus in front of the popliteal tunnel (Fig. 1.30).

When the transverse tear is in front of the popliteal tunnel, the rim should not be trimmed aggressively, to avoid instability of the meniscal bridge opposite the tunnel.

Vertical Longitudinal Tear

The vertical longitudinal tear, whether short, long, or bucket-handle, can be managed with the two-portal approach (Figs. 1.31, 1.33-1.35). Partial division of the posterior attachment of the tear is done with straight scissors, followed by complete section of the anterior attachment with angled scissors and avulsion of the mobile meniscal fragment with grasping forceps. Occasionally, with a dis-

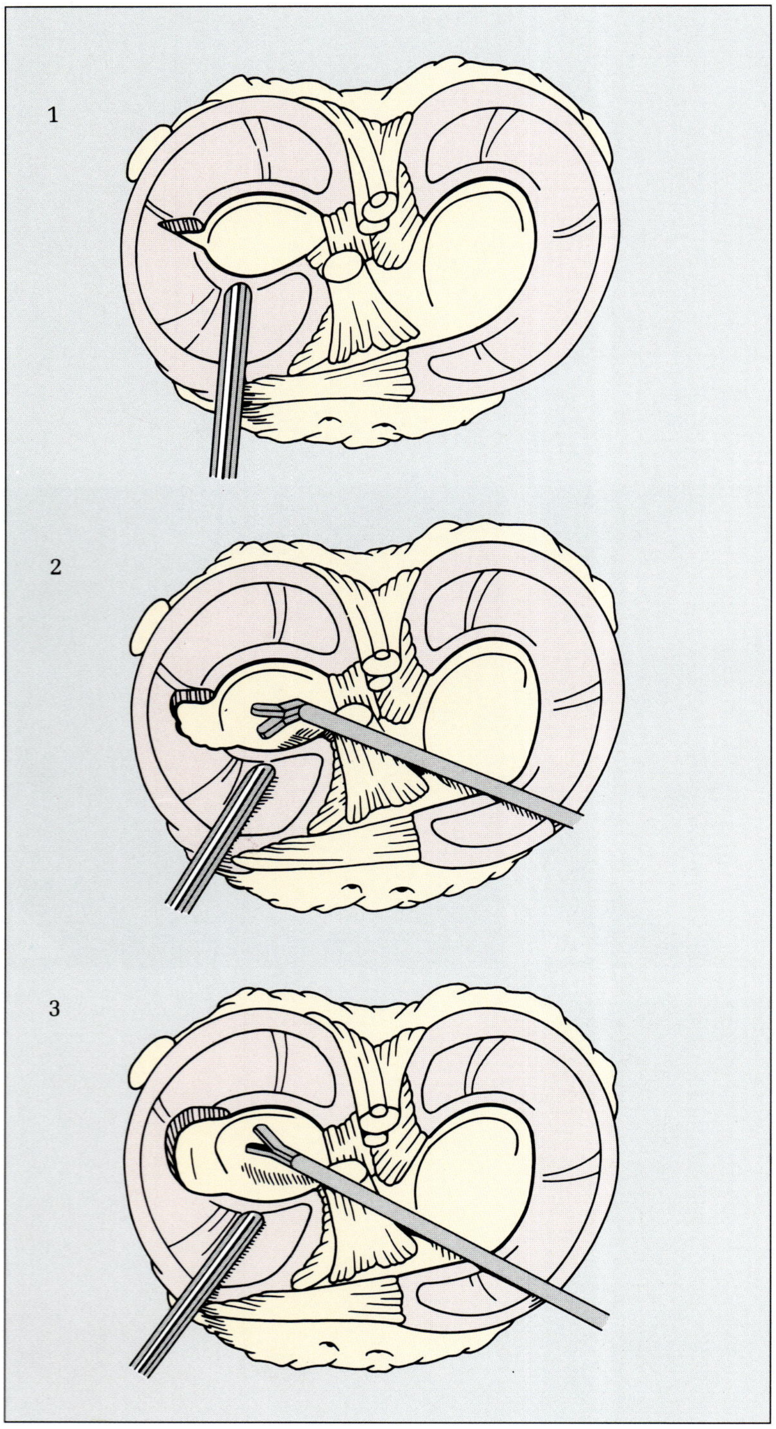

Figure 1.30
The steps of excision of a radial tear in the lateral meniscus right knee.

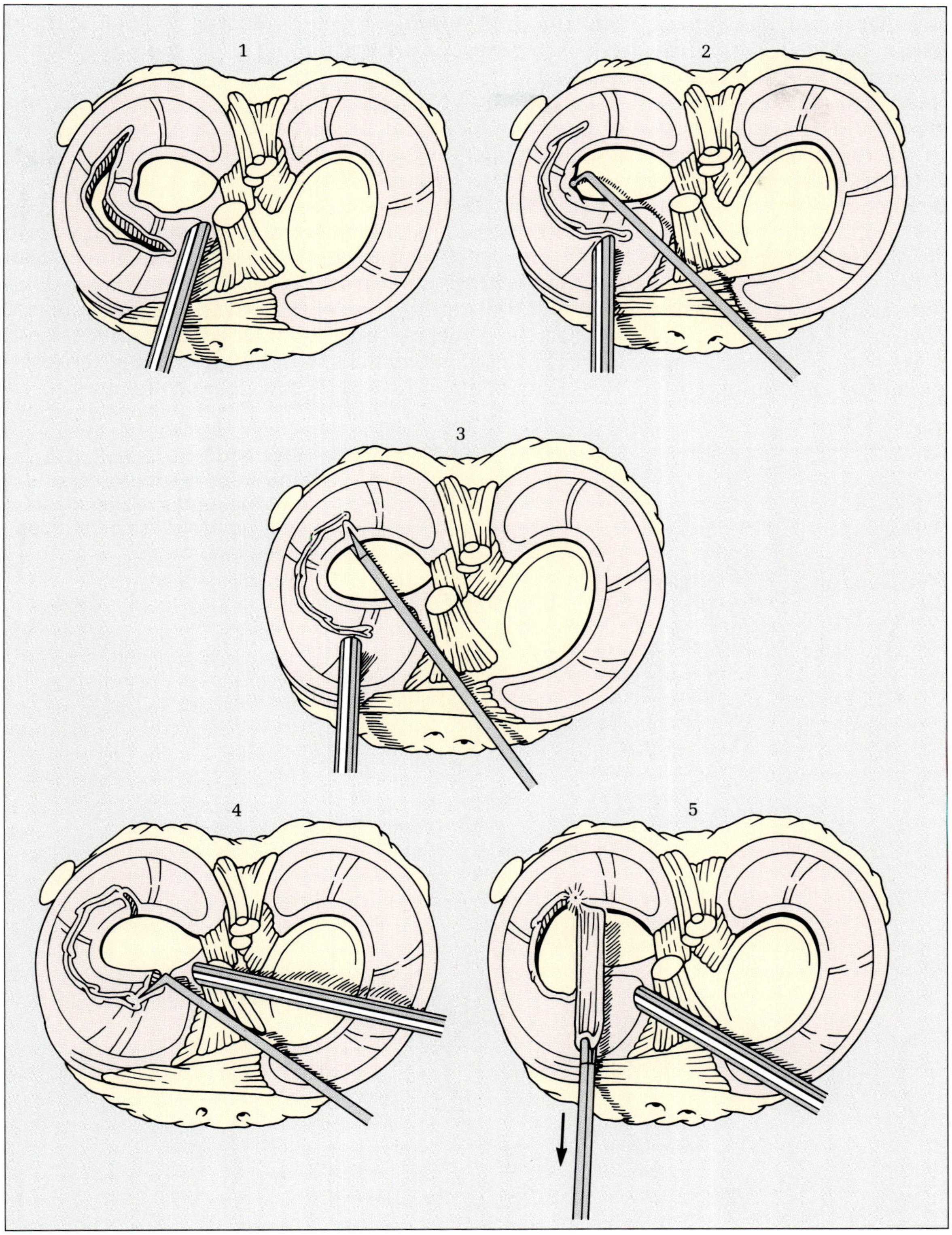

Figure 1.31

The steps of excision of a bucket-handle tear in the lateral meniscus using the two-portal approach.

placed chronic bucket-handle tear that cannot be reduced, a three-portal approach is necessary (Fig. 1.32). While viewing through a central or a midpatellar lateral approach, two instruments are placed through the inferior portals (medial and lateral) to grasp the previously sectioned anterior fragment and to cut the posterior attachment with a meniscotome or scissors. A switch of portals may be desirable to facilitate the manipulation of surgical instruments. The final steps are probing the remaining rim for instability and gentle trimming of the meniscal irregularities.

Again, extreme caution is necessary to avoid aggressive trimming of the "popliteal corner" of the remaining meniscal ring. If the fascicles are torn, causing a very unstable situation with the remaining rim subluxating into the joint anterior to the midcoronal plane, a more extensive resection with trimming of the posterior horn is necessary.

Longitudinal peripheral tears of the meniscus are candidates for meniscal preservation, provided that the mobile fragment is intact and not degenerated.

Horizontal Tear

When the horizontal tear involves less than half the width of the meniscus, saucerization of the torn fragments can be done with basket forceps. If the tear involves more than half the width of one of the leaves, it is preferable to salvage the superior one, provided it is stable. If both leaves have secondary tears with involvement of the fascicles, a subtotal meniscectomy may be unavoidable.

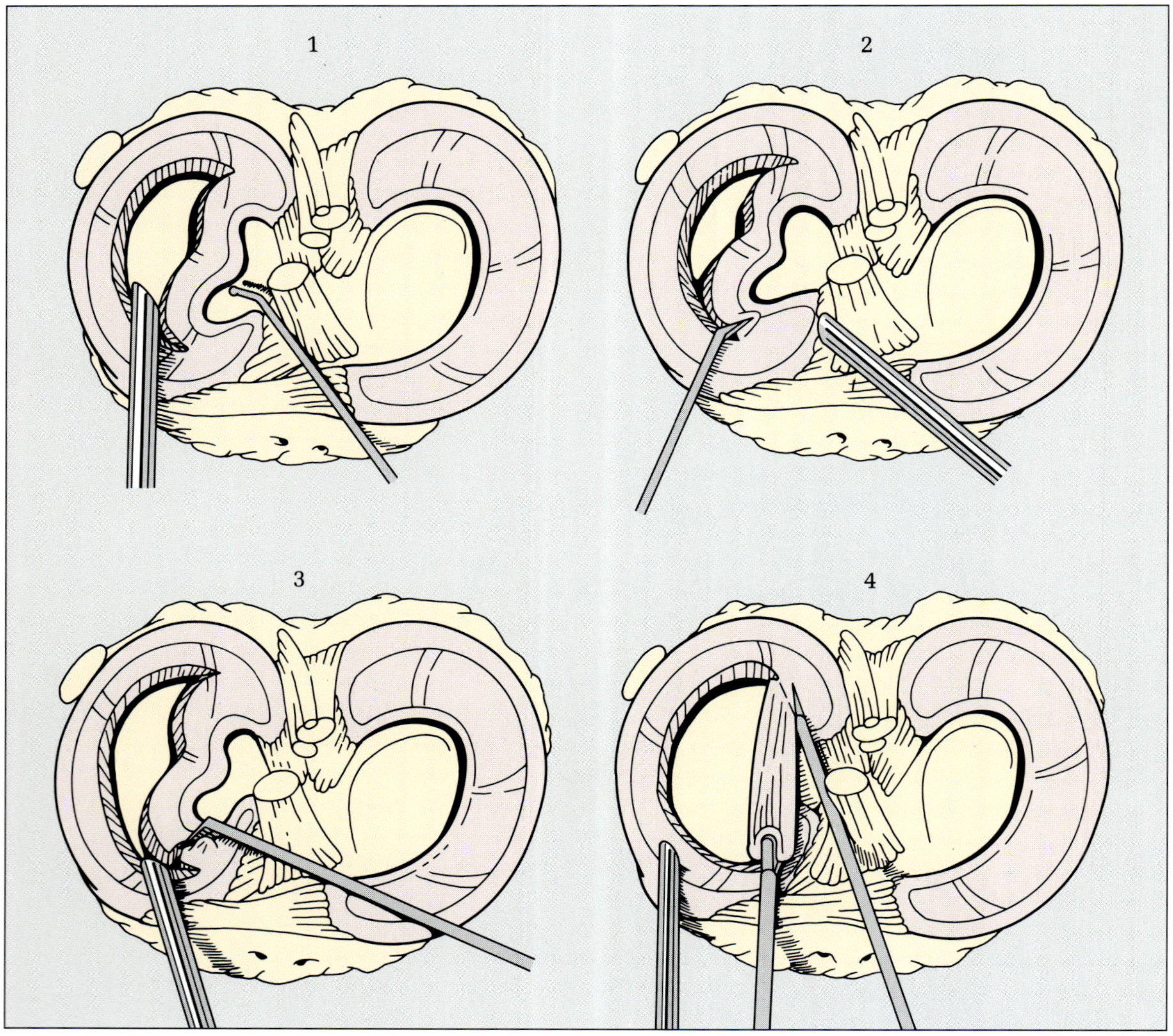

Figure 1.32 The steps of excision of a bucket-handle tear in the lateral meniscus using the three-portal approach.

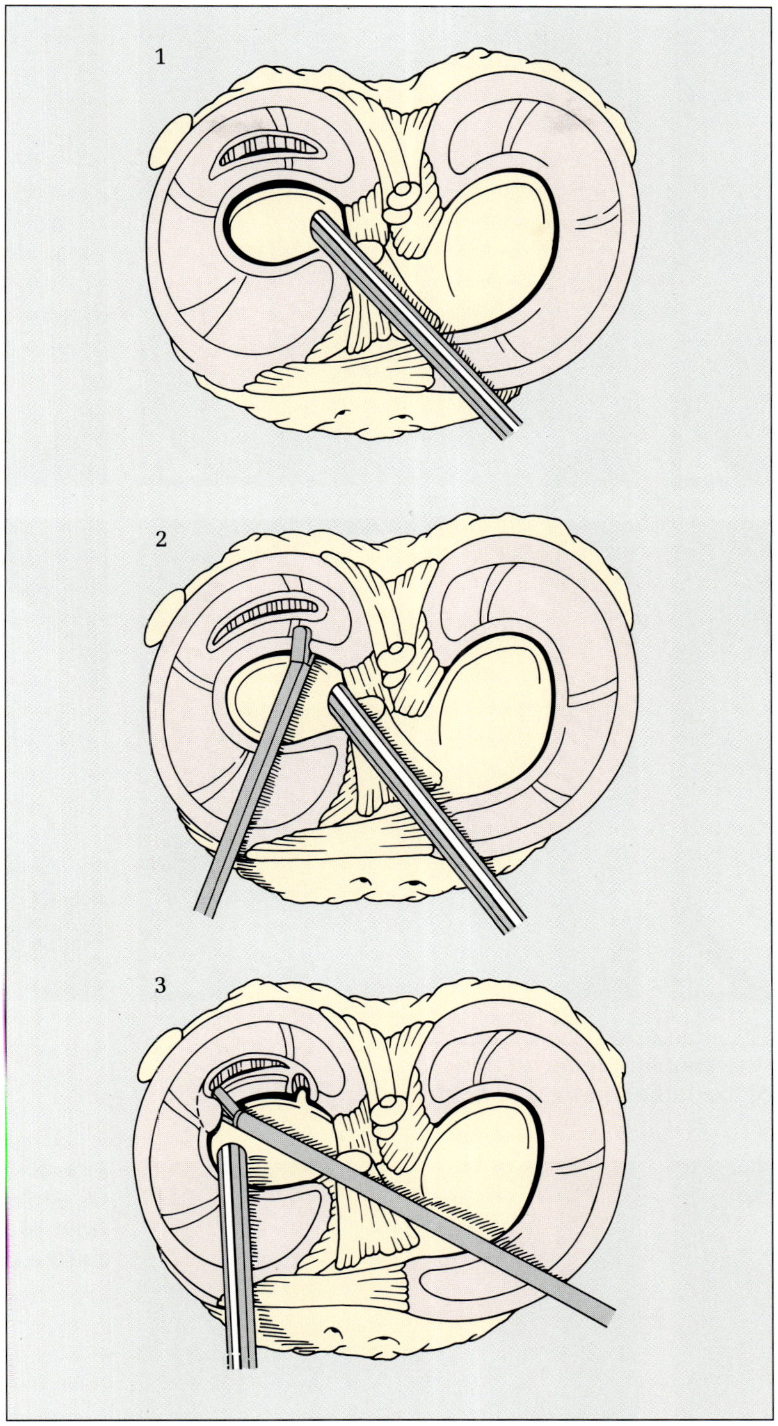

Figure 1.33
Schematic illustration of the various steps of excision of a vertical tear in the lateral meniscus right knee using the two-portal approach.

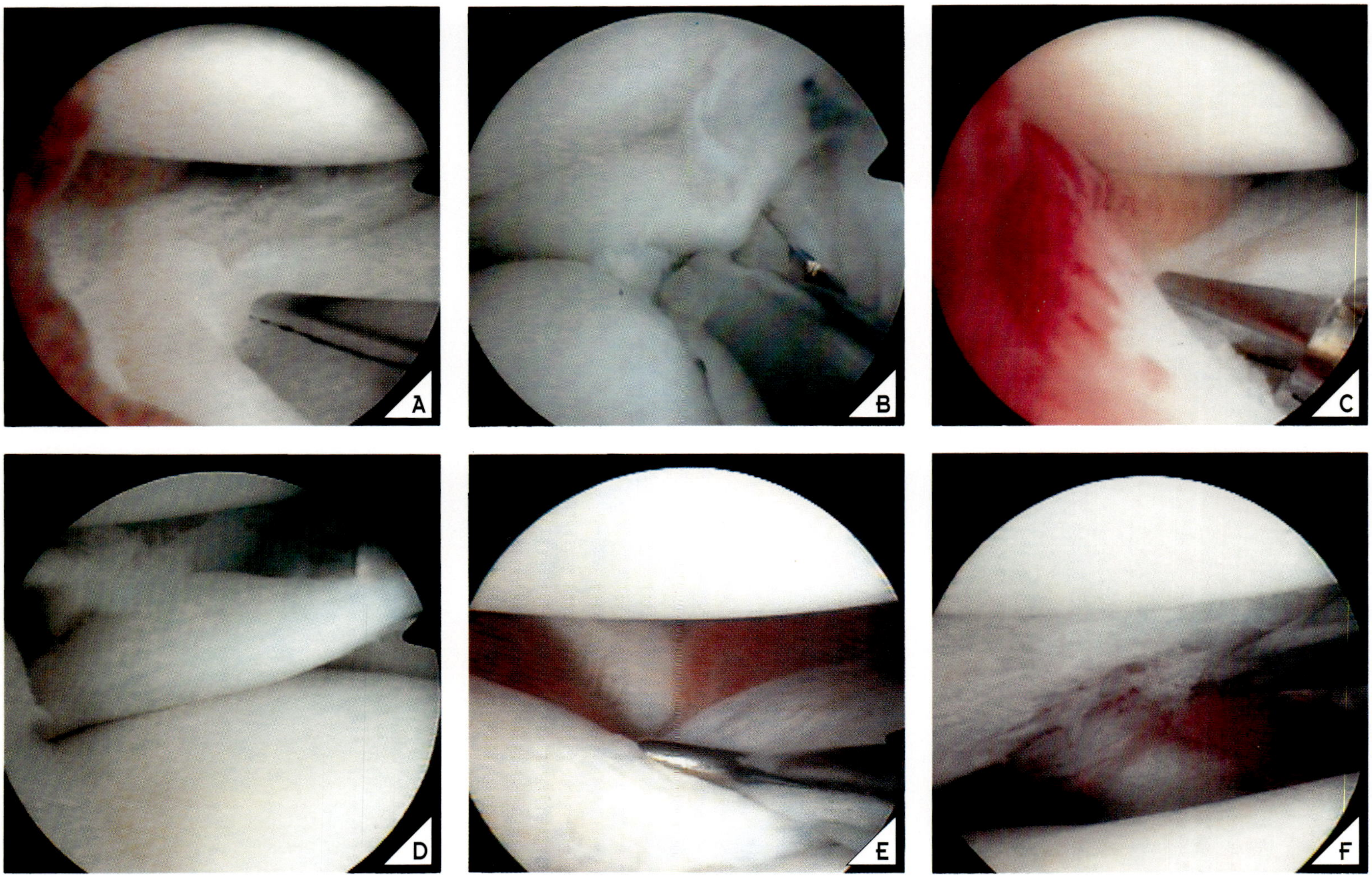

Figure 1.34
(A–F) Arthroscopic visualization of the steps for removal of a vertical tear in the posterior horn of the lateral meniscus right knee.

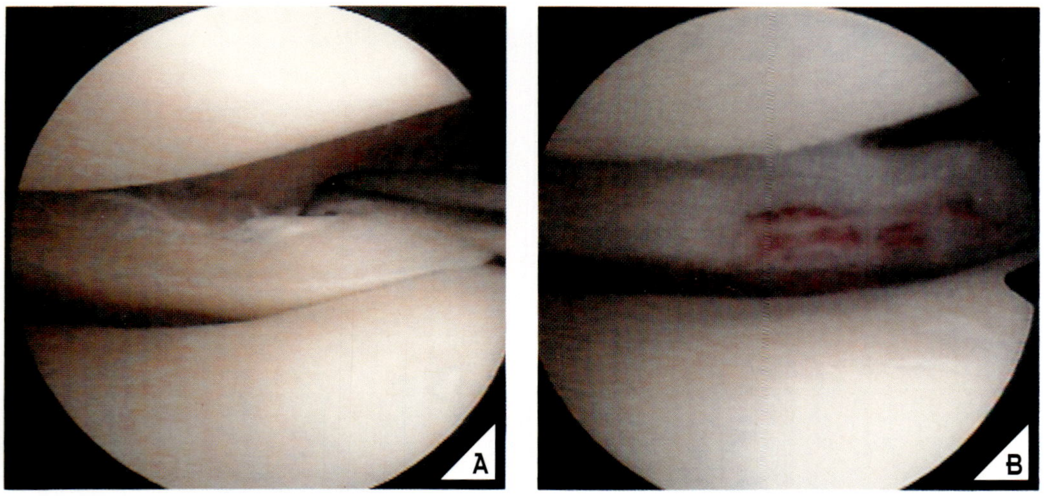

Figure 1.35
(A, B) Small vertical tear in the posterior horn of the lateral meniscus right knee before and after excision.

FLAP TEAR

The base of the posteriorly located long flap tear can be divided partially, leaving a few fibers of attachment to enable easy avulsion with grasping forceps. Small posterior tears can be excised with basket forceps. Small flap tears of the anterior horn can be easily handled with rotary basket forceps. A large flap can be placed under tension with a grasper or spinal needle while its base is divided with a knife or rotary scissors (Figs. 1.36, 1.37). A three-portal approach may also be necessary in this situation. Double oblique flap tears of the lateral meniscus, if stable, can be trimmed back to normal meniscus. However, if they are located in front of the popliteal tunnel, these tears can be quite unstable, and more generous excision may be needed.

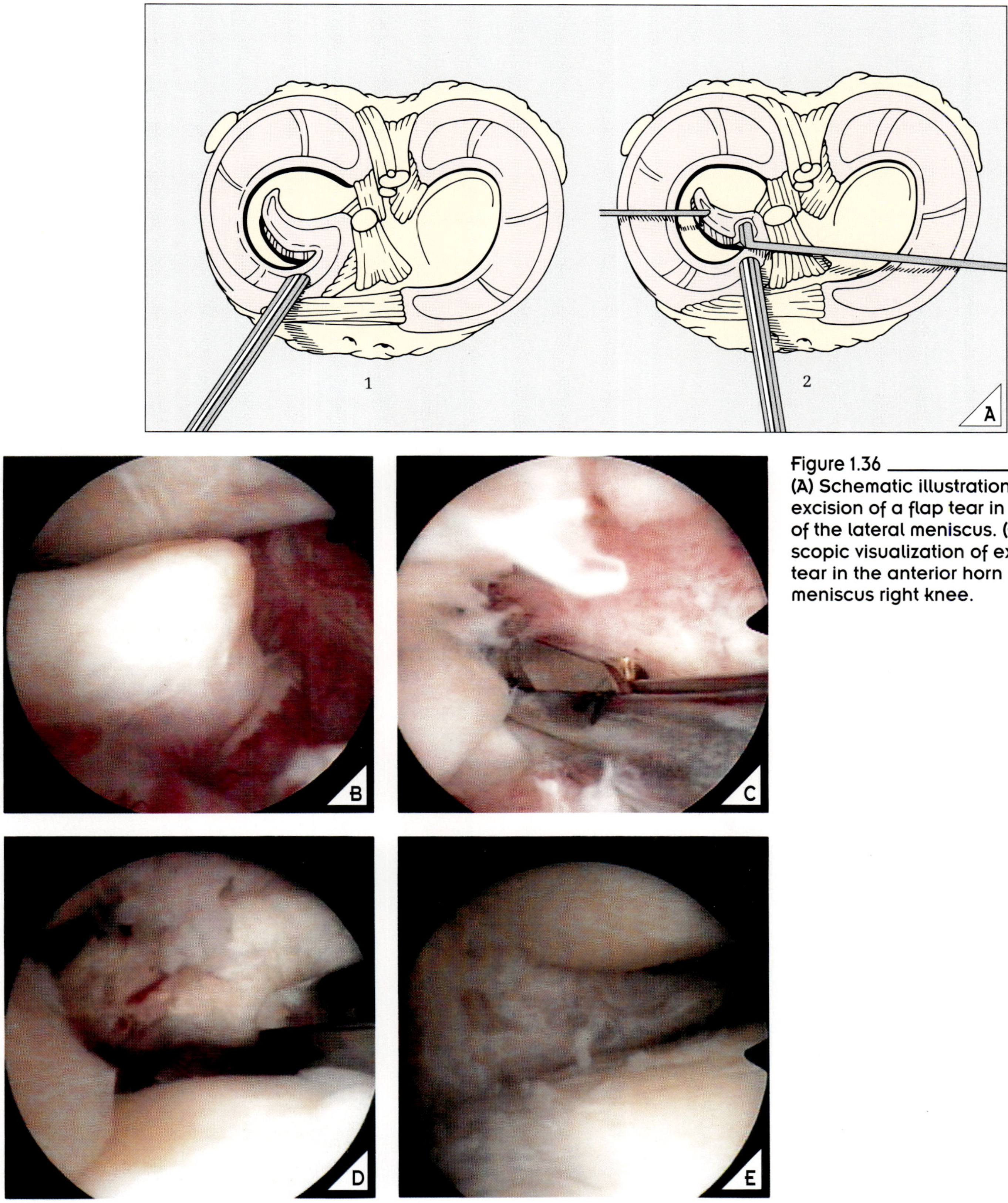

Figure 1.36
(A) Schematic illustration of steps for excision of a flap tear in the anterior horn of the lateral meniscus. (B–E) Arthroscopic visualization of excision of a flap tear in the anterior horn of the lateral meniscus right knee.

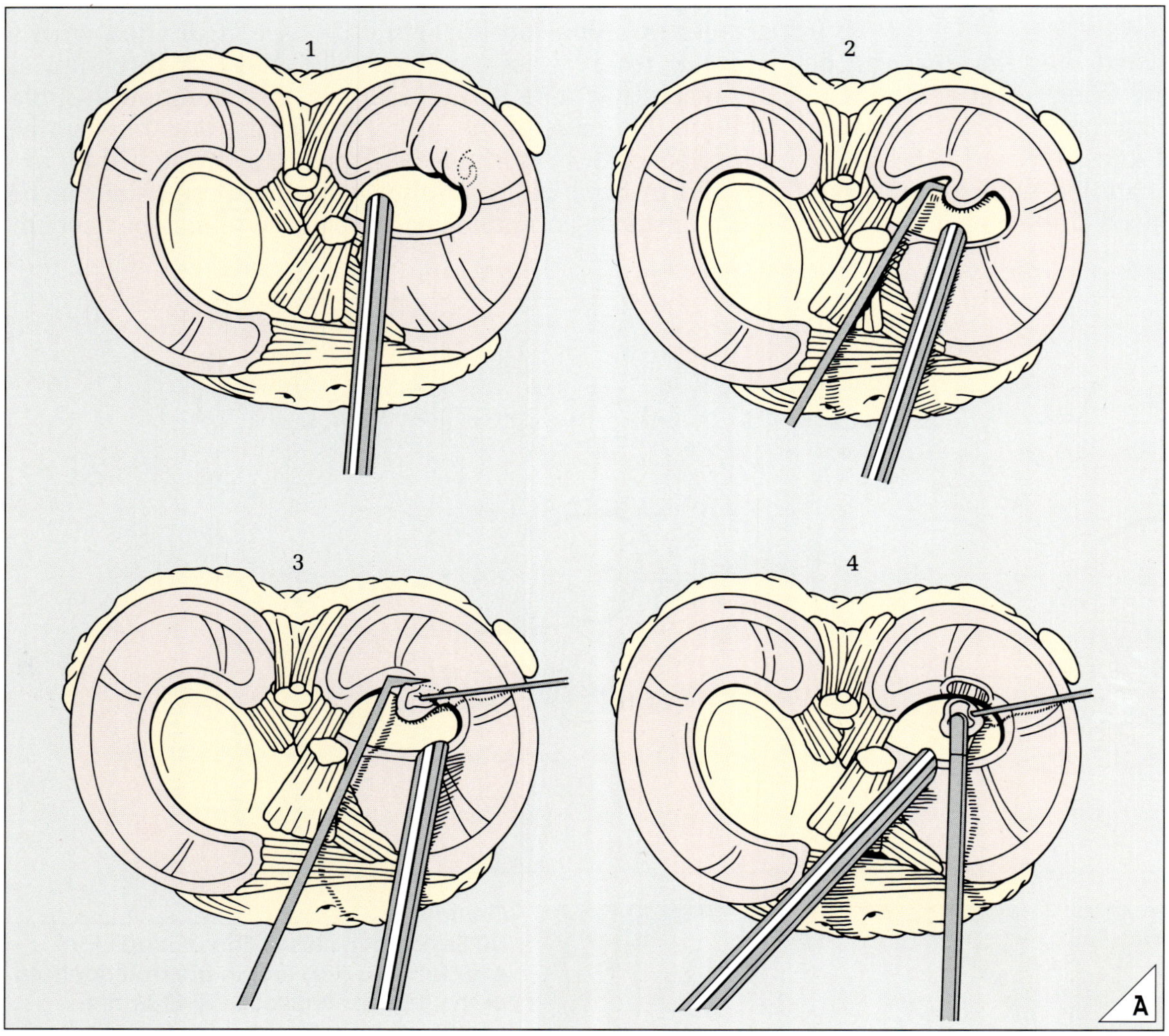

Figure 1.37

(A) Schematic illustration of steps for excision of an inverted flap tear in the posterior horn of the lateral meniscus left knee. (B–I) Arthroscopic visualization of some steps of excision of an inverted flap tear in the lateral meniscus left knee.

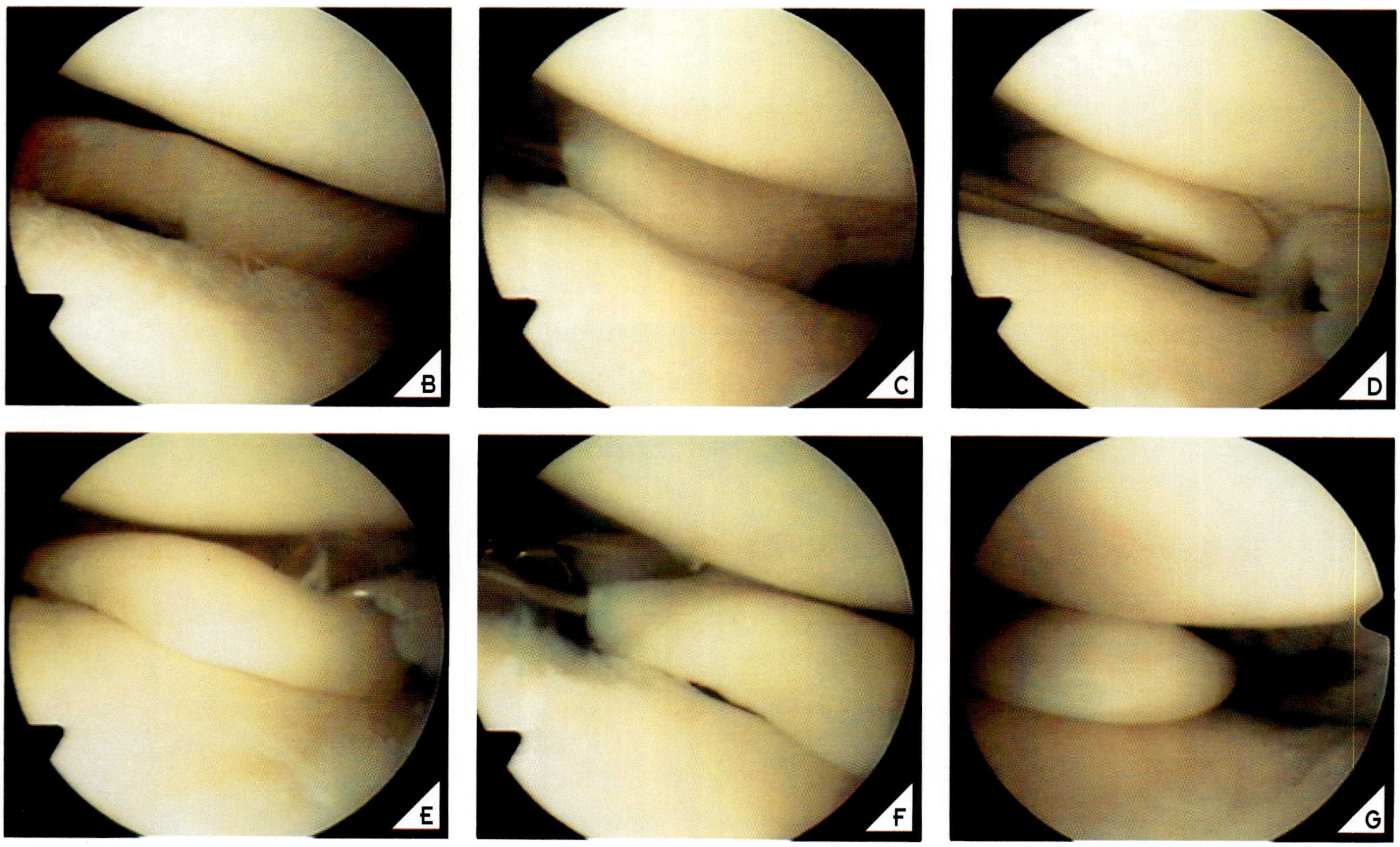

Cystic Degeneration of the Meniscus

Cysts of the menisci are more common on the lateral meniscus, and their etiology is still controversial.[16] Traumatic, congenital, and degenerative theories have been advocated in the literature. Such cysts are usually located in the midportion of the lateral meniscus and are palpated anterior to the lateral collateral ligament. The cysts, contrary to Smillie's assertion, are not always associated with meniscal tears. When a tear is present it is usually oblique or transverse with horizontal components (Fig. 1.38). The accepted treatment in the symptomatic patient is to excise the meniscal tear, when present, and to perform a closed cyst decompression.[16] If there is no association with a tear, the cyst needs only to be excised through a small arthrotomy incision.

Surgical Technique

With the arthroscope placed in the anterolateral portal, a curved knife or rotary basket is used to excise the anterior segment of the tear. A straight basket is then used to remove the posterior aspect of the tear. A small motorized

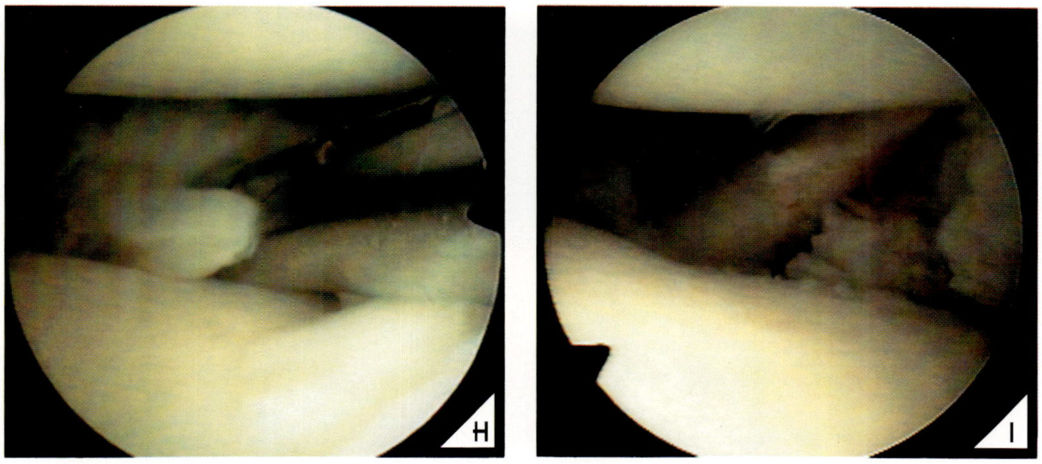

Figure 1.37 (continued)

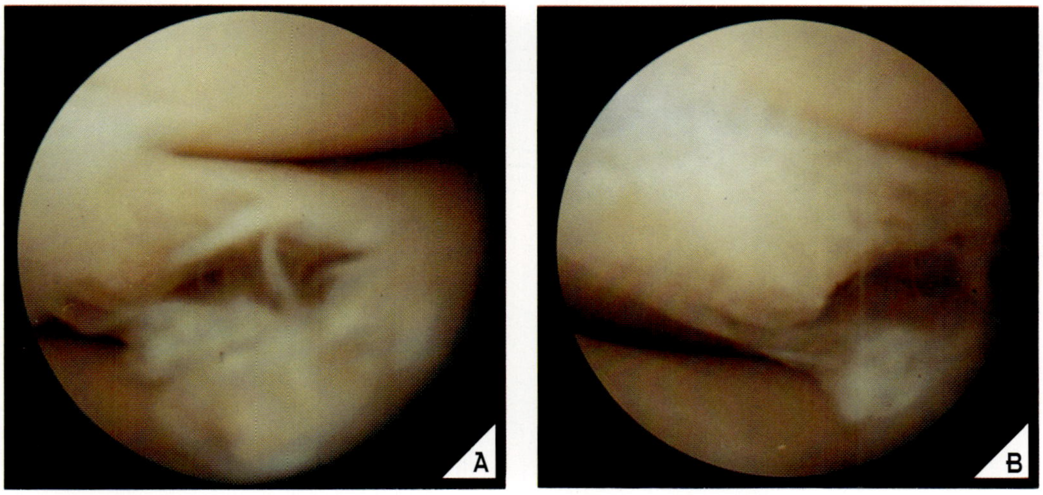

Figure 1.38
(A, B) Cleavage tear associated with a cystic lateral meniscus of the left knee.

cutter is introduced through the cyst opening from inside the knee to complete the debridement of the meniscal tissue and cyst material (Fig. 1.39). A spinal needle positioned from the outside through the cyst will indicate the exact placement of the instrument into the cyst (Fig. 1.40). If a peripheral tear is present, excision of the degenerative portion of the meniscus can be performed, followed by reattachment by closed or open means.

DISCOID MENISCI

Discoid menisci, when present, usually involve the lateral meniscus. From an arthroscopic standpoint, there are three types: complete, incomplete, and the Wrisberg ligament type (Fig. 1.41).[17] The complete type of discoid meniscus covers the lateral tibial plateau entirely and is

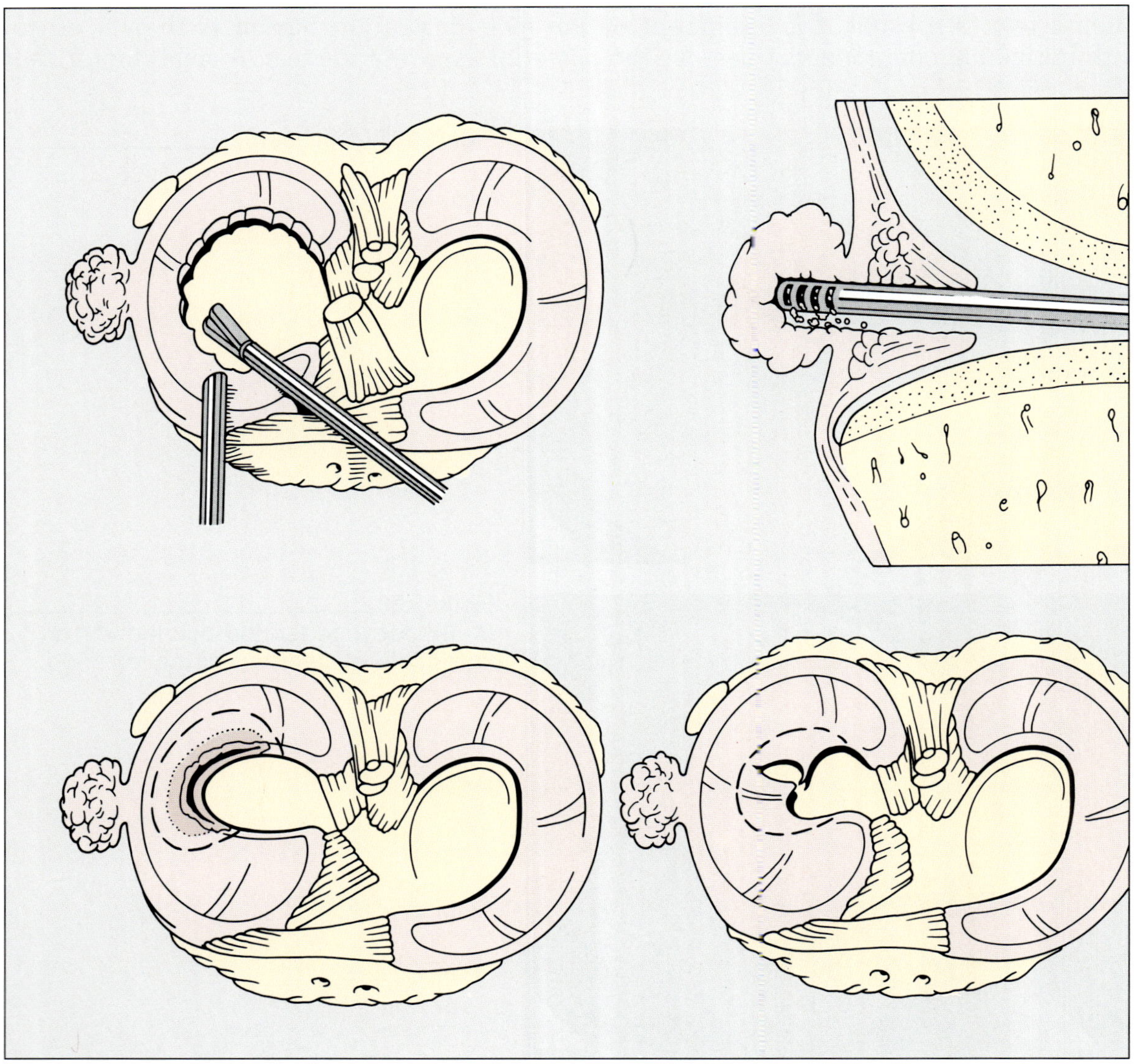

Figure 1.39
Schematic illustration of some steps of excision of various tears that may be associated with a cyst of the lateral meniscus.

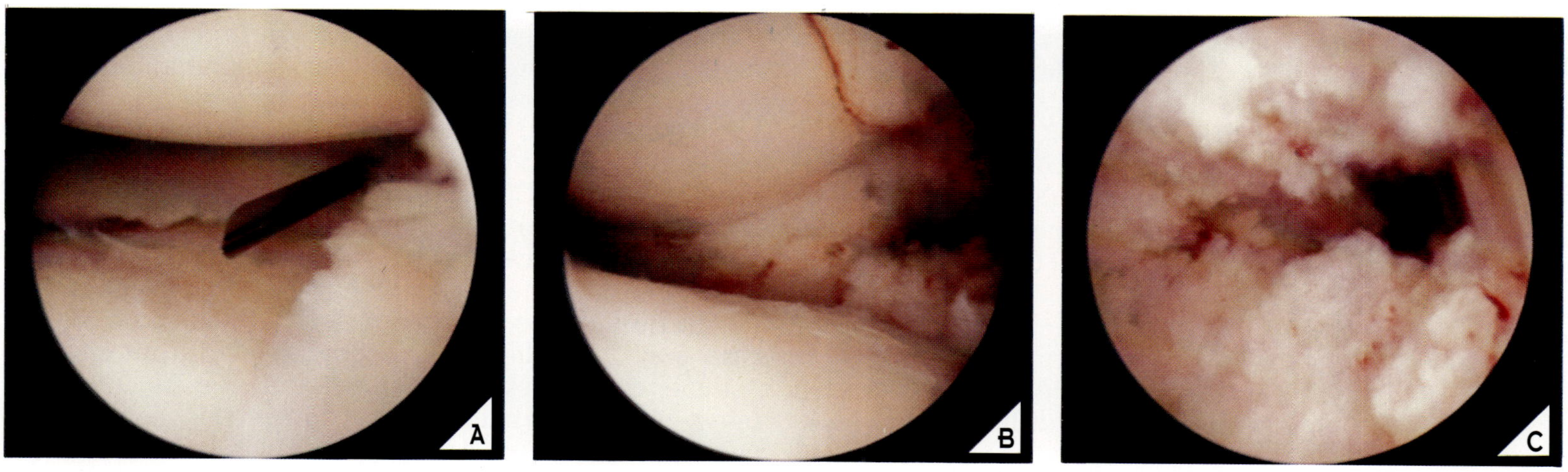

Figure 1.40
(A–C) Arthroscopic visualization of a cyst of the lateral meniscus of the left knee. A spinal needle is through the tear. After excision, the cyst track is visualized.

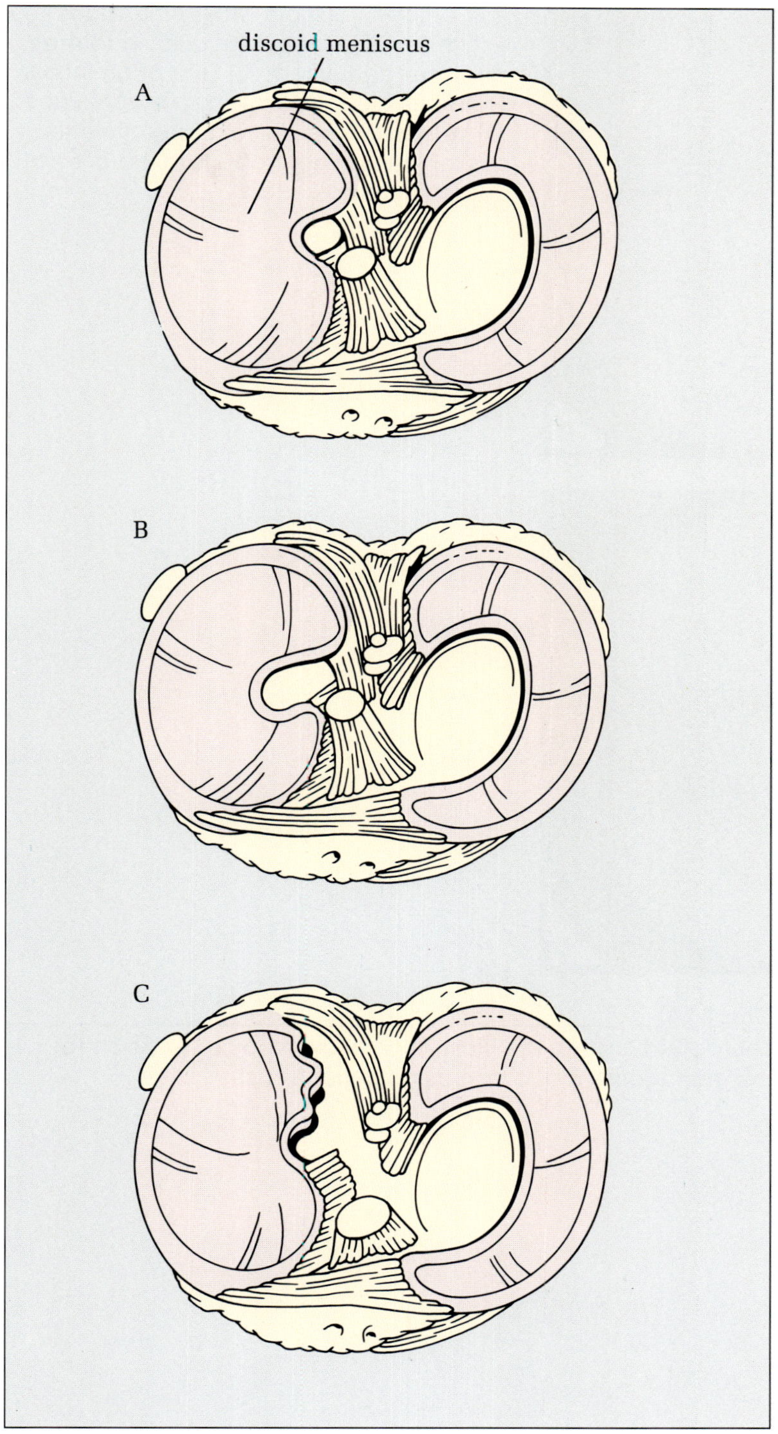

Figure 1.41
The three types of discoid lateral meniscus: complete (A), incomplete (B), and Wrisberg (C).

stable, without abnormal motion on flexion and extension of the joint (Fig. 1.42A). The incomplete type is slightly different in that it does not entirely cover the tibial plateau and is very stable (Fig. 1.42B,C). The Wrisberg ligament type, as originally described by Kaplan,[18,19] is unstable because the lateral meniscus is posteriorly attached only by the Wrisberg ligament, owing to the absence of the normal tibial attachment (Fig. 1.42D).

Surgical Technique

Tears in the incomplete type of discoid meniscus can be resected easily. The technique is no different from that used for the torn lateral meniscus.

The complete type, when it is torn, may be a challenge to the arthroscopist. The tear can be longitudinal, oblique, or transverse. A cleavage-type tear, detected only by probing, may also be present. If the tear is longitudinal and is located at the posterior aspect, the scope is placed through the lateral portal and basket forceps or scissors through the medial portal will divide the posterior attachment completely. Curved rotary scissors can then be used to detach the meniscus anteriorly. Taking care to leave a peripheral meniscal rim, the anterior cut is continued posteriorly until the axilla of the tear is reached. Grasping forceps through the anteromedial portal will complete the extraction. After the usual probing, further trimming can be done with a basket or motorized instrument. An alternative method of excision is to move the scope to the medial portal and use a 45° or 90° angled knife to reshape the anterior aspect of the discoid meniscus. The remainder of the excision is performed with a combination of

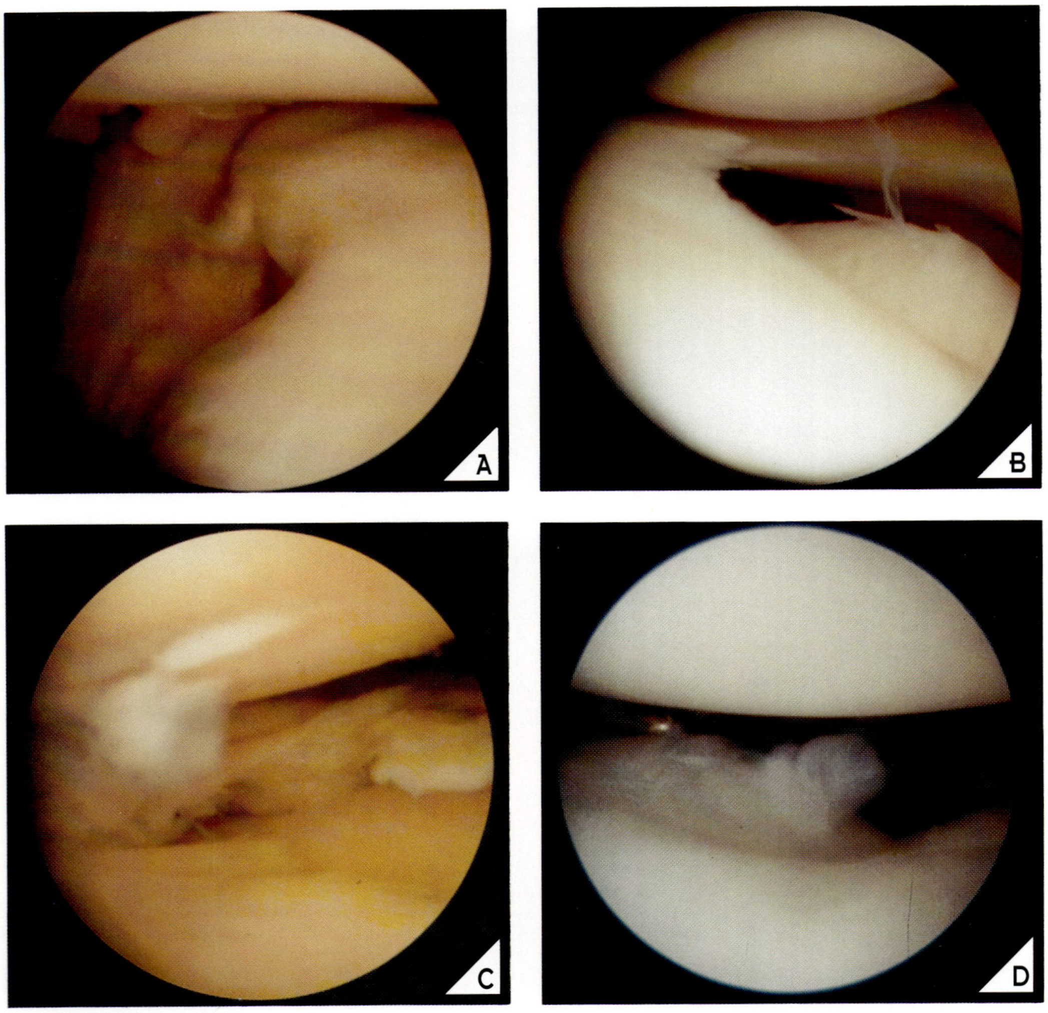

Figure 1.42
(A) Complete discoid lateral meniscus left knee. (B) Incomplete discoid lateral meniscus right knee. (C) Tear of an incomplete discoid lateral meniscus right knee. (D) Wrisberg-type discoid lateral meniscus left knee. The probe is in the area of detachment posteriorly.

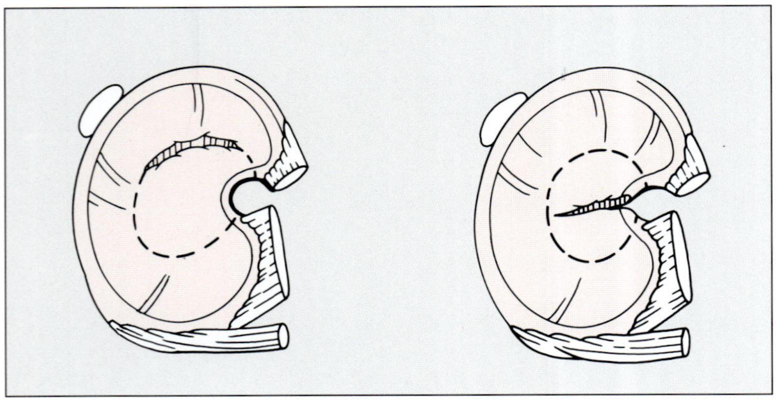

Figure 1.43
The dotted lines in the illustration show areas of excision for the management of a torn discoid meniscus.

instruments (basket and motorized meniscal cutter). A transverse or oblique tear can be handled with the basket forceps and motorized instrument placed medially. If the lateral discoid meniscus is torn at the periphery in a very young individual, a combination of partial resection and meniscal repair can be done.

With a Wrisberg-type discoid meniscus, subtotal meniscectomy may be the only alternative because of the hypermobility of the posterior horn (Figs. 1.43–1.48).

POSTOPERATIVE MANAGEMENT

After arthroscopic meniscectomy the portals are closed with a 3-0 nylon suture or a 5-0 subcuticular Dexon suture. A compression dressing is applied to the knee. Full weight-bearing with a cane or crutches is permitted as tolerated by the patient, who is encouraged to start straight leg raising as well as isometric and active range-

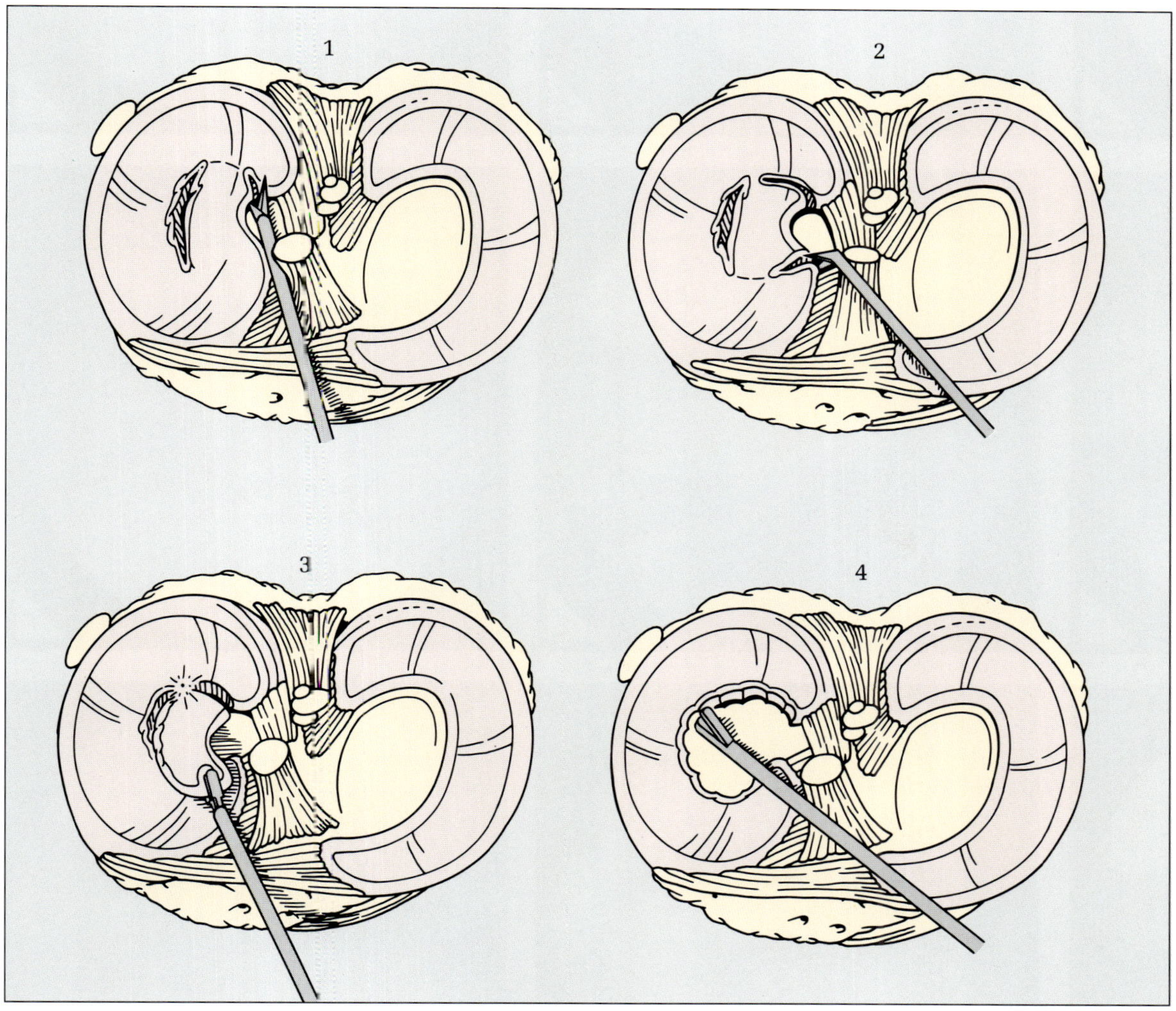

Figure 1.44
Schematic illustration of steps of excision of a torn discoid lateral meniscus.

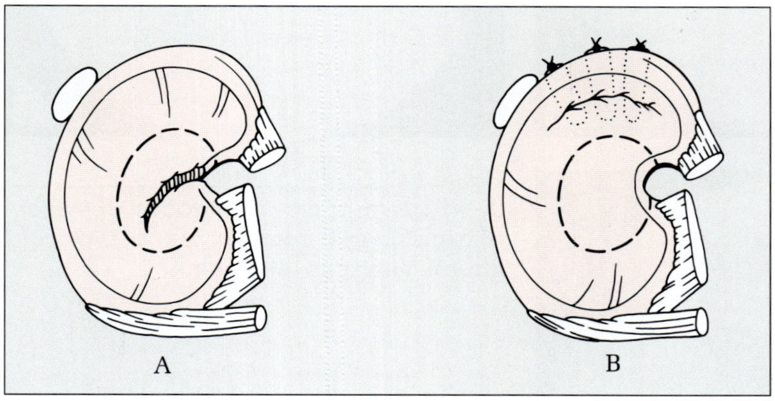

Figure 1.45
(A) Partial resection of a torn discoid lateral meniscus. (B) Combination of a partial excision and repair.

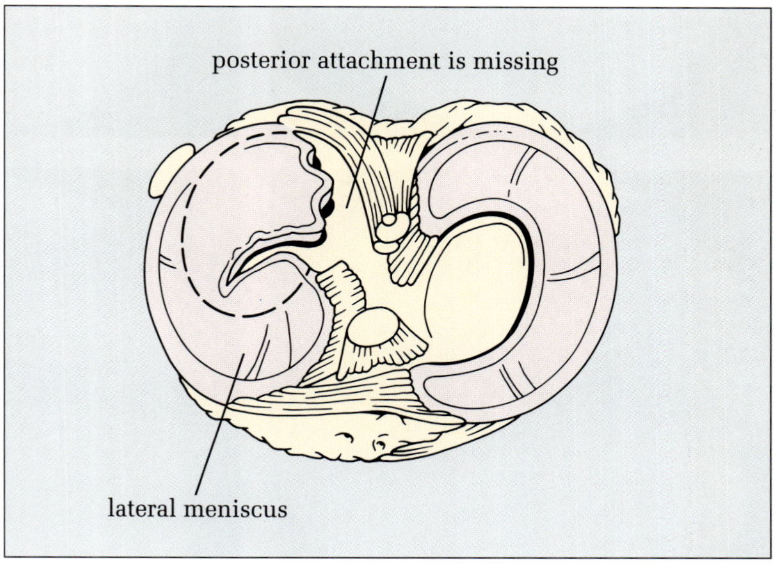

Figure 1.46
Schematic illustration of a subtotal meniscectomy for an unstable torn discoid meniscus (Wrisberg type).

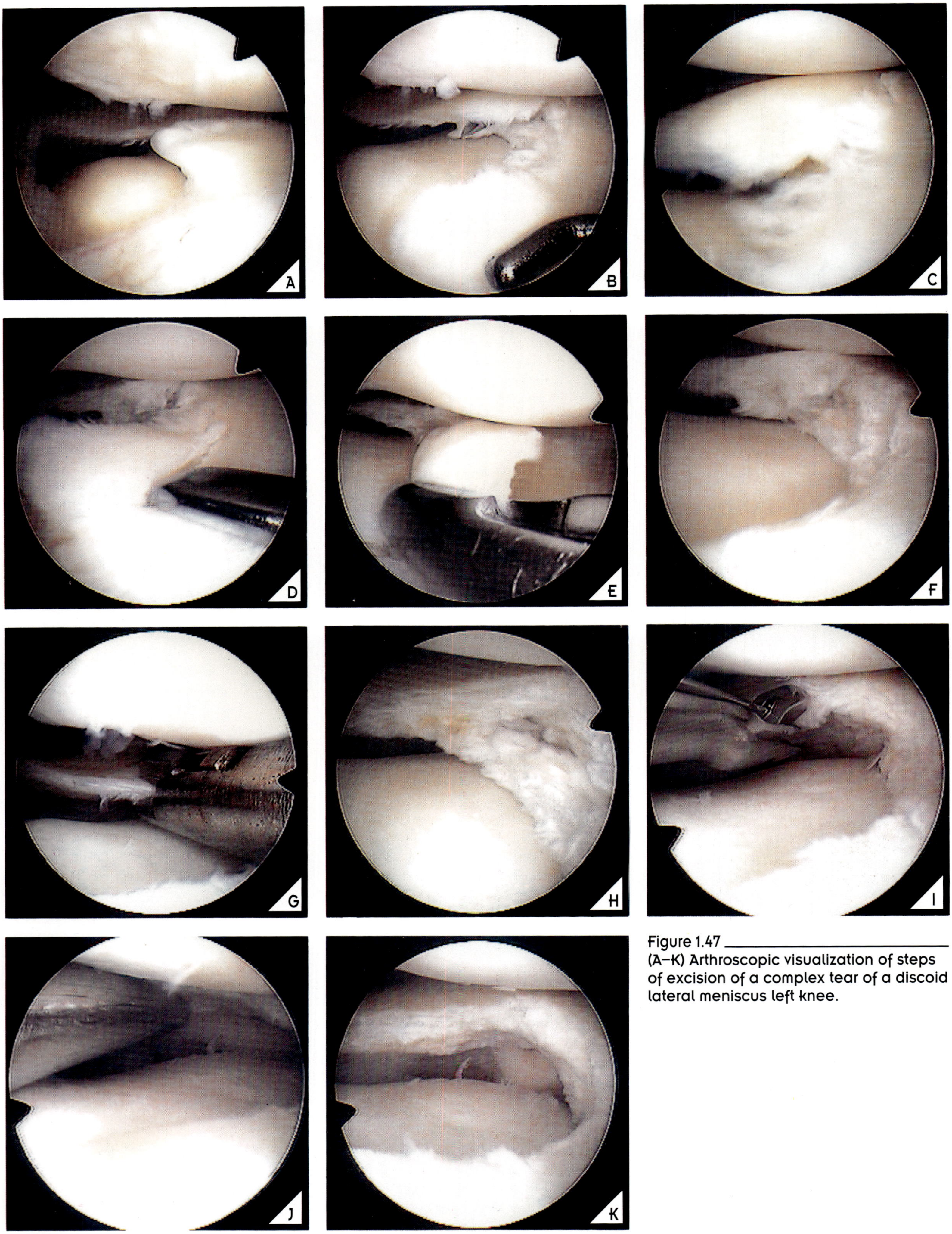

Figure 1.47
(A–K) Arthroscopic visualization of steps of excision of a complex tear of a discoid lateral meniscus left knee.

of-motion exercises immediately. Two or 3 days after discharge, a light dressing consisting of Band-Aids on the wounds and a single Ace bandage is applied.

COMPLICATIONS AND PITFALLS

Placement of the leg holder not too proximal to the knee is important to prevent abnormal rotation of the lower extremity. On the other hand, placement too close to the knee may hamper manipulation of surgical instruments through the superior portals. Abnormal and undue stresses on the knee in valgus or varus position can cause injury to the medial or lateral structures of the knee.

Unlike placement of the anterolateral portal, which is usually developed at the start of the arthroscopic examination, placement of the anteromedial portal is usually done under direct visualization by means of a percutaneous spinal needle. Although its location may be convenient for management of pathology affecting the posteromedial aspect of the knee, it may not be useful for the posterior aspect of the lateral meniscus. When arthroscopic exploration reveals pathology only of the lateral meniscus, the spinal needle should be placed more proximal to the anterior horn of the menisci and closer to the patellar tendon so that it can reach the posterior aspect of the lateral meniscus. If both menisci are torn and the anteromedial portal provides access only to the posteromedial aspect of the knee, an accessory medial portal should be developed for instrumentation within the lateral compartment.

With a tight knee, it may be very difficult to visualize the posteromedial aspect of the knee. The 70° scope can be placed through the intercondylar notch into the posteromedial compartment of the knee, medial to the anterior cruciate ligament. The posteromedial portal, as described earlier, can also be used for instrumentation or visualization. This portal can be developed directly while the distended knee is kept at approximately 90°, by making an incision posterior to the medial collateral ligament at the level of or just above the joint line. The portal placement is done indirectly with a spinal needle while looking from inside with a 70° arthroscope placed through the intercondylar notch.

In many instances, manual pressure on the posterior

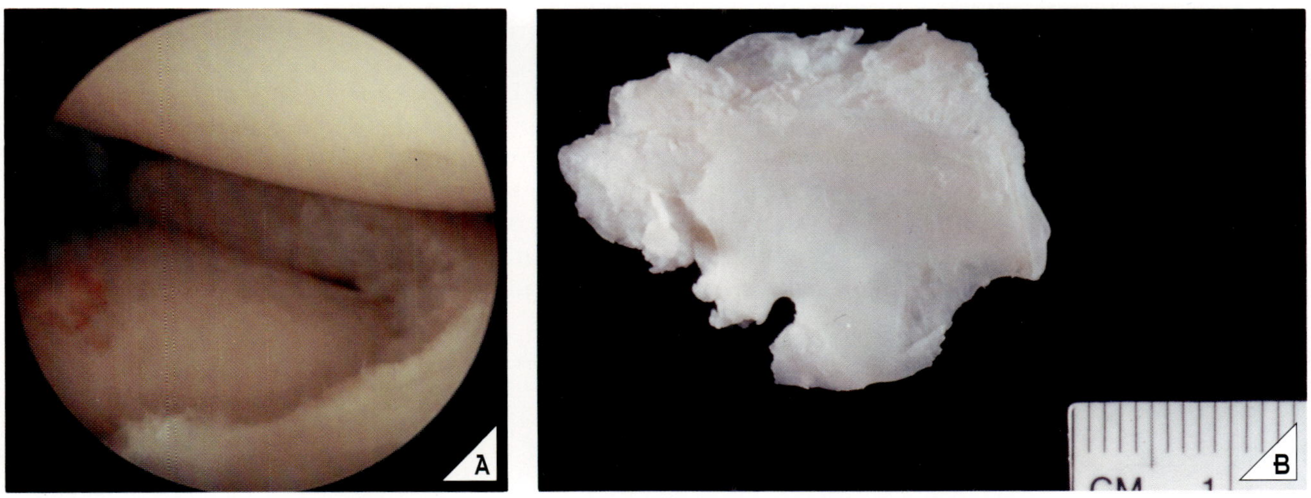

Figure 1.48
(A) Arthroscopic visualization of a resected discoid lateral meniscus left knee.
(B) Pathology specimen.

aspect of the knee while the knee is in full extension will bring the posterior horn forward into view (Fig. 1.49). A spinal needle placed into the posterior horn of the meniscus not only will stabilize the posterior aspect but will also bring a torn unstable area into view for trimming or excision.

During excision of a displaced bucket-handle tear of the meniscus and after reduction of the mobile fragment, when the posterior axilla is divided only a few fibers of attachment should be left, to facilitate avulsion with grasping forceps. If the posterior axilla is inadvertently cut off completely, a percutaneous spinal needle can be used to stabilize the mobile fragment. If the fat pad obscures visualization of the anterior attachment of the tear, use a motorized shaver to excise the hypertrophic synovial villi. Do not perform an aggressive synovectomy, since this invariably causes postoperative hemarthrosis. If the division of the anterior horn of a medial meniscus is difficult through the anteromedial portal, a switch of portals is advisable. Once the scope has been moved medially, always use the probe through the anterolateral portal to insure that the route to the meniscal fragment is direct, without impingement on the tibia or femur. If the position is incorrect, it may be necessary to use an accessory lateral portal to reach the anterior segment of the meniscus with a surgical instrument. If that is the situation, use a percutaneous spinal needle before making the skin incision.

Sometimes, the displaced fragment of a bucket-handle tear is so unstable that it must be stabilized before the posterior or anterior attachments can be divided. This can be done with a suture through the midsegment of the mobile fragment, by means of the meniscal repair cannula system. In this way it is possible not only to reduce the meniscus but also to maintain proper tension on it so as to divide the axillae of the tear.

Making a cut either anteriorly or posteriorly through a displaced fragment will leave an anterior or posterior meniscal stump that may be very difficult to remove in a tight knee. If this situation arises, use the spinal needle posteriorly to stabilize the stump, while the en-bloc excision is done with scissors or piecemeal excision is performed with a basket or motorized instrument. The anterior horn stump can be excised with a rotary basket forceps placed through the opposite portal, and a motorized shaver can smooth out the rim.

When a radial tear is located anteriorly in the middle third of the lateral meniscus, the excision is easier with rotary basket forceps placed medially. It is sometimes necessary to use a 45° or 90° angled knife through the anterolateral portal. In this situation, great skill is needed to avoid damaging the underlying articular cartilage.

In dealing with a large oblique tear with the flap sequestered beneath the meniscus, before making a cut through the rounded base make sure that the flap can be dislodged. Then reduce it under the meniscus, divide the base with meniscal scissors, and avulse the few remaining intact fibers with grasping forceps.

Tears of the posterior horn of the medial meniscus are often associated with an anterior cruciate-deficient knee. In handling this type of tear it is important to have an assistant hold the leg in valgus and external rotation, because of the tendency of the tibia to subluxate anteriorly while valgus is applied to the extended knee, resulting in a loss of visualization (Fig. 1.50).

It is important to remember that good visualization of the operative field is of critical importance for the perfor-

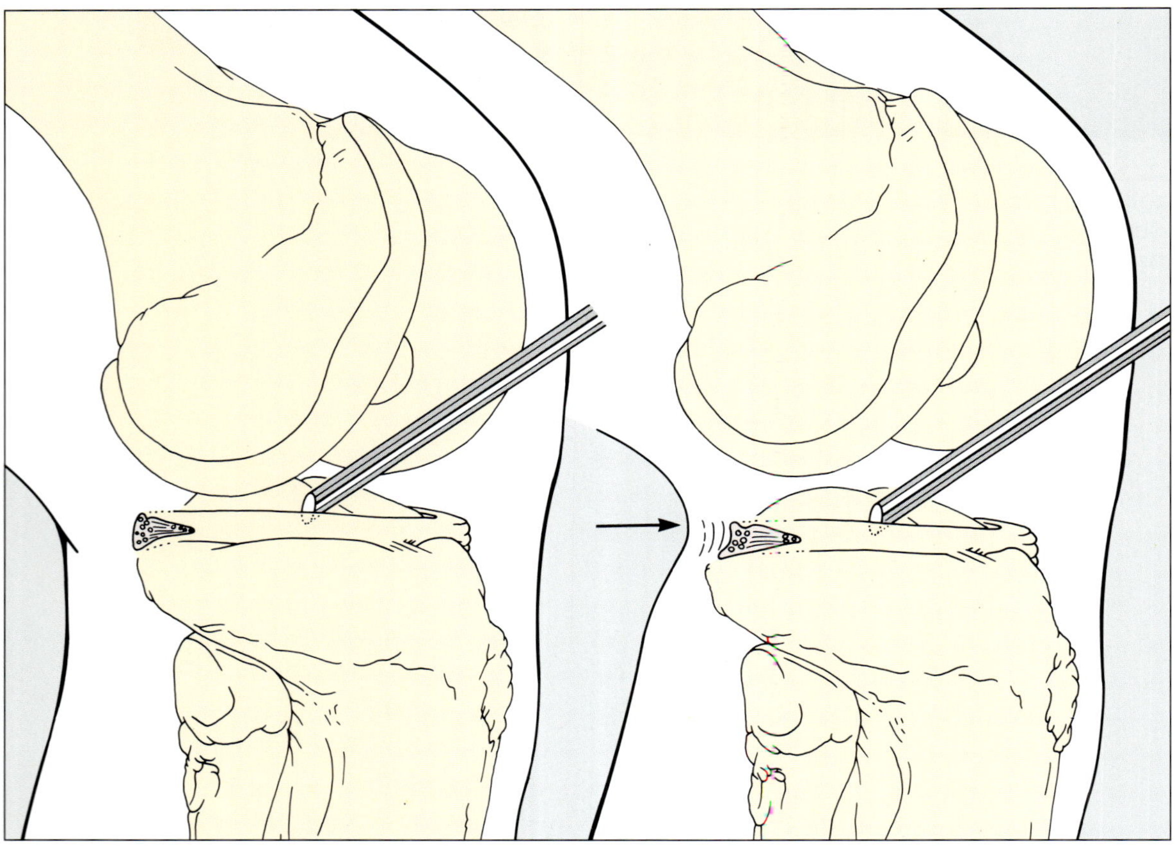

Figure 1.49
Manual pressure applied to the posterior aspect of the knee brings the posterior horn of the meniscus into view.

mance of any surgical procedures on the menisci. Optimal visualization requires not only an adequate optical system but also the proper amount of joint distention. Many arthroscopists prefer an automated mechanical pumping system over the gravity-feed method for fluid delivery, so that the use of a tourniquet can be avoided. The ideal pump can deliver constant pressure to the intraarticular vessels and regulate the flow rate on demand and has a safety device for avoidance of high intraarticular pressure. However, extreme care should be taken to insure that the inflow cannula is inside the joint cavity and thus to avoid extravasation of fluid into the adjacent soft tissue.

The arthroscopic management of a torn discoid lateral meniscus is not easy because of its increased thickness and size. Although in most situations the procedure can be performed through anteromedial and anterolateral portals, to avoid crowding of instruments the addition of midpatellar medial portal, can be very helpful by affording visualization while the triangulation technique is achieved with instruments through the two anterior portals.

Rates of complication for medial and lateral meniscectomies have been reported in a multicenter study as 1.8% and 1.6%, respectively.[20] Complications can be general or technically related.[21]

Complications such as infection can be avoided by the use of good preventive measures, such as prophylactic administration of antibiotics in patients with increased risk factors, in situations where there has been a break in surgical technique, or when the procedure has been of long duration.

Instrument-related complications can be prevented if the microsurgical arthroscopic instruments are manipulated gently, without excessive force, and are properly maintained. A magnetic retriever should always be available for retrieval of broken metal pieces from a knee joint.

Hemarthrosis after lateral meniscectomy can be avoided if the arthroscopic surgeon keeps in mind that the inferolateral geniculate artery and veins are at risk, since they are located along the border of the lateral meniscus.

Epinephrine solution and electrocautery are of great help in control of bleeding during arthroscopic surgery on the meniscus. Some physicians use a few milliliters of bupivacaine with 1:200,000 epinephrine solution at the portal locations. Others inject a small amount of the same solution into bleeding areas to achieve hemostasis. Electrocautery can also be used to effectively coagulate bleeding vessels under direct vision.

Portal fistula can be prevented by closing a large capsular incision with a deep capsular stitch.

Loss of meniscal fragments is a potential complication during arthroscopic surgery. After a large meniscal fragment is grasped, it is important to stretch the capsular incision with a clamp to facilitate removal of the fragment. In the event that the fragment is set free during extraction, it will usually follow the direction of the fluid flow and can be retrieved in the suprapatellar pouch, next to the outflow cannula.

Sensory nerves, such as the saphenous nerve and its infrapatellar branch, are at risk with the posteromedial and anteromedial portals. A superficial skin incision coupled with the use of an obturator may minimize injury to the nerves, as well as the subsequent risk of neuroma formation.

If a well-leg support is used, it should be well padded, with the peroneal nerve well protected. As shown by Rosenberg and coauthors,[22] this device, by keeping the hip flexed at 60°, abducted at 45°, and externally rotated 20°, allows posteromedial exposure of the operated knee. Most importantly, it avoids hyperextension at the hip, thus elimating the possibility of femoral nerve compression and traction. In high-risk patients, the nonoperated lower extremity is also wrapped with an Ace bandage to prevent venous stasis.

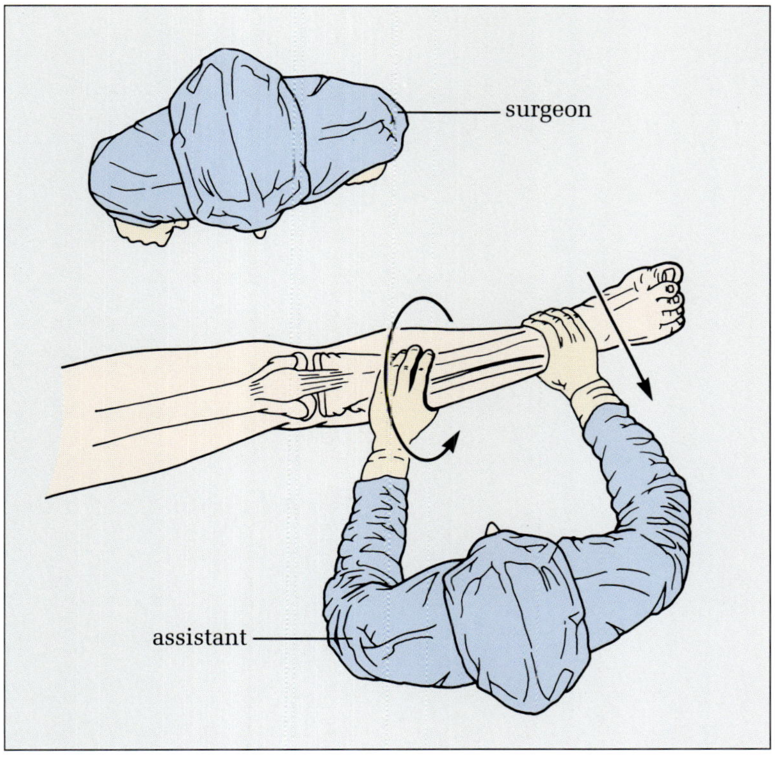

Figure 1.50
Schematic illustration of an assistant holding the leg in valgus and external rotation to prevent anterior subluxation of the tibia.

REFERENCES

1. Ahmed A, Burke DL. In vitro measurements of static pressure distribution in synovial joints, I: tibial surface of the knee. *J Biomech Eng.* 1983;105:216–225.
2. Baratz M, Fu F, Mengat R. Meniscal tears—the effect of meniscectomy and of repair in the intra-articular contact areas and stress in the human knee. *Am J Sports Med.* 1986;14:270–275.
3. Baratz M, Fu F, Rehak D, Rudert M. Peripheral tears of the meniscus—the effect of open versus arthroscopic repair on intra-articular contact stresses in the human knee. *Am J Sports Med.* 1988;16:1–6.
4. Dehaven K. The role of the meniscus. In: Ewing W, ed. *Articular Cartilage and Knee Joint Function.* New York, NY: Raven Press; 1990.
5. Levy IM, Torzilli P, Warren R. The effect of medial meniscectomy on anterior-posterior motion of the knee. *J Bone Joint Surg.* 1982;64:883–888.
6. Levy IM, Torzilli P, Gould J, Warren R. The effect of lateral meniscectomy on the motion of the knee. *J Bone Joint Surg.* 1989;71:401–406.
7. MacConaill M. The movements of the bones and joints: synovial fluid and its assistants. *J Bone Joint Surg.* 1950;32:244–252.
8. MacConaill M. The function of intra-articular cartilages, with special reference to the knee and inferior radio-ulnar joints. *J Anat.* 1932;66:210–227.
9. Salter R, Field P. The effects of continuous compression on living articular cartilage: an experimental investigation. *J Bone Joint Surg.* 1960;42:31–49.
10. Shoemaker S, Markoff K. The role of the meniscus in the anterior–posterior stability of the loaded anterior cruciate-deficient knee. *J Bone Joint Surg.* 1986;68A:71–79.
11. Arnoczky S, Warren R. Microvasculature of the human meniscus. *Am J Sports Med.* 1982;10:90–95.
12. O'Connor RL. *Arthroscopy.* Philadelphia, Pa: JB Lippincott; 1977.
13. Basmajian JV. Lovejoy JF Jr. Functions of the popliteus muscle in man. *J Bone Joint Surg.* 1971;53:557–562.
14. Cohn AK, Mains DB. Popliteal hiatus of the lateral meniscus. *Am J Sports Med.* 1979;7:221–226.
15. Last RJ. The popliteus muscle and the lateral meniscus. *J Bone Joint Surg.* 1950;32B:93.
16. Parisien JS. Arthroscopic treatment of cysts of the menisci—a preliminary report. *Clin Orthop Rel Res.* 1990;257:154–158.
17. Watanabe M. Arthroscopy of the knee joint. In: Helfet AJ. *Disorders of the Knee.* Philadelphia, Pa: JB Lippincott; 1974:145.
18. Kaplan EB. The embryology of the menisci of the knee joint. *Bull Hosp J Dis Orthop Inst.* 1955;16:111–124.
19. Kaplan EB. Discoid lateral meniscus of the knee joint: nature, mechanism and operative treatment *J Bone Joint Surg.* 1957;39A:77–87.
20. Small NC. Complications in arthroscopic surgery performed by experienced arthroscopists. *Arthroscopy.* 1988;4:215–221.
21. Sprague NF III. *Complications in Arthroscopic Surgery.* New York, NY: Raven Press; 1989.
22. Rosenberg TD, Paulos LE, et al. The well leg support. *Arthroscopy.* 1988;4:41–44.

chapter Two

Meniscus Repair

James S. Mulhollan

Meniscus repair is an accepted component of a knee arthroscopist's armamentarium. Although technique selection is variable and indications for use controversial, there is little doubt that many meniscus tears can be repaired. Repair is especially helpful in arthroscopic management of anterior cruciate ligament instability.

Meniscus Repair Methods

Open Suture

The first successful meniscus repairs were by direct open suture.[1,2] This method (Fig. 2.1), which is described because of its historical significance, is applicable for tears located within either the posteromedial or the posterolateral compartment. The same type of repair can now be accomplished by arthroscopic methods (see below). Recognition of tears suitable for open repair requires direct viewing of the posterior compartment with a 70° telescope passing through the intercondylar notch.[3] A tear located posteriorly is potentially missed without this examination. Tears in this location are most common in cruciate ligament cases.

Inside-Out Repair

Inside-out meniscus repair (Fig. 2.2) is applied more commonly than other methods.[4–6] In this procedure, the meniscus tear is visualized from the anterior compartment, usually with a 30° arthroscope.

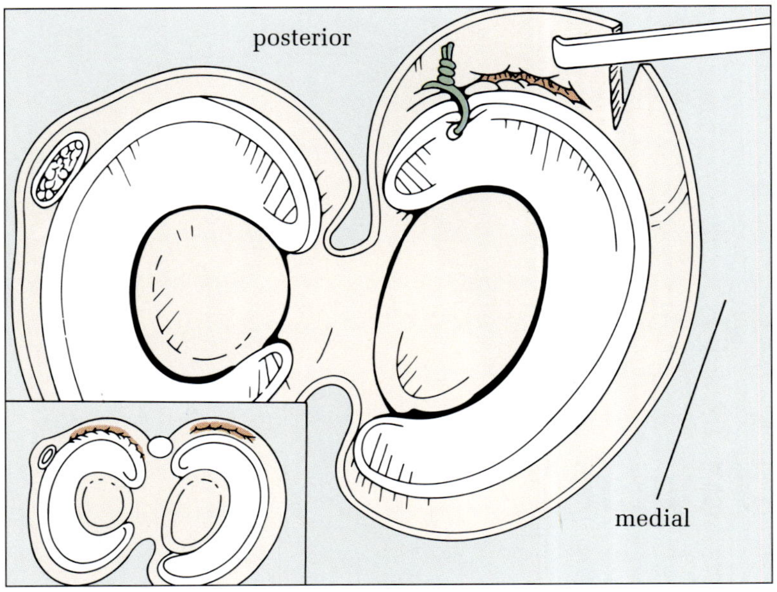

Figure 2.1

Open suture technique. This is the classic method of meniscus repair. It can be used for tears in both the posteromedial and posterolateral compartments. Tears at the meniscosynovial junction and those more peripheral are accessible by this method. The popliteal tendon causes difficulty laterally, but open approaches to this region are still possible.

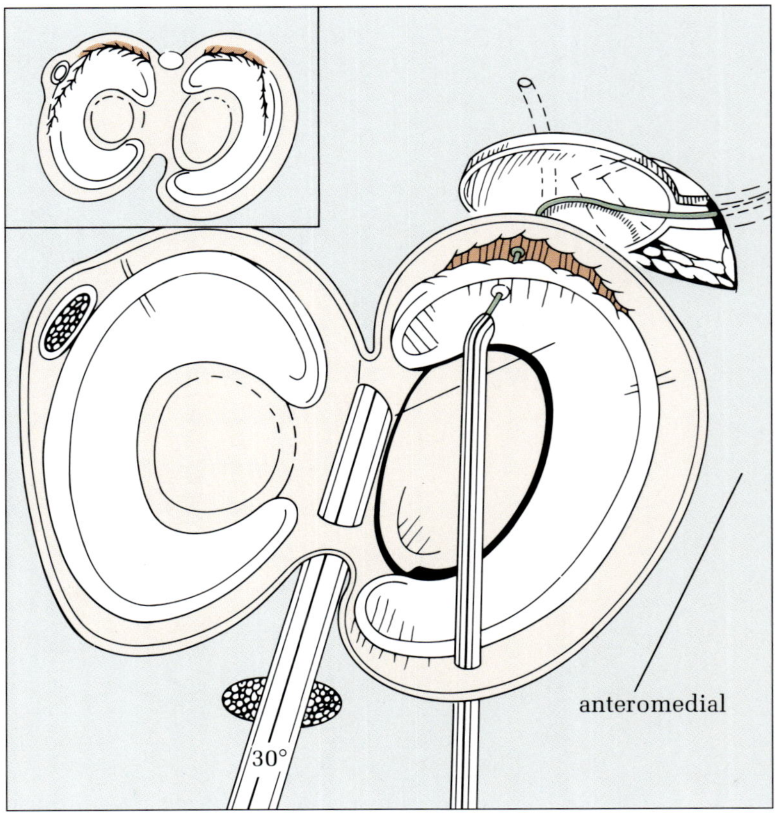

Figure 2.2

Inside-out technique. This meniscus repair system has the broadest application of available methods. It is equally appropriate in both the posterior and middle thirds of the meniscus. As needles are passed through the posterior meniscus, a prepositioned retractor is hit. In the middle third, incisions are made as the sutures are passed.

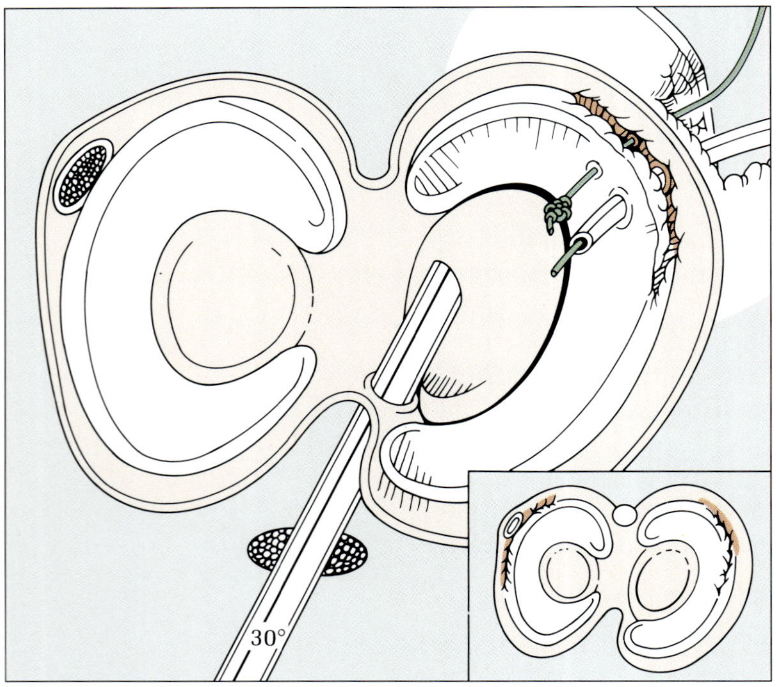

Figure 2.3

Outside-in technique. This method is most helpful within the middle third. Though proponents of this system use it posteriorly, I find the inside-out technique or wholly intraarticular technique more useful for posterior tears.

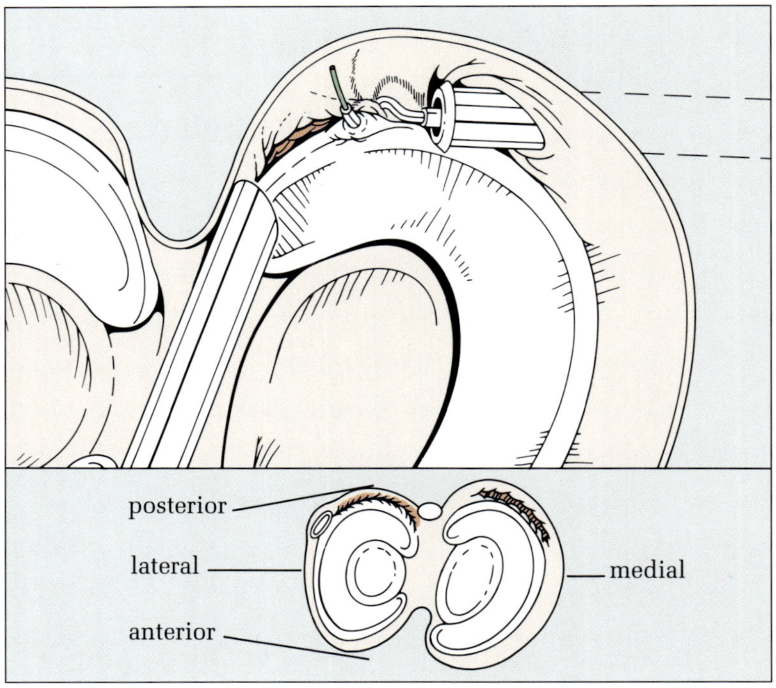

Figure 2.4

Wholly intraarticular technique. A posterior tear is visualized by passing through the intercondylar notch and using a 70° arthroscope (Swedish method). The cannula used to introduce the stitching device is placed posteromedially. It is possible to place sutures across vascular meniscal tears and tie them using only a single puncture incision.

A cannula is introduced through an anterior portal and positioned so that a needle can be passed through the cannula, across the tear, and into a posterior incision. Vessels and nerves located posteriorly are protected with a prepositioned metallic retractor. The inside-out meniscus repair method has the broadest application of all meniscus repair techniques and should be used in every surgical theatre. It is appropriate for tears at the meniscosynovial junction as well as for tears within the meniscal substance. It can be used successfully for both the posterior third of each meniscus and for tears that extend into the middle third.

Outside-In Repair

Outside-in meniscus suturing (Fig. 2.3) is quite easy and highly suitable for middle third lesions. Proponents of this type of repair also use it within the posterior third[7]; however, for this portion of the meniscus my opinion is that it is safer to use a posterior incision and retractor with the previously described inside-out method or, alternately, the wholly intraarticular method described below.

Wholly Intraarticular Repair

Wholly intraarticular meniscus repair (Fig. 2.4) has been recently reported,[8] and is commonly applied in my practice. This type of repair is appropriate for tears at the meniscosynovial junction or more peripherally, especially within the posterior medial compartment. Its range of application is identical to open meniscus repair and has generally replaced that technique. Its advantages are the puncture incision, the accuracy of tissue approximation, and the ability to do the procedure without a tourniquet. Since immobilization is not necessary, modern anterior cruciate ligament reconstruction can be done simultaneously and knee movement started immediately.

Anatomy of Meniscus Tears

There is a significant anatomic difference between the medial and the lateral meniscus, especially in the posterior one third, where most meniscus tears occur (Fig. 2.5).

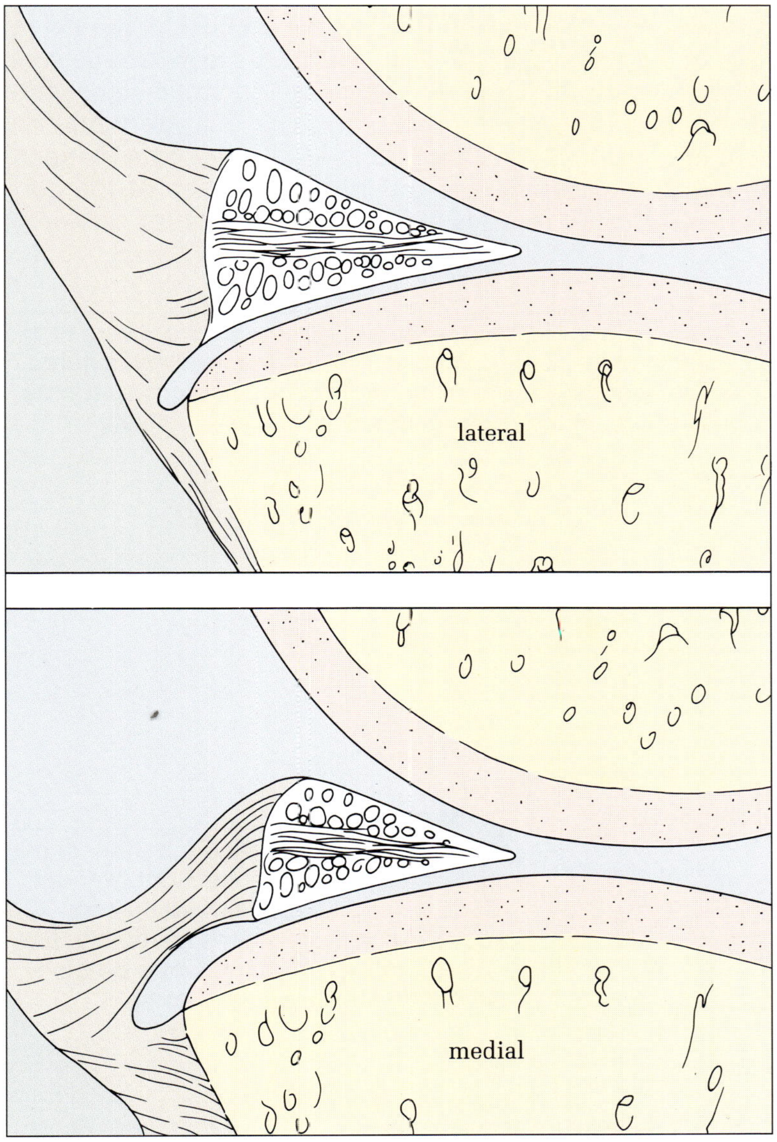

Figure 2.5
The medial meniscus is attached posteriorly by a thin stalk. Tears in this region often contain grossly visible vascularity, but do not heal unless sutured. Laterally the meniscus attachment is over a broad area and is highly vascular. Tears of the lateral meniscal attachment are inclined to heal spontaneously.

Medial Meniscus

Medially the meniscus is attached by a thin stalk. Tearing often occurs through this attachment when the anterior cruciate ligament fails. This part of the meniscal complex is best viewed with a 70° arthroscope that has passed through the intercondylar notch.[3] Tears within the medial meniscus attachment do not heal spontaneously with any reliability so they need to be sutured. Open, inside-out, and wholly intraarticular repair methods can be applied to these tears.

A tear at the meniscosynovial junction or in the stalk of the meniscus attachment medially is often visibly vascular (Fig. 2.6). When viewed arthroscopically, red circulation is visible often on one side and sometimes on both sides of the meniscus tear. The tear shown in Figure 2.7 is perfect for meniscus repair. This type of lesion is found in cases of anterior cruciate ligament loss. If sutured, it almost always heals. It is very important that meniscus repair is performed in anterior cruciate ligament cases since loss of the meniscus would worsen instability.

Lateral Meniscus

Laterally the meniscus is attached by a very broad base. Tears at the meniscosynovial junction occur with cruciate ligament injury. Because of the broad vascular lateral meniscus attachment, tears in this region frequently heal spontaneously. Tears can be repaired by the inside-out or the wholly intraarticular method. The open approach to this region is possible,[1] though difficult due to the popliteus tendon. It is my opinion that repair of vascular lateral meniscal tears is rarely necessary since abundant circulation usually yields spontaneous healing.

Indications for Resection and Repair

Numerous meniscus tears have little, if any, potential for healing and are resected. Vascular tear patterns are uncommon in stable knees. Figure 2.8 shows some common tear patterns that have no potential to heal. For example, a lateral radial tear is most appropriately resected, as are flap tears of the medial meniscus. Prevalence of meniscal substance tearing is commonly associated with aging. Most meniscus tearing in stable knees seems to have an attritional basis. There is little debate about the advisability of resection in cases such as these.

There is an intermediate group of tears for which repair is debatable but probably applicable in certain cases. The most peripheral portion of meniscus, even though grossly avascular, has a significant microcirculation.[9] This region of significant but limited vascularity can extend from between one fifth to one third of the meniscus diameter. In selected cases, grossly white meniscus tears can be successfully sutured. Numerous other factors must be considered before undertaking repair in tears that are white on both edges (Fig. 2.9). These include the age of the patient, extremity alignment, the technical expertise of the surgeon, associated injuries, willingness to accept postopera-

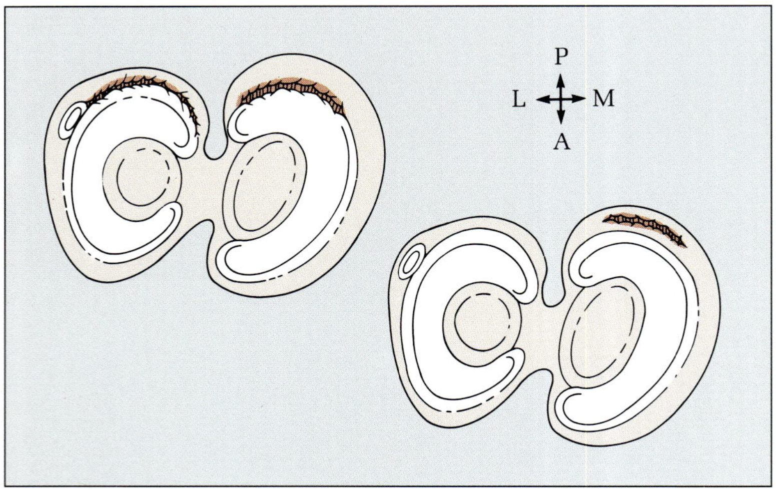

Figure 2.6
Tears are usually red on a least one side and have a very high probability of healing by a fibrovascular mechanism if sutured. Although spontaneous healing tends to occur laterally, spontaneous healing of the posteromedial meniscus is unlikely.

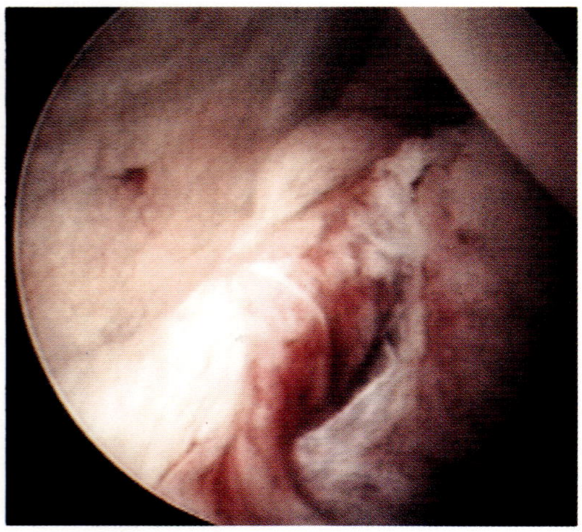

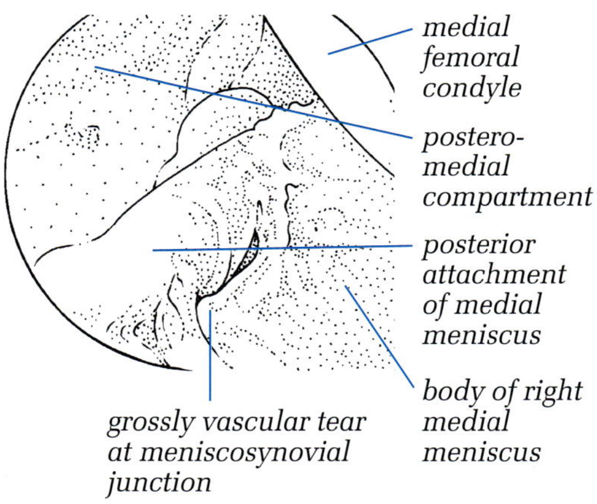

Figure 2.7
Medial meniscus avulsion type tear in a right anterior cruciate ligament. Without repair it will probably extend. Repair would lessen the patient's instability. This view is with the 70° arthroscope passing through the intracondylar notch.

tive restrictions, tourniquent time, etc. The tear illustrated in Figure 2.10 is an example of a lesion that might be repaired in some cases and resected in others.

The most frequent indication for meniscus repair is when anterior cruciate ligament loss has occurred. Displacement of the femur posteriorly during cruciate ligament rupture pulls the knee capsule away from the meniscus. This tearing occurs within the meniscus body or within its attachment, through one or several planes. In a fresh cruciate injury, the tear is almost always limited to the posterior one third of the meniscus. Up to one third of these lesions are visibly vascular and involve a single tear

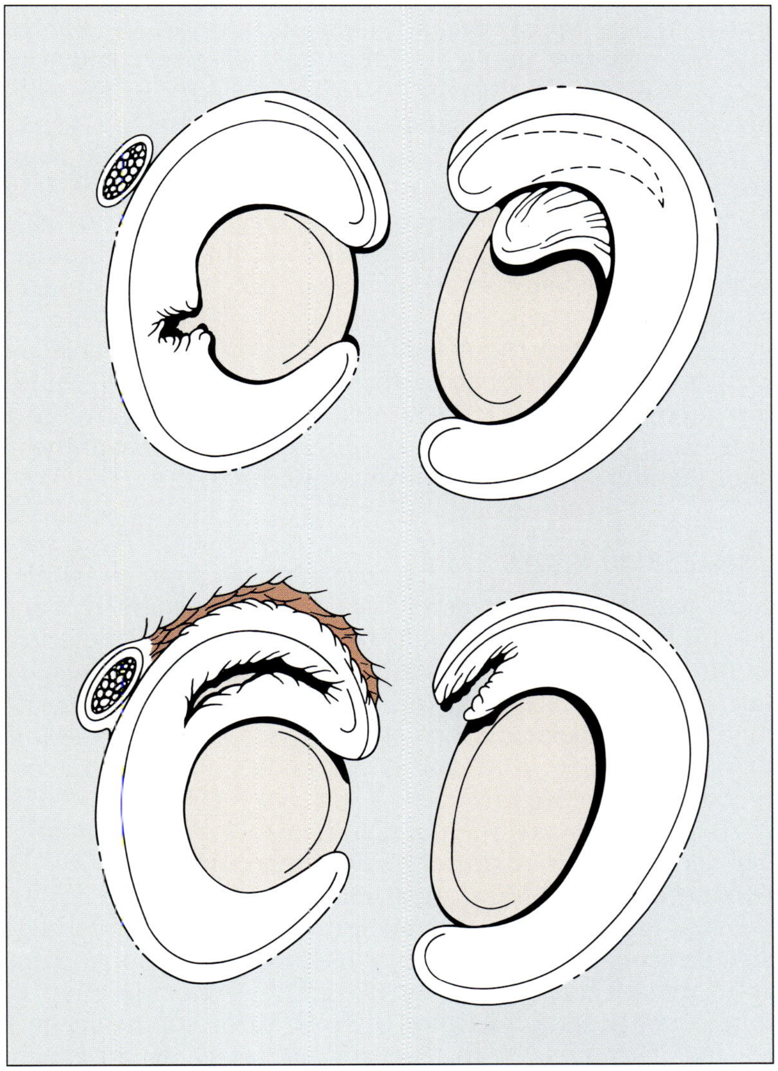

Figure 2.8

Irreparable tear patterns. Radial tears of the lateral meniscus are appropriately treated by partial meniscectomy as are flap tears of the medal meniscus. In general, tears associated with degeneration are more appropriately treated by excision than by repair.

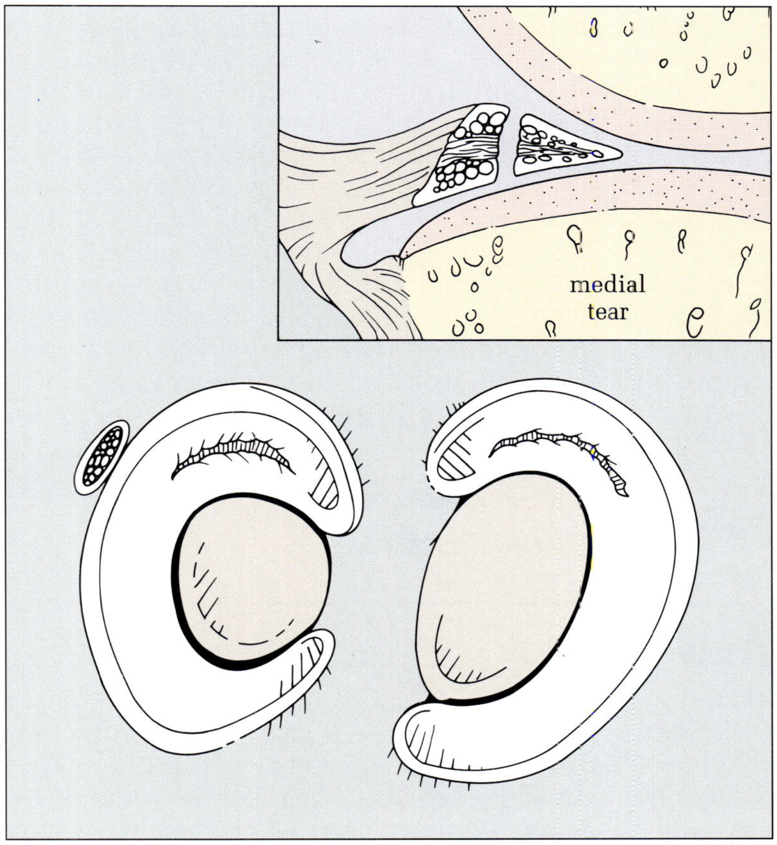

Figure 2.9

Tears within the white part of the meniscus have questionable vascularity and heal with less certainty. Factors besides the location of the tear probably should be taken into account before deciding whether to try to repair a lesion of this type.

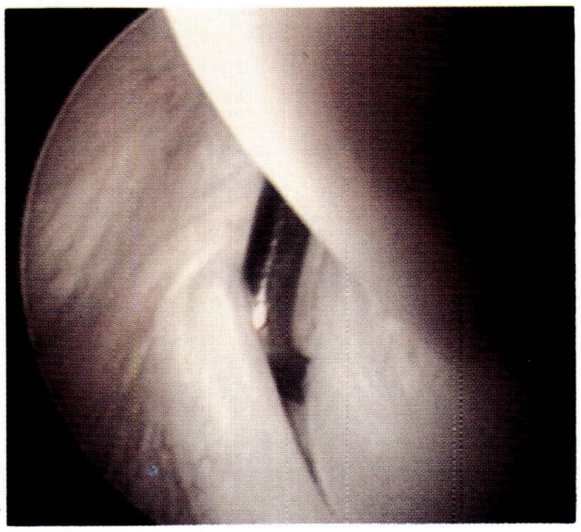

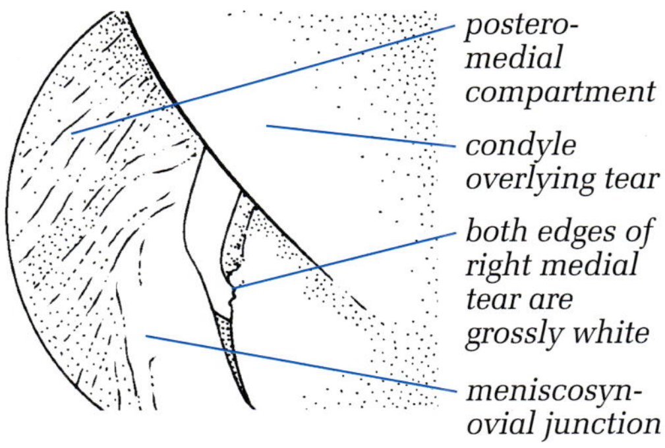

Figure 2.10

This medial meniscus tear is inside the meniscosynovial junction and both edges of the tear are white. There is circulation on the outer edge of this tear, but the tear itself eliminates circulation on the other side. In this view the probe enters through a posteromedial puncture and the 70° telescope passes through the intracondyle notch. The repairability of this lesion is, in my opinion, debatable.

plane (Fig. 2.11). It is very important that tears of this type are repaired since the meniscus is a secondary ligamentous restraint. Meniscectomy unquestionably worsens instability in cruciate cases.

Untreated meniscus tears in cruciate cases eventually extend anteriorly. Increasing meniscus instability usually causes symptoms, resulting in displacement into a bucket-handle configuration (Fig. 2.11). Extension of a tear past the collateral ligament into the anterior meniscus is inevitably associated with chronic cruciate syndrome. Time between the initial cruciate injury (and probably meniscus tear) and arthroscopic intervention for bucket-handle displacement has in my experience averaged 3 years. When chronic cruciate cases are examined arthroscopically, about one half of the tears will still be limited to the posterior one third while about one half will have extended anteriorly. A tear that has not yet extended forward is easiest to repair. Often a tear that has extended anteriorly as a bucket can still be repaired, but it may require a combination of the repair techniques described. Frequently the meniscus is too damaged to justify an attempt at repair.

Technical Considerations

Anatomy at Risk

Medially, the sartorial branch of the saphenous nerve is the structure at greatest risk.[7] During inside-out or outside-in meniscus repair medially, the knee is positioned in practically complete extension. This displaces the nerve forward.[7] When a posteromedial incision is made with the knee in flexion, a protective retractor passes anteriorly to the saphenous nerve. The nerve is held behind the retractor and not trapped when knots are tied. If a retractor is placed anteriorly to the nerve with the knee in flexion, stretching the nerve is possible when the knee is extended in order to pass an inside-out needle. This should be done with great care. Hypesthesia sometimes occurs, but significant saphenous injury is unlikely.

With the outside-in technique, the posteromedial incision is made behind the palpable pes with the knee in extension,[7] which is posterior to the nerve. Blunt dissection is carried down to the joint capsule. Two needles are passed from within the same area of dissection and, whether posterior or anterior to the nerve, the nerve is missed when knots are tied.

When a posteromedial incision is made, care must be taken not to carry the dissection across the midline laterally. The popliteal vessels and the sciatic nerve are located lateral to the midline but can be injured by metallic retractors inserted from the medial aspect. The popliteal structures do not appear to be at risk when a posteromedial puncture is made, at least if it is done under direct view with a 70° arthroscope passing through the intercondylar notch. It is helpful to plan a posteromedial puncture by transilluminating with a 70° arthroscope. A hypodermic needle is first passed into the compartment under direct view. Once the plane of approach is known, the sharp obturator is inserted. The popliteal vessels are protected during this maneuver by the tip of the arthroscope.

Posterolaterally, the peroneal nerve is at risk. It is intimately associated with the biceps tendon and posterior to it at the level of concern. A posterolateral puncture should be made above the biceps tendon with the knee in flexion. The appropriate site for the puncture can be trans-illuminated, using the 70° arthroscope passing through the notch. When a posterolateral incision is made, the biceps and the peroneal nerve are retracted posteriorly and protected. Seemingly there is less risk of injury to the peroneal nerve than to the saphenous nerve medially, because a flexed knee position is normally used when lateral tears are instrumented. Lateral repair is performed much less frequently than medial repair. The biggest concern with lateral repairs is the popliteal artery-sciatic nerve bundle, which lies just behind the posterocentral end of the posterior lateral meniscus.

Small reported the complication rate in 310 meniscus repairs by 21 experienced arthroscopists in 1988.[11] Inside-out medial repairs had a 1.52% complication rate and outside-in repairs a 1.89% complication rate. Few of these complications involved neurovascular injury.

Associated Issues

Most meniscus repair cases also involve instability; successful treatment of meniscus tears includes consideration of the cruciate ligament injury. When repaired, meniscus healing probably occurs independently of specific treatment of the associated ligament laxity. Lasting success of meniscus repairs, however, is no doubt enhanced by correction of instability.[1,6,10]

If ligament reconstruction is indicated, repairable meniscal lesions need treatment simultaneously. Stability is enhanced by successful meniscus repair. The need for an incision to accomplish the repair must be considered in ligament reconstruction cases, since early motion is mandatory in most modern techniques. Another consideration is tourniquet time. Sometimes there is too much to do in a reasonable interval. If the incision necessary for the repair is going to interfere with knee motion, or if the repair requires excessive tourniquet time, the ligament reconstruction should be performed as a separate second intervention.

If meniscus repair is performed as an isolated procedure, immobiliziation for 4 to 6 weeks after operation seems logical. Weight-bearing is allowed. I discourage squatting or sports for 3 to 4 months following surgery. When meniscus repair is performed along with ligament reconstruction, protocol for the ligament procedure is applied.

Surgical Technique

In most cases, meniscus repair is possible with several of the described methods. Virtually any repairable lesion is amenable to the inside-out technique using a posterior corner incision and a retractor. In my opinion, a tear within the attachment of the posteromedial meniscus is repaired more accurately with the wholly intraarticular method, which allows anatomic approximation of tear edges. The open method requires retraction (and distortion) to provide exposure. Also, procedure selection is based on the experience of the surgeon. For example, the outside-in technique is easy for some surgeons and difficult for others. Regardless of the technique selected, however, there will be no discernable difference in outcome.

Open Technique

Open meniscus repair, which I used for a decade, requires a small circumference sturdy needle swaged onto the suture material. Since slick suture material eases tying, we selected Prolene (polyprophylene) (Ethicon), which could be easily located during a possible repeat examination. A variety of retractors is necessary, especially with muscular or obese patients. Because of the depth of the posteromedial compartment, the incision needs to be over 5 cm in length.

It helps to have identified the posterior compartment during the preceeding arthroscopy. The lesion is viewed with a 70° arthroscope, room lights are dimmed, and transillumination is used to puncture the compartment with a spinal needle. The needle hole is easily seen when the skin incision is made. When the capsule is reached, the surgeon should dissect on its surface so it can be located as a layer for subsequent closure. It seems easiest to place all stitches and tag them prior to tying. Typically, for posteromedial tears, three vertical interrupted sutures are placed. Posteromedial incisions cause moderate discomfort that is reduced by immobilization.

Limited movement may enhance the success of this type of repair. Since cruciate ligament reconstructive procedures currently in use require an immediate arc of motion, I have abandoned open repair. The two procedures should not be performed simultaneously.

Inside-Out Technique

Meniscus repair cannulae are available from several manufacturers. A repair cannula with a mild curve of between 15° and 30° and a single bore has proven appropriate for almost all tears. The curve compensates for the convexity

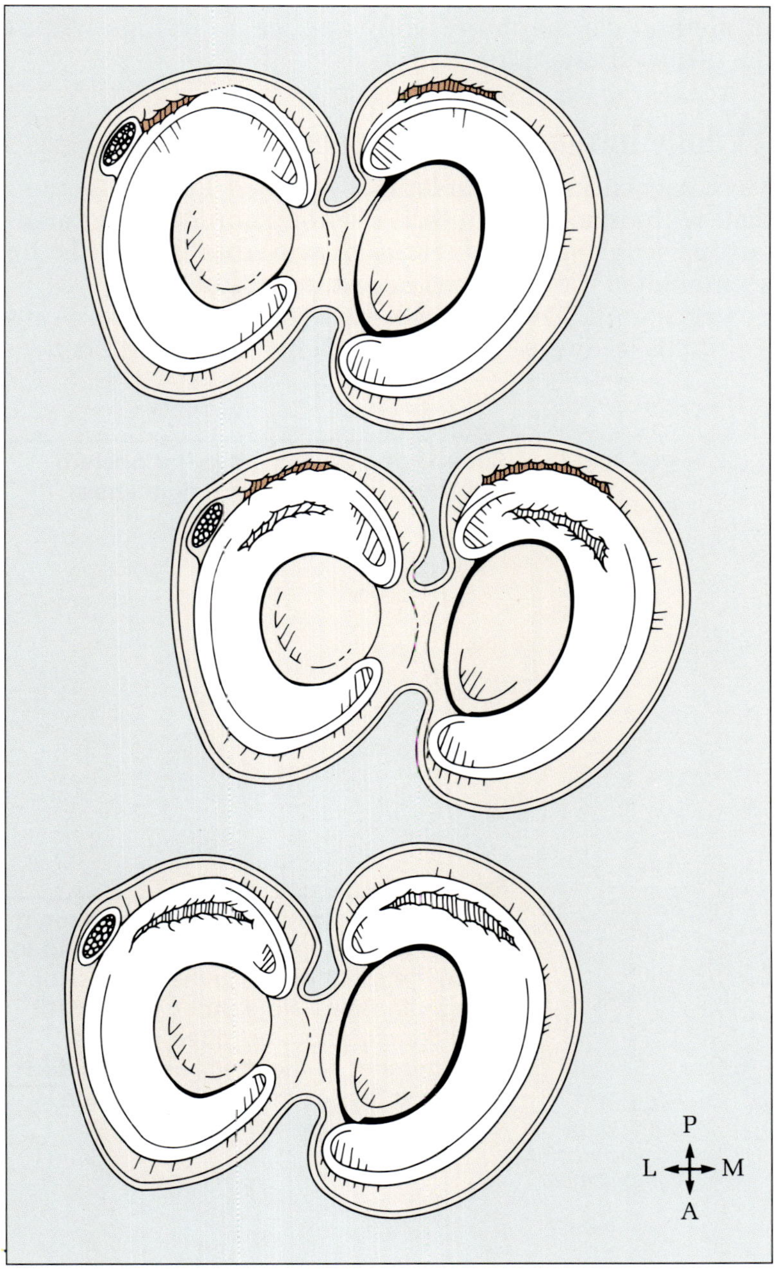

Figure 2.11

These are common meniscus tear patterns seen in fresh anterior cruciate ligament patients. Note that vascular tear patterns occur in both the medial and lateral meniscus. These meniscus tears represent injury to secondary retrants and should be repaired if there is sufficient vascularity. Untreated, tears eventually extend anteriorly and displace.

of the femoral condyle and allows the needle to be directed toward the previously placed metallic retractor. Multiple variations of this technique are described. The fine points of each individual procedure are best determined by reading the literature that accompanies the instrument by the manufacturer. I see no particular advantage to many of the devices.

When the posterior approaches are made for insertion of the metallic retractor, dissection should be carried bluntly down to the capsular level. Blunt dissection is then carried deeper with the fingertip, all the while palpating the posterior meniscus at the joint interval. Various manufacturers provide metallic retractors specifically designed for this type meniscus repair situation. Half of an adult small-sized vaginal speculum can be used.[12] A large kitchen spoon, bent to deflect the repair needle, is preferred by some surgeons. A thimble is a helpful adjunct at the instant of needle penetration and has increased significance in this era of HIV awareness. A knot-tying device helps with suture tying in the depths of small incisions (see below). When meniscus repair is performed in the middle third, needles will not exit through the posterior incision. It helps to push the needle through until the skin is tented, retract the needle, and make a short incision in the desired location. Then the surgeon should bluntly dissect down to the capsule and push the needle through into the dissected area. When the second needle is passed, the incision should be displaced so both needles exit the incision close together. The incision must be large enough to permit knot-tying by fingers, but it can be smaller if the knot-tying device is used. Suture placement is appropriately outside the capsule. It is not desirable to tie externally over a buttress, since this is associated with an unacceptable rate of sepsis.

Outside-In Technique

The outside-in approach has proven especially helpful for the middle one third of both menisci. Dimming the room lights helps conceptualize this repair. The arthroscope is used to visualize the tear and a small incision is made on the transilluminated light spot. Blunt dissection should be used to reach the capsule. Both spinal needles should enter the capsule very close together within the same region of dissection. Sutures can be passed through both the needles simultaneously. The ends should be pulled from an anterior portal and bulky knots tied in each. Both sutures are then pulled simultaneously and satisfactory apposition of the tear surfaces confirmed. A slip knot is used to tighten the first loop, then it is fixed with a knot-tier (Fig. 2.12). The knot on the meniscus surface is quickly covered and does not cause scuffing.

Morgan advocates use of the outside-in technique for tears located in the posterior thirds. He makes a short posteromedial puncture behind the palpable pes with the knee in extension. This approach is behind the saphenous nerve since it moves anteriorly with knee extension. It is my opinion that repair techniques other than the outside-in method can be more safely applied to lesions within the posterior one third.

Wholly Intraarticular Technique

More special instrumentation is required for this method than with other procedures. A set of complete instrumentation is not yet commercially available but could be accumulated. Components necessary include:

- A cannula sized to fit the suture-carrying devices. A lip on its leading edge helps hold it in the compartment.

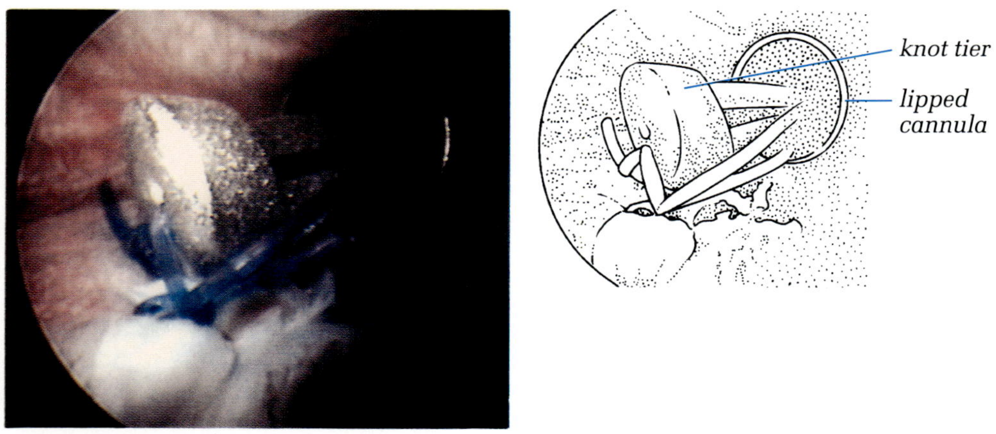

Figure 2.12
Suture tying device within the posteromedial compartment of a right knee.

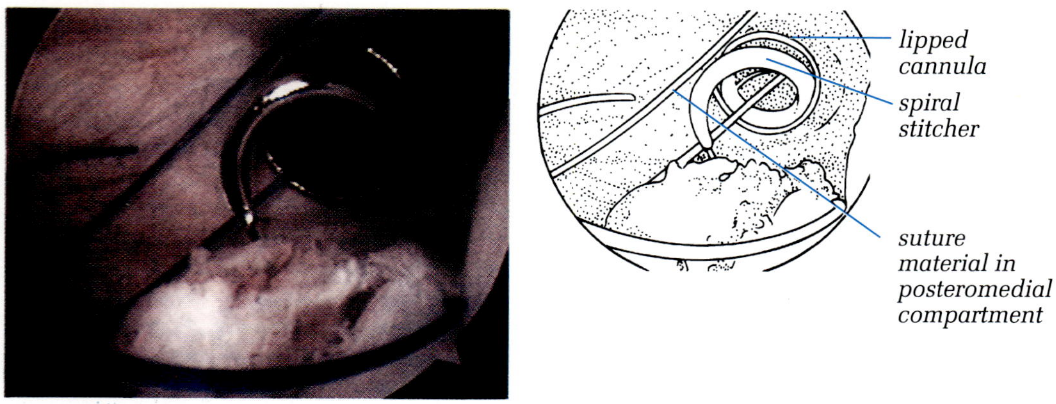

Figure 2.13
Wholly intraarticular meniscus repair in a right knee. The spiral stitcher was used to place the stitch and is in the process of being withdrawn. Note that a great deal of suture material was rolled into the compartment so that it will not be pulled out of the tear as the stitching device is retracted from the cannula.

- Suture carriers of either spiral or angular configuration (Fig. 2.13). The basic construction of a suturing device is simply a spiral needle shaped to direct a contained suture across a posterior tear.
- The 70° arthroscope is practically mandatory for this type of repair. The tear is visualized with the arthroscope passing through the notch and with the instrument cannula entering posteriorly.[3]

Suturing is easiest from outside the tear toward the meniscus and overlying condyle. Start near the tip of the cannula and proceed toward the arthroscope. When a stich is placed, roll a large amount of suture material into the compartment before the needle is backed out of the tear. The suture carrier must be pulled out of the cannula before introducing the grasper used to catch the suture end. Each stitch should be tied when it is placed. Suture cutting, although a function of some knot-tiers, can be easily performed with a straight basket.

Since the puncture incision used for wholly intraarticular meniscus repair requires neither immobilization nor a tourniquet, it can be used with ligament reconstruction.

Knot-Tying Devices

A knot-tying device was developed by the author in 1986 (U.S. Patent No. 4,602,635, Mulhollan and Starr, Baxter). Equivalent knot-tying devices are available from several manufacturers.

The most important step with knot tying devices is the first stitch, which is a slip knot. A simple knot is tightened around the second suture strand and then pulled down to the tear. Tension on the second suture strand holds tension on the knot until it is fixed by subsequent loops (Fig. 2.14). This works equally well through a cannula or through a puncture, since the knot tier is directed by the suture strand to the site of the knot. If the two suture strands do not pass through the same hole of a fascia plane, the knot tied will lie outside the capsule. This is especially useful in suture repair of the middle third of the meniscus (Fig. 2.15). The knot tier can place sutures outside the capsule through a very short superficial incision. To prevent failure, it is important to follow the exact technique described in manufacturer literature.

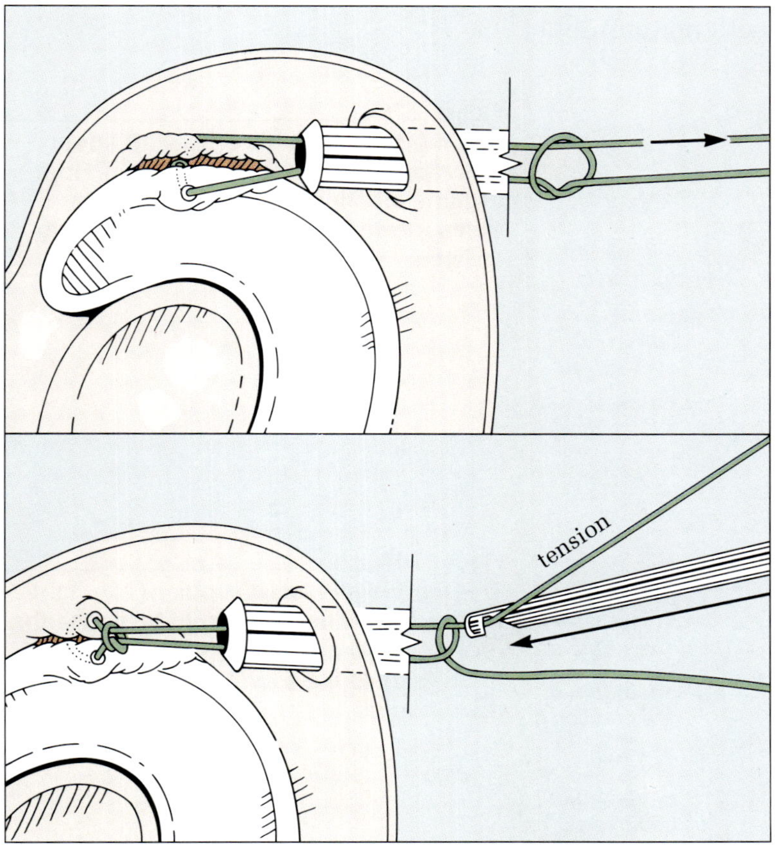

Figure 2.14
Knot-tying techniques. The first knot is a simple one placed around the second strand and then tightened and pulled down to the sight of the stitch. Tension on the strand holds the knot until fixed with subsequent knot loops.

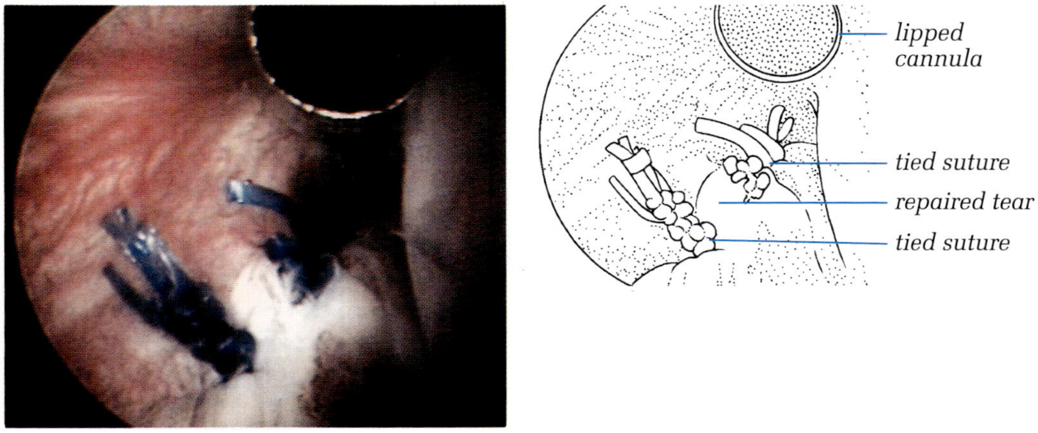

Figure 2.15
Typical appearence of a suture line placed by the wholly intraarticular meniscus repair technique in the medial meniscus of a right knee.

RESULTS

Varying success rates have been reported after meniscus suturing. In my own series, open repair of the medial meniscus was performed in 80 cases between 1980 and 1990. To date, five of these cases have been reoperated for recurrent tears. Wholly intraarticular meniscus repair, first applied in 1989, has been performed 25 times. Two of these patients have been operated for recurrent tears. The overall success rate with these grossly vascular lesions is, therefore, in excess of 90%. When meniscus repair is performed inside the meniscosynovial junction, that is, within the white part of the meniscus, healing is less likely. It is not clear at this date when repair at these inner levels should be undertaken. Small reported 3,927 meniscus cases performed by 21 experienced arthroscopic surgeons in 1988.[11] Repair was elected in approximately 8% of these cases. Most reports on meniscus repair group peripheral or visibly vascular tears with tears within the meniscal substance. A wide range of application of these techniques is reported, and reported success rates are equally inconsistent.

Assessment of results is difficult for many reasons. An MRI of a meniscus might show a tear signal when the lesion is healed by arthroscopic and clinical criteria.[13] A torn meniscus can be asymptomatic. Untreated, a meniscus tear can take years to become long enough for displacement to occur. It is possible to repair a meniscus unsuccessfully and have it remain silent for a long interval.

Repeat arthroscopic assessment is sometimes possible. A repair performed percutaneously within a vascular region was rearthroscoped at 6 months and is shown in Figure 2.16. A failed case of meniscus repair is shown in Figure 2.17. In failed cases the new tear develops inside the plane of the original meniscus repair.

CONCLUSION

Meniscus repair should be used by all arthroscopic knee surgeons. Justification for its application is not debatable; it is obligatory in management of the unstable knee. Only the range of its application is controversial. Inside-out techniques can be applied to virtually any repairable situation. In many cases, the newer intraarticular technique facilitates meniscus repair through a puncture incision with no tourniquet.

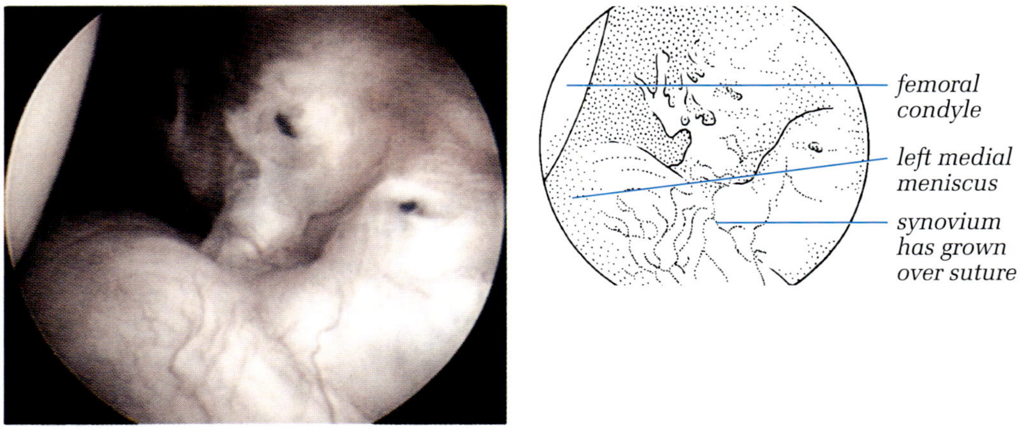

Figure 2.16 This medial meniscus of the left knee was repaired 6 months previously. Note that the stitches have been overgrown with synovial tissue and are practically invisible.

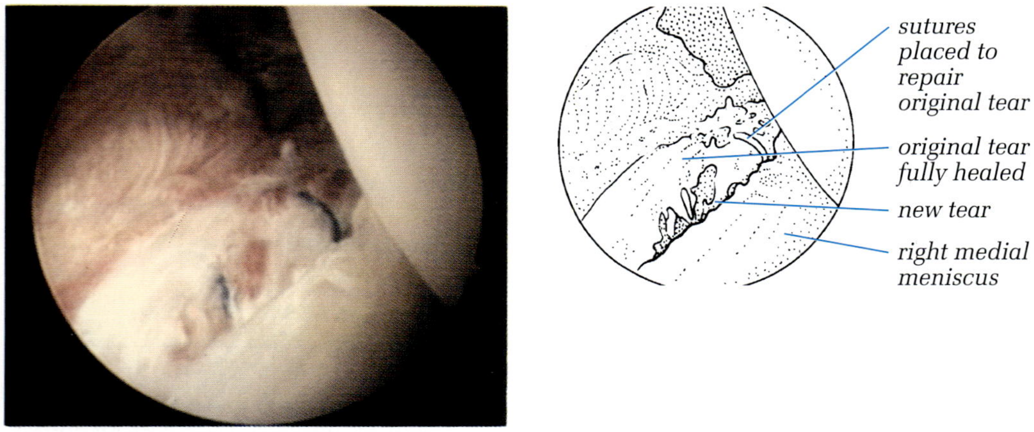

Figure 2.17 This medial meniscus repair of the right knee failed after 2 years. In this case the tear occured adjacent to the suture line. In all failures the tear itself appears to have healed.

REFERENCES

1. DeHaven KE, et al. Technique and two to nine year results. *Am J Sports Med.* 1989;17:788–795.
2. Hamberg P, et al. Suture of new and old peripheral meniscus tears. *J Bone Joint Surg.* 1983;65A:193–197.
3. Mulhollan JS. The Swedish system. *Orthop Clin North Am.* 1982;13:349.
4. Stone RG, Miller GA. A technique of arthroscopic suture of torn menisci. *J Arthro Rel Surg.* 1985;4:226–232.
5. Hanks GA, et al. Repair of peripheral meniscal tears: open versus arthroscopic technique. *J Arthro Rel Surg.* 1991;7:72–77.
6. Rosenberg TD, et al. Arthroscopic meniscal repair evaluated with repeat arthroscopy. *J Arthro Rel Surg.* 1986;2:14–20.
7. Morgan CD, Casscells SW. Arthroscopic meniscus repair: a safe approach to the posterior horns. *J Arthro Rel Surg.* 1986;2:3–12.
8. Morgan CD. The "all-inside" meniscus repair. *J Arthro Rel Surg.* 1991;7:120–125.
9. Arnoczky SP, Warren RF. Microvasculature of the human meniscus. *Am J Sports Med.* 1982;10:90–95.
10. Stone RG, et al. Long-term assessment of arthroscopic meniscus repair: a two to six-year follow-up study. *J Arthro Rel Surg.* 1990;6:73–98.
11. Small NC. Complications in arthroscopic surgery performed by experienced surgeons. *J Arthro Rel Surg.* 1988;4:215–221.
12. Bach BR. A modified soft tissue retractor for meniscal repair. *J Arthro Rel Surg.* 1988;4:295–296.
13. Deutsch AL, et al. Peripheral meniscus tears: MR findings after conservative treatment or meniscal repair. *J Radiol.* 1990;176:485–488.

Chapter Three

Arthroscopic Procedures on Bone and Articular Cartilage of the Knee Joint

James W. Stone
James F. Guhl

Arthroscopic surgical techniques have revolutionized knee surgery by allowing procedures to be performed with less operative trauma and faster rehabilitation than previously possible. In this chapter we discuss methods of surgical treatment of bone and articular cartilage abnormalities of the knee joint. We focus on technical issues, although the procedure's historical aspects and radiologic evaluation of the condition are also discussed.

SET UP FOR KNEE ARTHROSCOPY

We place the patient in the supine position with a lateral post for application of valgus stress for standard knee arthroscopy (Fig. 3.1). The patient should be positioned on the table so that the knee can be flexed if the foot of the table is lowered. Placing the leg in a figure 4 position facilitates application of varus stress to enable viewing of the lateral compartment. We do not use a leg holder because it limits access to the distal thigh and intraoperative mobility of the extremity. It may also cause complications such as a tourniquet effect. An arthroscopic fluid pump facilitates the procedure by maintaining both flow and distention pressure. With the fluid flowing through the arthroscopic cannula, debris is directed away from the field of view.

Positive pressure minimizes bleeding and a tourniquet is rarely required. A radiolucent operative table is used for intraoperative image intensification during procedures on bone, such as those required for osteochondritis dissecans or reduction and fixation of fractures.

A 30°, 5 mm arthroscope is used for most procedures, but a 70° arthroscope should be available for posterior viewing. An interchangeable cannula system allows the operating surgeon to switch portals without repetitive joint entry. This feature minimizes extravasation of fluid into soft tissues. Routine manual instruments—graspers, basket forceps, and knives—along with a power shaver and abrader system are the mainstays of instrumentation. Recently we have used the holmium:YAG (Ho:YAG) laser, particularly for procedures on articular cartilage and menisci. Its specific applications are discussed below.

LOOSE BODIES

Loose bodies in the knee joint frequently arise after trauma. Acute patellar dislocation or subluxation can result in chondral or osteochondral fracture of the patella or lateral femoral condyle.[1] Chondral or osteochondral fracture can also result from direct trauma to the articular surface from a force applied externally to the joint (Fig. 3.2). With the development of degenerative joint disease, loose bodies can result when an osteophyte fractures off the articular margin. A further source of loose bodies is osteochondritis dissecans, which usually occurs on the medial femoral condyle and, less commonly, on the lateral femoral condyle.[2]

Clinically, the patient frequently perceives an object floating within the joint or may instead experience a "giving way" of the knee joint. Most have evidence of internal derangement with effusion and pain. If the loose body is osteochondral, it will usually be evident on routine radiographs. However, a chondral loose body may be invisible on routine radiographs and be seen only with special studies, such as an arthrogram or magnetic resonance imaging (MRI).

Surgical Technique

The arthroscopic approach to loose bodies is routine. The arthroscope is inserted into the joint through the anterolateral approach, and adequate inflow and outflow of fluid are established. A systematic examination of the joint is performed, beginning in the suprapatellar pouch, followed by examination of the patellofemoral joint. The medial gutter and then the medial joint are inspected next, followed by examination of the intercondylar notch, the lateral joint, the lateral gutter, popliteal tendon, and the posterior joint via the intercondylar notch.

If at any point during the examination a loose body is seen, the surgeon should concentrate on its removal rather

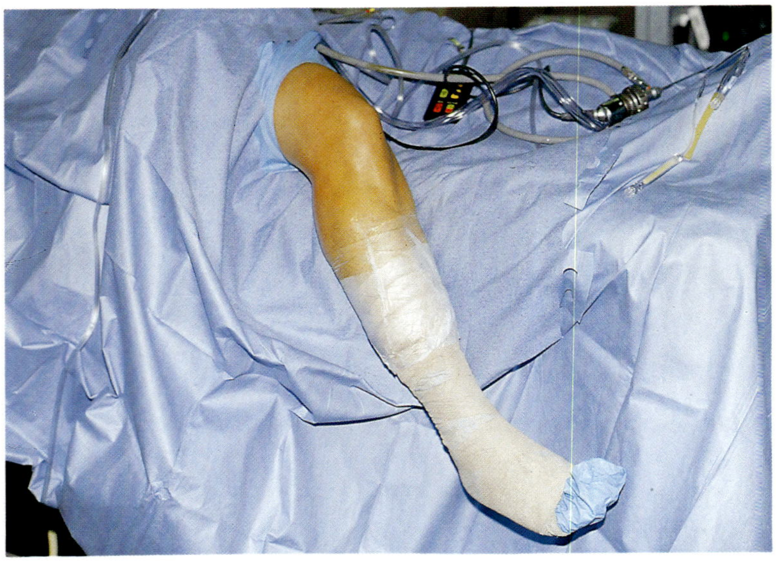

Figure 3.1
Patient prepped and draped for arthroscopic knee surgery. A lateral post rather than a knee holder is used for application of valgus stress. The knee may be lowered over the side of the table, or the foot of the table may be lowered and the leg allowed to hang free.

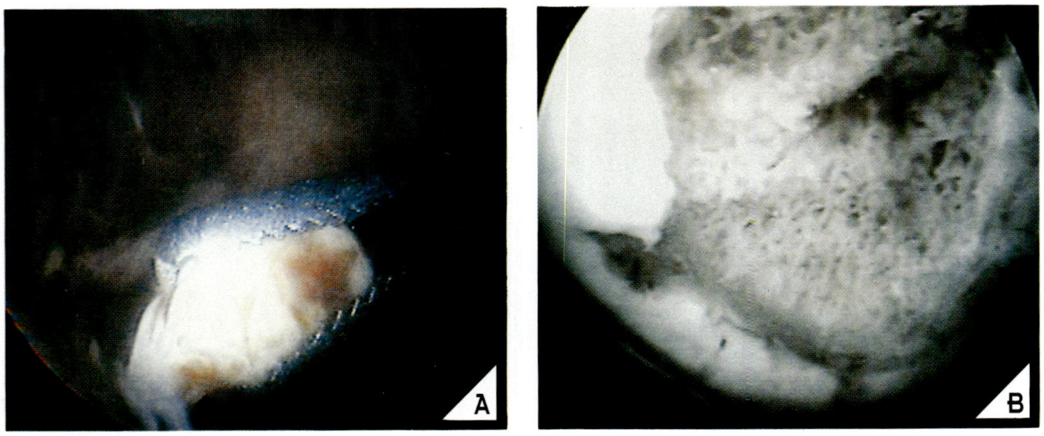

Figure 3.2
(A) Arthroscopic view of a loose body in the jaws of a grasping forceps. The patient had sustained a patellar dislocation. (B) A complete survey of the knee joint revealed the area of the lateral femoral condyle from which the loose body arose.

than further joint surveillance. Decreasing or stopping the inflow, if it is directed through the arthroscope, prevents the loose body from being pushed away from the field of view. The loose body may be stabilized with a spinal needle and then grasped with a loose body forceps. An accessory portal medially, laterally, or in the suprapatellar pouch may be used. If the loose body is found in the posterior joint compartment, an accessory portal posteromedially or, less commonly, posterolaterally may be used.

After the loose body is removed, and the remainder of the joint has been inspected, the origin of the loose body must be located and treated. If the source is an osteophyte, remaining osteophytes should be debrided using pituitary rongeurs or a motorized burr. If the loose body is an osteochondral fragment with a significant piece of attached bone and the result of either direct or indirect trauma, treatment is internal fixation rather than removal. Internal fixation requires the presence of adequate bone and a precise fit into the defect. With time, the site of origin and the fragment itself become deformed, making internal fixation impossible. If the loose body can be replaced and held with a Kirschner wire, internal fixation can be with screws or additional wires. Arthrotomy may be required for accurate internal fixation, especially for lesions of the posterior aspect of the lateral femoral condyle or undersurface of the patella.

Osteochondritis Dissecans

Osteochondritis dissecans is a focal abnormality of articular cartilage and underlying subchondral bone that can result in fragment separation, detachment, and loose body formation. Its etiology is uncertain, but direct and indirect trauma, or primary ischemia to a segment of bone and cartilage, are most frequently implicated. The disorder can occur in any joint, but most commonly occurs in the knee, ankle, and elbow. Patients usually present in the second or third decade for evaluation of joint swelling, catching, pain, or sensation of instability.

Plain radiographs generally reveal a well-circumscribed lesion of the articular surface, sometimes with a clearly defined fragment of subchondral bone (Fig. 3.3). The Berndt and Harty staging system, developed to evaluate ankle joint osteochondritis dissecans, divides lesions into intact, separated, detached, or loose bodies.[3] Unfortunately, plain radiographs do not accurately predict the actual type of lesion found on arthroscopic examination. Tomography, arthrotomography, and CT also fail to predict the relative intactness of the articular surface reliably. MRI holds promise as an effective imaging tool for the articular cartilage and may give us the best noninvasive assessment as to whether the surface is intact and unbroken, or whether the fragment and its underlying bone are separated or detached (Fig. 3.4).

Surgical Technique

After the history, physical examination, and preoperative radiographic evaluations, surgical assessment should be performed arthroscopically. If the lesion is difficult to detect, it can be outlined by light-dimming techniques, tangential viewing, or instillation of methylene blue dye. The lesion must be carefully probed to determine the intactness of the articular cartilage and to assess whether the underlying bone is intact or loose.

Osteochondritis dissecans lesions may be approached in a variety of ways. Detached lesions, particularly those

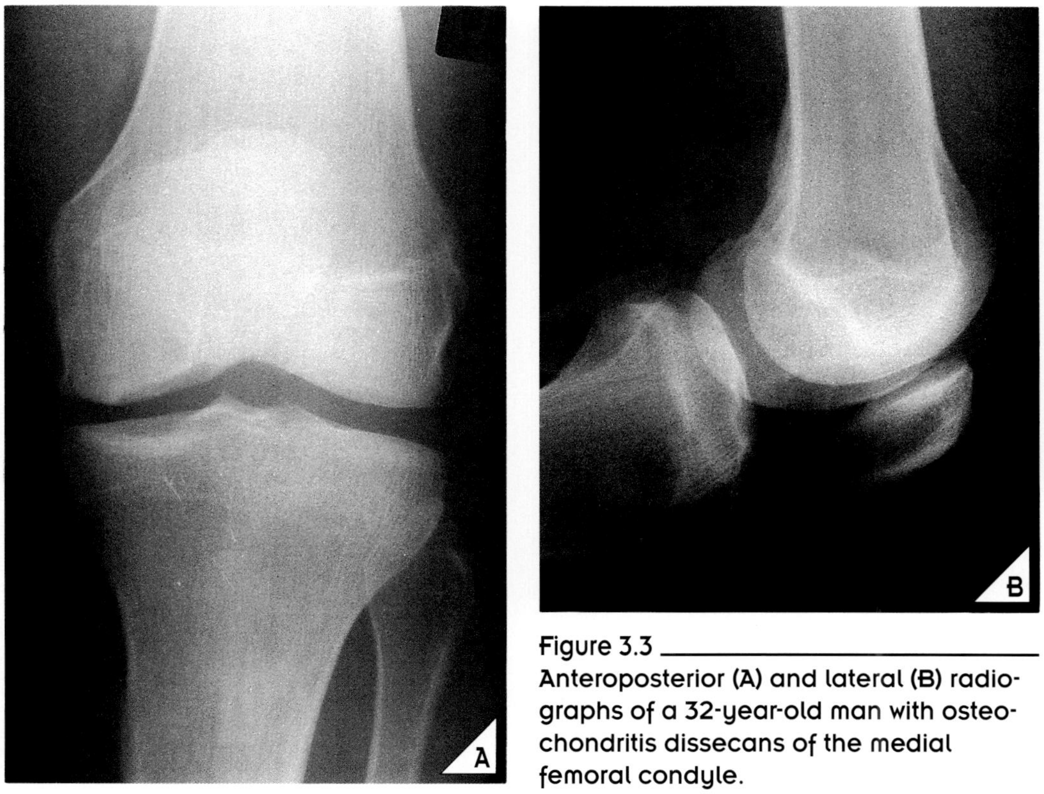

Figure 3.3
Anteroposterior (A) and lateral (B) radiographs of a 32-year-old man with osteochondritis dissecans of the medial femoral condyle.

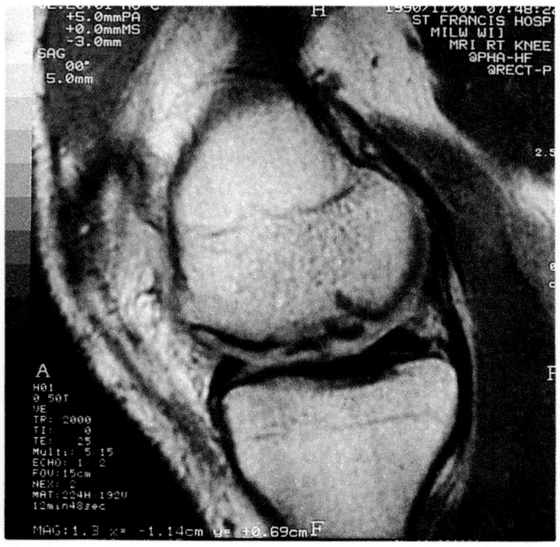

Figure 3.4
Sagittal MR image of the patient in Figure 3.3 reveals the lesion to be thin with little attached subchondral bone.

with minimal or no subchondral bone, are generally debrided (Fig. 3.5). With the arthroscope in the lateral parapatellar portal, the more common lesions of the lateral aspect of the medial femoral condyle can be approached from the medial parapatellar portal with a pituitary rongeur or similar grasping instrument. After removing the lesion, the rim of articular cartilage should be debrided to stable cartilage with edges perpendicular to the surface of the subchondral bone. Treatment of the exposed subchondral bone is subject to debate. Most authorities recommend either abrasion or drilling of the surface. We generally recommend placement of multiple drill holes using a .062 inch Kirschner wire that is advanced through a small cannula, so as not to bend or break the wire, to a preset depth.

Internal Fixation

An attempt should be made to salvage intact or separated lesions. Once again, the actual technique for salvage of these lesions is open to debate. Internal fixation is one alternative. In the simplest technique, smooth Kirschner wires are advanced from distal to proximal under arthroscopic control (Fig. 3.6).[4] The pins should exit the metaphysis in adults, or the epiphysis in patients prior to

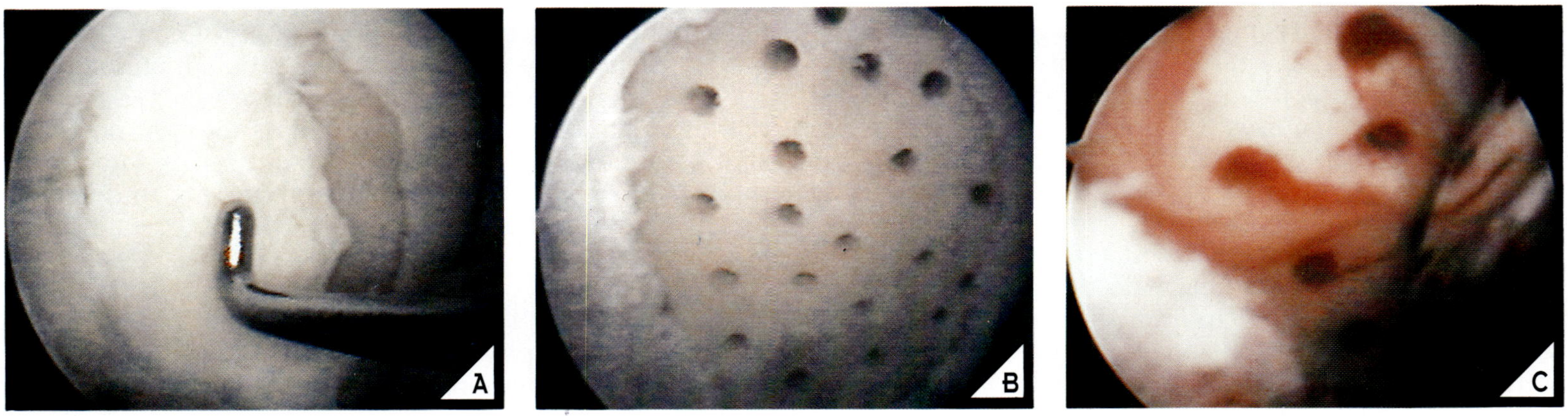

Figure 3.5
Intraoperative arthroscopic image of the patient in Figures 3.3 and 3.4. (A) The probe is palpating the loose fragment, which is noted to be comprised mainly of articular cartilage with minimal attached bone. (B) The lesion was debrided and multiple drill holes were placed in the bone bed using a 0.062 inch Kirschner wire. (C) As the tourniquet is deflated blood can be seen emanating from the drill holes.

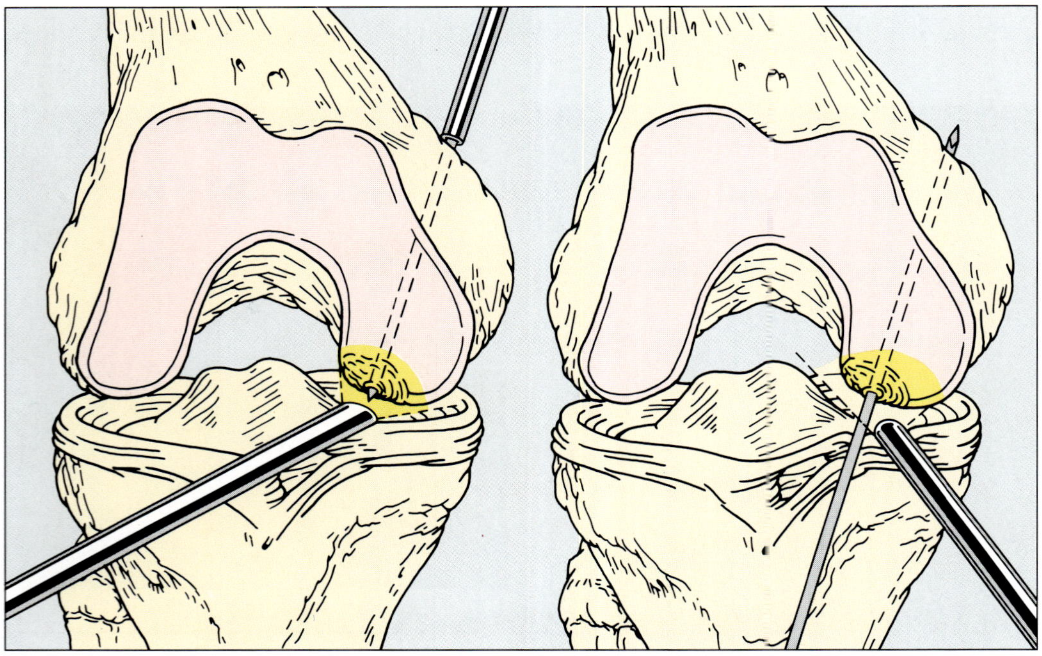

Figure 3.6
Arthroscopic internal fixation of osteochondritis dissecans lesion of the medial femoral condyle using Kirschner wires. The arthroscope is placed in the anteromedial portal and a Kirschner wire is advanced from distal to proximal under direct visualization. The Kirschner wire is advanced through a small cannula to prevent bending. (A) An accessory lateral parapatellar or transpatellar tendon portal may be used to obtain a perpendicular angle to the lesion. The wire is advanced through the medial femoral condyle and out the skin. (B) The drill is attached to the K-wire which is then backed out in a retrograde fashion under arthroscopic guidance to just below the articular surface.

skeletal maturity, to prevent injuring the physeal plate. Placing multiple pins assures improved rotational control of the lesion. The pins are positioned under the skin so removal can be performed in an outpatient setting. The primary advantage of this technique is its ease; its primary disadvantage is that the fixation device does not provide compression across the lesion.

Fixation with Cancellous Screws

The development of cannulated cancellous screws has facilitated internal fixation of osteochondritis dissecans fragments. A small guide pin is placed to temporarily fix the fragment. The cannulated screw is simple to place once the guide pin has been accurately positioned. There is little risk of the internal fixation screw becoming loose within the joint. After the lesion has healed, screw removal is facilitated by replacement of a wire into the screw prior to backing the screw out.

After determining suitability of the lesion for internal fixation, a guide pin is advanced across the lesion under arthroscopic guidance (Fig. 3.7). Accessory portals medially or laterally are frequently required to optimize the angle of approach and allow perpendicular placement of the screw. After guidewire placement, a screw of appropriate length is advanced over the guidewire. Some systems use a fragile, small-diameter guidewire, and care must be taken not to transect the wire with an advancing screw that is not angled perfectly along the wire. The screw head must be countersunk below the articular cartilage surface to avoid subsequent injury to the adjacent tibial plateau. Although a well countersunk screw could be left in place, we generally recommend screw removal approximately 12 weeks after placement.

We allow initiation of motion in a brace approximately 4 to 6 weeks postoperatively, if good fixation and compression have been achieved. However, we do not allow greater than toe-touch weight-bearing while the screws are in place. Advantages of this technique compared to simple Kirschner wire fixation include more rigid fixation of the fragment and possibly better healing potential. Disadvantages include the loss of articular cartilage surface required by the size of the screw head, along with the need for a secondary surgical procedure to remove the hardware. On the other hand, a second examination helps assess healing, and the tracts left by the screws may provide channels for healing across the lesion.

Fixation with Herbert Screws

An alternative fixation device with advantages over simple compression screws is the Herbert screw.[5] Compression across the bone fragments is achieved as the screw is tightened based on the differential pitch of the two screw ends. The head is completely buried under the articular cartilage. We believe that the screws should be removed prior to weight-bearing, but that early range of motion can be initiated with the screws in place. The Herbert screw is available in both a cannulated and a noncannulated version. We recommend use of the cannulated type as its

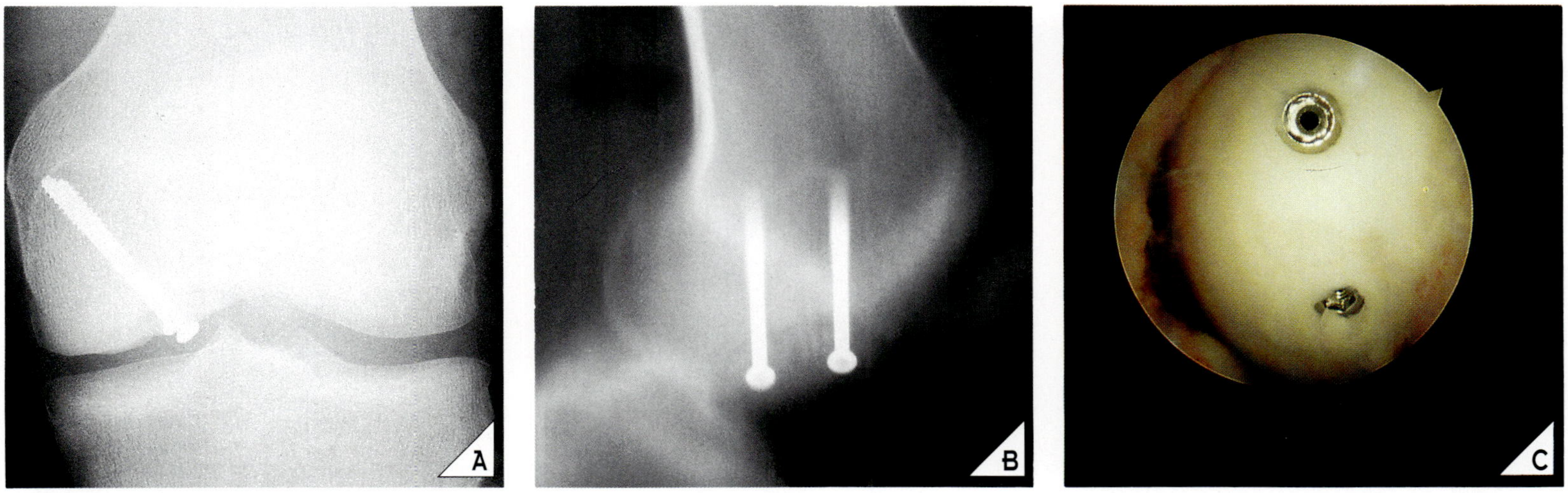

Figure 3.7
Anteroposterior radiograph (A) and lateral tomogram (B) showing osteochondritis dissecans fragment of the medial femoral condyle fixed with two cannulated cancellous screws. Intraoperative arthroscopic view (C) of the two cancellous screws countersunk below the articular surface.

placement and removal are facilitated with a guidewire (Fig. 3.8). Fixation with the Herbert screw is performed as described above for cannulated cancellous screws, except that the drill sizes for the proximal and distal portions of the hole must be appropriate for the two ends of the screw.

A detached fragment must be prepared prior to internal fixation in order to optimize healing. An attempt is made to maintain a hinge of bone and/or articular cartilage so that the majority of the lesion can be elevated without creating a loose fragment. The subchondral bone on the undersurface of the lesion is gently curetted to remove any loose fibrous tissue. The base of the lesion is similarly debrided to bleeding cancellous bone. If a significant defect has been produced so replacement of the lesion results in incongruity of the articular surface, a bone graft is placed in the base prior to replacement of the fragment and subsequent fixation. Lesions that appear to be intact or separated but have fibrous tissue protruding from the margins will be found to have significant amounts of fibrous tissue beneath the bone fragment. Such a lesion should be treated as a detached fragment and the base debrided. Performing these techniques arthroscopically can be very demanding. The surgeon should not hesitate to perform an arthrotomy if a technically more adequate procedure can be executed. Do not perform a procedure arthroscopically if it can be done with greater accuracy via an open incision.

Bone Grafting

An alternative to internal fixation for intact osteochondritis dissecans lesions is bone grafting. The use of bone pegs accomplishes both the goal of internal fixation and bone grafting. Small corticocancellous matchstick grafts are harvested from the proximal tibia and placed across the lesion arthroscopically or via a small arthrotomy incision (Fig. 3.9). As stated above, the base of the lesion must be appropriately prepared to maximize the chances of success of the procedure.

Alternatively, cancellous bone grafting from proximal to distal can be accomplished with relative ease arthroscopically (Fig. 3.10). The intact lesion is localized arthroscopically, and an anterior cruciate ligament reconstruction guide is used to place a guidewire from the femoral metaphysis into the lesion. The guidewire is then overdrilled with a 6 to 7 mm reamer, being careful not to breach the articular cartilage. Cancellous bone graft harvested from the iliac crest is then packed down the tunnel. Image intensification or intraoperative radiographs are useful to assure accurate placement of the guidewire and the reamer. Once again, protected weight-bearing is enforced for the first 6 to 12 weeks, although controlled range of motion exercises can be instituted at approximately 6 weeks.

Acute Chondral and Osteochondral Fractures

Acute osteochondral fractures usually occur in adolescents and young adults in contrast to pure chondral fractures, which are seen almost exclusively in adults. Johnson-Nurse and Dandy proposed that in the younger age group, the articular cartilage was so firmly attached to

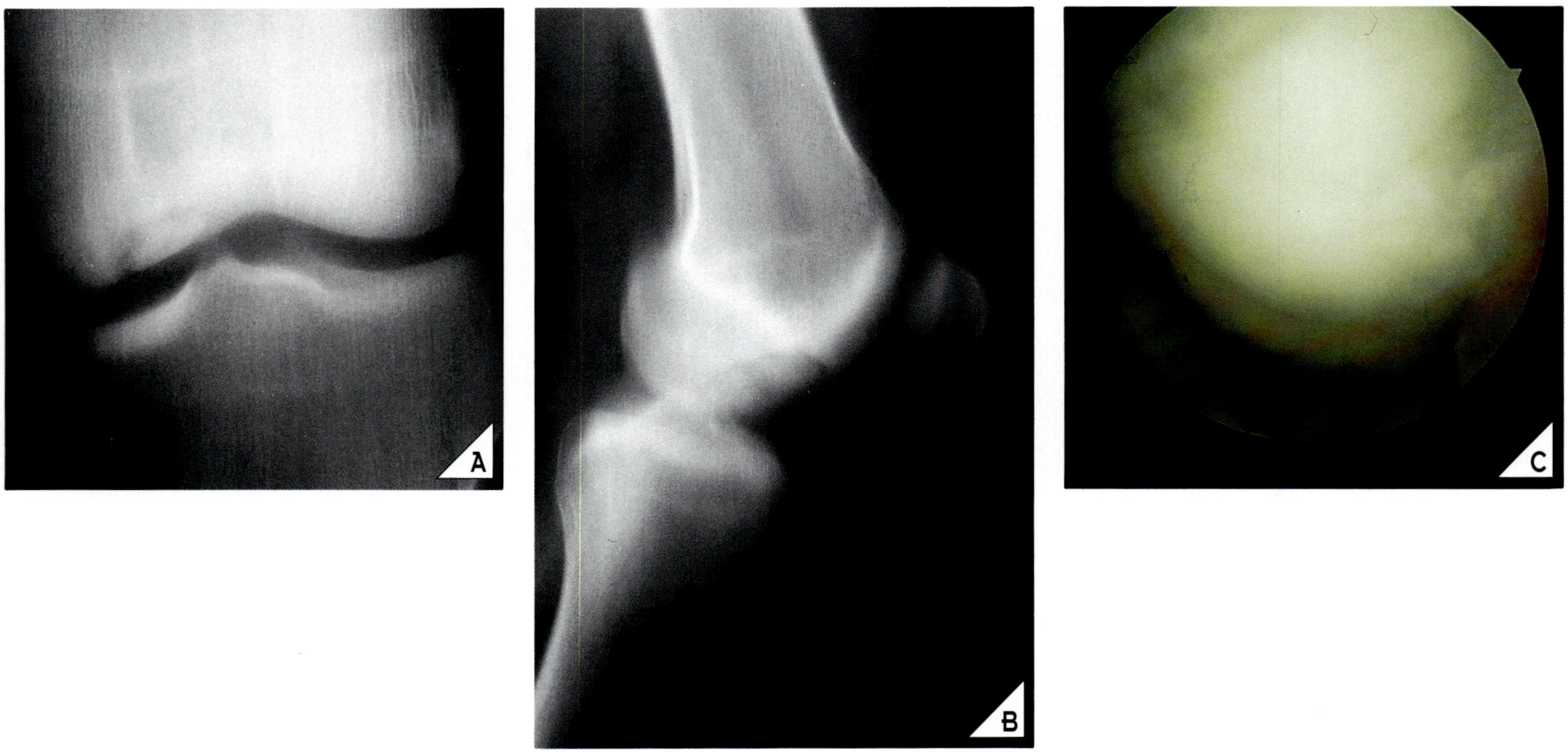

Figure 3.8
Anteroposterior (A) and lateral (B) tomograms of a large osteochondritis dissecans lesion of the medial femoral condyle. The lesion is comprised of two large bone fragments. (C) Arthroscopic view shows the articular surface to be intact with slight elevation of the fragment. The lesion was fixed with two cannulated Herbert screws, one in each major bone fragment. Multiple drill holes were also placed at the periphery of the lesion using 0.062 inch Kirschner wire.

the underlying bone that the subchondral bone constituted the weaker area.[6] In contrast, the basal zone of articular cartilage becomes calcified in adults, and there is separation between the calcified and uncalcified zones. This area represents the weak link in the articular cartilage, explaining the relatively greater frequency of chondral fractures in the adult patients.

These chondral and osteochondral fractures can occur secondary to patellar subluxation and dislocation, twisting injuries to the knee in the absence of patellar dislocation that result in shear forces across the articular cartilage, or direct trauma to the joint. Patients frequently describe a twisting injury, possibly associated with the sensation of a "pop" in the joint. A hemarthrosis generally develops with osteochondral fractures, although not necessarily with pure chondral injuries. The patient may complain of locking or catching, with a sensation of giving way. The physical examination will reveal no evidence of ligament laxity in the patient with isolated osteochondral or chondral fracture. However, these injuries may coexist with meniscus tears and ligament injuries.

The radiographic examination must at a minimum consist of anteroposterior, lateral, tunnel, and tangential patellar views. Additional oblique radiographs may be obtained for further definition.

Surgical Technique

Arthroscopy provides the most accurate assessment of the size and character of an osteochondral or chondral injury. A complete examination of the joint must be performed in an organized fashion. The anterolateral parapatellar portal is used to perform the initial evaluation. The suprapatellar pouch, undersurface of the patella, and the femoral groove are evaluated first with the knee in full extension. The medial gutter is then visualized and the knee flexed to examine the medial compartment. The intercondylar notch is assessed, followed by the lateral compartment with the knee in the figure 4 position. The lateral gutter and popliteus recess are then examined in knee extension. Finally, the posteromedial and lateral compartments are examined through the intercondylar notch. The 70° or 90° arthroscope can be useful in the posterior examination. Accurate assessment of an injured area may require viewing through multiple portals, including the anteromedial and anterolateral portals, the lateral suprapatellar portal to evaluate the undersurface of the patella, and the posteromedial or posterolateral portals for the posterior joint.

In the case of osteochondral fractures, the decision to replace the loose fragment depends on the size of the

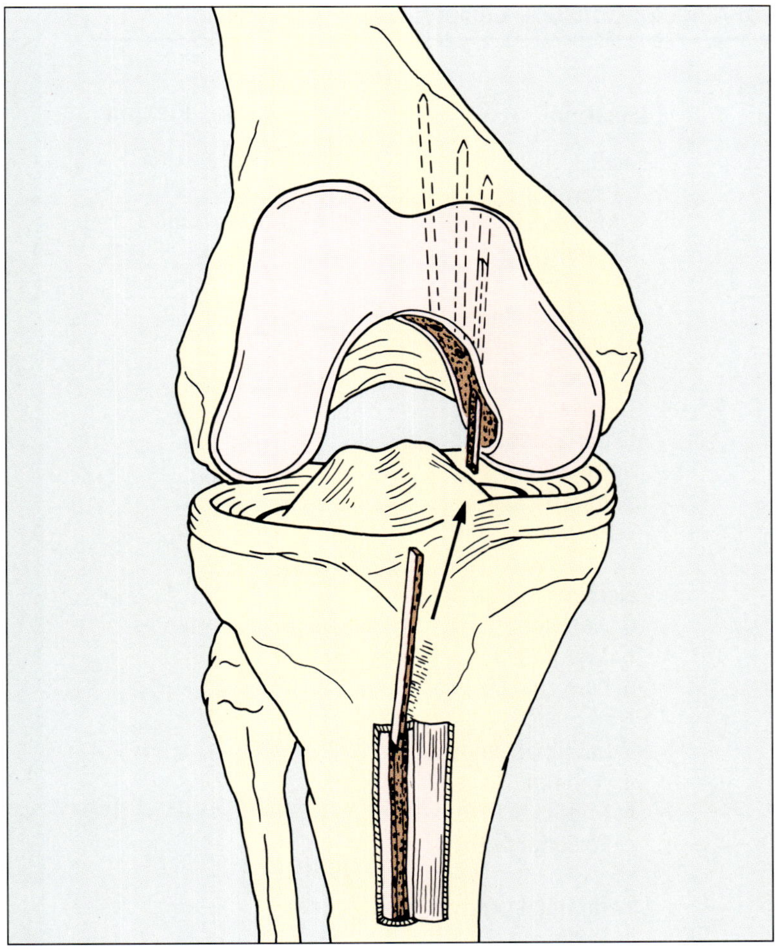

Figure 3.9

The procedure for matchstick corticocancellous bone grafting of osteochondritis dissecans. The procedure can be performed arthroscopically or by arthrotomy. Small corticocancellous strips are harvested from the proximal tibia and fashioned into matchstick grafts. They are advanced through a small cannula into holes predrilled into the lesion.

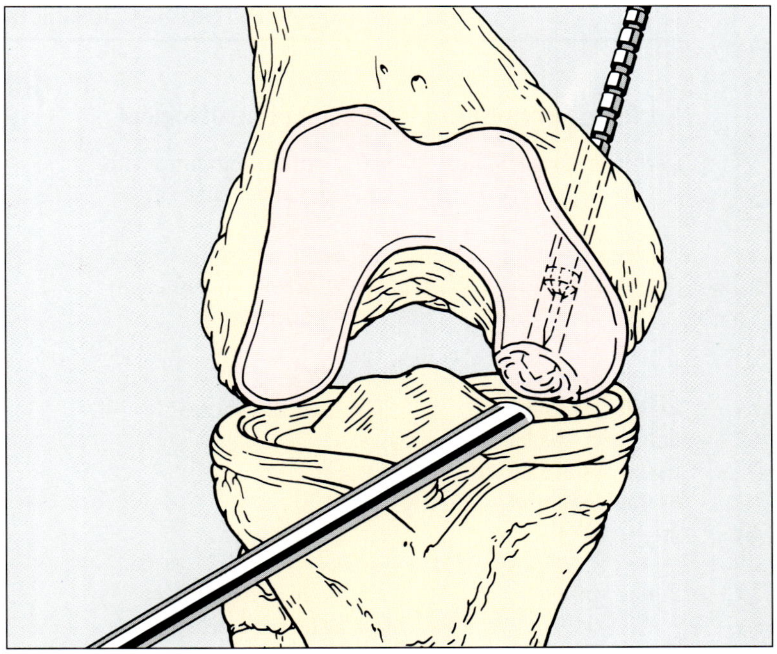

Figure 3.10

Arthroscopically assisted cancellous bone graft procedure for osteochondritis dissecans. The anterior cruciate ligament guide helps place a pin from the medial femoral condyle into the center of the lesion. The cannulated reamer (5 to 6 mm) is then used to create a channel to the lesion, being careful not to penetrate the articular surface. Cancellous bone graft is then packed down the channel.

lesion, the presence of multiple fragments, the time since the injury, the quality of the bone attached to the articular fragment, and the accessibility to arthroscopic internal fixation. The acute injury with a large single fragment on the weight-bearing surface of the medial or lateral femoral condyle should be replaced. Cases with multiple fragments or attached bone insufficient to accept internal fixation must undergo fragment removal. Large fragments from inaccessible areas, such as the undersurface of the patella or posterior aspect of the lateral femoral condyle, should be internally fixed by arthrotomy if necessary. Internal fixation can be accomplished with any of the devices discussed above, including Kirschner wires, cannulated cancellous screws, or Herbert screws.

Lesions of Articular Cartilage

Numerous systems exist to classify articular cartilage lesions. Noyes and Stabler present a succinct review of these classifications and propose a more comprehensive system of their own design (Table 3.1).[7] Their system includes an assessment of the articular cartilage surface appearance, the depth of involvement, and the size and the location of the lesion. More recently, Tippett has proposed an eight-stage system for classification of articular cartilage defects (Table 3.2).[8]

When there is softening of the articular cartilage without flaps or fissures, conservative management is the most prudent approach. One should not debride these lesions and create a large area of iatrogenic injury. Fissures that on probing are felt to extend down to the level of subchondral bone can be carefully drilled using a .062 inch Kirschner wire to encourage ingrowth of fibrous tissue that may stabilize the lesion. With increasing involvement, flaps of articular cartilage may exist with delamination of the articular cartilage. The unstable flaps of cartilage should be debrided, but remaining intact cartilage at the base should be left alone.

When the articular cartilage lesion extends down to the level of the subchondral bone, the unstable flaps of tissue must be debrided to a stable rim of articular cartilage with edges perpendicular to the bone surface. Treatment of the resulting defect is controversial. Some authors suggest placement of multiple drill holes using a small Kirschner wire, while others suggest abrasion of the subchondral

TABLE 3.1
Noyes and Stabler Classification of Articular Cartilage Lesions

Surface Description	Extent of Involvement	Diameter (mm)	Location	Degree of Knee Flexion
Cartilage surface intact	A. Definite softening with some resilience remaining B. Extensive softening with loss of resilience (deformation)	<10 ≤15 ≤20 ≤25 >25	Patella A. Proximal 1/3 Middle 1/3 Distal 1/3 B. Odd facet Middle facet Lateral facet	Degree of knee flexion where the lesion is in weight-bearing contact (e.g., 20°–45°)
Cartilage surface damaged: cracks, fissures, fibrillation, or fragmentation	A. <1/2 thickness B. ≥1/2 thickness		Trochlea Medial femoral condyle a. Anterior 1/3 b. Middle 1/3 c. Posterior 1/3	
Bone exposed	A. Bone surface intact B. Bone surface cavitation		Lateral femoral condyle a. Anterior 1/3 b. Middle 1/3 c. Posterior 1/3	
			Medial tibial condyle a. Anterior 1/3 b. Middle 1/3 c. Posterior 1/3	
			Lateral tibial condyle a. Anterior 1/3 b. Middle 1/3 c. Posterior 1/3	

Reprinted with permission from Noyes FR, Stabler CL, 1989

bone. After either treatment, we recommend 6 weeks of non-weight-bearing with early range-of-motion exercises.

A recent study in rabbits investigated articular cartilage repair after a 3 mm patellar chondral shaving or subchondral abrasion was performed.[9] After 12 weeks, there was no evidence of reparative tissue in the chondral shaving group, and degeneration of the remaining underlying cartilage was noted. In contrast, full-thickness defects treated with subchondral abrasion healed with regeneration of a "hyaline-like" cartilage, and continuous passive motion appeared to enhance this healing. This study included only a single-sized lesion with follow up of 12 weeks maximum so the durability of the healing tissue is impossible to assess. This study, along with previous studies by Salter, suggest that continuous passive motion may enhance healing in the presence of full-thickness defects of articular cartilage.

Lasers in the Treatment of Chondral Lesions

Use of laser technology in arthroscopic surgery has increased in recent years. Several types of laser systems are available, each with advantages and disadvantages. A detailed discussion of laser physiology is beyond the scope of this chapter. However, a few comments regarding laser technology and its usefulness in arthroscopic procedures on the knee should be made.

There is considerable pressure to adopt new technology such as the laser. This pressure is exerted from outside the medical community by sales-motivated manufacturers. There is also pressure from within the medical community to be up-to-date and competitive with other orthopedists. Prior to embracing this new technology, more basic research must be performed to investigate the long-term effects on bone, articular cartilage, and meniscal cartilage, and to determine whether results are improved when using this technique versus standard mechanical instrumentation.

The carbon dioxide (CO_2) laser was the first approved for arthroscopic applications but suffers because it requires a gas medium. It also requires an articulated arm for delivery, and poses potential complications in the free-beam mode of use. Lasers that function in a fluid medium include the Ho:YAG, neodymium:YAG (Nd:YAG), KTP, and Excimer lasers. The arthroscopic Nd:YAG laser uses a special tip that is heated by the laser energy. It is used in a contact mode rather than free-beam mode in a fashion similar to electrocautery. In this configuration, it has no ability to ablate tissue and has little effect on articular cartilage. Limited use of this laser in our practice suggested that it offered little if any advantage over standard instrumentation.

The Ho:YAG laser operates at a wavelength of 2.1 μm, a position between the Nd:YAG laser and the CO_2 laser. The laser energy is delivered via a fiberoptic cable enclosed in a small diameter metal handpiece that is considerably less fragile than other devices. It is used in a near-contact or contact mode, and the amount of energy transmitted to the tissue is adjusted by defocusing the beam by varying the distance from the tissue. Another advantage is its ability to photocoagulate vessels during the cutting or ablation procedure.

TABLE 3.2
Classification of Cartilaginous Lesions

Grade	Description
Grade I	Softening of the hyaline articular cartilage with no disruption of the surface layers
Grade II	Linear fissures into the cartilaginous surface of varying depths and number
Grade III	Fissures associated with multiple thin fasciculations on the surface of the cartilage
Grade IV	A fibrillated cartilaginous lesion varying from 20% to 50% in depth of surface cartilage irrespective of area size
Grade V	A more advanced fibrillation involving depths of 50% to 90% from the surface area
Grade VI	A defect down to subchondral bone of an area measuring 1 cm or less after trimming the adjacent chondral flaps to a stable cartilage-bone interface, but involving only one articular surface
Grade VII	A full-thickness defect greater than 1 cm in area after debridement still involving only one articular surface
Grade VIII	An eburnated bony lesion on adjacent cartilaginous surfaces of varying sizes.

Adapted with permission from Tippet JW, 1991

Early unpublished reports by Dillingham have suggested that this laser is well suited to debridement of articular cartilage lesions.[10] It offers advantages over standard instrumentation such as shavers. The beam is quite precise, and there is excellent proprioceptive feedback so debridement is performed without injury to adjacent areas of uninvolved bone and cartilage. This laser has a short absorption length so there is minimal thermal effect in the adjacent tissues. The frayed cartilage appears to "melt" under the effect of the laser, and the margins of the lesion can be made perfectly smooth. Our own experience supports the findings of Dillingham. However, there are no long-term follow-up studies in humans, nor are there animal studies to document definite advantages over standard instrumentation.

Degenerative Joint Disease

The role of arthroscopy in the treatment of degenerative joint disease is controversial. Conservative treatment consists of activity modification, nonsteroidal antiinflammatory medications, weight loss, weight relief with a cane, shoe cushioning, and judicious use of corticosteroid injections. Although corticosteroid injections may give significant symptomatic improvement, the effect is transient, and the potential adverse effects on the metabolism of remaining articular cartilage make it less appealing.

Open Debridement

Surgical alternatives include open debridement as advocated by Magnuson, tibial or femoral osteotomy, hemiarthroplasty, and total joint arthroplasty.[11] The advent of arthroscopy has provided an additional opportunity for a minimally invasive procedure to perform lavage, debridement of torn menisci and impinging osteophytes, synovectomy, and drilling or abrasion. Jackson's approach to degenerative arthritis includes debridement of loose fragments of articular cartilage and trimming of degenerative meniscus tears.[12] Osteophytes that cause impingement on soft tissues are trimmed. Joint lavage allows removal of loose articular fragments in addition to removal of irritating substances such as degenerative enzymes and substance. Jackson affirms that the procedure is a temporizing one and that patients accept this concept to try to delay more invasive procedures. His study of patients undergoing debridement for degenerative arthritis suggested that 80% to 85% achieved significant symptomatic improvement. The presence of bone-on-bone articulation made success less likely.

Abrasion Arthroplasty

Johnson has asserted that abrasion arthroplasty can stimulate repair of articular cartilage in patients with a "sclerotic lesion."[13] The lesion represents complete loss of articular cartilage over the subchondral bone. Johnson found that intracortical blood vessels could be exposed with simple abrasion of the superficial 1 to 2 mm of subchondral bone.[14] A second arthroscopic examination revealed coalescing reparative tissue when the abrasion was carried out over the entire condyle. Postoperative management included 8 weeks of non-weight-bearing ambulation.

Details of the abrasion procedure, as described by Johnson, include associated synovectomy, loose body removal, meniscus debridement, chondroplasty, and the abrasion procedure itself. Areas of intact articular cartilage, although significantly thinned, are not debrided down to bone. Only the "sclerotic lesion" is abraded. A motorized burr is used to abrade only the superficial 1 to 2 mm of subchondral bone. Debridement is not carried down to the level of cancellous bone.

Johnson suggests that postoperatively the initial fibrocartilaginous covering may eventually develop increased levels of type II collagen, characteristic of hyaline cartilage.

Tippett suggests placement of multiple drill holes 3 to 4 mm deep in the femoral condyle using a 2 mm burr.[15] The tibial surface is decorticated to the level of cancellous bone. A tibial osteotomy is then performed to correct (over-correct by 3°) varus malalignment. Johnson also advocates osteotomy in unicompartmental degenerative arthritis with significant varus angulation.[13]

Some investigators have suggested that optimization of joint loading by osteotomy alone can result in regeneration of cartilage over a period of years.[16,17] Coventry points out that in order for articular cartilage regeneration to occur, angular overcorrection must be performed to decrease stress on the involved condyle and transfer stress to the uninvolved side.

Tibial Plateau Fractures

Intraarticular fractures of the proximal tibia have been classified by Hohl according to the degree of depression, association of split fragments, and bicondylar involvement (Fig. 3.11).[18] The goals of operative treatment of these fractures include reduction of displaced fragments, stabilization of the fracture to allow early motion, and treatment of associated ligament or meniscal injury. Although nondisplaced or minimally displaced fractures can be managed without surgery, it is generally agreed that fractures demonstrating significant compression or displacement should undergo open reduction and internal fixation to restore anatomic position of the fragments.

Open treatment of these fractures is associated with significant operative morbidity and potential postoperative complications. To gain exposure of the fracture site, significant stripping of soft tissues from the proximal tibia is necessary. The meniscus must be elevated from the plateau and carefully reattached at the conclusion of the procedure.[19] Postoperative complications such as deep vein thrombosis, pulmonary embolus, restricted knee motion, failure of fixation with displacement or collapse of fracture fragments, and infection can occur. Several investigators have suggested that arthroscopic evaluation or arthroscopy-assisted internal fixation may be appropriate for some fractures and can achieve an equal quality of reduction and fixation with less operative morbidity.[20,21]

Initial evaluation of the patient with a tibial plateau fracture includes clinical assessment of the knee for alignment and evidence of concomitant injury to ligament supports or other intraarticular injury. The assessment of

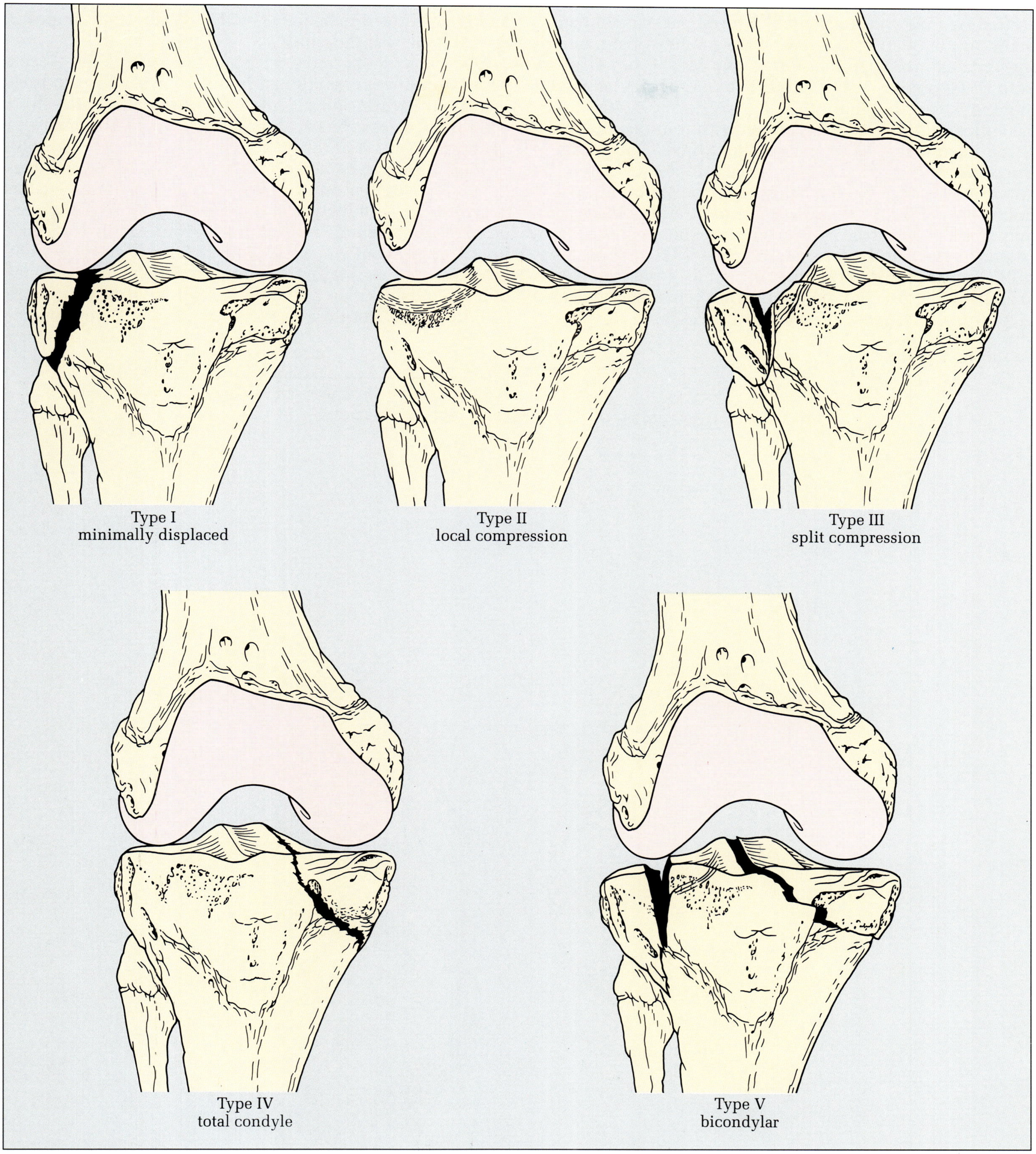

Figure 3.11

Classification of tibial plateau fractures according to Hohl.

coexisting injury in the acutely injured patient can be difficult and is often hampered by the patient's pain, guarding, hemarthrosis, and interference by the bone injury with the ligament examination. The neurovascular assessment must be complete.

Radiographic evaluation begins with routine anteroposterior, lateral, and tangential patellar x-rays. Angulation of the x-ray tube approximately 10° posteriorly for the anteroposterior view may provide a better detail of the fracture.[22] The degree of displacement and compression may not be clear from routine studies such as the anteroposterior view, and lateral tomograms or CT may be helpful.[23] Computed tomograms are usually obtained with axial cuts that parallel the joint surface, making the degree of plateau compression difficult to assess. New techniques of three-dimensional reconstruction may improve the usefulness of this study.

Once the preoperative radiographic studies have been performed, the surgeon must first decide whether to treat the fracture nonoperatively or operatively, and then whether arthroscopic evaluation may have a role in the treatment plan. Arthroscopy can be useful in the assessment of the concomitant soft tissue injury, including ligament and meniscal injury. Certain fractures are amenable to arthroscopic reduction and internal fixation, particularly split fractures or split-compression fractures. Significant comminution with loss of lateral support that requires buttress plating to obtain sufficient fracture stability mandates open reduction and internal fixation. One should not substitute a less adequate arthroscopic proce-

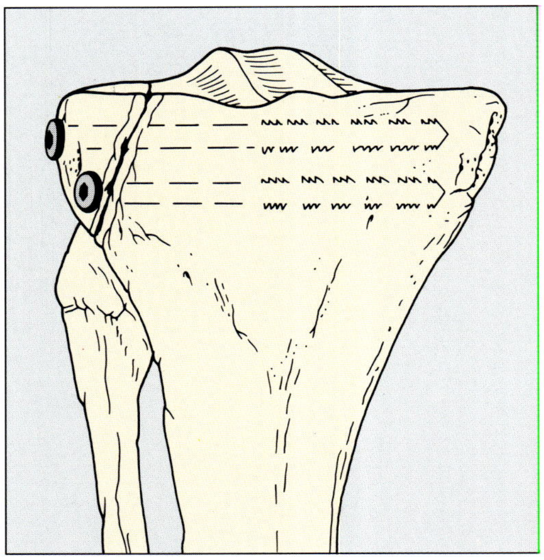

Figure 3.12
Fixation of type I fracture with two transverse cancellous screws

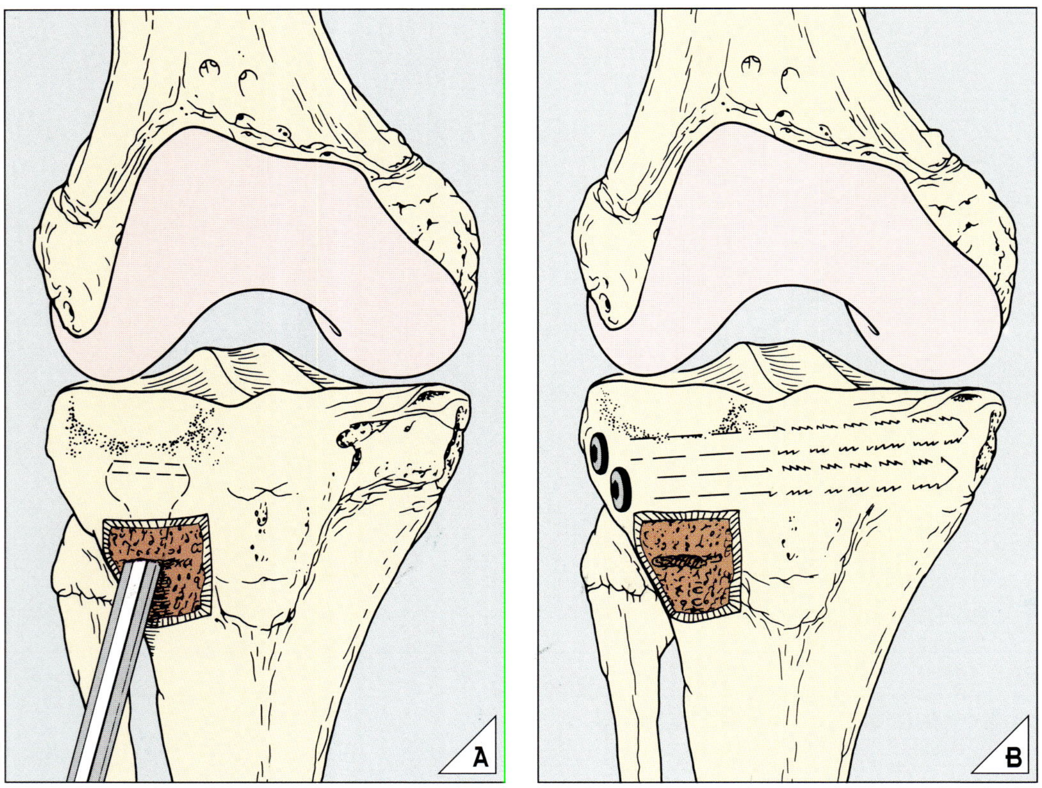

Figure 3.13
(A) Fixation of a type II fracture after the depressed tibial plateau is elevated and the bone is grafted. (B) The fracture is fixed with cancellous screws.

dure for an open procedure that provides greater accuracy of reduction and stability.

Surgical Technique

The patient is positioned supine on the operating table with a tourniquet applied to the thigh. A radiolucent board is used for the image intensifier. We prefer to use a lateral thigh post rather than a constricting leg holder, as the post allows optimal intraoperative mobility of the extremity for manipulation and positioning of internal fixation devices. After induction of general or spinal anesthesia, a careful physical examination of the knee is performed to evaluate associated ligament injury.

We recommend the arthroscopic fluid pump for high-flow, low-pressure irrigation and clearing of the hemarthrosis. A complete examination of the knee includes special attention to the medial and lateral menisci along with the cruciate ligaments. The fracture compartment is usually easily visualized owing to depression of the plateau and concomitant enlargement of the compartment. The fracture itself is assessed with an arthroscopic probe. The image intensifier can assist in estimating the degree of articular cartilage depression and the need for elevation. The fracture site must be cleansed of clot and debris using the probe or a small curette.

Hohl type I (minimally displaced) fractures can be reduced and fixed with cancellous bone screws after the fracture site has been debrided (Fig. 3.12). Cannulated screws offer the easiest way to stabilize a fracture with intraoperative radiographic confirmation of anatomic alignment. The guide pins are placed across the fracture site and accurate position is confirmed by fluoroscopy. Self-drilling, self-tapping screws are available and provide the most direct means of internal fixation. In bone of poor quality, the opposite cortex may be engaged by the screw, and a washer can be used if the cortex will not support the screwhead.

Hohl type II (local compression) fractures must be elevated to restore anatomic alignment of the articular surface. The elevated segment usually requires support by a bone graft. This maneuver can be accomplished by making a small cortical window in the tibial metaphysis and inserting an osteotome or small bone tamp to elevate the depressed fragments. The procedure is monitored by direct arthroscopic visualization of the articular surface, and the adequacy of the reduction is confirmed radiographically. Bone graft is obtained from the iliac crest and is inserted to support the tibial plateau and fill the defect. In some situations in which the cortical support is intact with central depression of the plateau, internal fixation may not be required. However, increased support for the plateau in the face of depression can be achieved with Steinmann pins or screws placed just beneath the subchondral plate (Fig. 3.13).

Hohl type III (split compression) fractures are more challenging but can be fixed in a similar fashion. After debridement of clot and debris from the fracture site, the depressed fragments are elevated, and then provisional reduction is obtained with compression of the plateau and placement of guide pins. The meniscus may be caught in the fracture and must be removed before reduction can be achieved. Once anatomic alignment has been obtained, the depressed fragment is supported with a bone graft, and fixation is achieved with interfragmentary screws as described above. If the meniscus is torn peripherally, then an arthroscopic repair should be performed after fixation of the fracture (Figs. 3.14, 3.15).

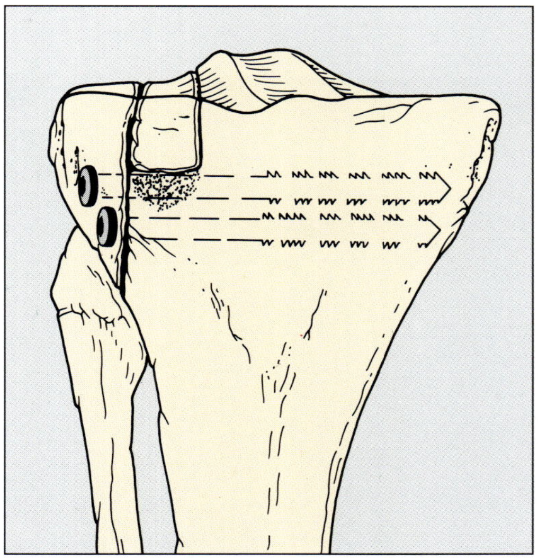

Figure 3.14
A split compression type III fracture is elevated, the bone is grafted, and it is fixed with cancellous screws.

Although Hohl type IV (total condylar depression) fractures can involve either plateau, they frequently involve the medial side, with the fracture line entering the joint near the intercondylar eminence. If arthroscopic interfragmentary compression screw fixation is used, the construct must have adequate strength to resist shear forces that could cause postoperative displacement (Fig. 3.16). If this cannot be achieved arthroscopically, open reduction and buttress-plate fixation should be performed (Fig. 3.17).

Hohl type V (bicondylar) fractures are usually best treated by open reduction and internal fixation (Fig. 3.18). Arthroscopic assessment may be useful for evaluation of associated injury.

When adequate internal fixation is achieved, then early range-of-motion exercises can be begun postoperatively. However, we recommend limitation of weight bearing for 12 weeks after fixation of a fracture that exhibits a significant degree of compression. If fixation is felt to be too tenuous to tolerate postoperative motion, then immobilization for 4 to 6 weeks is used until early healing has taken place and simple range-of-motion exercise is safe. Once again, an open procedure should be performed if it will result in improved fixation with the ability to institute early postoperative motion.

Ischemic Necrosis of the Femoral Condyle

Idiopathic osteonecrosis of the femoral condyle was first described by Alback et al.,[24] who delineated the classic radiographic lesion and its characteristic increased uptake on bone scan. The lesion is more common in the medial femoral condyle but can also occur in the lateral femoral condyle. It is most common in women over age 60 years and is not associated with trauma or other preexisting disease. Pain is usually well localized to the side of the lesion and is characteristically worse at night. Tenderness is present over the involved condyle and may be accom-

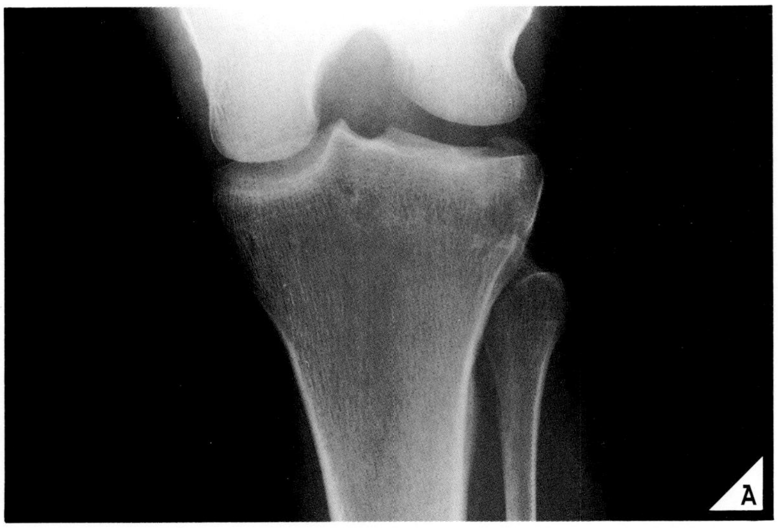

Figure 3.15
Anteroposterior (A) and lateral (B) radiographs of a 43-year-old woman who sustained a split-compression fracture of the lateral tibial plateau when she fell while cross country skiing. Tomograms confirmed a significant degree of compression of the articular fragment with minimal displacement of the split fragment. Anteroposterior (C) and lateral (D) postoperative radiographs after elevation of the depressed fragment, iliac crest bone grafting, and internal fixation with a single cancellous screw. Joint motion was instituted immediately postoperatively and she was kept non-weight-bearing for 12 weeks.

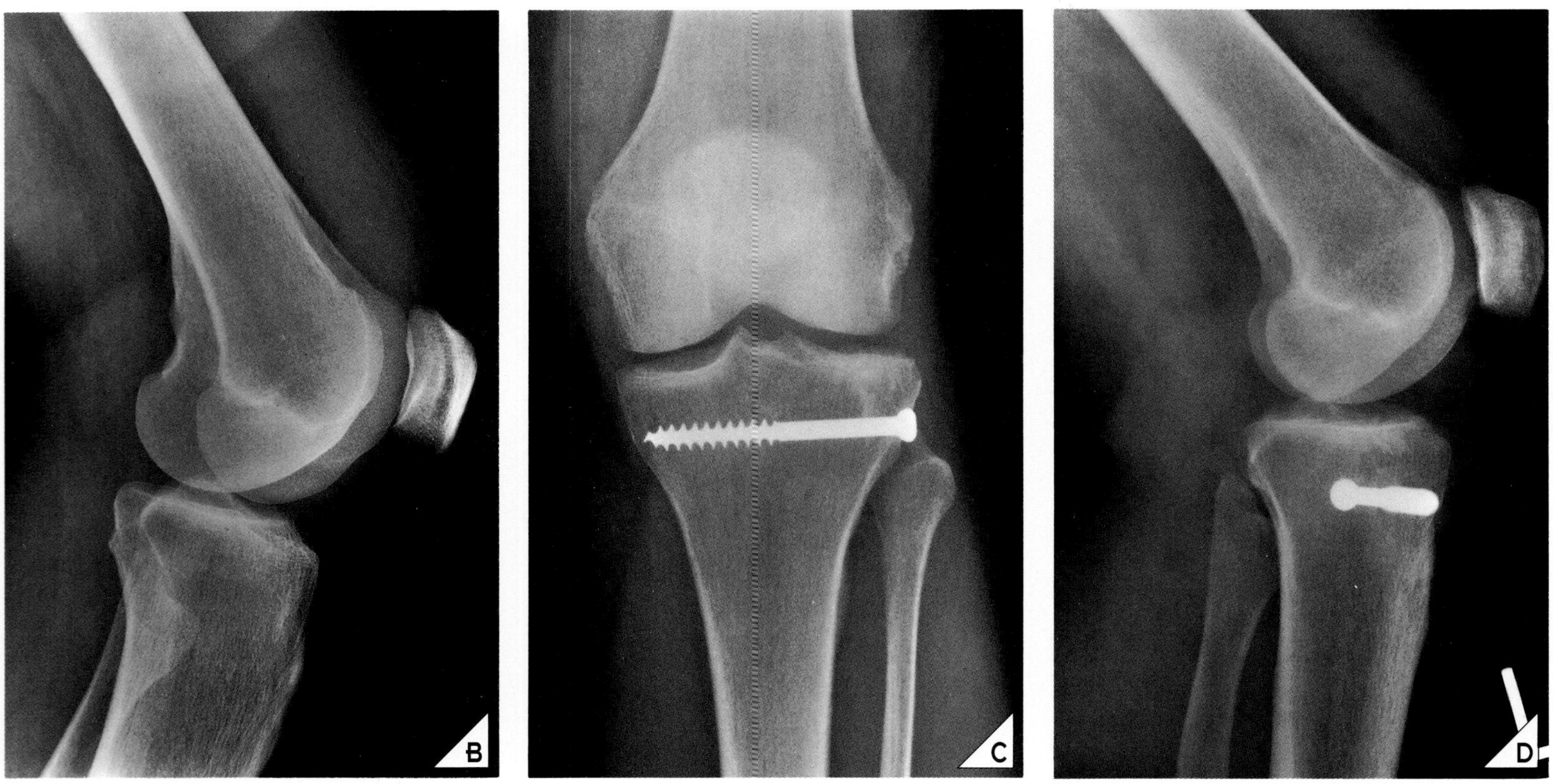

panied by effusion and evidence of synovitis and joint inflammation.

Other causes of osteonecrosis of the femoral condyle that are not idiopathic include corticosteroid administration, alcohol abuse, caisson disease, sickle cell anemia, Gaucher's disease, renal transplantation, and trauma.[25]

Radiographs may be normal in the case of a small lesion in the early stages of the disease process (stage I). In stage II disease there is flattening of the normal contour of the femoral condyle (Fig. 3.19A). Radiographic stage III disease shows the characteristic area of radiolucency over the involved condyle on both the anteroposterior and lateral views with bone sclerosis at the base of the lesion (Fig. 3.19B). In stage IV osteonecrosis there is increased sclerosis around the lesion (Fig. 3.20), and stage V disease exhibits joint space narrowing with osteophyte production and further collapse.[25]

The bone scan is the most sensitive and least expensive examination for consistent demonstration of the lesion with increased uptake in the involved condyle. The MRI study will also show abnormal areas on both T1- and T2-weighted images.[25]

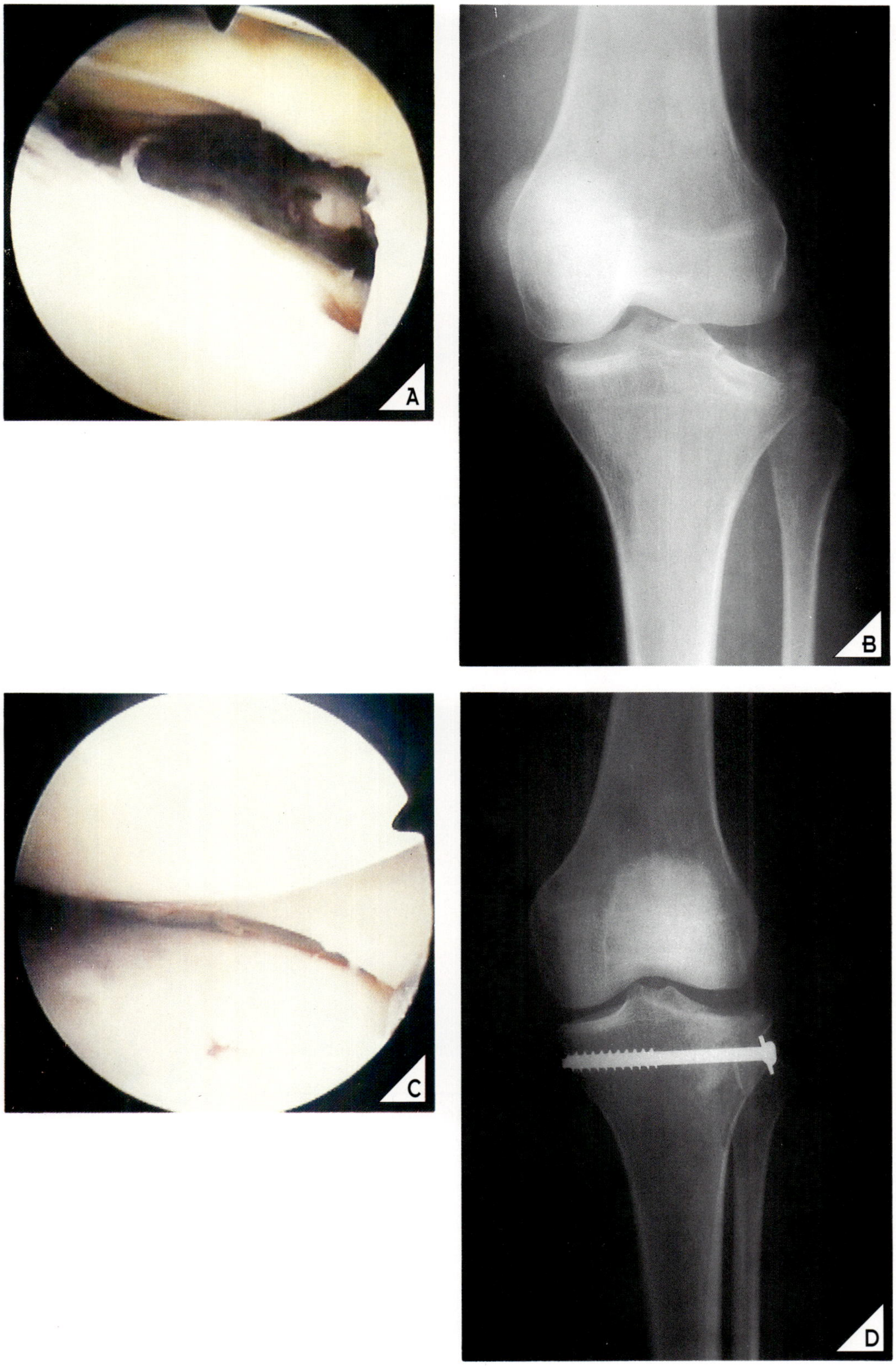

Figure 3.16

Arthroscopic visualization (A) and radiograph (B) of a depressed lateral tibial plateau fracture left knee. Arthroscopic visualization (C) and radiograph (D) after reduction and fixation. (Courtesy of Donald Rose, MD)

The prognosis for patients with idiopathic osteonecrosis depends on the degree of femoral condyle involvement. Lesions that occupy more than 40% to 50% of the width of the involved condyle, or that occupy an area of more than 3.5 to 5.0 cm^2, have a poor prognosis and a high likelihood of progressive joint destruction.[26–29]

Treatment of osteonecrosis of the femoral condyle is controversial, and the role of arthroscopic intervention is not well defined by controlled clinical studies. In general, patients with small lesions in the early stage of the disease should be treated conservatively with activity limitation, restricted weight bearing, and antiinflammatory medications. It may be difficult to determine the actual size of the lesion for several months after the disorder is initially diagnosed. Small lesions, as defined above, often do not require further intervention and symptoms will subside. Large lesions usually require treatment as pain will persist and progressive degenerative changes will occur.

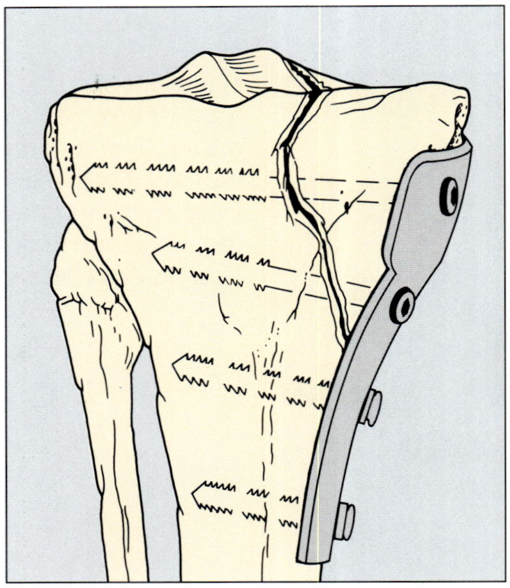

Figure 3.17
A total condyle type IV fracture is fixed with a medial buttress plate and cancellous screws after open reduction.

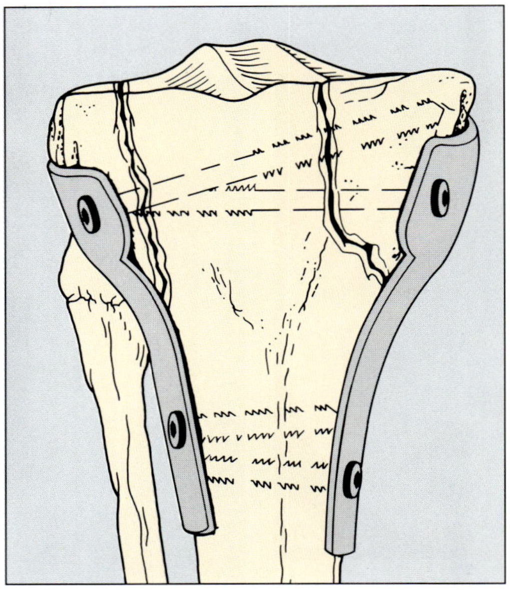

Figure 3.18
A type V fracture is protected on both sides with buttress plates after open reduction.

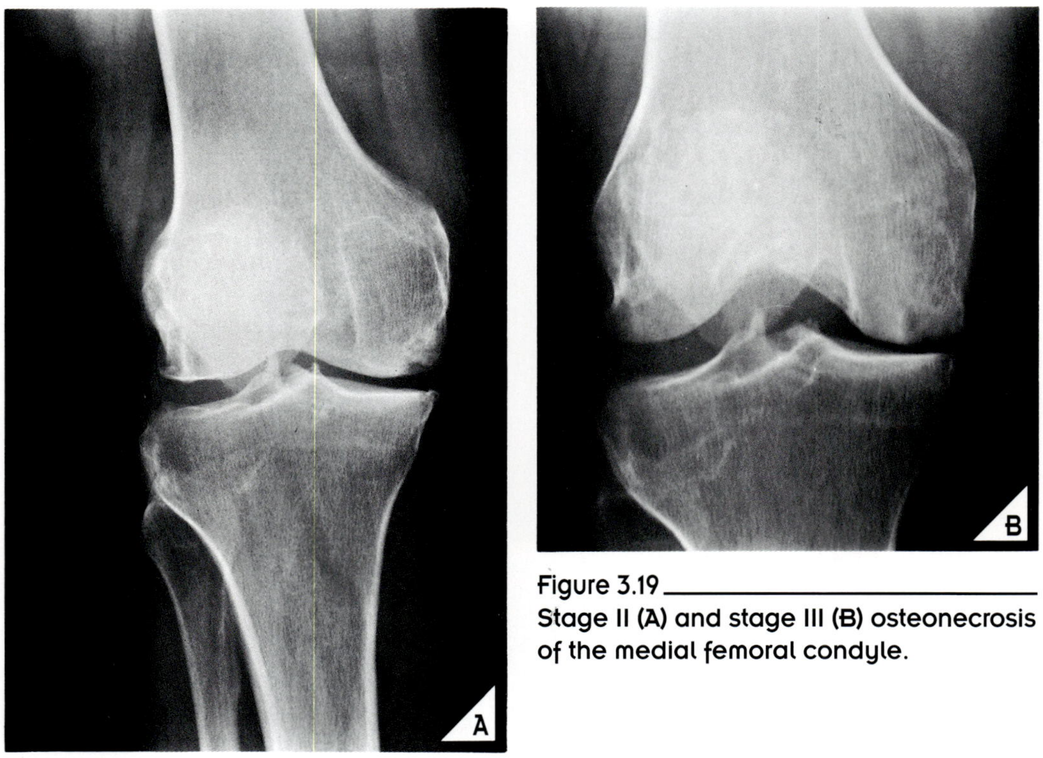

Figure 3.19
Stage II (A) and stage III (B) osteonecrosis of the medial femoral condyle.

Koshino et al. performed arthroscopic examinations on eight knees with spontaneous femoral osteonecrosis and correlated their arthroscopic findings with findings at arthrotomy, which was performed in seven of the knees.[29] They suggested that arthroscopy be performed to evaluate the condition of the articular surface before committing the patient to other procedures such as open drilling, bone grafting, or osteotomy.

With the development of more sophisticated arthroscopic surgical techniques, other authors have performed debridement procedures for spontaneous femoral osteonecrosis. Miller et al. reported the cases of five patients with the condition who underwent arthroscopic examination with debridement and abrasion of the base of the lesion.[28] Debridement involved removal of all loose pieces of articular cartilage and abrasion of the base until bleeding bone was noted under direct visualization. The patients remained non-weight-bearing for 6 weeks and then advanced to full weight bearing by 8 weeks postoperatively. At an average of 31 months postoperatively, pain was decreased or eliminated in four of the five patients. Longer-term results could not be estimated from this study.

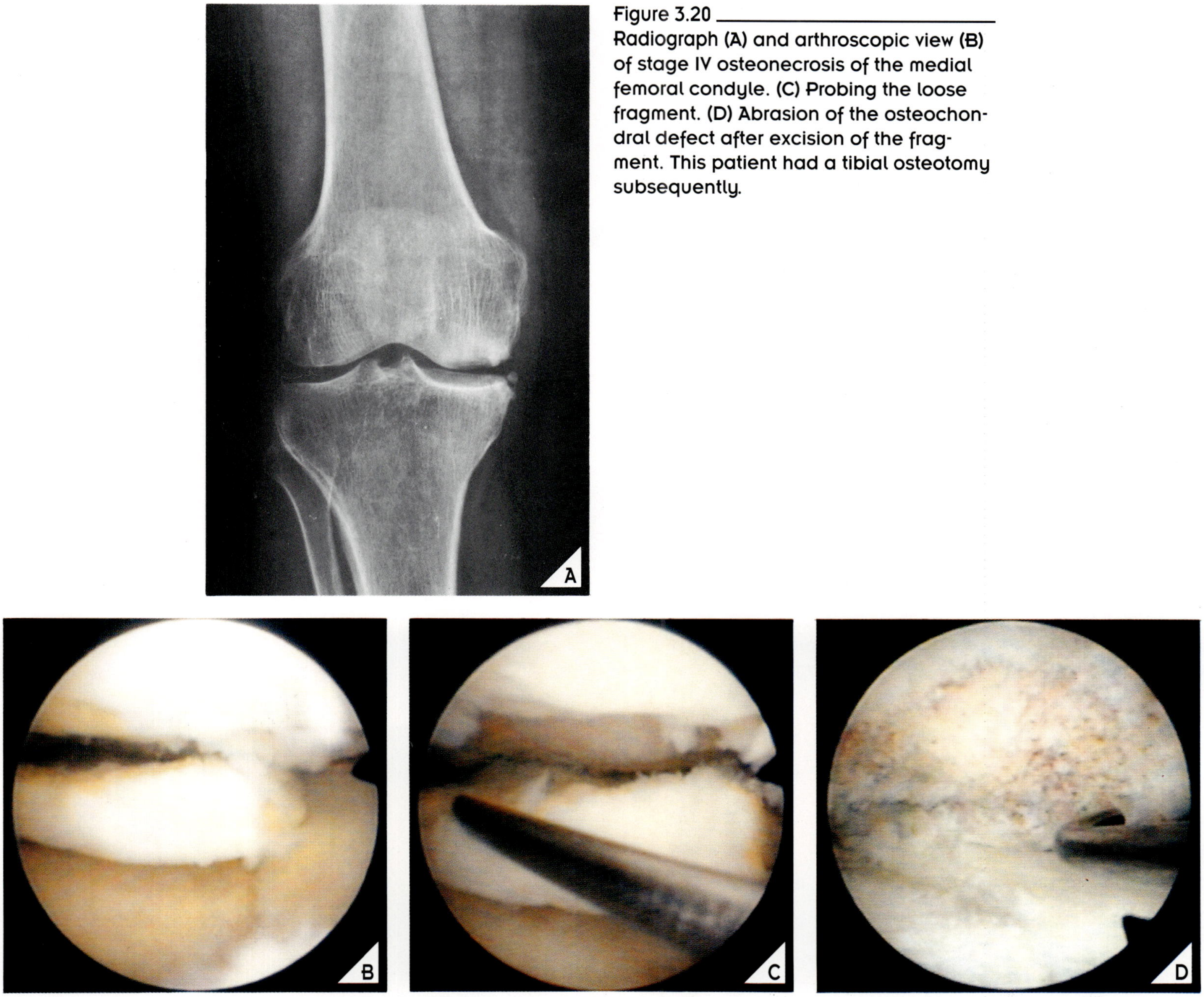

Figure 3.20
Radiograph (A) and arthroscopic view (B) of stage IV osteonecrosis of the medial femoral condyle. (C) Probing the loose fragment. (D) Abrasion of the osteochondral defect after excision of the fragment. This patient had a tibial osteotomy subsequently.

Wiedel reported the results of arthroscopic treatment of corticosteroid-induced osteonecrosis of the femoral condyle in ten knees that failed to respond to conservative treatment measures.[30] Treatment included debridement of loose flaps of articular cartilage, removal of loose bodies (Fig. 3.21), and excision of torn meniscal fragments with abrasion of full-thickness surface defects. Patients were allowed to bear weight as tolerated postoperatively. The procedure appeared to provide good relief of symptoms related to internal derangement at an average 14-month follow up. The results of treatment of steroid-induced osteonecrosis should not be extrapolated to idiopathic osteonecrosis, since different pathophysiologic mechanisms may be contributing to the development and progression of the disorder and its response to treatment.

We agree that patients with idiopathic osteonecrosis of the femoral condyle should be treated initially with conservative measures as outlined above. A bone scan or MRI examination should be obtained to confirm the diagnosis and appropriate medical work-up pursued to rule out other causes of osteonecrosis. Serial radiographs should be obtained to follow the course of the lesion and determine its ultimate size, which most accurately predicts the natural history of the disorder.

Surgical Technique

Patients with persistent symptoms despite conservative treatment, who present with small lesions and physical signs of internal derangement, are the best candidates for arthroscopic intervention. A routine arthroscopic knee set up with either a leg holder or a post for application of intraoperative valgus stress, along with an arthroscopic fluid pump, is recommended. Complete evaluation of the knee joint, starting in the suprapatellar pouch, should be performed with specific evaluation of the articular surface of the patella, femoral groove, medial gutter, medial joint, intercondylar notch, lateral joint, lateral gutter, and posterior joint. The area of femoral condyle involvement should be carefully probed, and areas of loose, flaking

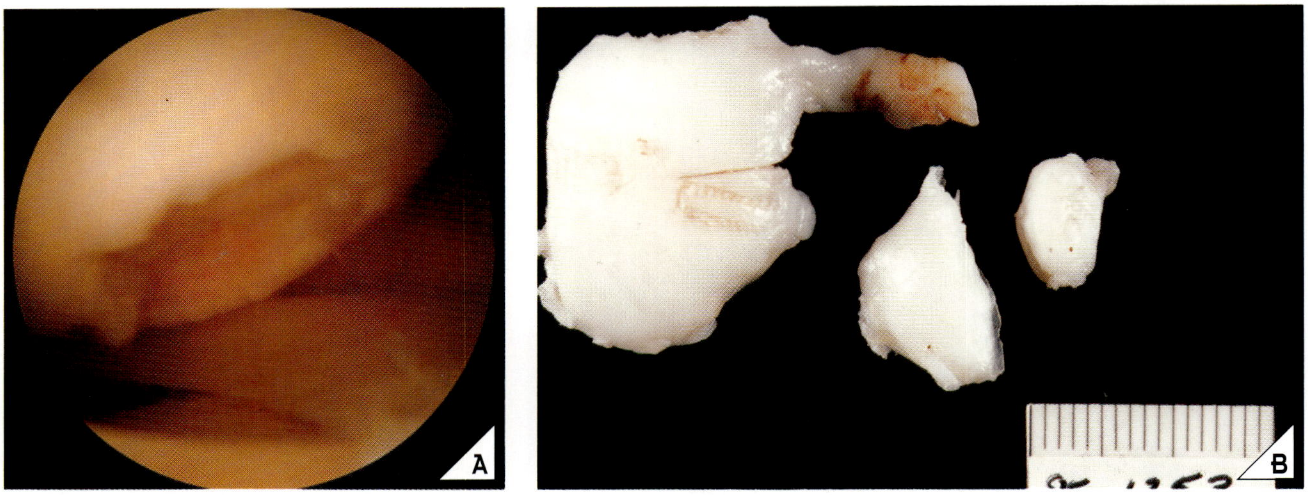

Figure 3.21
(A) Osteonecrosis of the medial femoral condyle right knee. (B) Loose fragments were found in the joint.

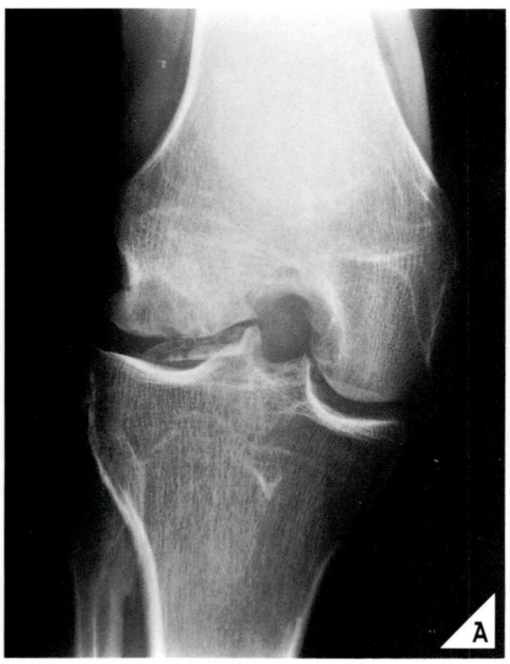

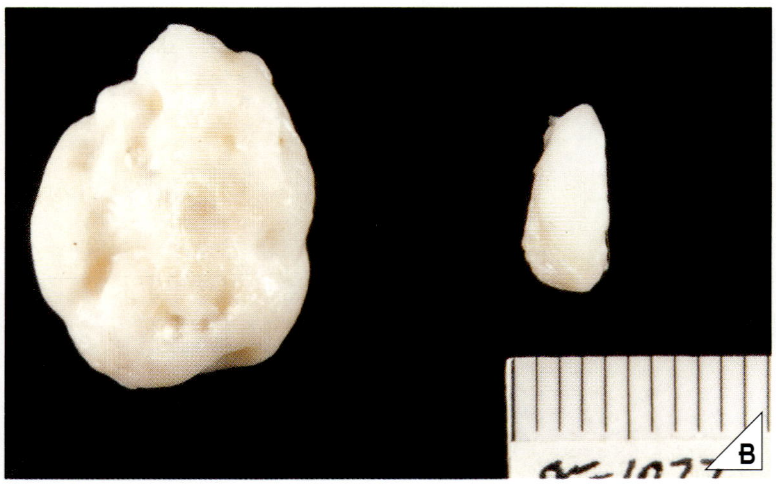

Figure 3.22
(A) Radiograph of an old lesion of osteonecrosis of the lateral femoral condyle. The patient became asymptomatic after removal of loose fragments. (B) Loose fragments that were removed arthroscopically.

articular cartilage should be debrided to stable edges. This procedure can be performed with basket forceps, curettes, motorized shavers, or with the laser. The Ho:YAG laser allows precise debridement of articular cartilage and contouring of the margins. The base of the lesion should also be carefully probed to remove any loose pieces of subchondral bone. This bone should be gently abraded until punctate bleeding can be seen arthroscopically when the fluid pressure is decreased. Finally, meniscal tears should be debrided to a stable rim, and loose bodies should be removed. Postoperatively, we recommend non-weight-bearing ambulation with crutches or a walker for 6 weeks, with gradual resumption of full weight-bearing status afterward.

Patients with large lesions who demonstrate more advanced radiographic changes with joint collapse and osteophyte formation should be considered for tibial osteotomy (possibly in conjunction with arthroscopic debridement), unicompartmental joint arthroplasty, or total joint arthroplasty (Figs. 3.22, 3.23).

COMPLICATIONS

As with open surgical procedures, complications of arthroscopic surgery on the knee can be related directly to the procedure itself or indirectly to an associated aspect of the procedure, such as anesthetic complications. We will discuss complications directly related to the procedure.

In attempting to remove loose bodies, some may prove difficult to locate. The surgeon must perform the examination in an organized fashion. Small loose bodies may be hidden beneath the medial or lateral meniscus or posterolaterally in the popliteus hiatus. Posterior examination via a posteromedial or posterolateral portal may be required if a loose body resides deep in the posterior joint. Even after a single loose body is found, further examination must be performed to insure that additional ones are not present. An adequate portal to accommodate a large loose body should be made to prevent loss of the loose body in the soft tissues and the need for an even larger incision.

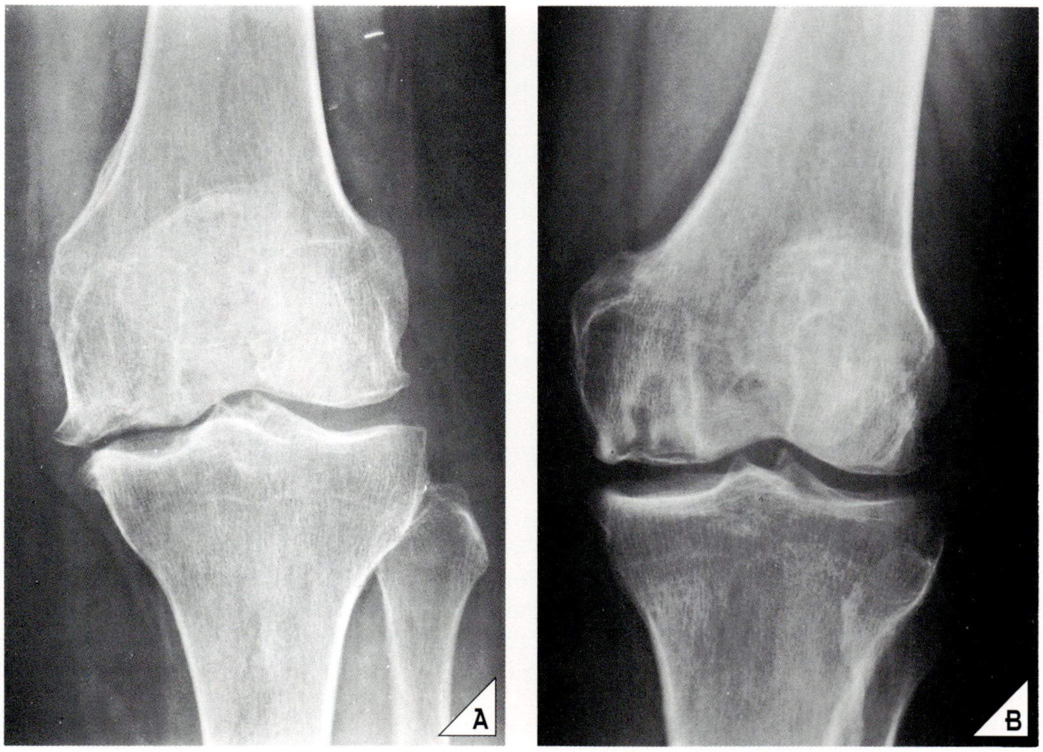

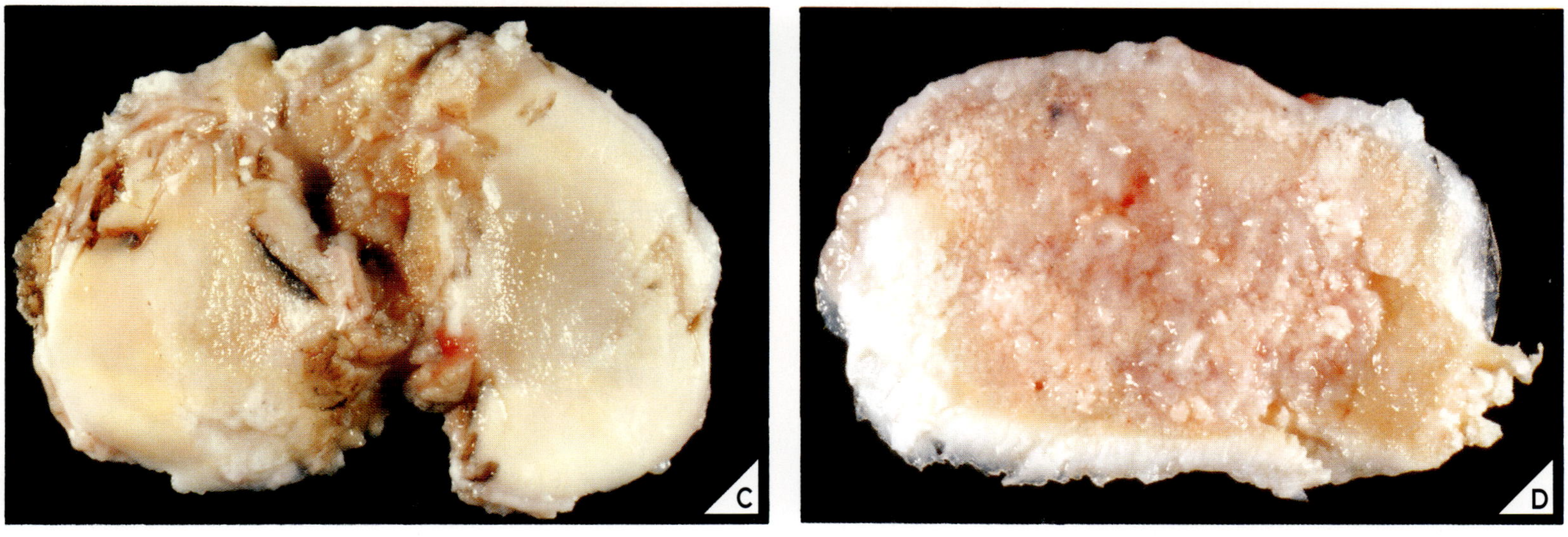

Figure 3.23
(A, B) Two examples of stage V osteonecrosis of the medial femoral condyle. Both patients had a joint replacement for complete relief of their pain. (C) Pathology specimen of the osteonecrotic femoral condyle showing the articular surface. (D) Pathology specimen showing area of subchondral bone necrosis.

Osteochondritis dissecans lesions may be difficult to localize, and the incorrect areas can be drilled, bone grafted, or internally fixed. If there is any question, intraoperative radiographs and confirmation of correct placement of internal fixation devices should always be obtained. If small Kirschner wires are used for fixation, care must be taken not to bend a wire, making removal difficult and risking breakage. In skeletally immature patients, insertion of fixation should not cross the physis as injury could cause growth abnormality.

If screws are used for fixation, the heads must be countersunk. Prior to starting motion of the joint, radiographs should be obtained to confirm that the screws have not backed out, risking damage to adjacent articular surfaces. Upon removal, screws, washers, or small Kirschner wires that become loose in the joint may be difficult to locate and extract. If bone pegs or cancellous graft is harvested from the tibia or femur, the extremity should be protected to avoid fracture through a stress riser.

Replacement of detached osteochondritis dissecans fragments or acute osteochondral fractures may be unsuccessful with loss of fixation, nonunion, and formation of loose bodies. If this occurs, the fragment and the internal fixation device must be removed.

The major complication of treatment of chondral injuries and degenerative joint disease is failure to obtain symptomatic improvement. When patients with degenerative joint disease are counseled preoperatively they must be made aware that the procedure may give only partial, temporary relief of symptoms, and other operative procedures, such as joint replacement or osteotomy, may be necessary.

REFERENCES

1. Dainer RD, Barrack RL, Buckley SL, Alexander AH. Arthroscopic treatment of acute patellar dislocations. *Arthroscopy* 1988;4:267–271.
2. Guhl JF. Arthroscopic treatment of osteochondritis dissecans of the knee. *Clin Orthop.* 1982;67:66–74.
3. Berndt AL, Harty M. Transchondral fracture of the talus. *J Bone Joint Surg.* 1959;41:988–1022.
4. Guhl JF, Johnson RP, Stone JW. The impact of arthroscopy on osteochondritis dissecans. In: McGinty J. *Operative Arthroscopy.* New York, NY: Raven Press; 1991:297–317.
5. Thomson NL: Osteochondritis dissecans and osteochondral fragments managed by Herbert compression screw fixation. *Clin Orthop.* 1987;224:71–78.
6. Johnson-Nurse C, Dandy DJ. Fracture–separation of articular cartilage in the adult knee. *J Bone Joint Surg.* 1985;67B:42–43.
7. Noyes FR, Stabler CL. A system for grading articular cartilage lesions at arthroscopy. *Am J Sports Med.* 1989;17:505–573.
8. Tippett JW. In: McGinty, ed. *J Operative Arthroscopy.* New York, NY: Raven Press; 1991:325–338.
9. Kim HKW, Moran ME, Salter RB. The potential for regeneration of articular cartilage in defects created by chondral shaving and subchondral abrasion. *J Bone Joint Surg.* 1991;73A:1301–1314.
10. Dillingham M. Personal communication, 1991.
11. Magnusen RB. Joint debridement: surgical treatment of degenerative arthritis. *Surg Gynecol Obstet.* 1941;73:1–9.
12. Jackson RW. Arthroscopic treatment of degenerative arthritis. In: McGinty J, ed. *Operative Arthroscopy.* New York, NY: Raven Press; 1991:319–323.
13. Johnson LL. Arthroscopic abrasion arthroplasty. In: McGinty J, ed. *Operative Arthroscopy.* New York, NY Raven Press; 1991:341–359.
14. Johnson LL. Arthroscopic abrasion arthroplasty historical and pathologic perspective: present status. *Arthroscopy.* 1986;2:54–69.
15. Tippett JW. Articuliar cartilage drilling and osteotomy in arthritis of the knee. In: McGinty J, ed. *Operative Arthroscopy.* New York, NY: Raven Press;1991:325–338.
16. Coventry MB. In: Ewing JW, ed. *Articular Cartilage and Knee Joint Function, Basic Science and Arthroscopy.* New York, NY: Raven Press; 1990:311–317.
17. Fujisawa Y, Masuhara K, Shiomi S: The effect of high tibial osteotomy on osteoarthritis of the knee: an arthroscopic study of 54 knee joints. *Orthop Clin North Am.* 1979; 10:585–608.
18. Hohl M. Tibial condylar fractures. *J Bone Joint Surg.* 1967; 49A:1456–1467.
19. Perry CR, Evans LG, Rice S, Fogarty J, Burdge RE. A new surgical approach to fractures of the lateral tibial plateau. *J Bone Joint Surg.* 1984;66A:1236–1240.
20. Jennings, JE. Arthroscopic management of tibial plateau fractures. *Arthroscopy.* 1985;1:160–168.
21. Caspari RB, Hutton PMJ, Whipple TL, Meyers JF. The role of arthroscopy in the management of tibial plateau fractures. *Arthroscopy.* 1985;1:76–82.
22. Moore TM, Harvey JP Jr. Roentgenographic measurement of the tibial plateau depression due to fracture. *J Bone Joint Surg.* 1974;56A:155–160.
23. Elstrom J, Pankovich AM, Sasoon H, Rodriguez J. The use of tomography in the assessment of fractures of the tibial plateau. *J Bone Joint Surg.* 1976;58A:551–555.
24. Alback S, Bauer GCH, Bohne WH. Spontaneous osteonecrosis of the knee. *Arthritis Rheum.* 1968;11:705–733.
25. Lotke PA, Ecker ML. Osteonecrosis of the knee: current concepts review. *J Bone Joint Surg.* 1988;70A:470–473.
26. Muheim G, Bohne WH. Prognosis in spontaneous osteonecrosis of the knee: investigation by radionuclide scintimetry and radiography. *J Bone Joint Surg.* 1970; 52B:605–612.
27. Lotke PA, Abend JA, Ecker ML. The treatment of osteonecrosis of the medial femoral condyle. *Clin Orthop.* 1982;172:109–116.
28. Miller GK, Maylahn DJ, Drennan DB. The treatment of idiopathic osteonecrosis of the medial femoral condyle with arthroscopic debridement. *Arthroscopy.* 1986;2:21–29.
29. Koshino T, Okamoto R, Takamura K, Tsuchiya K. Arthroscopy in spontaneous osteonecrosis of the knee. *Orthop Clin North Am.* 1979;10:609–618.
30. Wiedel JD. Arthroscopy in steroid-induced osteonecrosis of the knee. *Arthroscopy.* 1985;1:68–72.

Chapter Four

Arthroscopic Procedures on Synovium and Joint Capsule

J. Serge Parisien

Pathologic Conditions Associated with Plicae of the Knee Joint

With an incidence varying from 20% to 60%, three types of plicae[1–3] are commonly described and are named according to their location inside the knee (Fig. 4.1).

The *suprapatellar plica* or *plica synovialis suprapatellaris* is located in the suprapatellar pouch. This plica varies in shape, size, and thickness. An unusually large, thickened suprapatellar plica can be clinically significant. When the suprapatellar plica is complete it can divide the joint into two separate compartments. Synovial fluid can therefore collect above the plica, causing a painful suprapatellar mass.

The *medial patellar plica* or *medial shelf* is located along the medial wall of the knee joint and inserts into the infrapatellar pad area (Fig. 4.2). While four configurations of medical plicae have been described[4] depending on their size, width, and fenestration, the majority are thin, pliable synovial folds that are asymptomatic. The pathologic changes are usually secondary to trauma, strenuous exercise, or any inflammatory process of the knee joint. The plica becomes a thickened, fibrotic band that either can impinge on the medial femoral condyle if large enough or can cause pain due to its tethering effect on its synovial insertion, rich in nerve endings.

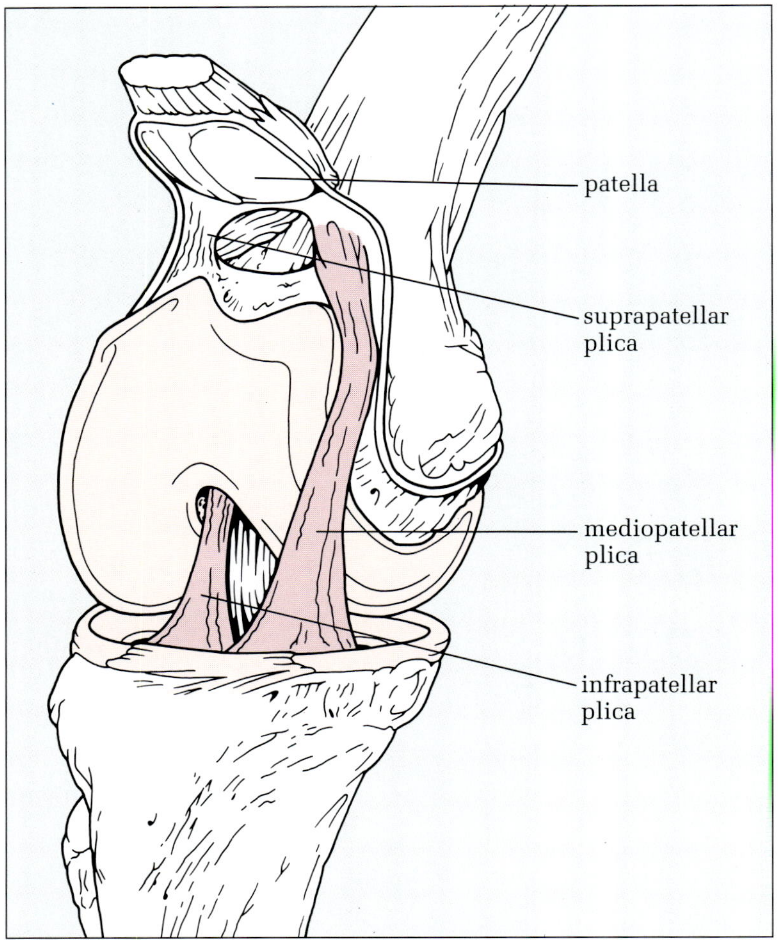

Figure 4.1
The three common plicae of the knee joint.

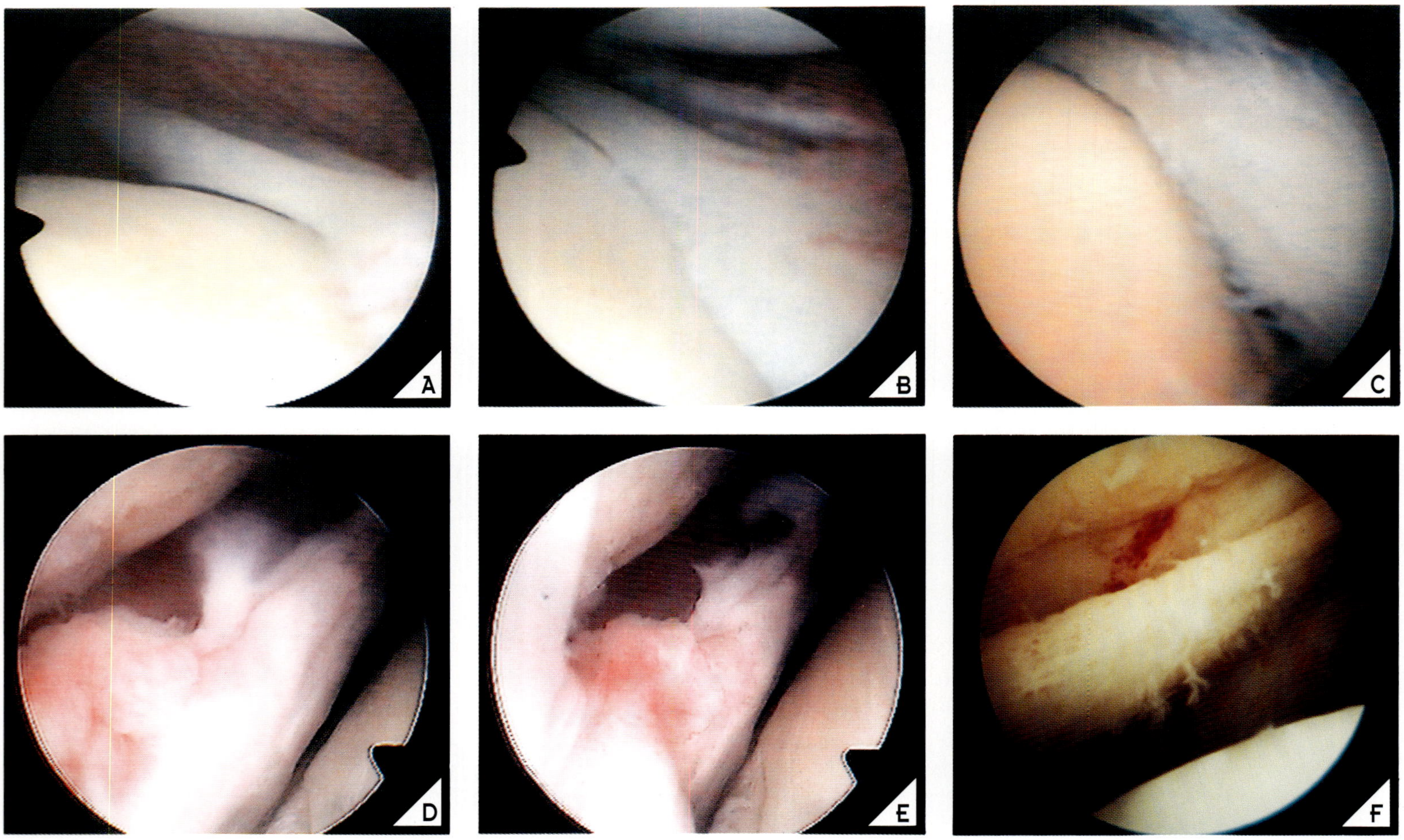

Figure 4.2
(A) Medial shelf right knee. (B) Medial shelf with fenestration. (C) Fibrotic medial shelf. (D, E) Thickened, fibrotic medial plica left knee. (F) Another example of a thick symptomatic medial shelf with chondromalacia of the patella above.

The typical patient with plica syndrome is a young athlete who complains of intermittent dull, aching pain at the superior aspect of the knee over the femoral condyle. Examination discloses localized tenderness on the medial femoral condyle, with a palpable or an audible snap between 45° and 60° of flexion of the knee joint. Arthroscopically, localized chondromalacia on the medial femoral condyle and patella can be observed as well as an inelastic and fibrotic plica.

The *infrapatellar plica,* also called the *ligamentum mucosum,* is the most common of the synovial folds of the knee joint. Superiorly, it originates from the anterior aspect of the intercondylar notch and its distal insertion is in the infrapatellar fat pad. At times, a complete septum can hamper manipulation of the arthroscope and surgical instruments within the joint.

Surgical Technique

Excision of a pathologic suprapatellar plica can be performed from the anteromedial portal with the arthroscope placed through the anterolateral portal.

Excision of a medial shelf can also be performed easily by use of two portals (Fig. 4.3). The anterolateral portal is used for the arthroscopic examination and a superolateral portal is used for resection of the proximal aspect of the plica, with either a basket forceps, suction punch basket, or motorized shaver. Subsequently, a switch of portals is

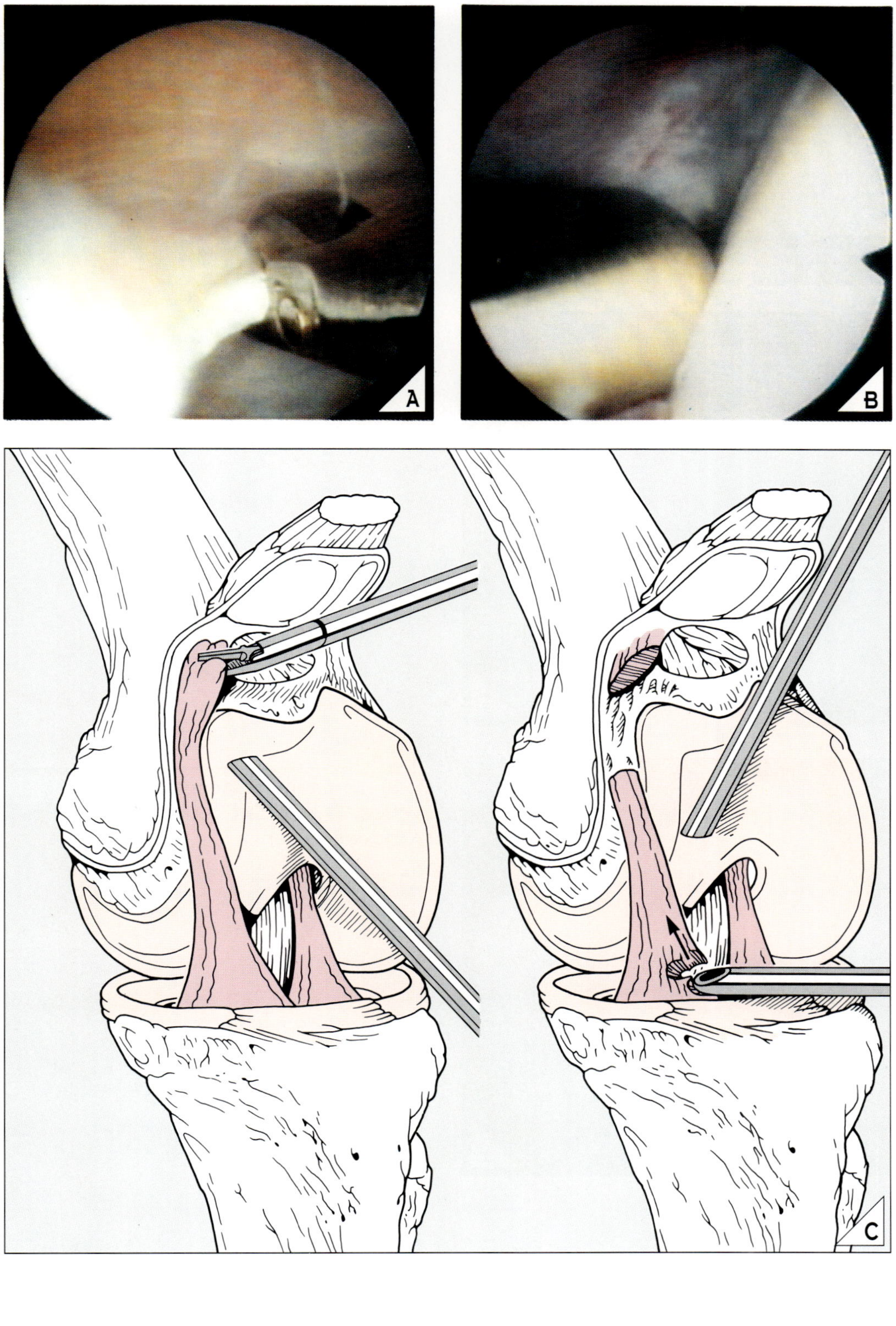

Figure 4.3
(A) The basket forceps from the superolateral portal excising a thick medial shelf left knee. (B) The shaver through the inferolateral portal completing the excision. (C) Schematic illustration of the steps for excision of a medial shelf.

made, with the arthroscope placed through the superolateral portal[5] and the surgical instrument, preferably the shaver, through the anterolateral portal. The remaining distal aspect of the plica that is inserted on the infrapatellar pad is then resected (Fig. 4.4).

If an infrapatellar plica or ligamentum mucosum must be resected, the procedure can be performed with the surgical instrument placed through the anteromedial portal (Fig. 4.5).

LOCALIZED LESIONS OF THE SYNOVIUM

Localized lesions of the synovium,[6,7] such as the localized form of pigmented villonodular synovitis, synovial hemangioma, and ganglia, can be removed arthroscopically (Fig. 4.6).

The localized synovial lesion encountered in a large arthroscopy practice is the localized form of pigmented

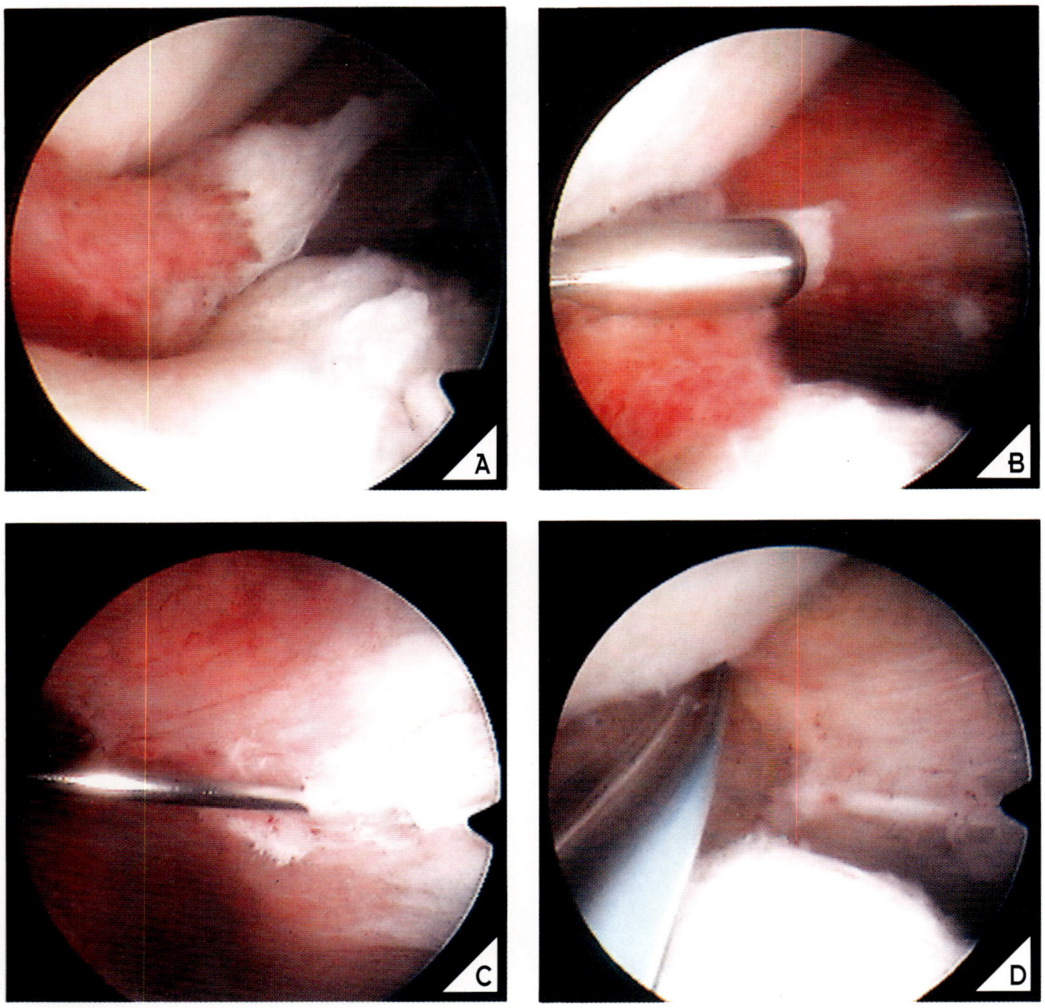

Figure 4.4
(A–D) Steps of excision of the distal aspect of a medial shelf. Chondromalacic changes of the femoral condyle are noted at the bottom of the picture.

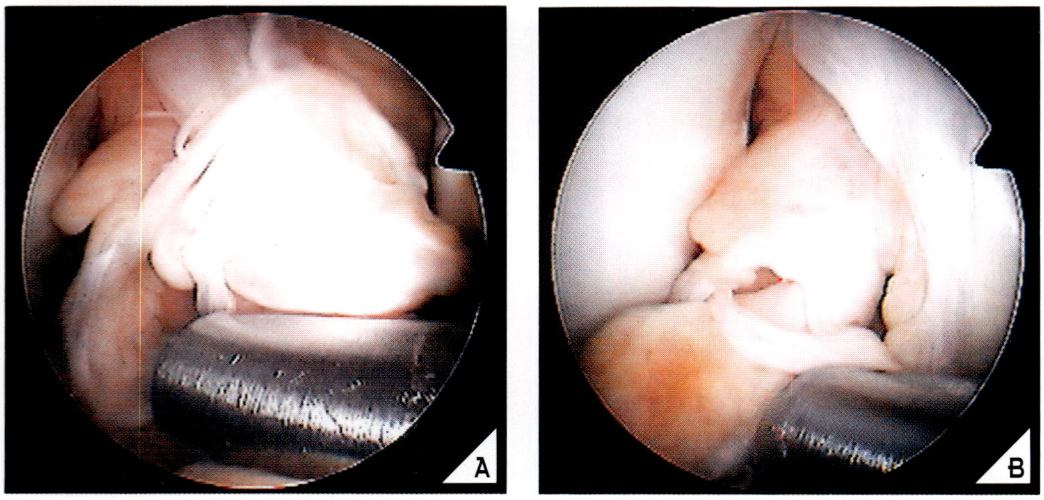

Figure 4.5
(A, B) Ligamentum mucosum being excised to expose a tear of the anterior cruciate ligament.

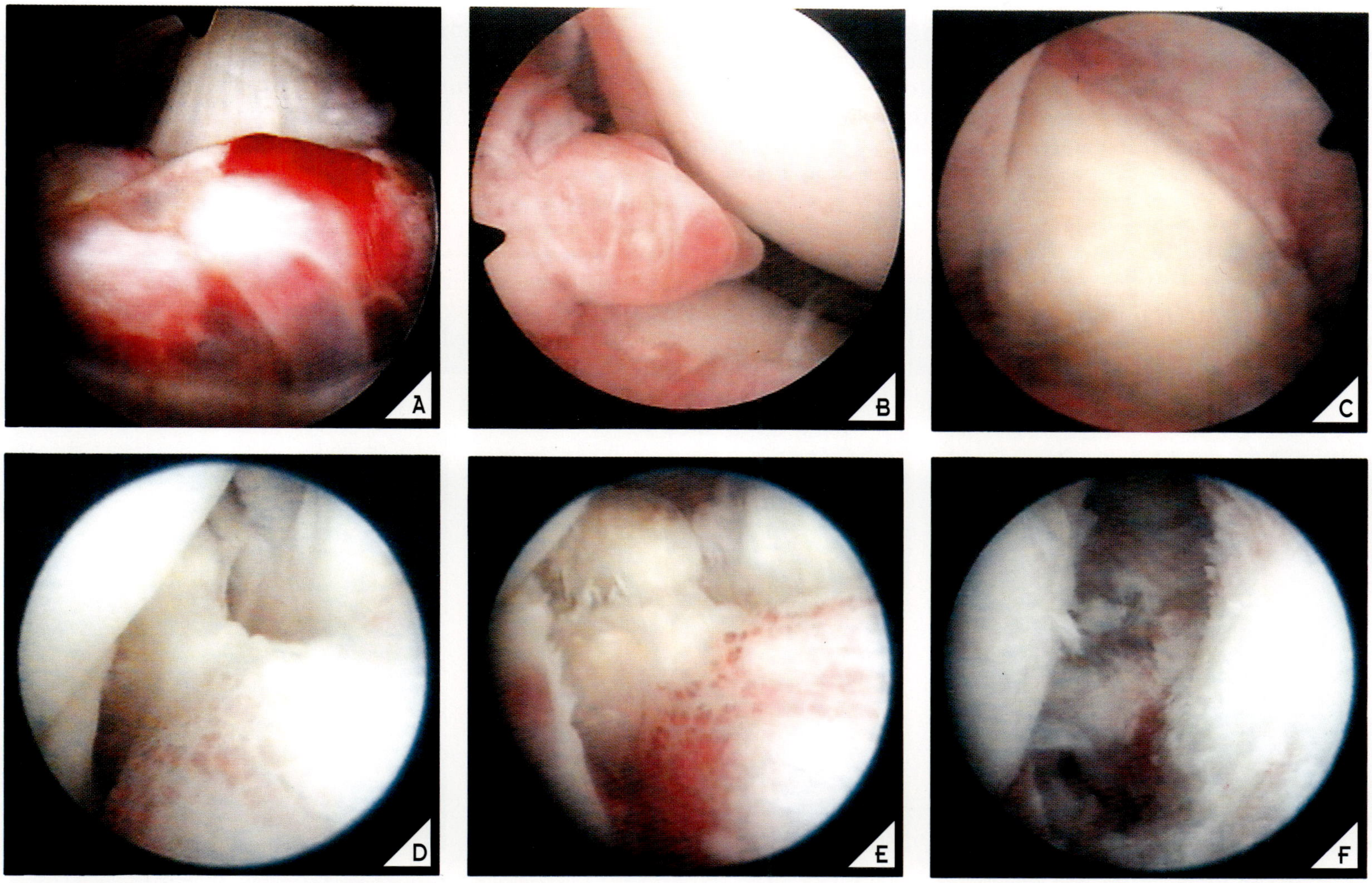

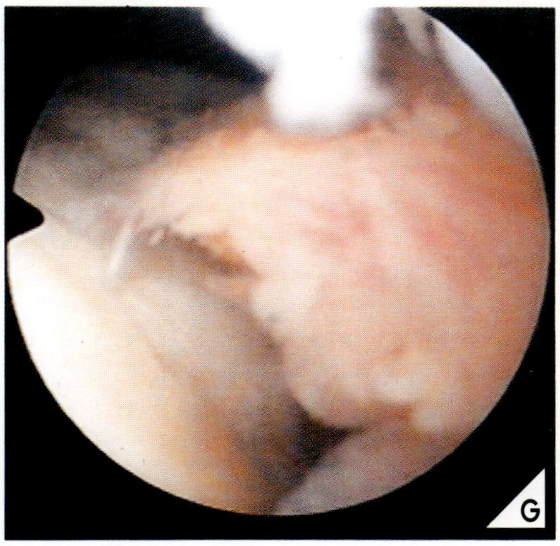

Figure 4.6

(A) Localized pigmented villonodular synovitis at tibial insertion of the anterior cruciate ligament. (B) Localized pigmented villonodular synovitis next to the medial femoral condyle right knee. (C) Ganglion cyst in the anterior cruciate ligament area. (D–F) Unusual location of localized pigmented villonodular synovitis in the popliteal tunnel left knee before and after arthroscopic excision. (G) Hypertrophic mass of aggregated synovial villi causing impingement in the patellofemoral joint. Chondromalacic changes of the trochlea are noted at the left side of the picture.

villonodular synovitis (PVNS). This lesion is rare. When present it occurs in the knee. Because of its rarity the diagnosis is rarely made before surgery. The patient usually presents with symptoms such as locking, giving way, and swelling, mimicking an internal derangement of the knee. Pain is not usually a prominent feature.

Surgical Technique

Two arthroscopic portals are necessary to remove the pedunculated or sessile synovial lesion (Fig. 4.7). An incision is made at the base of the lesion with a scissors, leaving a small attachment for avulsion of the mass with a grasping forceps. A partial synovectomy of the adjacent area of the synovium is done using a motorized shaver. Arthroscopic resection is usually successful in the few reported series, without evidence of recurrence.

Generalized Lesions of the Synovium

Among the generalized lesions of the synovium amenable to arthroscopic surgery, the most common forms are the inflammatory disorders such as rheumatoid arthritis, synovial chondromatosis, and generalized PVNS (Fig. 4.8).

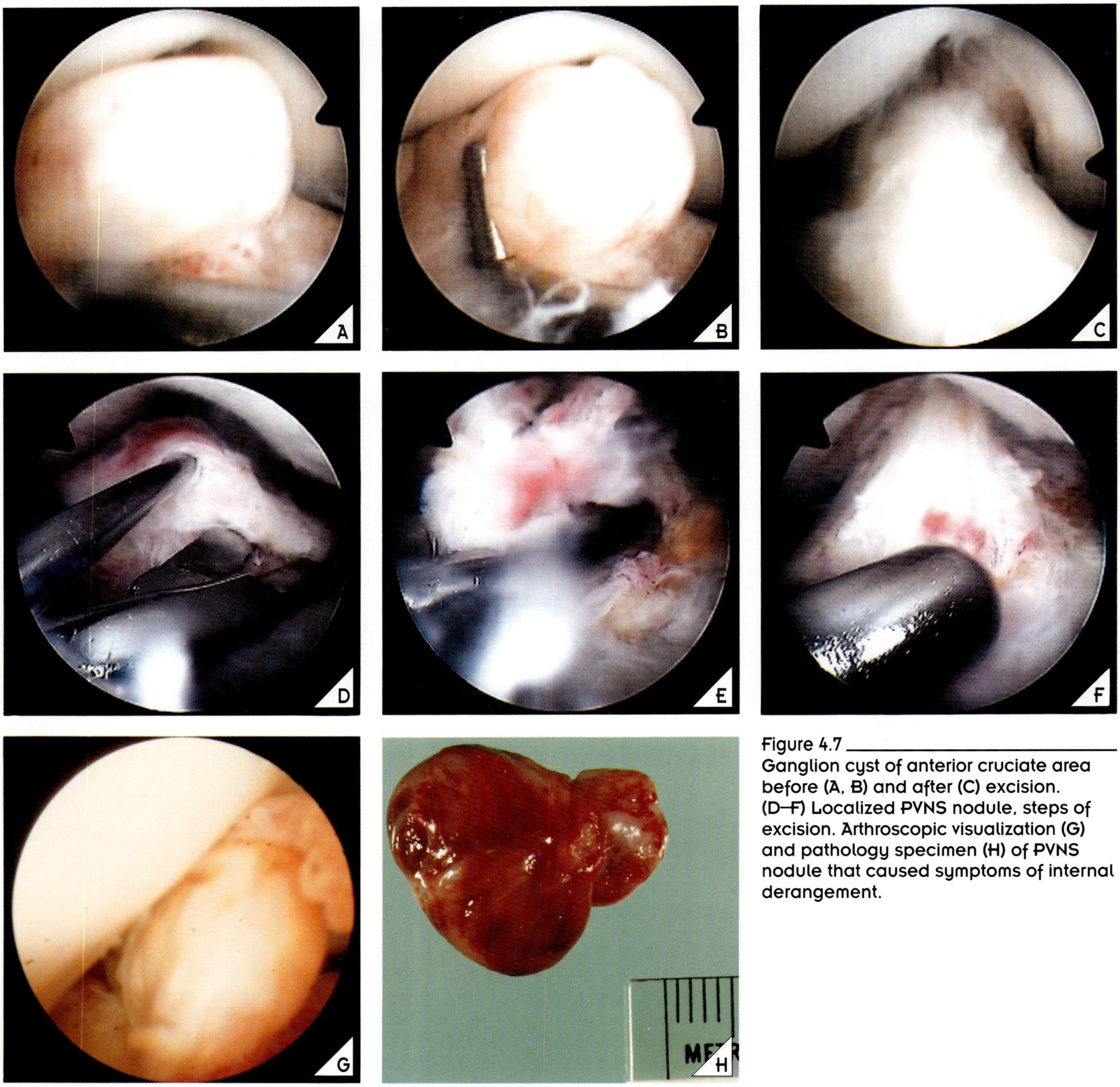

Figure 4.7
Ganglion cyst of anterior cruciate area before (A, B) and after (C) excision. (D–F) Localized PVNS nodule, steps of excision. Arthroscopic visualization (G) and pathology specimen (H) of PVNS nodule that caused symptoms of internal derangement.

Rheumatoid arthritis is the most common form of inflammatory arthritis with joint involvement.[8] Although initially this condition can often be managed medically, when it remains resistant to a period of at least 6 months of medical management synovectomy is indicated. Chemical or radioisotope synovectomy is now being used more frequently at some medical centers in the United States with gratifying results.[9,10] Recent reports have stressed that a previous surgical synovectomy enhances the outcome.[11]

Initially, synovectomy was performed through long arthrotomy incisions, with increased morbidity due mostly to loss of range of motion of the joint involved. With the advent of arthroscopy[12] and the availability of sophisticated high-speed motorized instruments, the procedure can be performed with less morbidity for the patient and obvious advantages, such as a more complete excision involving the posterior aspect of the joint and sparing of the meniscal tissue. Since the quadriceps mechanism is not violated, as in the traditional open procedure, manipulation of the joint is usually not necessary.

Synovial osteochondromatosis is a monoarticular condition characterized by formation of multiple loose bodies secondary to metaplastic transformation of the subintimal connective tissue of the synovium. Three phases of this process have been described by Milgram[13]: 1) an active intrasynovial phase, without formation of loose bodies; 2) a transitional phase, characterized by both active synovial

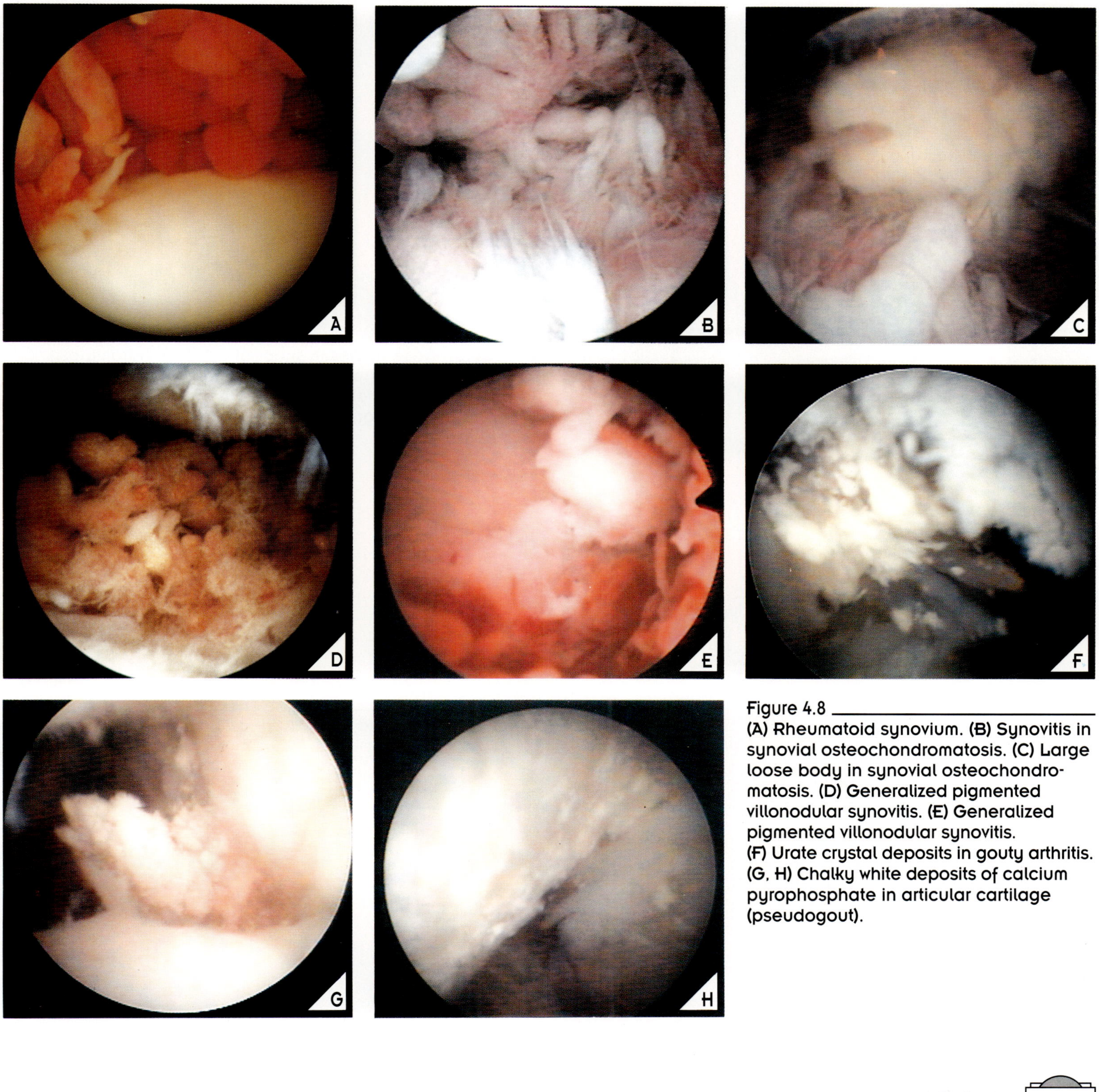

Figure 4.8

(A) Rheumatoid synovium. (B) Synovitis in synovial osteochondromatosis. (C) Large loose body in synovial osteochondromatosis. (D) Generalized pigmented villonodular synovitis. (E) Generalized pigmented villonodular synovitis. (F) Urate crystal deposits in gouty arthritis. (G, H) Chalky white deposits of calcium pyrophosphate in articular cartilage (pseudogout).

disease and formation of loose bodies; and 3) a "burned-out" phase in which there is no intrasynovial activity, with a joint filled with multiple osteochondral bodies. In stage 1, with increased synovial activity, arthroscopic synovectomy may be indicated. Its value is disputed in stage 2, and synovectomy is not justified in stage 3, when there is no synovial activity. Small loose bodies can be washed out easily from the joint through a large trocar cannula. The larger ones need to be removed with grasping forceps (Fig. 4.9).[14]

The *generalized form of PVNS* usually affects the knee and causes a diffuse synovial thickening of the joint. Although synovectomy can be performed by arthroscopic means, the high rate of recurrence has led some investigators to advocate chemical or radioisotope synovectomy, or even radiotherapy.[11,15] The six-portals approach, described later in the chapter, is used for the arthroscopic procedure.

Synovectomy has been advocated in *hemophilic arthropathy* to prevent recurrent joint bleeding and, perhaps, to slow the progression of the arthropathy. Recently, arthroscopic synovectomy has been used in hemophilic patients and has been shown to decrease postoperative morbidity and rehabilitation time. Wiedel[16] has used arthroscopic synovectomy for chronic hemophilia in five patients with the purpose of stopping recurrent bleeding and excising the hypertrophic synovial tissue. He report-

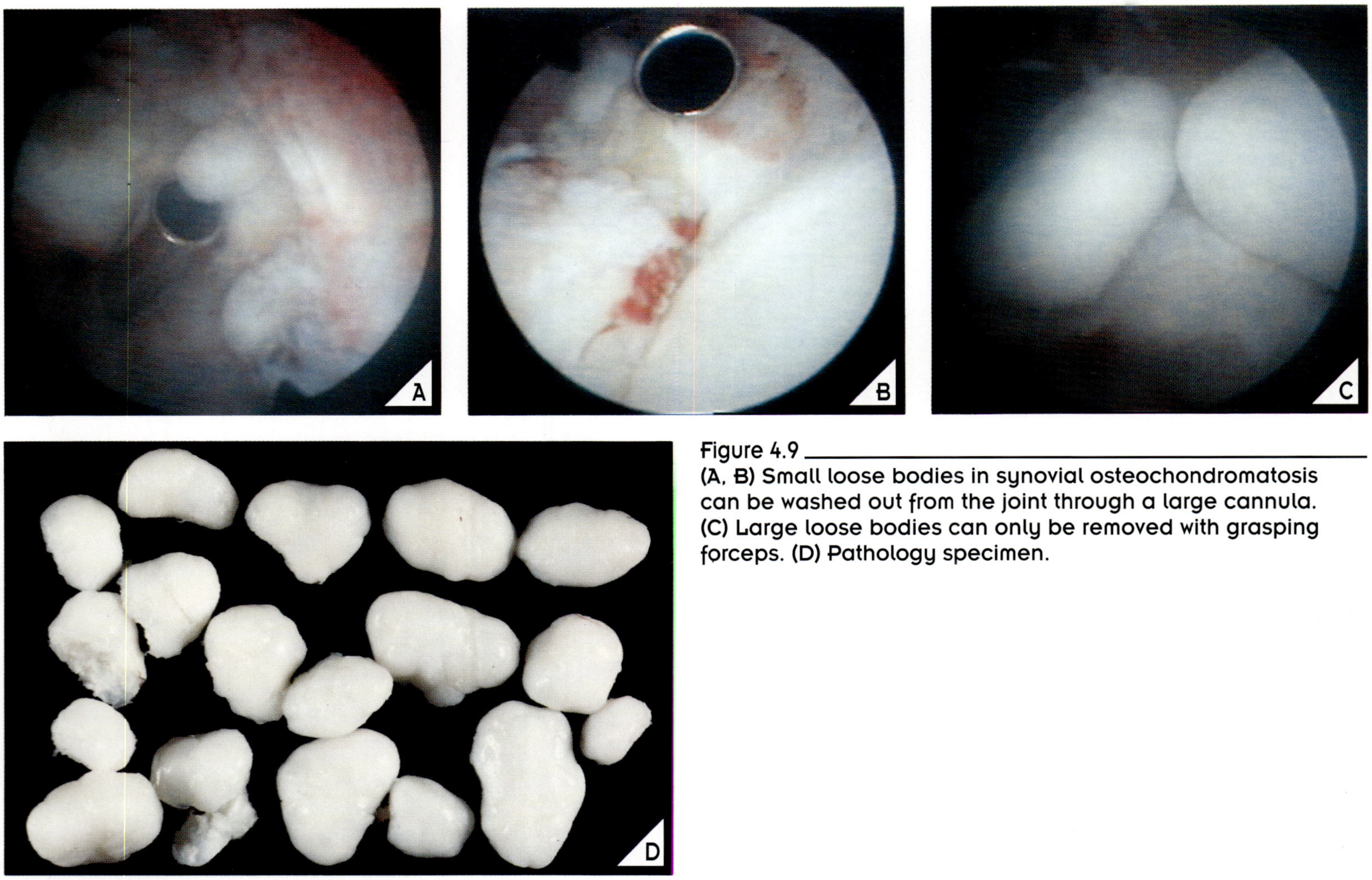

Figure 4.9

(A, B) Small loose bodies in synovial osteochondromatosis can be washed out from the joint through a large cannula. (C) Large loose bodies can only be removed with grasping forceps. (D) Pathology specimen.

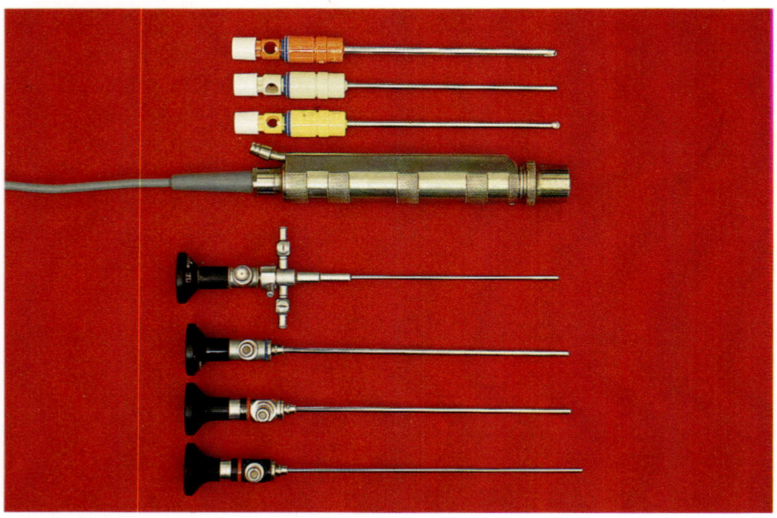

Figure 4.10

Synovial resector and 4 mm 25° and 70° arthroscopes.

ed no complications, and all patients regained their preoperative range of motion.

Surgical Technique

A tourniquet is advised for all patients. Procedures can be performed under general or epidural anesthesia. A power shaver system with 5.5 mm and 3.2 mm full radius resectors is necessary. Both 4 mm 25° and 70° arthroscopes are useful (Fig. 4.10). The use of a pump makes the procedure easier, but a gravity system can also be used. The resection should be done in systematic fashion to excise the diseased synovium from the various compartments of the joint. An almost complete synovectomy of the knee requires a minimum of six portals, four anterior and two posterior (Fig. 4.11).

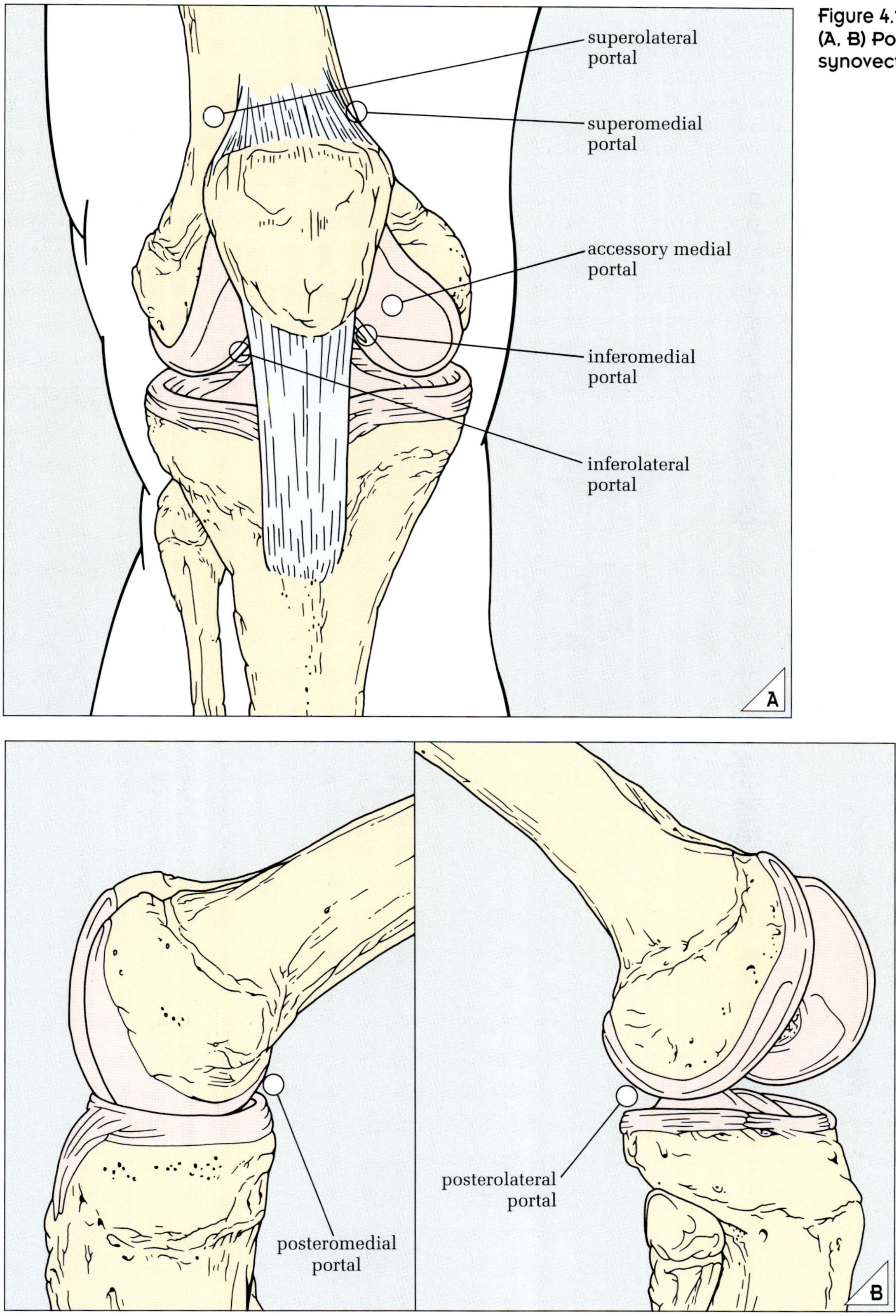

Figure 4.11
(A, B) Portals used for arthroscopic synovectomy. **(continued on next page)**

Excision of synovium must be done in a systematic way to achieve a successful result (Fig. 4.12). Through the anterolateral portal, the 4 mm 25° arthroscope is placed into the suprapatellar pouch. The motorized shaver is then introduced through the superolateral portal to excise the synovium from the lateral aspect of the pouch and the superior aspect of the lateral gutter. The surgical instrument is then passed from the superolateral to the superomedial portal to complete the synovectomy in the superomedial aspect of the pouch as well as in the superior part of the medial gutter.

Synovectomy of the lower part of the knee joint is done through the two anteroinferior portals. The arthroscope and the shaver should be switched to allow better visualization of the compartments as well as optimal excision of the diseased tissue. For instance, excision of the synovium from the lower aspects of the lateral or medial gutter is facilitated by visualizing from the superolateral or superomedial portal, while the shaver is placed on the same side of the knee through the corresponding anteroinferior portal.

A smaller synovectomy blade is required for debridement of the inferior aspect of the menisci and the posterior aspect of the femoral notch in the vicinity of the cruciate ligaments. Then the posteromedial corner of the knee is visualized by placing a 70° scope through the anterolateral portal into the posteromedial compartment. With the knee flexed at 90°, the posteromedial portal is developed by means of a spinal needle inserted in an area 1 cm posterior to the femoral condyle, for introduction of the motorized shaver. The same steps are performed in the posterolateral corner of the joint in order to complete the synovectomy. To summarize, when the excision is carried out in a systematic manner for a right knee the motorized resector is displaced clockwise, and for a left knee it is moved counterclockwise.

Postoperatively, a suction drain is left in the knee joint and a compression dressing is applied over the lower extremity. Full weight-bearing is allowed the same day of the surgery. Quadriceps exercises as well as knee flexion exercises are encouraged immediately. With this technique the risks and complications of open surgical synovectomy are avoided and the main goals of the arthroscopic technique, such as preservation of the range of motion with minimal morbidity and short hospital stay for the patient, are achieved.

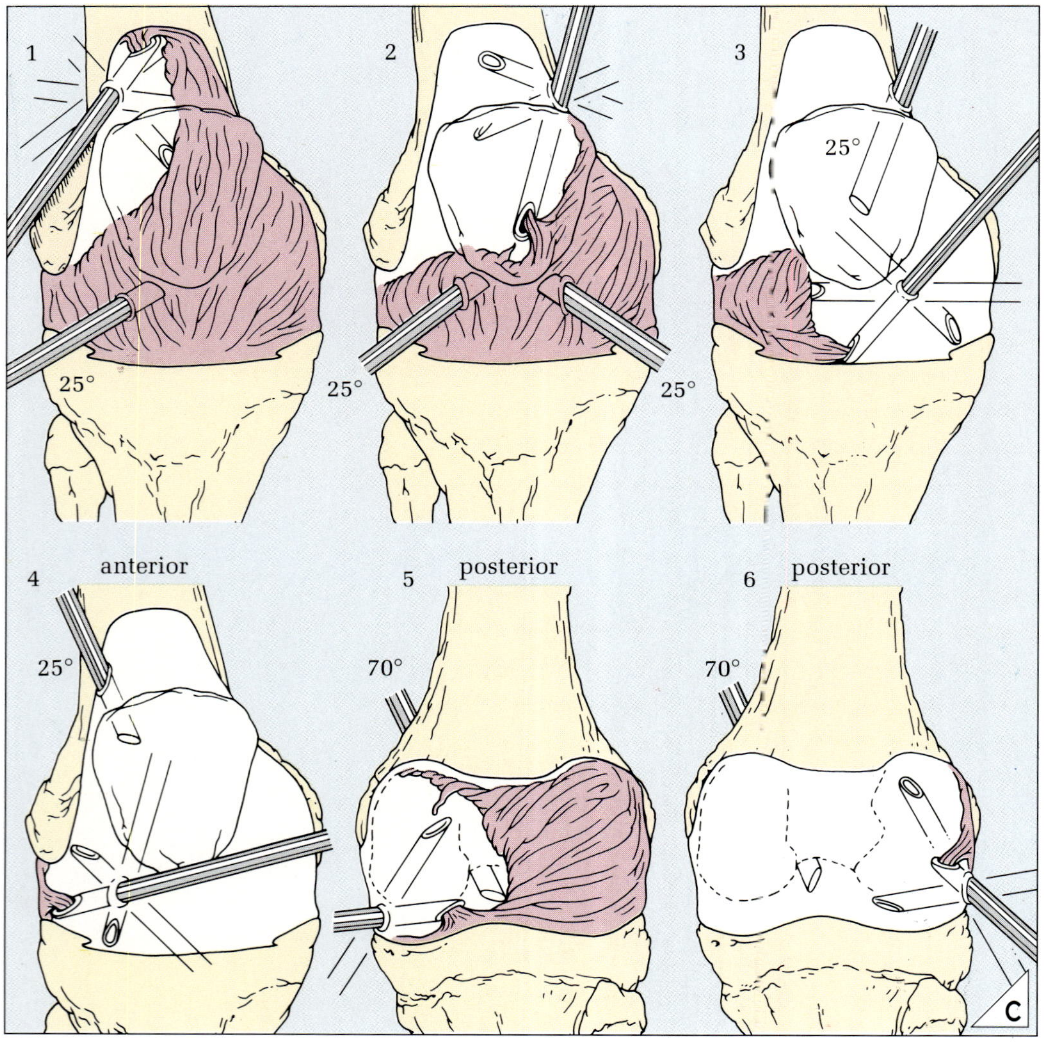

Figure 4.11 (continued)
(C) Steps of complete synovial excision.

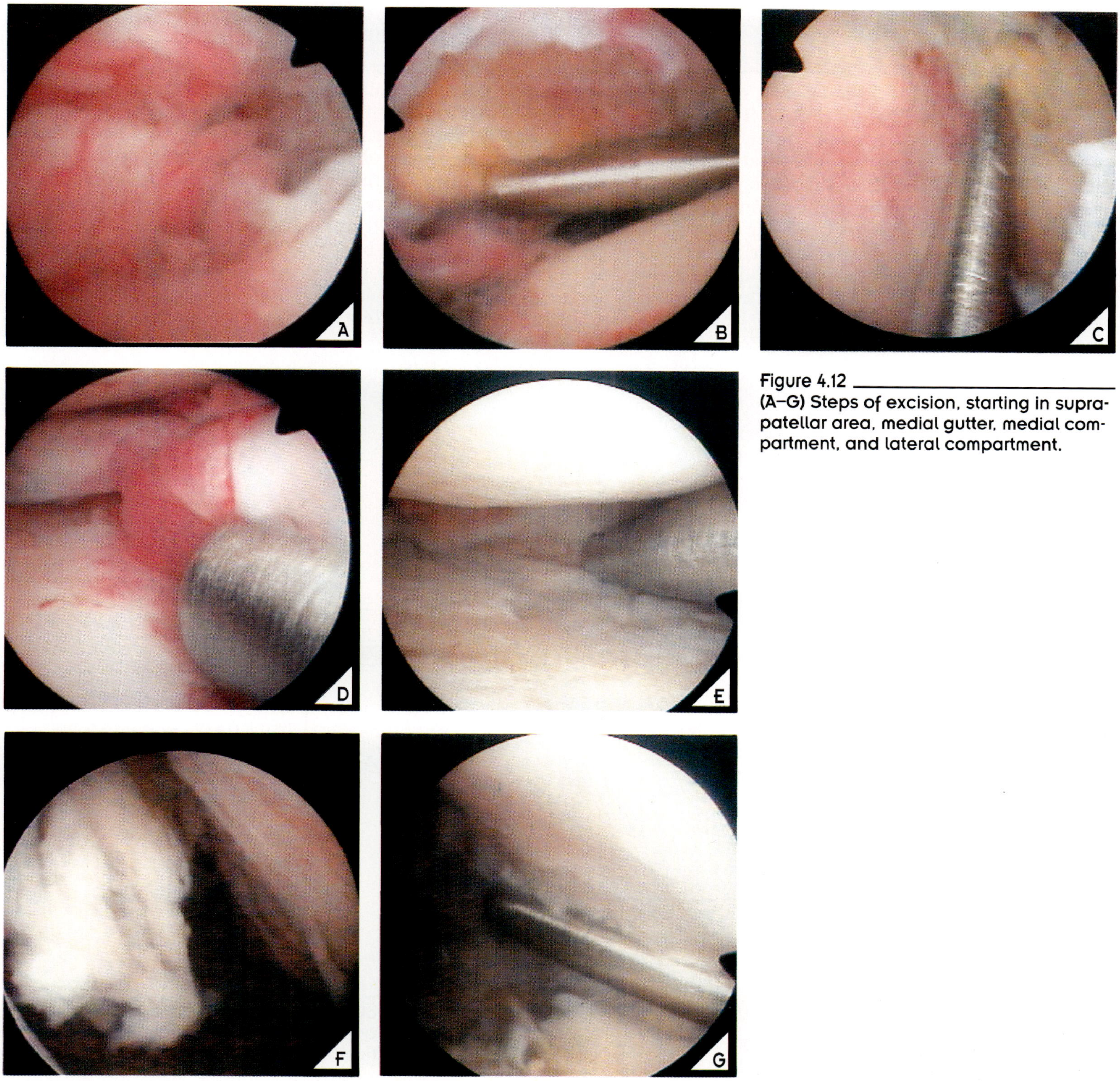

Figure 4.12

(A–G) Steps of excision, starting in suprapatellar area, medial gutter, medial compartment, and lateral compartment.

ARTHROFIBROSIS

Arthroscopic surgical technique is an established procedure for the treatment of arthrofibrosis (Fig. 4.13). Excision of adhesions under direct vision with gentle manipulation followed by an aggressive rehabilitation program has achieved good to excellent results in the few reported series, with marked improvement of range of motion.[17,18] The dreadful complications of the traditional forceful closed manipulation, such as indiscriminate tearing of intraarticular tissue, excessive patellofemoral compression, rupture of the patellar tendon, or even fracture of the femoral shaft, can be avoided.

Surgical Technique

Before the arthroscopic procedure, which is performed under general, spinal, or epidural anesthesia, the knee is examined to assess the range of motion and mobility of the patella. Limitation of extension and flexion of the joint, with impairment of patellar mobility, suggests the presence of infrapatellar contracture syndrome, originally described by Paulos.[19] The knee joint is entered superomedially with a large trocar and some adhesions in the suprapatellar pouch are broken with a blunt obturator. Then an inflow cannula is placed into the suprapatellar pouch. Through the anterolateral portal another blunt obturator is inserted into the joint to break more adhesions, followed

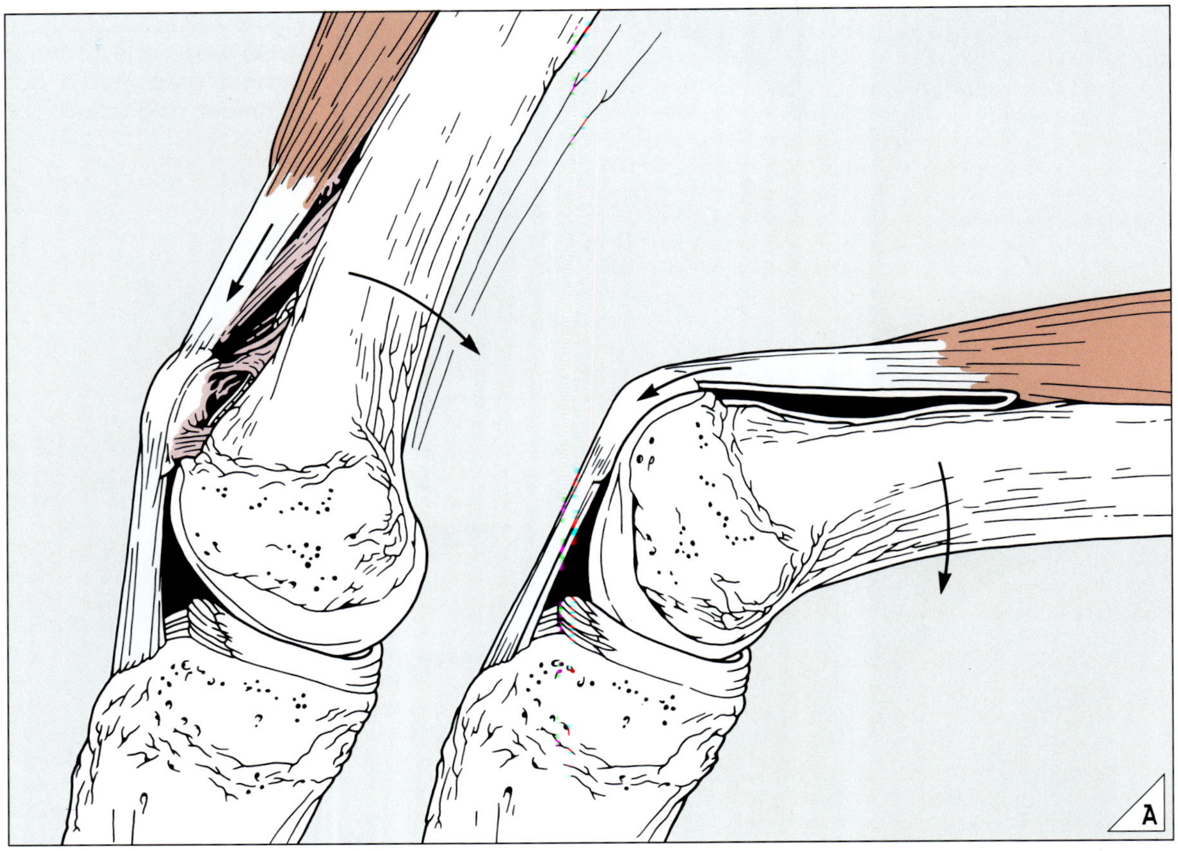

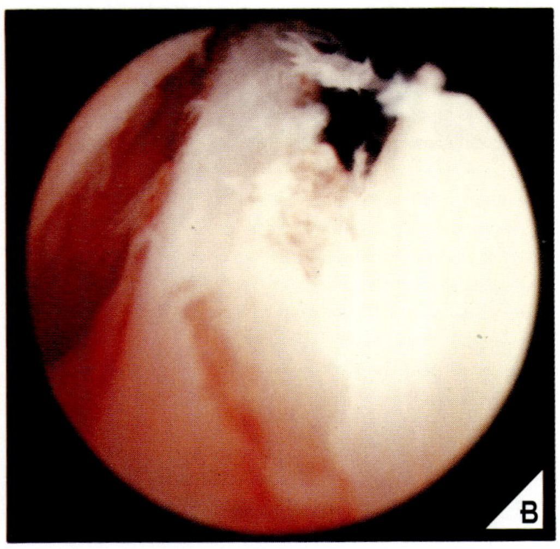

Figure 4.13
(A) Schematic illustration of arthrofibrosis in suprapatellar area before and after excision. (B) Arthroscopic visualization of arthrofibrosis in suprapatellar area.

by the 4 mm 25° arthroscope. A third superolateral portal is developed for placement of a 5 mm hook scissors. Adhesive bands are cut, followed by resection using a full-radius blade of the high-speed arthroplasty set.

A systematic removal of all intraarticular adhesions is performed, from the suprapatellar pouch, both gutters, intraarticular notch, and the fat pad area (Fig. 4.14). A lateral release using electrocautery is performed. A small periosteal elevator is then used in the suprapatellar pouch from any of the inferior portals to free the quadriceps muscle from the anterior aspect of the femur. At this point, gentle manipulation of the knee is performed. In patients with anterior cruciate ligament reconstruction, if impingement of the graft is present in full extension an anterior notchplasty may be necessary. Partial resection of the anterior fibers of the graft or complete section may have to be performed if the range of flexion cannot be improved with manipulation. A Hemovac is inserted into the joint before closure. The portals are then closed with nylon sutures and a compression dressing is applied. Immediate passive range of motion in a CPM machine is instituted in the recovery room.

The day after surgery the drain and the compression dressing are removed. Quadriceps tightening and straight leg raising exercises are started with a program of active assisted range-of-motion exercises under the guidance of a physical therapist. The patient is discharged on the third or fourth day with a CPM machine. Arrangements are also made for an intensive rehabilitation program on an outpatient basis under the close supervision of a physical therapist. The stitches are removed after a week or 10 days and full ambulation is allowed as tolerated by the patient. If progress in physical therapy is very slow, the physician should not hesitate to manipulate the knee under general anesthesia. The use of a Dynasplint may be necessary in long-standing, motion-limiting arthrofibrosis cases.

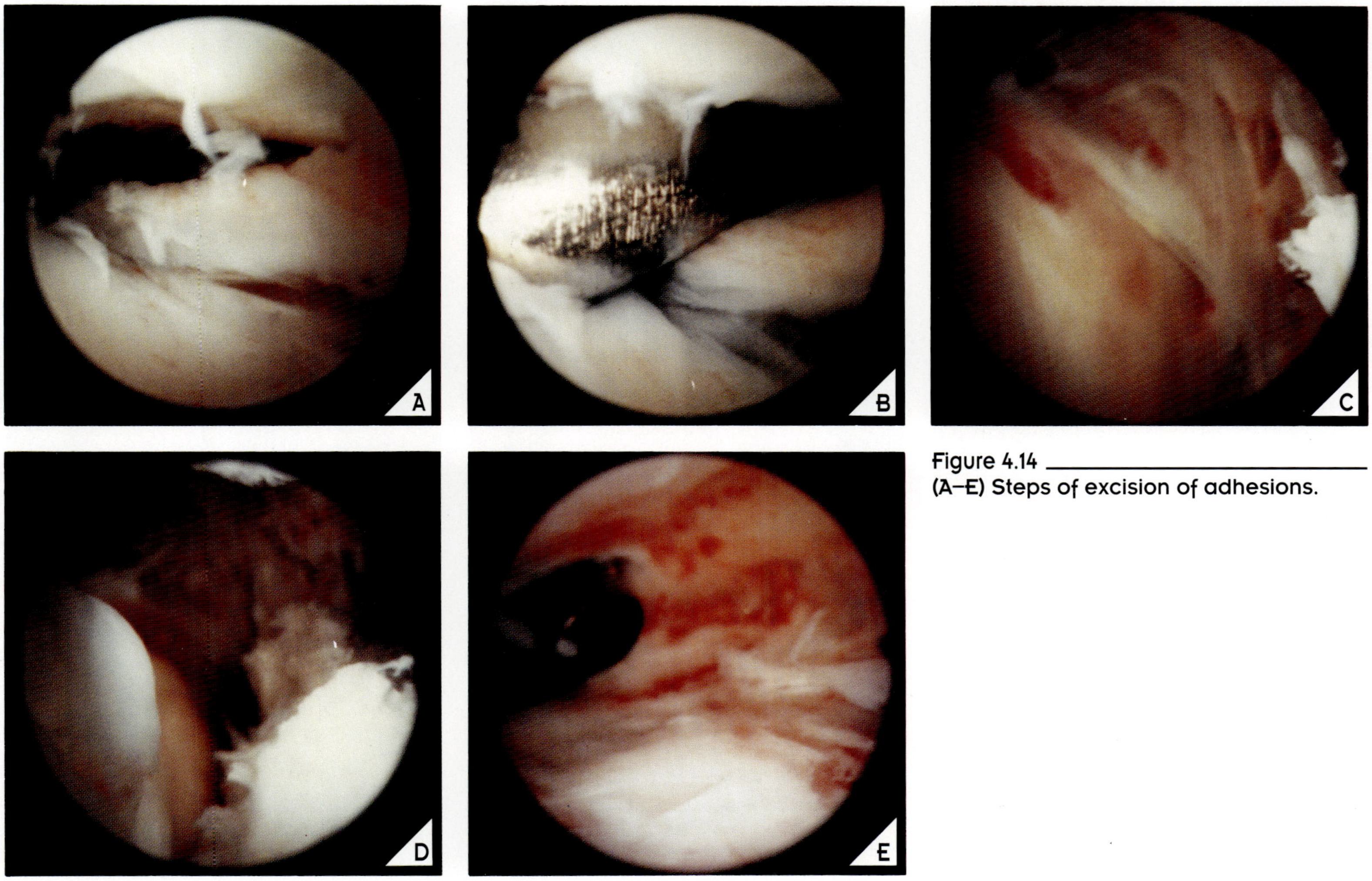

Figure 4.14
(A–E) Steps of excision of adhesions.

PYARTHROSIS

Although drainage by repeated needle aspiration combined with the appropriate antimicrobial therapy has been the traditional form of treatment in acute pyarthrosis, surgical drainage has been advocated in many instances (early by some, late by others) when the presence of fibrinous material is preventing adequate needle aspiration. With the advent of arthroscopy, arthrotomy, which carries the risk of significant limitation of range of motion, is no longer advocated.[20–22] Arthroscopic techniques allow debridement of the fibrinous debris, the necrotic synovium, and the loculated pockets of adhesions as well as the application of a continuous drainage system (Figs. 4.15, 4.16).

Surgical Technique

With the patient under general anesthesia, a large inflow cannula is placed through the medial suprapatellar portal and an arthroscopic exploration is performed. If the joint shows no evidence of fibrinous debris or loculations, it is irrigated with normal saline solution and a drainage catheter is inserted through the inferomedial portal (Fig. 4.17). When fibrinous debris and necrotic synovium are found, the motorized shaver is used to debride the involved compartments. *No synovectomy is necessary.* Continuous irrigation and continuous drainage are applied, using catheters placed into the medial and lateral gutters. When ingress/egress tubes are inserted into the joint, sterile precautions should be used to avoid contaminating the knee with a different organism by way of these tubes.

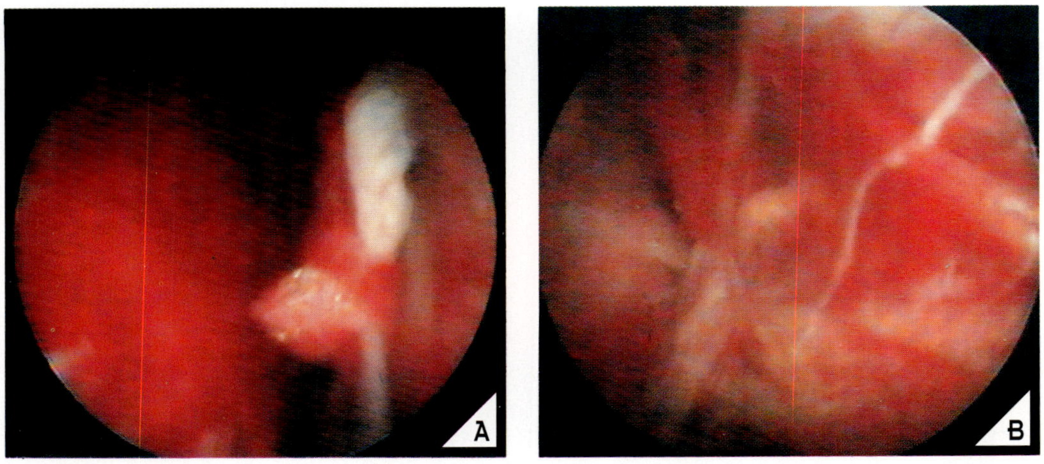

Figure 4.15
(A, B) Synovitis in pyarthrosis of the knee.

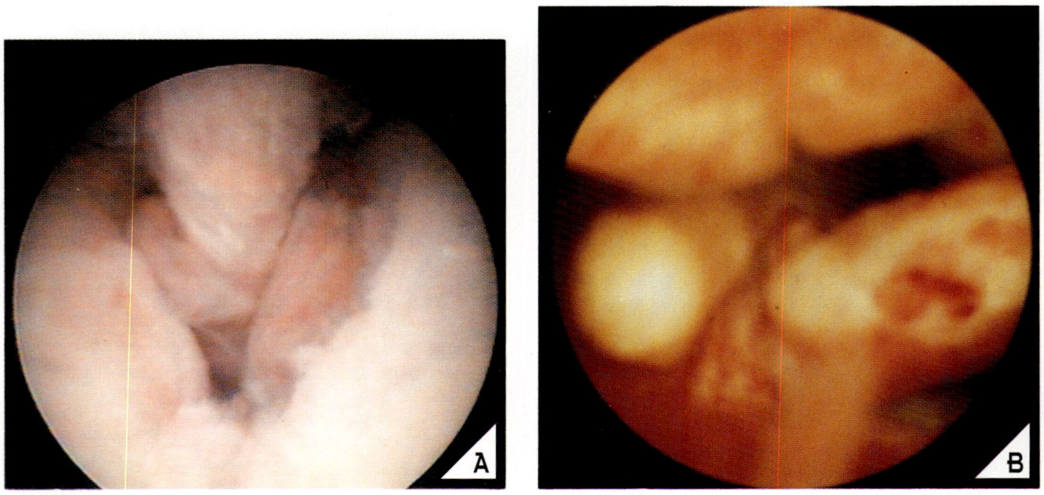

Figure 4.16
(A, B) Necrotic synovium in pyarthrosis of the knee joint.

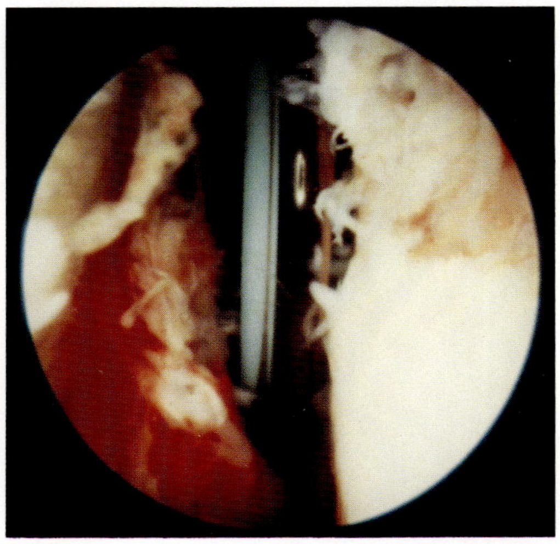

Figure 4.17
Catheter placed in lateral gutter after joint debridement of pyarthrosis right knee.

Appropriate antibiotics are given intravenously. No antibiotics are necessary in the irrigation solution, since previous data have conclusively demonstrated that adequate antibiotic concentrations in joint effusion can be achieved by parenteral administration. The final choice and duration of antibiotic therapy are best monitored by an infectious disease consultant. Continuous passive motion is begun on the same day or on the day after the surgery, as well as active motion under the supervision of a therapist. The drains are removed after 48 hours. Non-weight-bearing for a period of at least 6 weeks is advocated by many physicians.

Complications and Pitfalls of Synovectomy

For arthroscopic synovectomy the use of at least six portals is necessary for adequate debridement. A 70° arthroscope and small motorized instruments are added to the regular 25° scope and large 5 mm synovial resector. Synovial ingrowth and pannus formation under the menisci and around the cruciate ligaments should be resected carefully by means of a small shaver blade. The resection should be performed in a systematic way, and the technique requires frequent repositioning of the arthroscope and power instruments through the various portals. If the 70° arthroscope inserted through the intercondylar notch does not provide adequate visualization of the posterior compartments, a second posteromedial portal may be necessary. During debridement of the posterior compartment it is essential at all times to visualize the tip of the surgical instrument, to avoid the risk of penetrating the posterior capsule.

Lateral Retinacular Release

Lateral retinacular release is indicated in excessive lateral pressure syndrome and in selected cases of patellar malalignment, those that do not have a deficient medial capsule or an abnormal Q angle. The procedure can be performed in many ways. After a complete arthroscopic examination, with debridement of the chondromalacic articular cartilage of the patella when indicated, a Smillie meniscectomy knife or a retrograde knife can be used from the anterolateral approach, with the arthroscope in the anteromedial portal (Fig. 4.18). The incision in the cap-

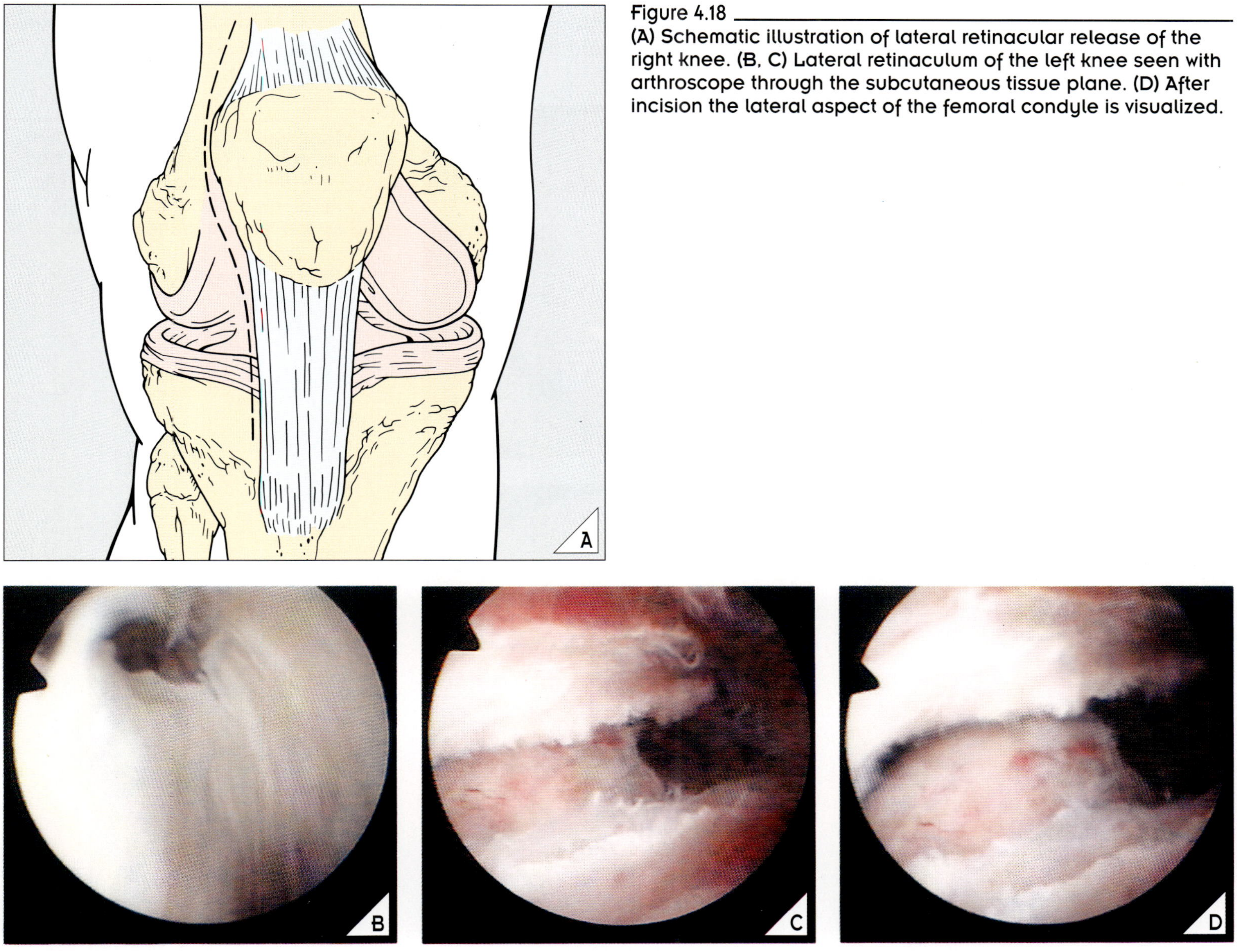

Figure 4.18
(A) Schematic illustration of lateral retinacular release of the right knee. (B, C) Lateral retinaculum of the left knee seen with arthroscope through the subcutaneous tissue plane. (D) After incision the lateral aspect of the femoral condyle is visualized.

sule is made close to the edge of the patella to minimize bleeding. The incision is made approximately 2 cm above the patella in order to cut the insertion of the vastus lateralis tendon. The release is carried out distally along the patellar tendon. Some physicians, instead, use an electrocautery knife for the release of the capsule (Fig. 4.19).[23]

Another arthroscopic technique, popularized by Metcalf,[24] can also be used, with Metzenbaum scissors placed through the anterolateral portal. Before incising the capsule a subcutaneous tissue plane is developed as far as the superior edge of the patella. A second skin incision can be made more proximally to carry the subcutaneous tissue plane above the patella if necessary. The Metzenbaum scissors are then used to divide the capsule as far proximally as possible. Arthroscopic basket scissors can also be used to complete the dissection more proximally.

Regardless of the techniques used, the lateral aspect of the capsule is infiltrated with a solution of Marcaine 0.5% containing epinephrine to minimize the possibility of bleeding and postoperative pain. Electrocautery under direct vision can cauterize the geniculate vessels to control bleeding. To be effective, the tourniquet, if inflated during the release, should be deflated at the time of the cauterization.

Postoperatively, a compression dressing is applied and the extremity is placed in a knee immobilizer for 2 to 3 days. Isometric exercises can be started the same day, and the patient can bear weight on the extremity as tolerated with a pair of crutches.

Medial Capsular Reefing

When the medial aspect of the capsule is compromised by subluxation or even dislocation, realignment can be performed with the arthroscope, provided the Q angle is not abnormal. With the arthroscope placed laterally, three or four curved large needles are placed posteriorly through the skin of the medial aspect of the knee to emerge anteriorly medial to the patella. Underneath the needles, inside the joint, a retrograde knife is used to perform a medial capsular release down to the subcutaneous tissue. A motorized synovial resector is used to create a defect in the medial capsule by excising the edges of the incision. Then the lateral release is performed, after switching the scope to the medial aspect of the knee, as described before. While the needles are still in place, the posterior puncture areas are incised slightly along the skin creases with #11 blade to facilitate burying the knots at the completion of the procedure. The needles carrying absorbable sutures are replaced through the anterior needle puncture subcutaneously and exit posteriorly through the posterior enlarged skin puncture. The joint is decompressed and the sutures are tied at the posteromedial aspect of the knee and the knots buried under the skin (Figs. 4.20, 4.21).

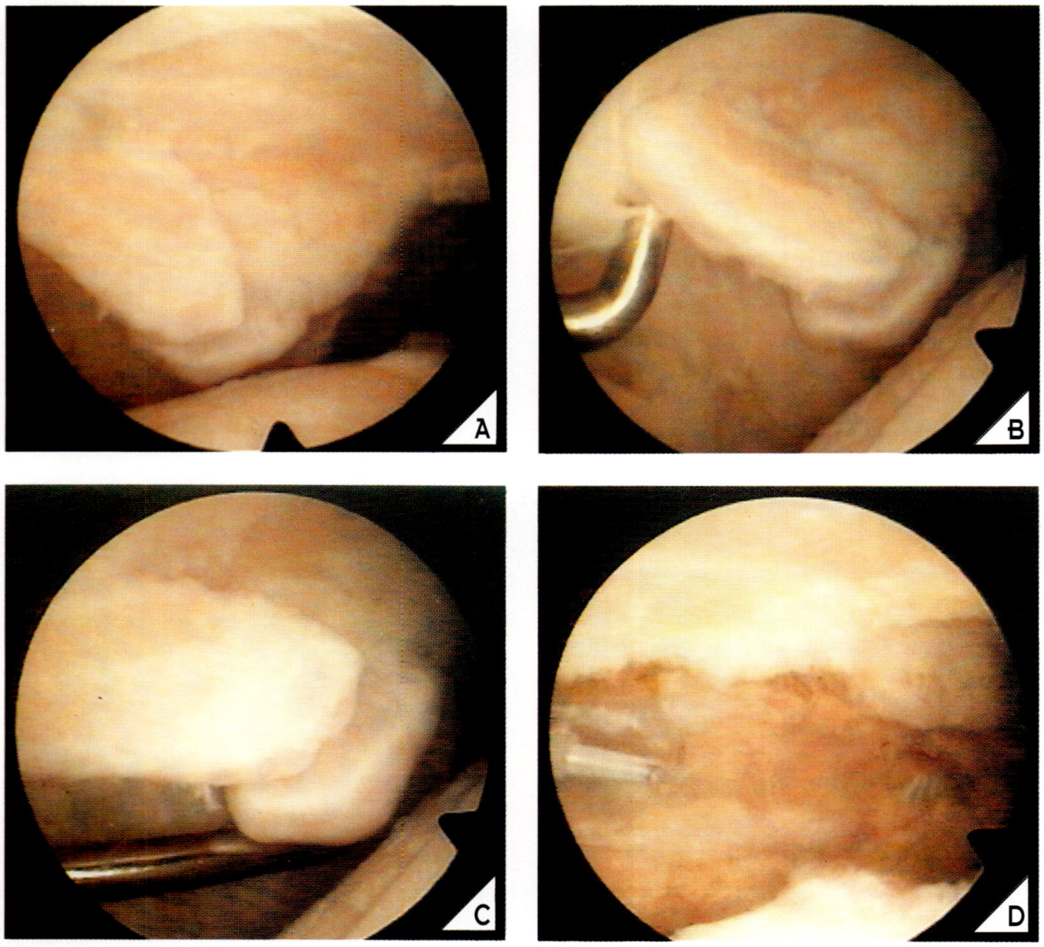

Figure 4.19
(A–D) Patellofemoral arthritis right knee. Steps of excision of osteochondral bodies on the lateral aspect of the patella, with lateral release. Cautery is being used for the release of the capsule.

Figure 4.20
(A–E) Schematic illustration of the various steps for medial reefing of the capsule of the right knee. (continued on next page)

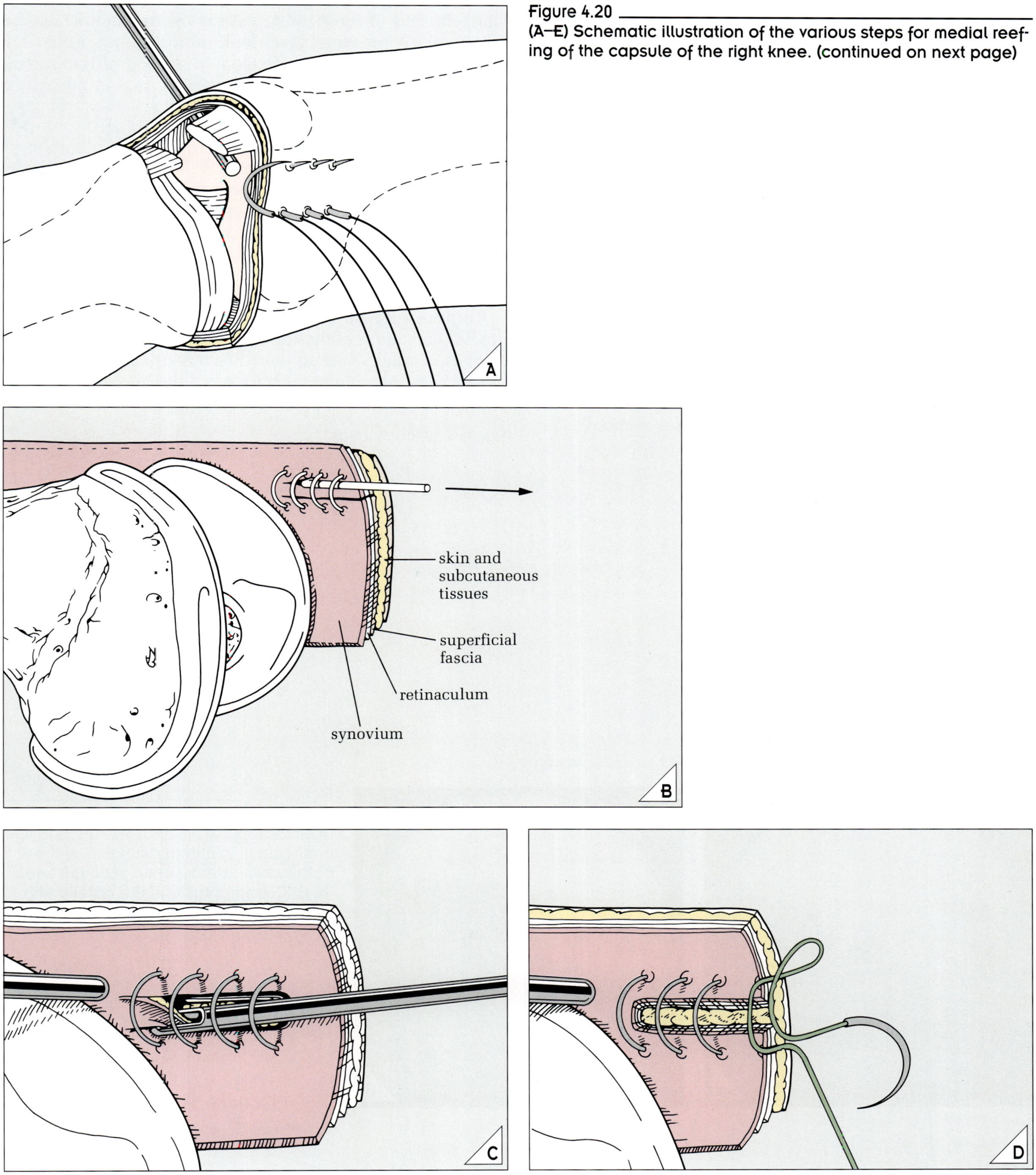

Postoperatively, the patient is placed in a knee immobilizer for 1 or 2 weeks and is discharged the same day on crutches. Following this period of immobilization, active assisted range of motion up to 45° of flexion is encouraged. At 6 weeks, the knee immobilizer is replaced by a patellar alignment brace allowing full knee flexion and an intensive program of rehabilitation is started. Complete recovery may take 5 to 6 months.

Complications and Pitfalls of Lateral Release and Medial Capsular Reefing

Arthroscopic lateral release is not an innocuous procedure and careful patient selection, as well as meticulous attention to the technical details, is paramount for a successful outcome. The ideal indication should be a patient with a tight lateral capsule with or without chondromalacic changes of the patella. Lateral release should not be systematic whenever any chondroplasty is performed for patellar chondromalacia. Extensive release of the vastus lateralis should be avoided as well as laceration of the quadriceps tendon. By placing the capsular incision closer to the patella, bleeding will be minimal. If the tourniquet is in use, it should be released in order to obtain control of the bleeding with electrocautery. A suction drain may or may not be used; however, it cannot be a substitute for good hemostasis. Quadriceps insufficiency with medial subluxation of the patella secondary to an aggressive release of the vastus lateralis and severe hemarthrosis with subsequent arthrofibrosis are serious potential complications of this procedure.

To avoid amputation of the suture material during medial capsule reefing, the skin around the needle punctures is incised while the needles are still in place, rather than during subcutaneous burying of the knots.

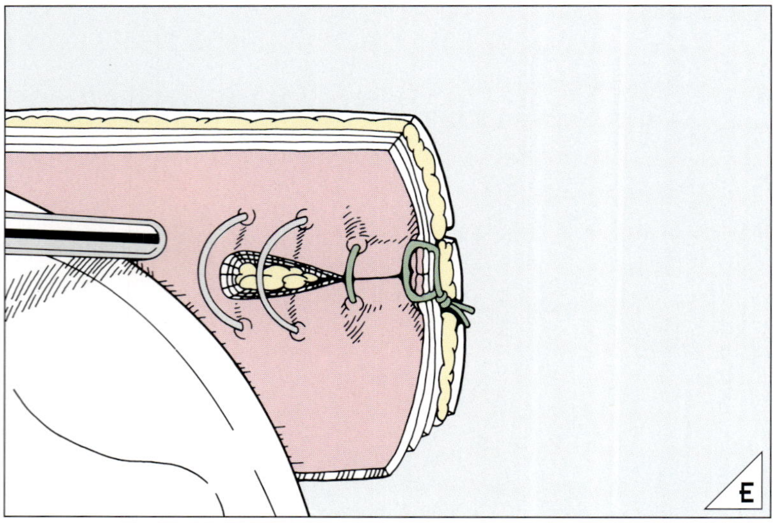

Figure 4.20 (continued)

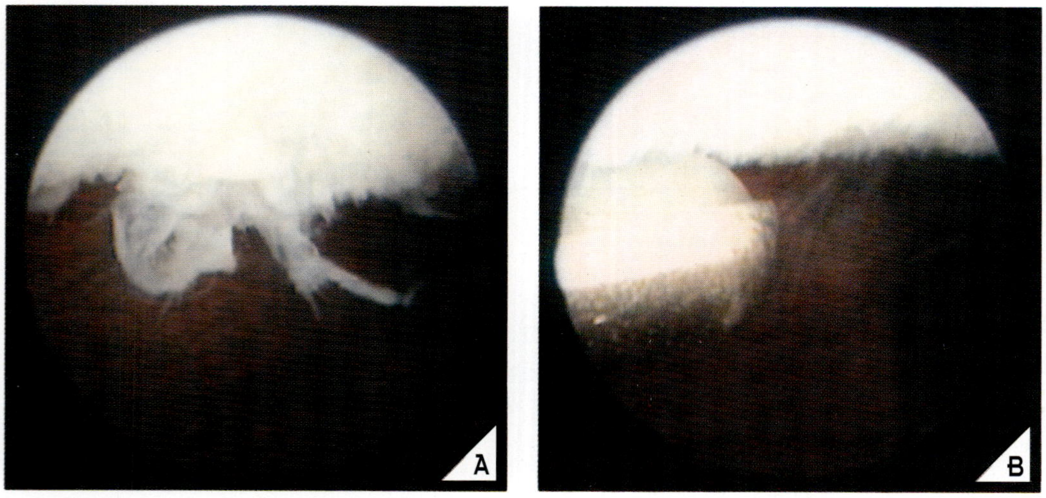

Figure 4.21
Arthroscopic visualization of various steps of chondroplasty, medial reefing, and lateral release in chondromalacia of the patella with lateral subluxation left knee. (A, B) Chondroplasty of the patella with motorized shaver. (continued on next page)

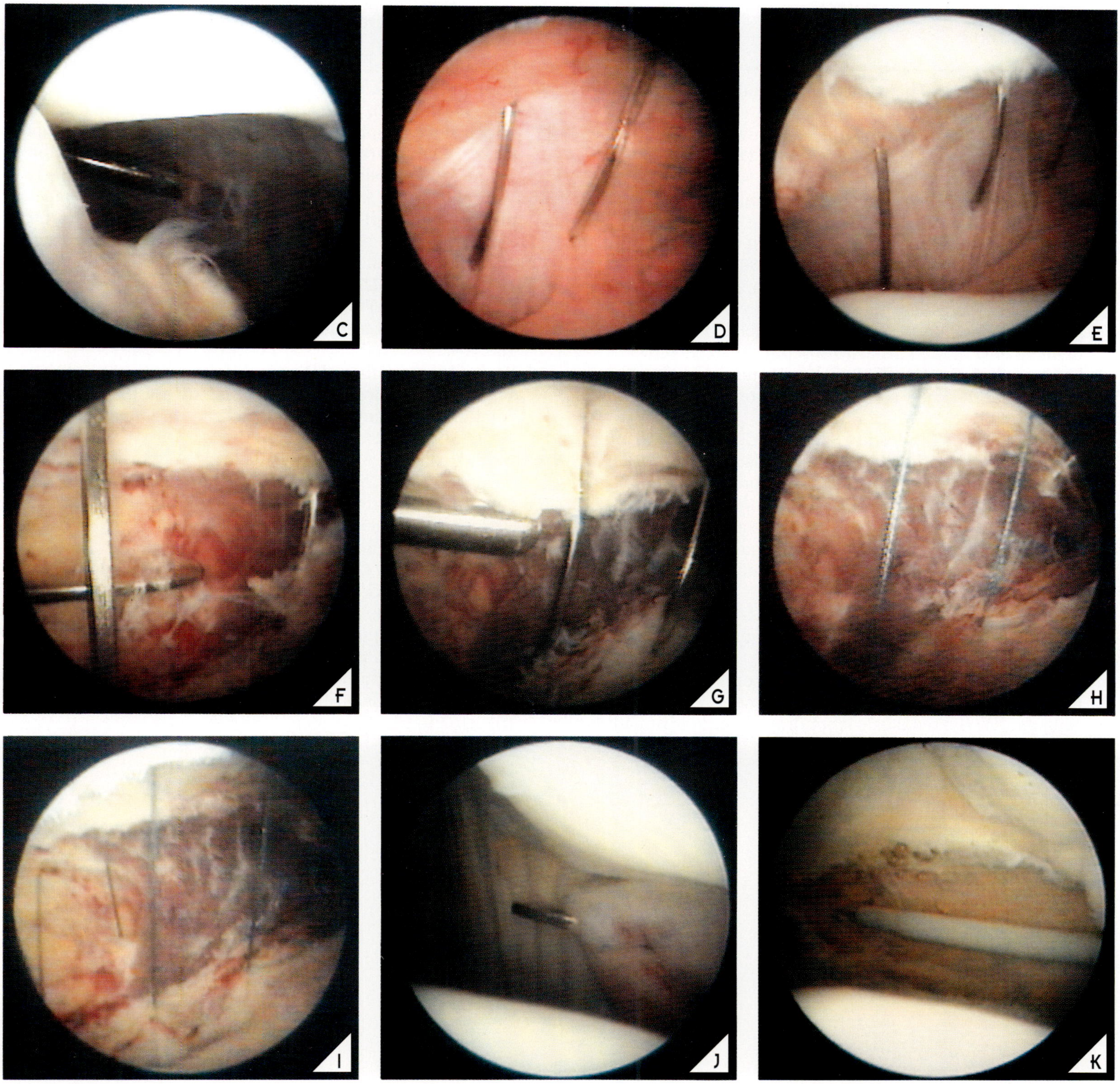

Figure 4.21 (continued)
(C) Lateral subluxation. (D–I) Steps of medial capsular reefing. (J, K) Lateral retinacular release.

REFERENCES

1. Jackson RW, et al. The pathologic medial shelf. *Orthop Clin North Am.* 1982;13:307.
2. Patel D. Arthroscopy of the plica—synovial folds and their significance. *Am J Sports Med.* 1978;6:217–225.
3. Pipkin G. Knee injuries: the role of the suprapatellar plica and suprapatellar bursa in simulating internal derangement. *Clin Orthop.* 1971;74:161.
4. Ilino S. Normal arthroscopic findings in the knee joint in adult cadavers. *J Jpn Orthop Assoc.* 1939;14:467.
5. Brief LP, Laico JP. The superolateral approach: a better view of the medial patellar plica. *Arthroscopy.* 1987;3:170–172.
6. Meislin R, Parisien JS. Arthroscopic excision of synovial hemangioma of the knee. *Arthroscopy.* 1990;6:64–67.
7. Moskovich R, Parisien JS. Localized pigmented villonodular synovitis of the knee: arthroscopic treatment. *Clin Orthop Rel Res.* 1991;271:218–224.
8. Kelley W, Harris ED, Ruddy S, Sledge CB, eds. *Textbook of Rheumatology.* Philadelphia, Pa: WB Saunders Co., 1989.
9. Guaydier-Souquieres C, et al. Knee arthroscopy after yttrium or osmic acid injection. *Arthroscopy.* 1989;5:70–75.
10. Sledge CB, Zuckerman JD et al. Synovectomy of the rheumatoid knee using intra-articular injection of dysprosium 165, ferric hydroxide macroaggregates. *J Bone Joint Surg.* 1987; 69(A):970–975.
11. Tsahakis PJ, et al. The role of radiation synovectomy in the treatment of pigmented villonodular synovitis of the knee. *Orthop Transactions.* 1991;15:701.
12. Ogilvie-Harris DJ, Basinski A. Arthroscopic synovectomy of the knee for rheumatoid arthritis. *Arthroscopy.* 1991;7:91–97.
13. Milgram JW. Synovial osteochondromatosis: a histopathologic study of thirty-one cases. *J Bone Joint Surg.* 1977; 59(A):792.
14. Dorfmann H, et al. Arthroscopic treatment of synovial chondromatosis of the knee. *Arthroscopy.* 1989;5:48–51.
15. Ogilvie-Harris DJ, McLean J, Zarnett ME. Pigmented villonodular synovitis of the knee: the results of total arthroscopic synovectomy, partial arthroscopic synovectomy, and arthroscopic local excision. *J Bone Joint Surg.* 1992;74(A):119–123.
16. Wiedel JD. Arthroscopic synovectomy for chronic hemophilic synovitis of the knee. *Arthroscopy.* 1985;1:205–209.
17. Parisien JS. Role of arthroscopy in the treatment of postoperative fibroarthrosis of the knee joint. *Clin Orthop Rel Res.* 1988;229:185–192.
18. Sprague NF III, O'Connor RL, Fox JM. Treatment of postoperative knee fibroarthrosis. *Clin Orthop Rel Res.* 1982; 166:165.
19. Paulos LE, Rosenberg TD, et al. Infrapatellar contracture syndrome, an unrecognized cause of knee stiffness with patella entrapment and patella infera. *Am J Sports Med.* 1981;15:331–341.
20. Ivey M, Clark R. Arthroscopic debridement of the knee for septic arthritis. *Clin Orthop Rel Res.* 1985;199:201.
21. Jackson RW. Arthroscopic treatment of the septic knee. *Arthroscopy.* 1985;1:194.
22. Parisien JS, Shaffer B. Arthroscopic management of pyarthrosis. *Clin Orthop Rel Res.* 1992;275:243–247.
23. Fox J, Sherman O, Pevsner D. Patello-femoral problems and malalignment. In: McGinty J, ed. *Arthroscopic Surgery Update: Techniques in Orthopedics.* Baltimore, Md: University Park Press; 1985:31–57.
24. Metcalf R. An arthroscopic method for lateral release of the subluxating or dislocating patella. *Clin Orthop Rel Res.* 1982;167:9–18.

chapter Five

Endoscopic Technique for ACL Reconstruction of the Knee

David S. Menche

Prior to arthroscopic intervention, assessment of total ligament instability should be performed by examination under anesthesia. If a diagnosis of anterior cruciate ligament instability is confirmed, harvesting the bone-patellar tendon-bone graft prior to arthroscopic intervention is preferred. Obviously, if there is any doubt regarding the diagnosis, initial arthroscopy should be performed to document pathology.

Preparing the Bone-Patellar Tendon-Bone Graft

A longitudinal skin incision is made, centered over the patellar tendon (Fig. 5.1A). The skin incision is carried down through the subcutaneous tissues to expose the paratenon. The paratenon is incised in line with the skin incision, exposing the medial and lateral border of the patellar tendon (Fig. 5.1B).

After the full width of the patellar tendon is identified, a 10 mm bone-patellar tendon-bone graft is outlined using methylene blue (Fig. 5.2A,B). Bone tendon junctions are identified and bone blocks 25 mm long and 10 mm wide are outlined with a knife. In marking the tendon graft, at least 10 mm of tendon must remain on both the medial and lateral borders in order to prevent patellar tendon rupture. Longitudinal cuts are made through the full thickness of the patellar tendon prior to obtaining bone blocks.

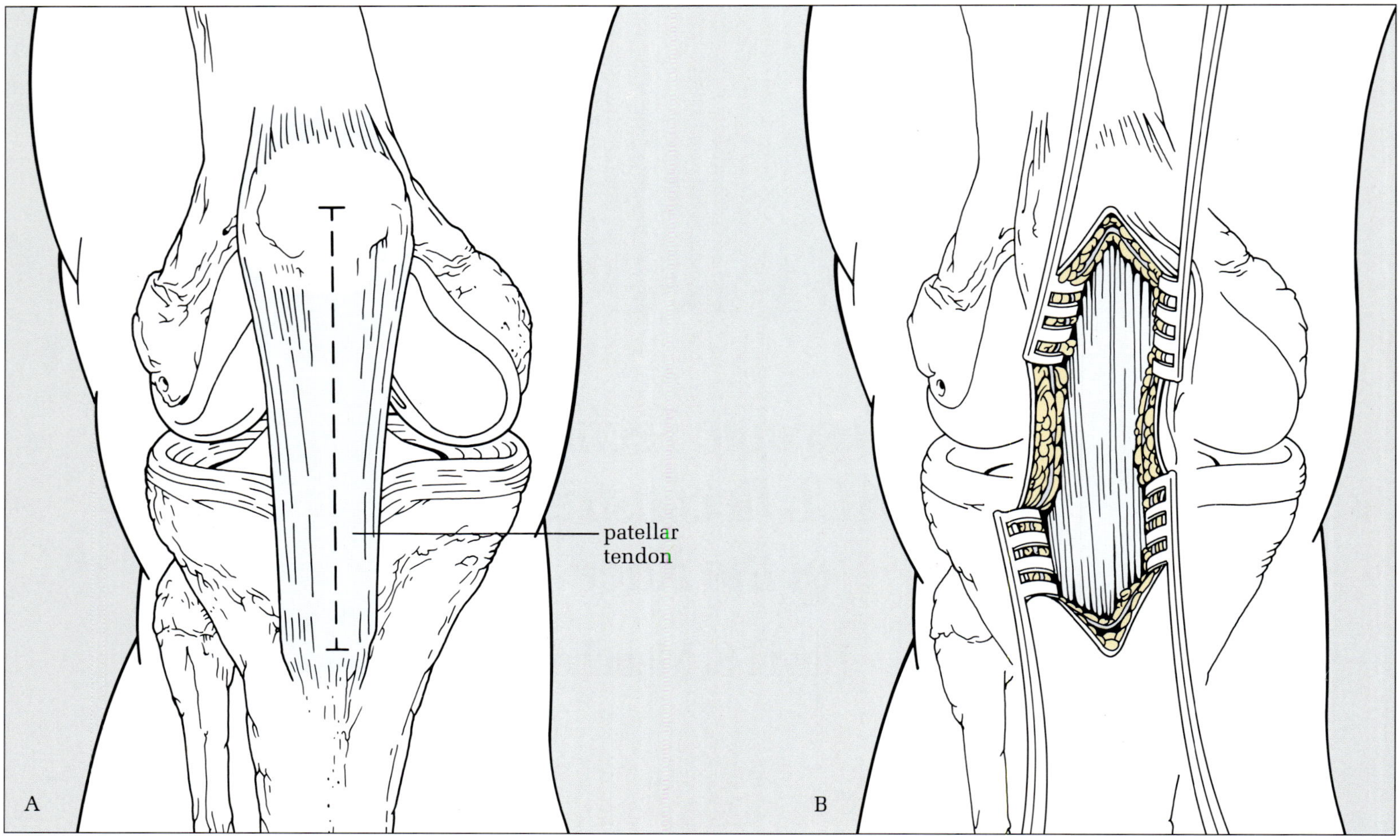

Figure 5.1

(A) Skin Incision. An incision is made centered over the patellar tendon and extends from the patella to the level of the tibial tubercle. (B) Exposing the patellar tendon. Self-retaining retractors are placed into the wound, retracting the paratenon in order to identify the full width of the patellar tendon.

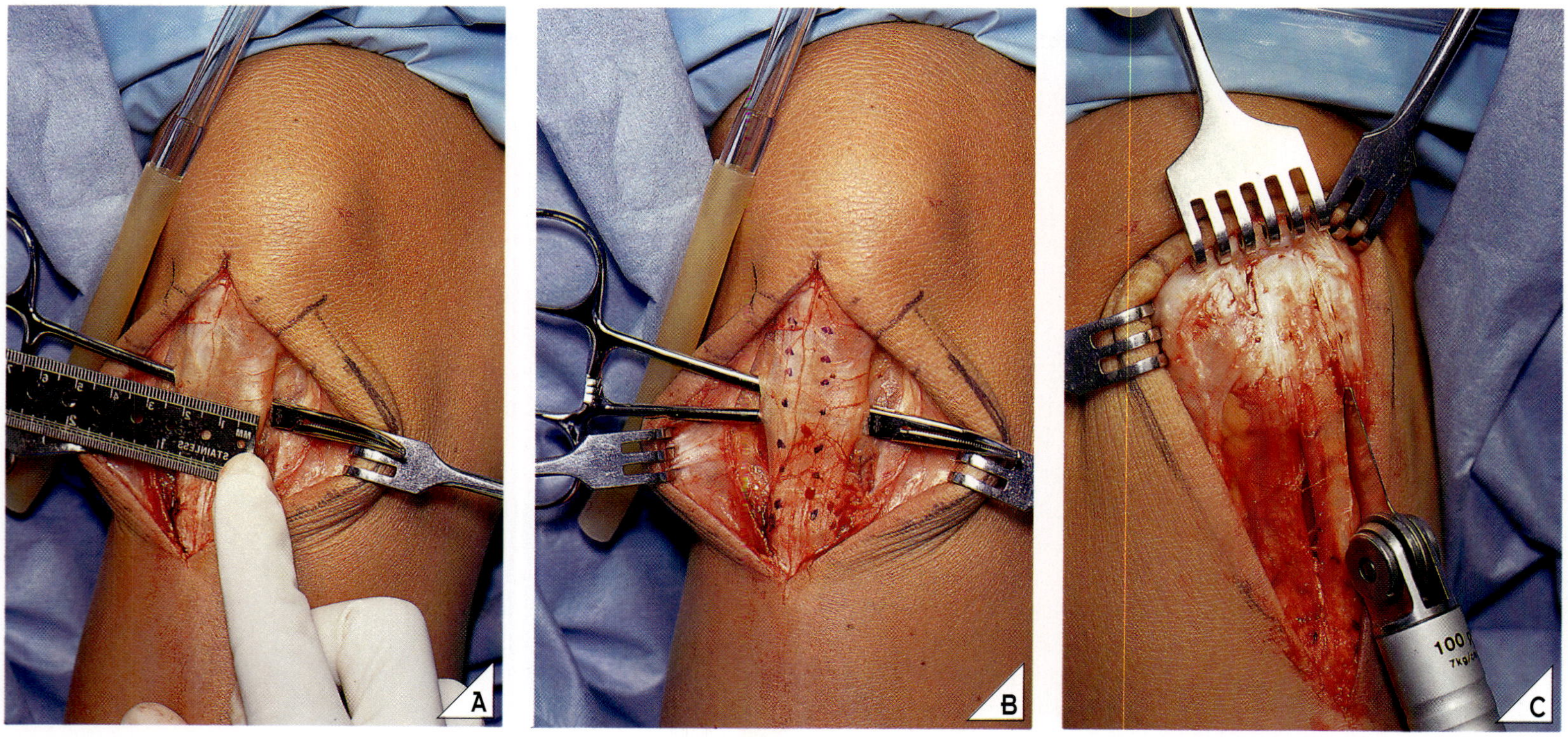

Figure 5.2

(A, B) Measuring the bone-tendon-bone autograft. Methylene blue is used to outline a 10 mm bone-tendon-bone autograft. (C) Harvesting the patellar bone block. Longitudinal cuts are made by placing the microsagittal saw at the bone-tendon junction and pushing the blade proximally until the transverse mark is reached.

When harvesting the bone block from the patella, the longitudinal cuts are made by placing the microsagittal saw at the bone-tendon junction and pushing the blade proximally until the transverse mark is reached (Fig. 5.2C). The transverse cut is then made to a depth of 4 to 5 mm. A triangular bone block is created by placing the saw in the longitudinal cuts at a 45° angle and aiming the saw towards the midline of the graft. Care should be taken not to penetrate the articular surface. A 1 inch curved osteotome is used to complete the osteotomy (Fig. 5.3). By paying careful attention not to torque the graft, fractures of the bone blocks are avoided. The tibial bone block is created at the level of the tibial tubercle with the microsagittal saw. A curved osteotome is used to deliver the tibial bone block. The bone blocks are removed, making sure to obtain the full thickness of the patellar tendon fibers and leaving the fat pad in place. Penetration of the fat pad creates unwarranted extravasation. Careful dissection is necessary at the bone-tendon junction in order to avoid violating this area.

On a separate table the bone block is prepared by removing extraneous tissue to allow clear visualization during graft passage. The bone blocks should pass snugly through a 10 mm sizer in both directions in case removal of the graft is necessary. The bone block, which is to be placed into the femur, is prepared from the larger tibial bone block. A 2 mm AP drill hole is made in this bone block approximately 4 mm from the distal end. A #1 Mersilene suture is placed through the hole but not tied. The bone-patellar tendon junction is marked with methylene blue for identification during graft passage.

The bone block obtained from the patella, which will be secured to the tibia, is prepared by drilling three equally spaced AP holes into the bone block. A #5 Tycron suture is placed through each drill hole and tied over the end of the bone block. Again, methylene blue is used to mark the bone-tendon junction (Fig. 5.4). A 3M

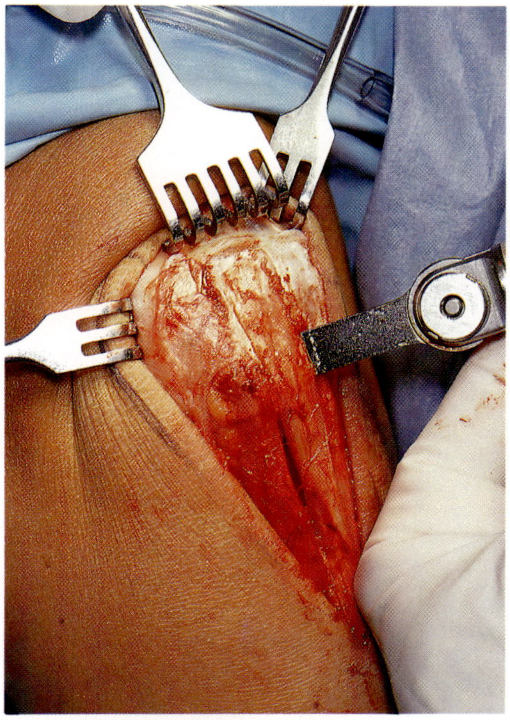

Figure 5.3

Completing the osteotomy. The microsagittal saw is placed at a 45° angle and aimed towards the midline of the graft.

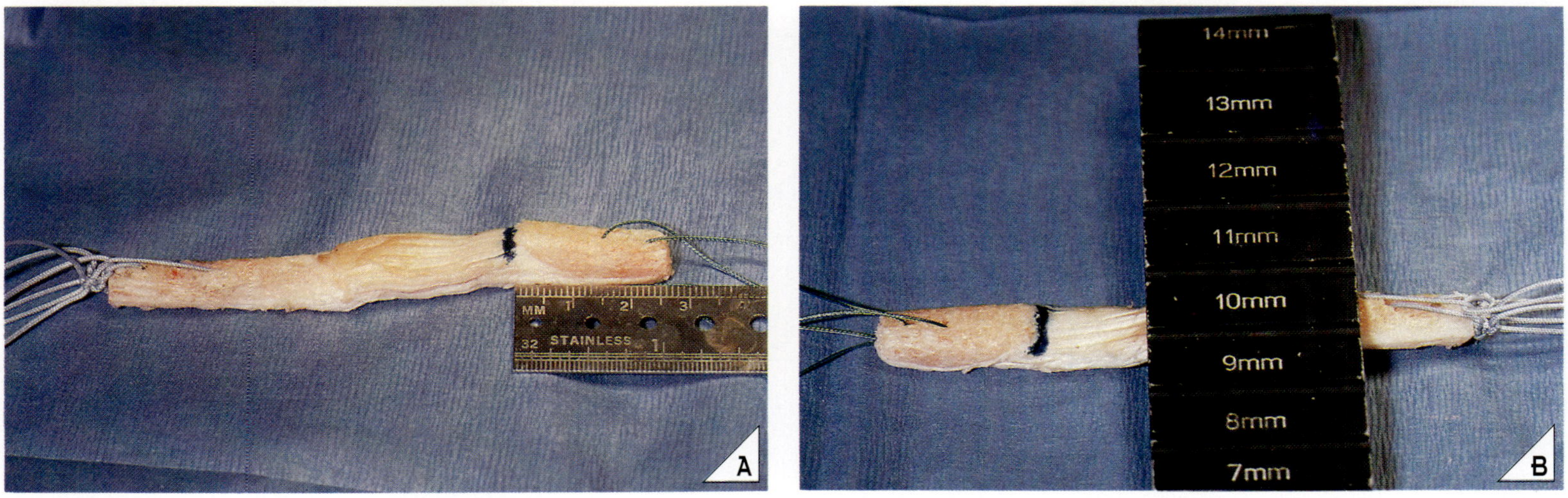

Figure 5.4

(A) Prepared graft. (B) The graft should fit snugly through a 10 mm sizer. The bone block obtained from the patella is used distally and three 2 mm AP drill holes are created. A #5 Tycron suture is placed through each drill hole and tied over the top. A 2 mm AP drill hole is placed through the bone block obtained from the tibia with a #1 Mersilene suture passed through it but not tied. Methylene blue is used to mark the bone-tendon junctions.

tensioner is used to prestress the graft prior to placing it within the knee (Fig. 5.5).

Surgical Technique

The superomedial and anterolateral portals are made using standard techniques. Arthroscopic evaluation is performed, identifying associated pathology. The anteromedial portal is selected by placing an 18-gauge needle directly over the anterior horn of the medial meniscus (Fig. 5.6). If a meniscal repair is necessary, the sutures are passed but not tied until the end of the procedure.

In performing the endoscopic technique, a significant archplasty (notchplasty) is required to visualize the anatomic femoral point adequately (Fig. 5.7). A combination of hand and power instrumentation is necessary to create an acceptable notch for this procedure. Initially, a 5.5 synovial resector is used to remove the remaining tibial stump down to bone (Fig. 5.8). This enhances visualization of the tibial tunnel and allows easy passage of the graft. In addition, it removes soft tissue debris that could create a cyclops lesion, which has been known to contribute to arthrofibrosis postoperatively. Next, all soft tissue along the medial aspect of the lateral femoral condyle should be removed. A half-moon rasp facilitates this aspect of the procedure (Fig. 5.9). An arthroscopic burr is then used to create a vertical wall, removing all ridges until the articular cartilage of the posterior aspect of the lateral femoral condyle is clearly identified (Fig. 5.10). As the arch is prepared posteriorly, the posterior cruciate ligament will become visible, and the instrumentation should lie between the posterior cruciate ligament and the lateral wall. The most important part of the archplasty/roofplasty

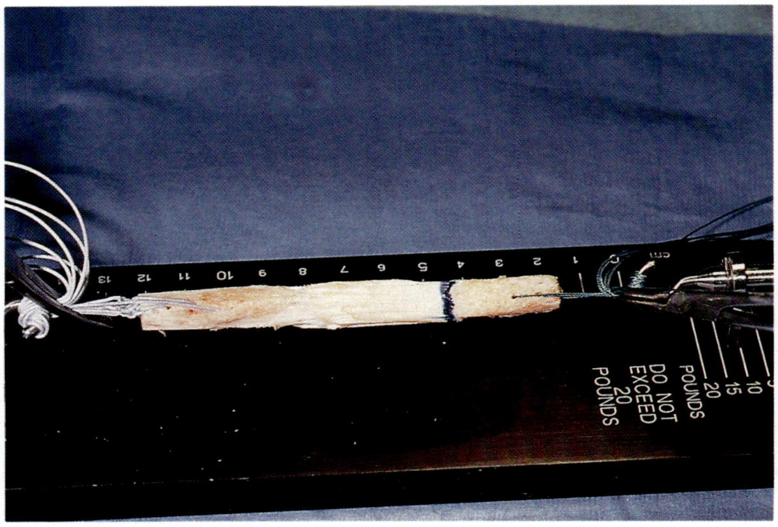

Figure 5.5
3M tensioning device. After the graft is prepared, the bone-tendon-bone graft is placed on the 3M tensioning device to prestress the graft.

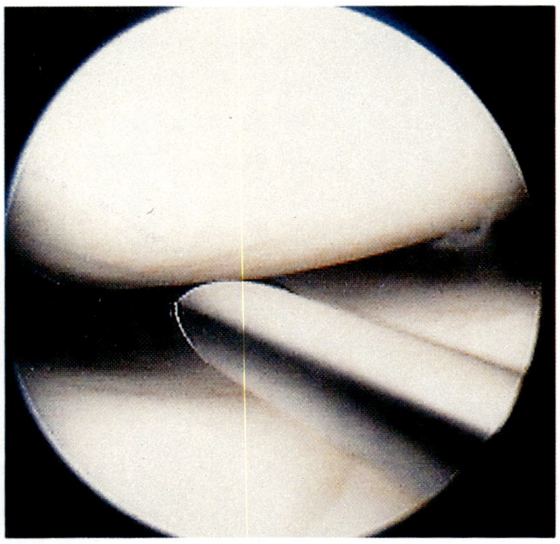

Figure 5.6
Anteromedial portal. The anteromedial portal is determined by placing an 18-gauge needle over the anterior horn of the medial meniscus. This portal site will provide better access to the intercondylar notch.

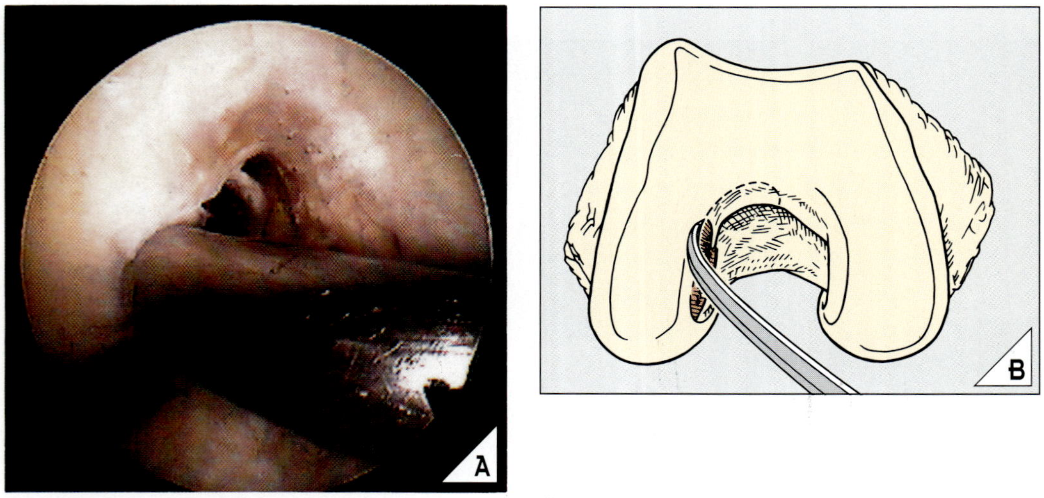

Figure 5.7
Anterior notchplasty. This arthroscopic view (A) and schematic illustration (B) show an outline of the notchplasty to be performed. The extent of the notchplasty varies, depending on the chronicity of the case and individual anatomic variations.

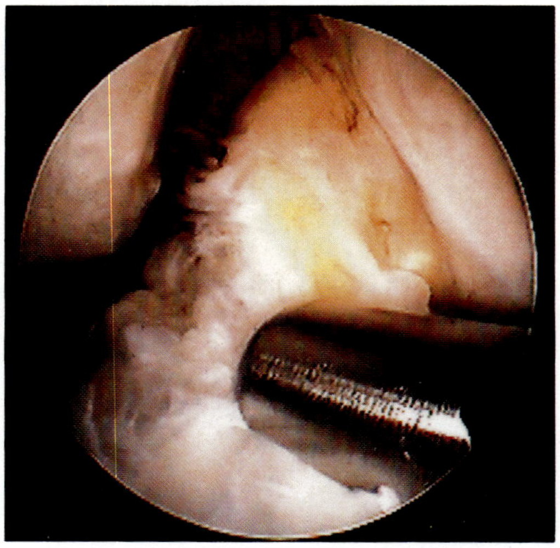

Figure 5.8
Synovial tibial stump. A 5.5 synovial resector is used to remove the tibial stump down to bone.

is insuring that there is enough room laterally as well as superiorly to avoid impingement. As the archplasty is being performed, the knee is taken from a relatively extended position to a flexed position greater than 90°. At the completion of the archplasty, excellent visualization of the over-the-top position as well as superior clearance for the graft should be obtained (Fig. 5.11).

The anatomic point on the femoral side is then chosen. Complete removal of the femoral anterior cruciate ligament stump and visualization of the articular cartilage on the most posterior aspect of the lateral femoral condyle are critical for proper placement. With increased flexion of the knee the anatomic point is easier to visualize (Fig. 5.12). A 5.5 mm burr or curette may be used to mark this

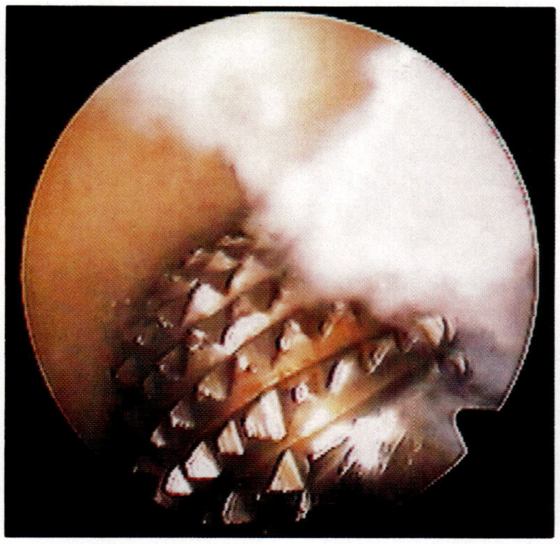

Figure 5.9
Half-moon rasp. A half-moon rasp is very effective for removing soft tissue and bony ridges along the medial aspect of the lateral femoral condyle.

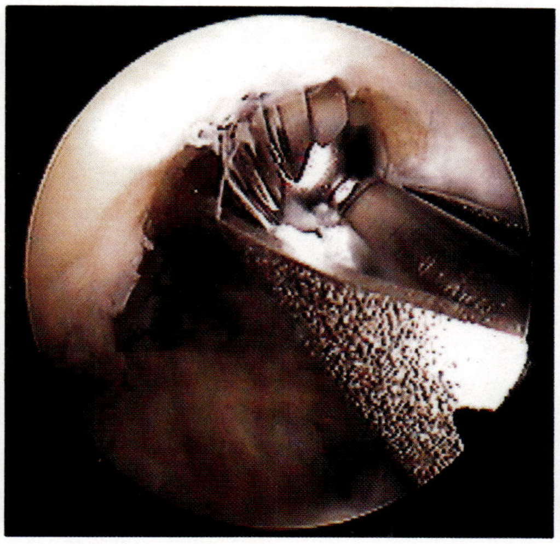

Figure 5.10
Use of the arthroscopic burr. The arthroscopic burr may be used in reverse as it will give the surgeon more control. All ridges should be removed until a vertical wall is created and the posterior aspect of the lateral femoral condyle is easily identified.

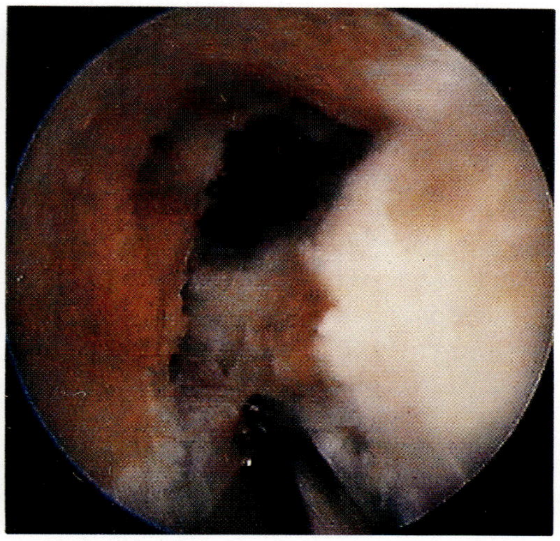

Figure 5.11
Complete archplasty. The archplasty is complete when the vertical wall is created and excellent visualization is obtained.

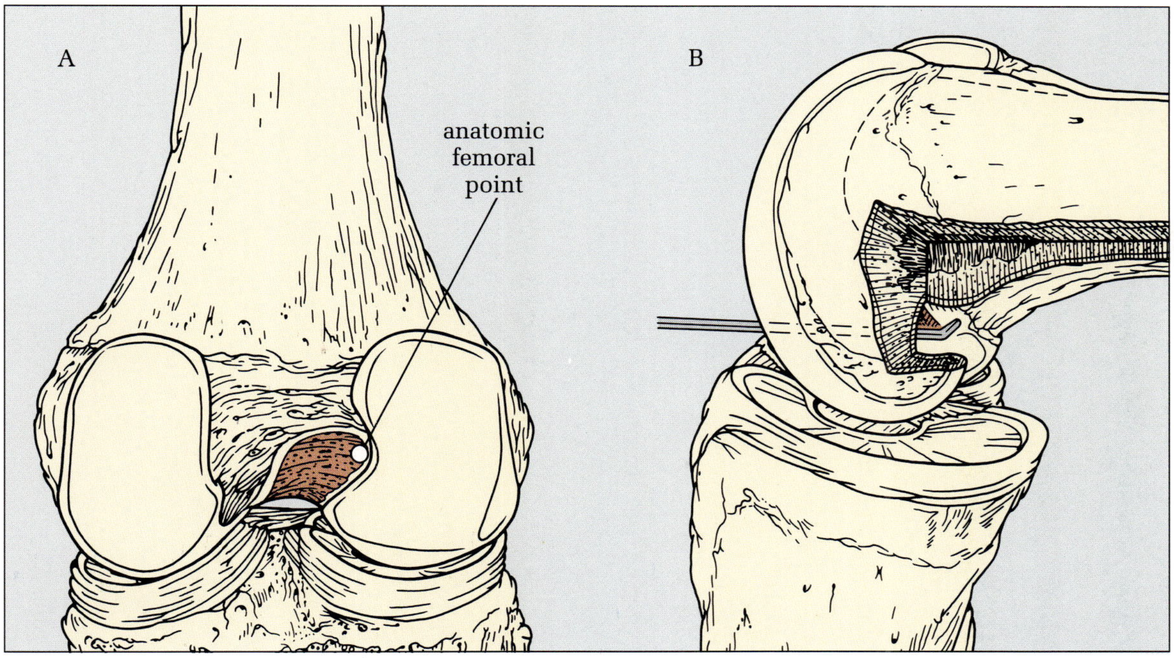

Figure 5.12
Anatomic femoral point, posterior view. (A) The anatomic femoral point shown in the diagram is high on the notch, close to the over-the-top position. (B) Cut-away view of the anatomic femoral point. (continued on next page)

area (Fig. 5.13). When marking the point with a 5.5 mm burr the knee should first be flexed to 90°. The burr is placed at the 9 o'clock position in the right knee or the 3 o'clock position in the left knee, and it is brought forward one burr width and then superior one burr width to lie at the junction of the wall and the roof of the notch. Since the surgeon is drilling a 10 mm hole, a 5 mm clearance from the posterior margin of the femoral condyle is necessary to avoid penetrating the posterior cortex. The point is then confirmed using a probe from the anteromedial portal to insure proper anatomic placement (Fig. 5.14). The most common error is anterior placement of the femoral hole in a nonanatomic position.

Next, the tibial anatomic point is identified using the Acufex endoscopic guide. The guide is placed through the anteromedial portal, and the location of the pin entry into the proximal tibia is identified. When performing the endoscopic technique, it is critical to make sure that the entry of the tibial pin is at the level of the tibial tubercle and not proximal to it. If, when placing the guide, a point proximal to the tibial tubercle is obtained, an accessory portal just medial to the patellar tendon and distal to the initial anteromedial portal should be created. This will place the guide in a more distal position and at the level of the tibial tubercle. Alternatively, using the new Acufex guide, adjustments in the angle of the guide may be made, thus maintaining the original anteromedial portal site. The point of the guide is placed in the tibial anatomic site central and just anterior to the posterior cruciate ligament. This posterior point has the advantage of preventing impingement in the postoperative period while still maintaining an anatomic position. Recent studies have shown an increased postoperative range of motion when choosing this more posterior point. A guide pin is then drilled through the guide into the proximal tibia. The intraarticular penetration of the pin is viewed arthroscopically (Fig. 5.15).

A closed-end curette is placed over the pin to prevent accidental protrusion into the posterior cruciate ligament. Next, a 10 mm cannulated reamer is advanced over the pin. A combination of hand and power instrumentation is used to remove the debris around the tibial tunnel (Fig.

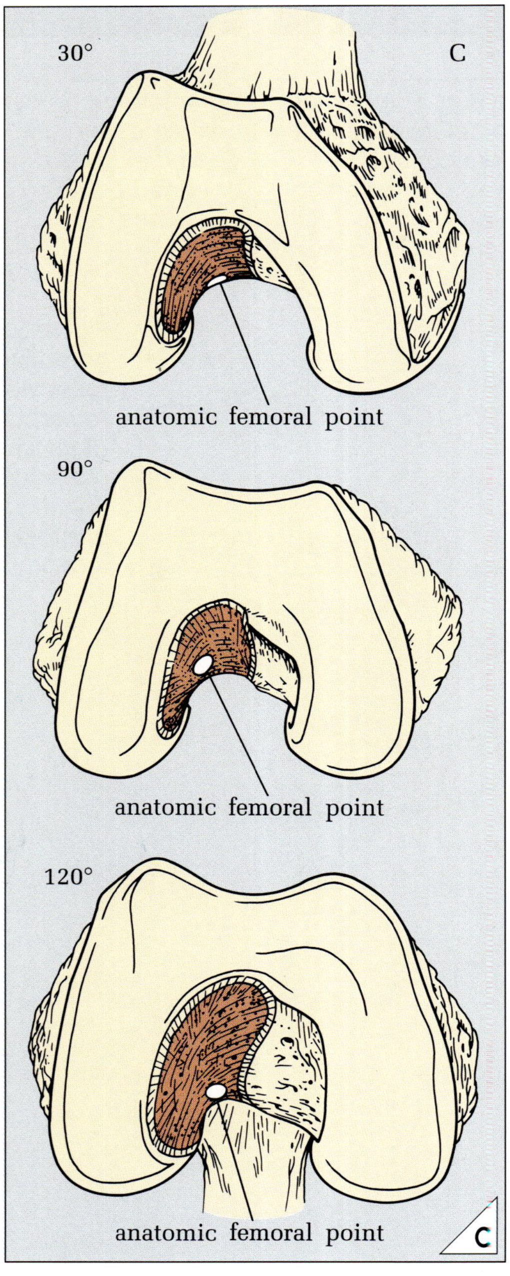

Figure 5.12 (continued)
(C) With increased flexion of the knee, the anatomic point is more directly in view.

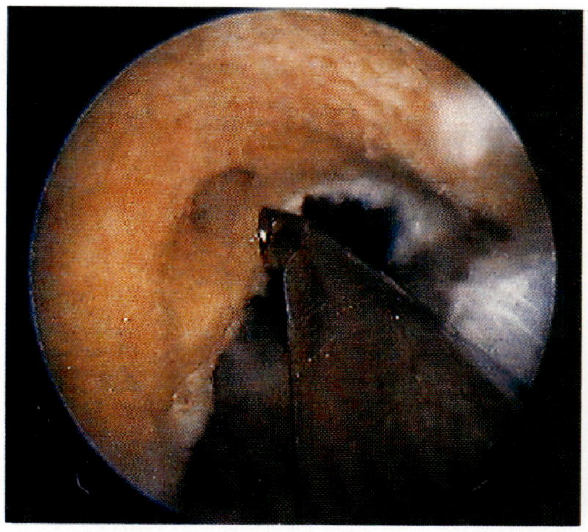

Figure 5.13
Marking the anatomic femoral point. After the femoral point is chosen, a burr or curette is used to mark this area for future reference.

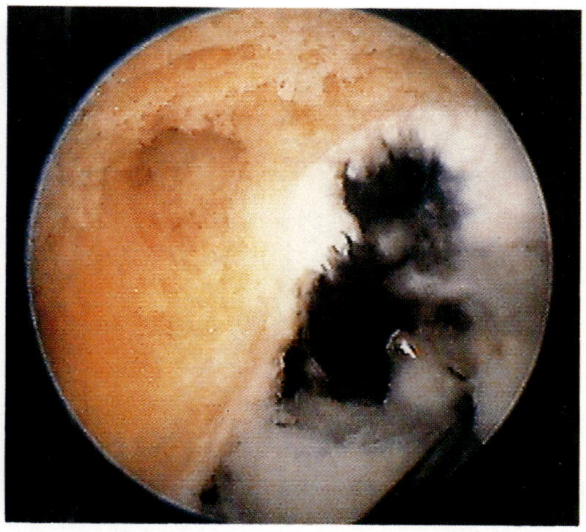

Figure 5.14
Confirming the anatomic point. The arthroscope is placed through the anteromedial portal to confirm the proposed placement.

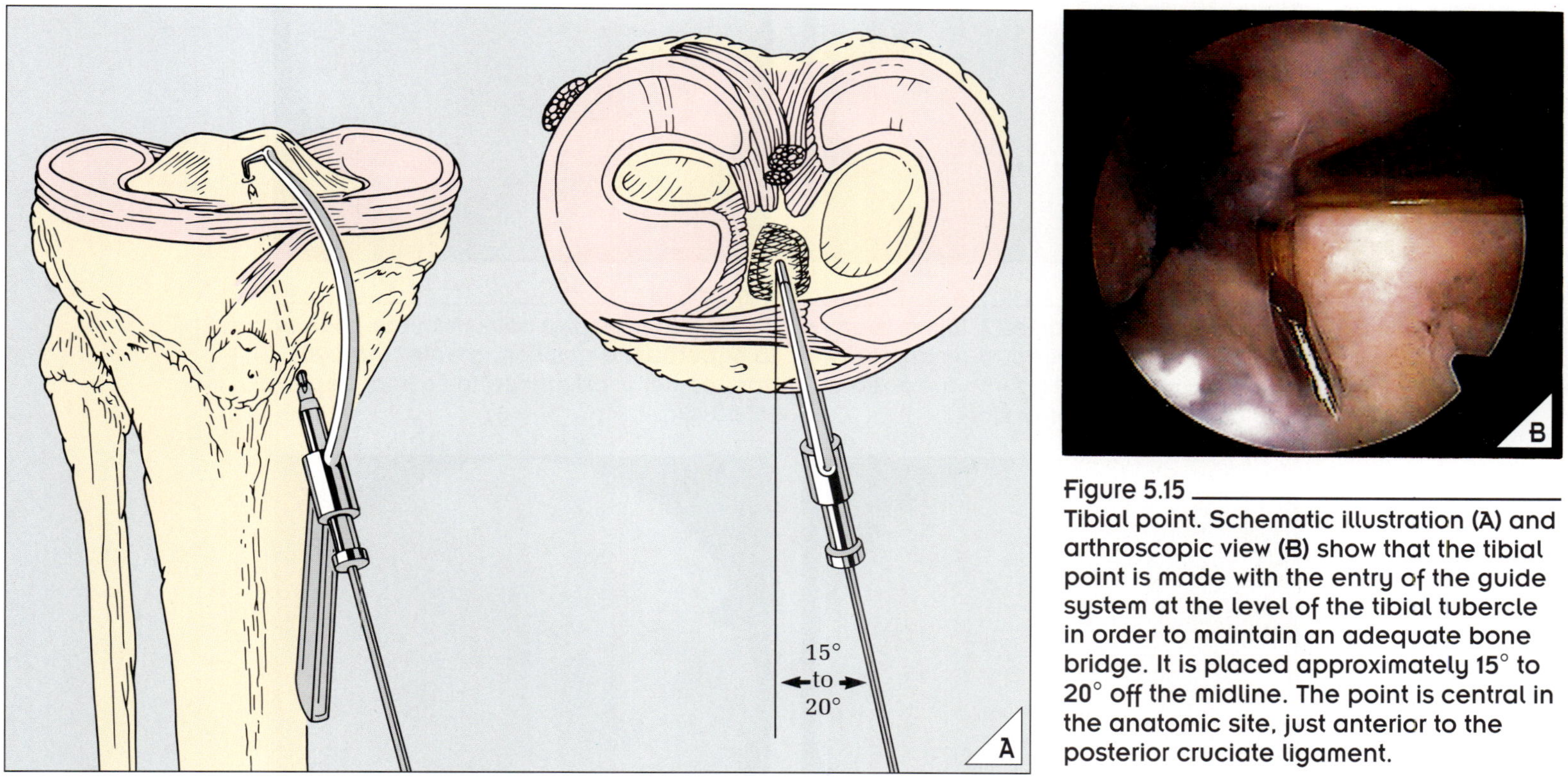

Figure 5.15
Tibial point. Schematic illustration (A) and arthroscopic view (B) show that the tibial point is made with the entry of the guide system at the level of the tibial tubercle in order to maintain an adequate bone bridge. It is placed approximately 15° to 20° off the midline. The point is central in the anatomic site, just anterior to the posterior cruciate ligament.

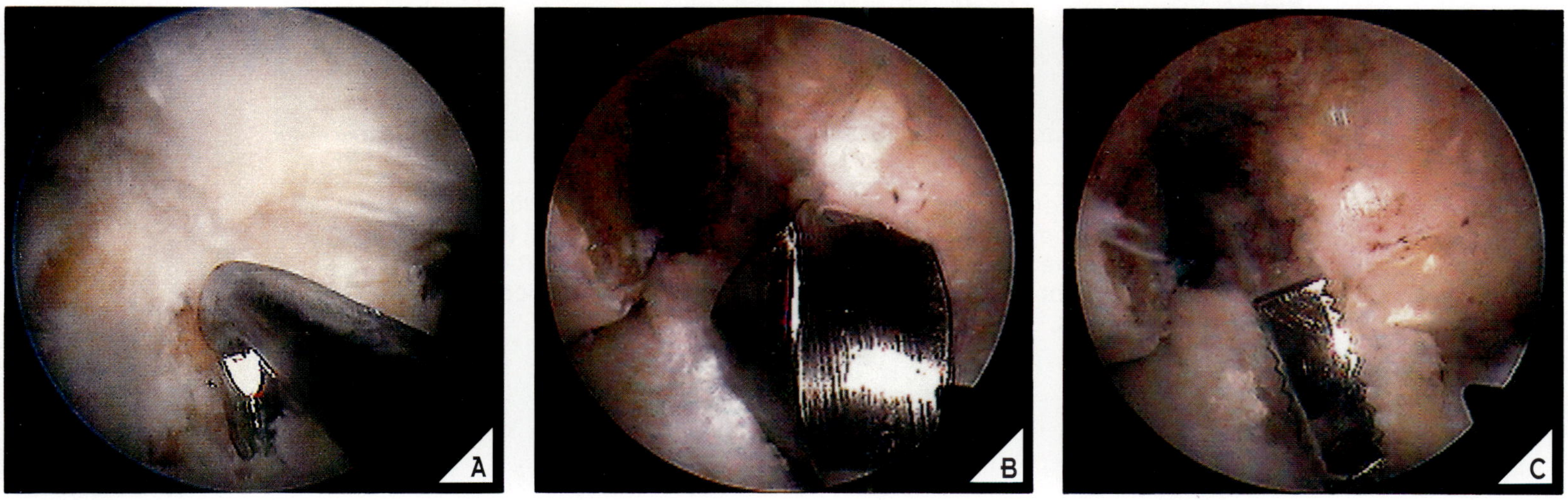

Figure 5.16
Creation of the tibial tunnel. (A) A closed-end curette is placed over the guide pin to prevent accidental protrusion. (B) The tibial tunnel is reamed. (C) The tibial tunnel is carefully chamfered.

5.16). With the knee flexed to approximately 30°, the 10 mm reamer is placed into the tibial tunnel and advanced to the predetermined point on the femur (Fig. 5.17). Once the reaming is started, the knee is hyperflexed and the reamer advanced to a final depth of 30 mm (Fig. 5.18). After the reaming is completed, debris is removed with the synovial resector, and the femoral hole is carefully chamfered.

The arthroscope is passed through the tibial tunnel, providing full visualization of the femoral hole (Fig. 5.19) and documenting that no posterior penetration has occurred. Posterior penetration is prevented by hyperflexion during reaming. In addition, the tibial tunnel may be visualized to confirm that no penetration of the anterior tibial wall has occurred (Fig. 5.20).

After the femoral hole is reamed with the knee in the hyperflexed position, it is critical that this position be maintained until femoral fixation is performed. The arthroscope is next placed back into the anterolateral portal. A Beeth-type pin is placed through the tibial tunnel into the femoral hole and drilled out the thigh superolaterally. The #1 Mersilene suture that was placed through

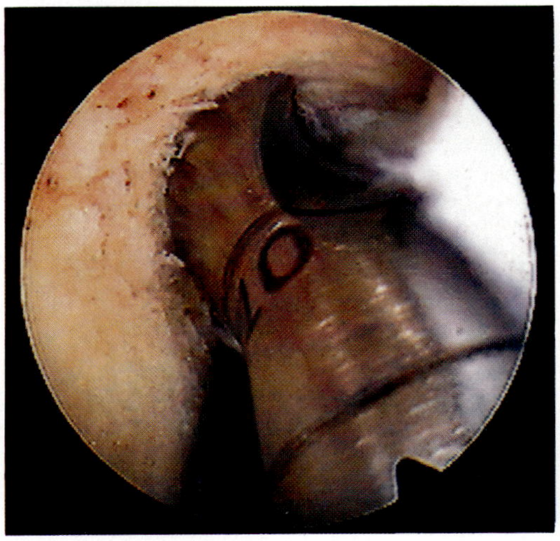

Figure 5.17
Placement of the reamer. A 10 mm reamer is placed into the previously marked anatomic point, starting with the knee at approximately 30° of flexion.

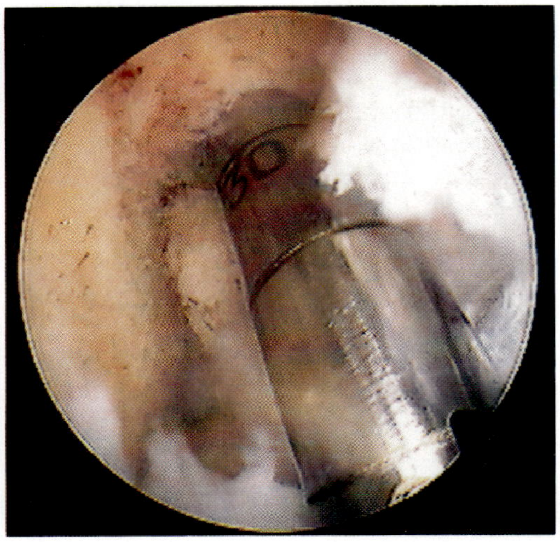

Figure 5.18
Drilling the femoral hole. With the knee in a hyperflexed position, greater than 90°, the reamer is advanced to its final depth of 30 mm.

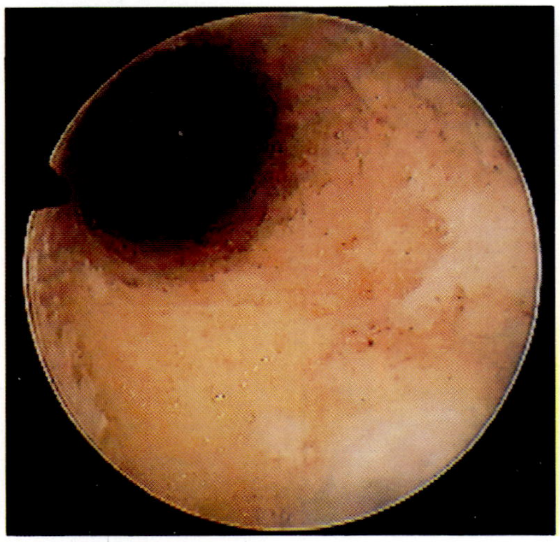

Figure 5.19
Visualization of the femoral hole. The arthroscope is placed through the tibial tunnel to visualize the femoral hole fully and to document that no posterior penetration has occurred.

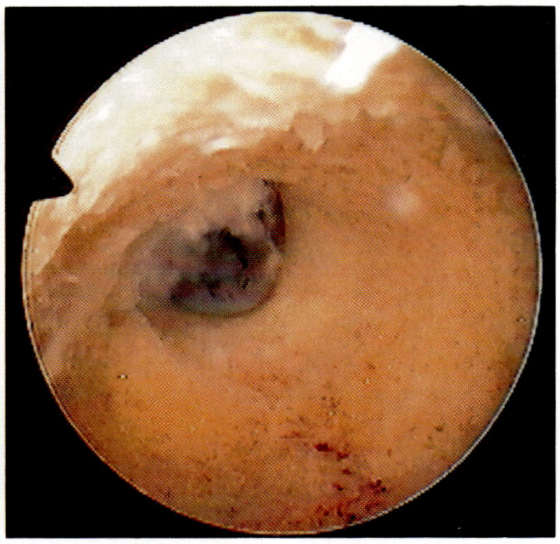

Figure 5.20
Visualization of the tibial tunnel. In a similar fashion, the tibial tunnel is fully visualized to confirm that no anterior tibial wall breakage has occurred.

the femoral bone block is placed into the eye of the Beeth pin. The Beeth pin is removed manually, pulling the Mersilene suture out through the skin (Fig. 5.21). The bone block is then passed through the tibial tunnel with simple traction on the Mersilene suture. A probe is placed into the knee joint to facilitate atraumatic passage of the graft into the femoral hole. With continued traction on the suture, the bone block is passed into the femoral hole with the cancellous portion of bone facing anteriorly (Fig. 5.22A). If the bone block is difficult to pass into the femoral hole, flexion of the knee should be checked. A bone tamp may be used carefully to assist in this part of the procedure.

The femoral bone block is advanced into the femoral hole until the bone-tendon junction is flush with the entrance of the hole (Fig. 5.22B). An 18-gauge needle is placed through the anteromedial portal to insure parallel endoscopic placement of the interference screw (Fig.

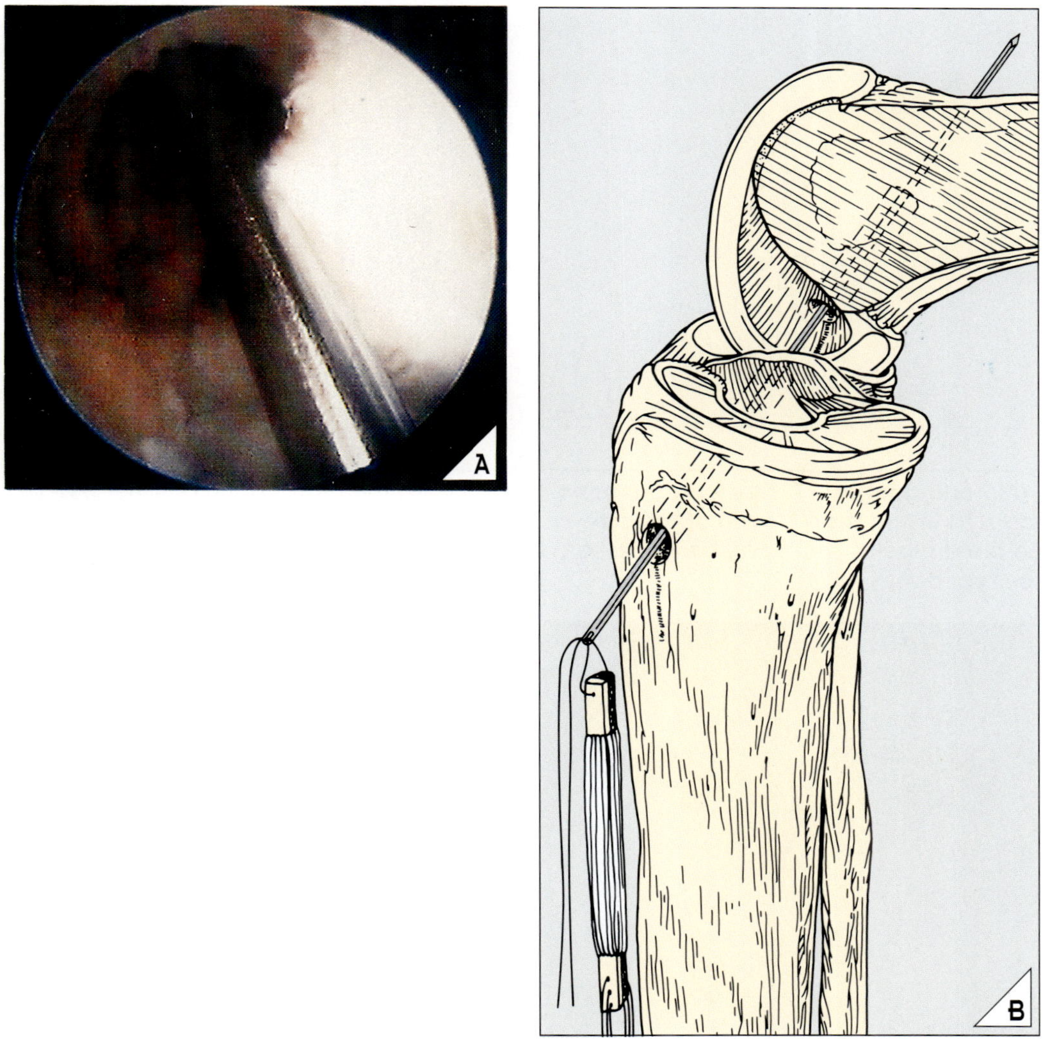

Figure 5.21
Beeth pin. (A) With the knee maintained in a hyperflexed position, the Beeth pin is placed through the tibial tunnel, into the femoral hole, and drilled out the skin superolaterally. (B) A #1 Mersilene suture attached to the femoral bone block is placed through the hole of the Beeth pin and the Beeth pin is subsequently removed manually. (Adapted with permission from Rosenberg TD. Endoscopic Technique for ACL Reconstruction With Pro-Trac Tibial Guide. Mansfield, Ma: Acufex Microsurgical, Inc; 1991:Figure 12)

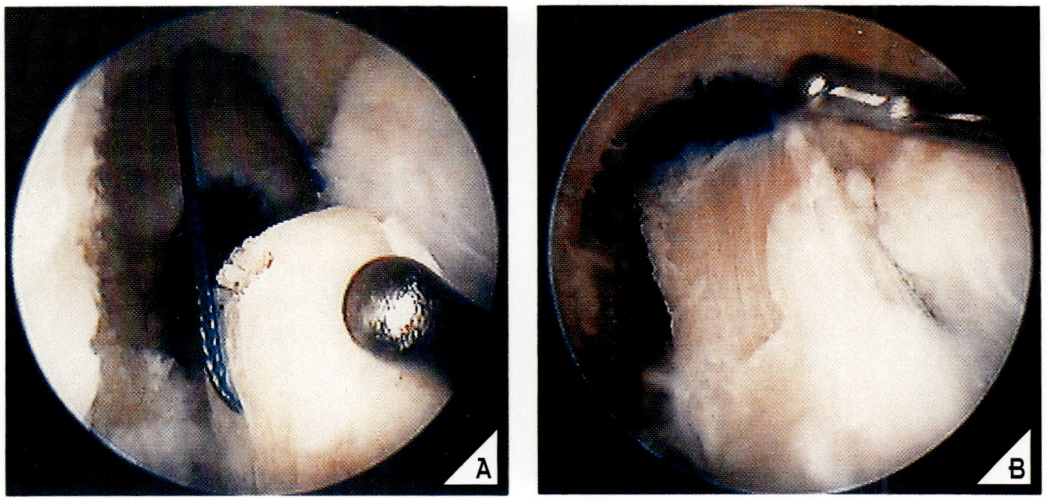

Figure 5.22
Passage of the graft. (A) The probe facilitates passage of the graft through the tibial tunnel. It is imperative to place the femoral bone block with the cancellous portion anteriorly in order to provide the visualization necessary to perform accurate endoscopic screw fixation. (B) The femoral bone block is advanced until the bone-tendon junction marked with methylene blue is at the entry point of the hole.

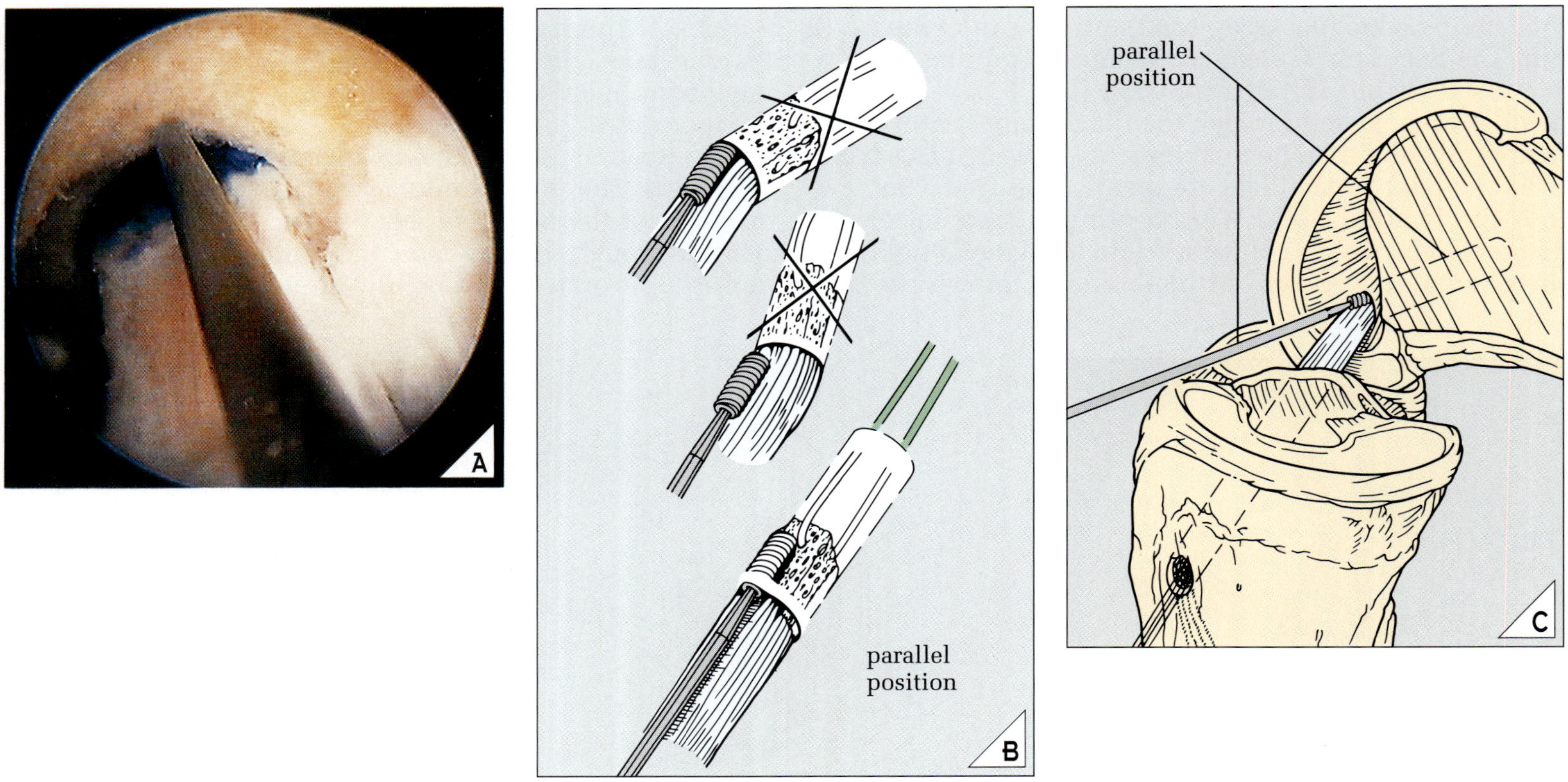

Figure 5.23

Parallel placement of the interference screw. (A) An 18-gauge needle is placed through the anteromedial portal to insure that the interference screw is placed parallel to the bone block. (B) In order to obtain optimal fixation on the femoral bone block and to prevent damaging the graft fibers, parallel placement of the screw is essential. (C) Increased flexion of the knee may be necessary to insure parallel placement.

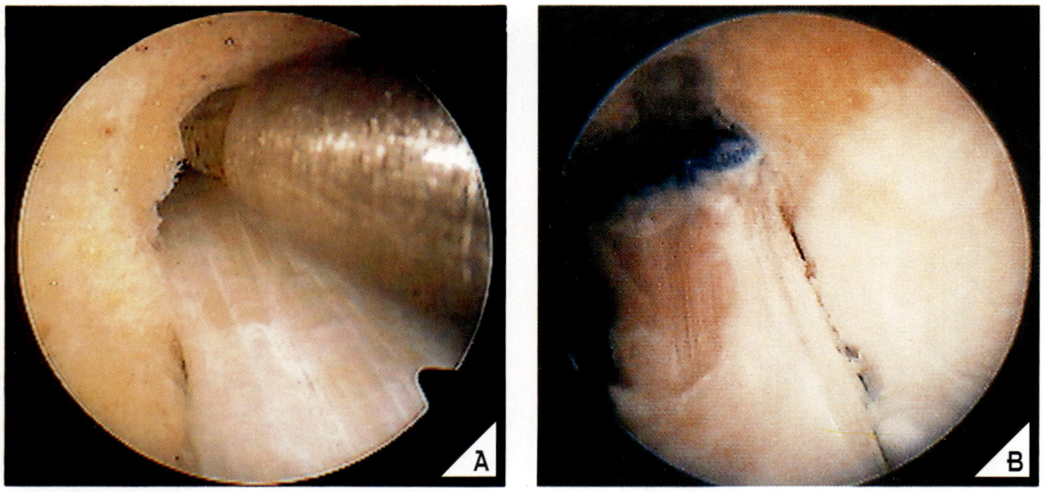

Figure 5.24

(A, B) Creation of the interference notch. An interference notch is created using an AO screwdriver.

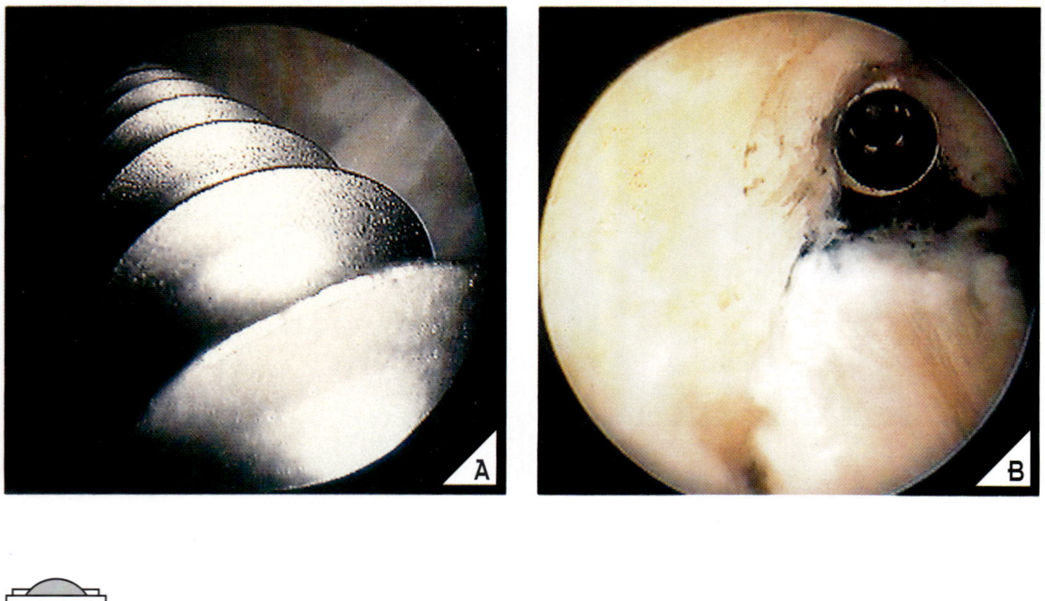

Figure 5.25

Final fixation. (A) The interference screw is placed into the interference notch and tamped lightly. (B) Under direct visualization the screw is then secured to the area of the bone-tendon junction marked with methylene blue, paying careful attention not to damage the graft fibers.

5.23A). Increased flexion of the knee may be necessary to insure parallel placement. Alternatively, it may be necessary to create an accessory portal that is adjacent to the patellar tendon and distal to the initial portal to obtain the parallel position. This can be accomplished by simply enlarging the existing portal (Fig. 5.23B,C). With the parallel position confirmed, an AO screwdriver is used to create an interference notch at the superior aspect of the femoral hole (Fig 5.24). A 7 mm diameter, 25 mm long interference screw is placed into the interference notch and tamped into place with a mallet. The interference screw is advanced with the screwdriver under direct visualization. Tension of the graft should be maintained both proximally and distally to prevent any possible rotation and/or advancement of the graft. The bone block should fit into the femoral hole snugly in order to prevent this complication. If a cannulated screw is used, the guidewire should be removed as soon as the screw is secure to prevent bending and possible breakage of the wire. Finally, the screw should be advanced until it is flush with the methylene blue mark indicating the bone-tendon junction (Fig. 5.25).

The ligament is then prestressed by flexing and extending the knee through a full range of motion while placing tension on the graft. Fixation of the graft to the tibia can be performed using alternative techniques. In approximately one half of cases, the tibial bone block will exit the tibial tunnel, in which case staple fixation may be used. This fixation may be augmented by tying the Tycron sutures around the staples. Alternatively, when the bone block fails to exit the tunnel, an AO screw and washer can act as a post to secure the #5 Tycron sutures, or an interference screw may be used. During tibial fixation, the graft should be tensioned with the knee in full extension. After fixation of the graft is completed, arthroscopic visualization of the anterior cruciate ligament is performed in order to observe appropriate tension throughout a full range of motion without impingement occurring either superiorly or laterally. Meniscal repair sutures may be tied at this time. The patella defect is bone grafted prior to closure. The patellar tendon and paratenon are closed using #0 vicryl and 2-0 vicryl suture, respectively, and the subcutaneous tissue and skin are closed in routine fashion.

Initial Postoperative Management

The patient may start CPM, early range-of-motion exercises, and weight-bearing with crutches as tolerated. The Bledsoe brace is locked at 0° and is worn during ambulation.

chapter Six

ACL Reconstruction Using the Semitendinosus and Gracilis Tendons

Mark I. Pitman

Various tissues continue to be used as autogenous grafts for reconstruction of the anterior cruciate ligament. These include the patellar tendon, commonly used as a bone-tendon-bone preparation, iliotibial band, and the medial hamstring tendons, either semitendinosus alone or semitendinosus and gracilis in combination.

It has been shown that the initial strength of the semitendinosus tendon approaches 70% of the normal anterior cruciate ligament, while the gracilis tendon approaches 49%.[1] It can be inferred, therefore, that their combined strength approaches 115% of the normal anterior cruciate ligament's strength.

PREPARING THE GRAFT

The surgeon selects the tissue to be used. Use of tissue other than patellar tendon is indicated when the patellar tendon mechanism is less than optimal. This would include patients with abnormal patellar mechanics, including a history of patellar subluxation or of recurrent dislocation; abnormal Q-angles, residual of Osgood Schlatter's disease with prominent tibial tubercle or ossicles within the patella tendon insertion; or patellofemoral arthrosis or anterior knee pain.

The semitendinosus and gracilis tendons provide easily obtainable and adequate sources for the autogenous tissue. It has been shown that the use of semitendinosus and gracilis tendons does not cause any significant measurable decrease in strength of knee flexion or internal rotation.[2]

We have been augmenting this composite gracilis and semitendinosus graft with the Kennedy Ligament Augmentation Device (3M).[3] The ligament augmentation device is a flat polypropylene braid 1.5 mm thick and either 6 or 8 mm wide and of varying lengths from 6 to 25 mm. The purpose of this device is to augment the strength of the biologic graft and to share the load with the biologic tissue during its period of weakness in the early healing period. It has been shown to be biomechanically strong and immune to degradation and to possess excellent mechanical properties. The device is anchored directly to bone at only one end, and therefore does not completely eliminate stress on the autograft. This theoretically stimulates the graft to hypertrophy and strengthen as it matures. As it does, load is gradually transferred from the ligament augmentation device to the tissue. It is estimated that at the time of surgery the device carries approximately 45% of the load. This increases during the period of early healing, then decreases during the period of intermediate and late healing as the autogenous tissues hypertrophy.[4–6]

Our technique is to expose, dissect, and harvest the semitendinosus and gracilis grafts, leaving them attached at the tibial end and harvesting them at the musculotendinous junction. The ligament augmentation device is sandwiched between the two tendons and sutured to the tendons starting 1 cm from the tibial end, and the composite graft is attached to the lateral femoral cortex with two barbed staples.

Surgical Technique

Preoperatively, before and after the onset of anesthesia, both knees should be examined to determine the amount and type of laxity present. It should involve, of course, the standard clinical tests for instability, tests for patellar stability, and instrumented arthrometry. It is important that results of the examination be recorded for future reference on the operative report.

Arthroscopy is performed using standard anterolateral and anteromedial portals for arthroscopy and for instrumentation. Diagnostic arthroscopy is performed first, starting in the supratellar pouch, examining the patellofemoral joint for abnormalities of tracking and chondral abnormalities. The synovial wall, especially the medial synovial wall, should be examined for plica. Both the

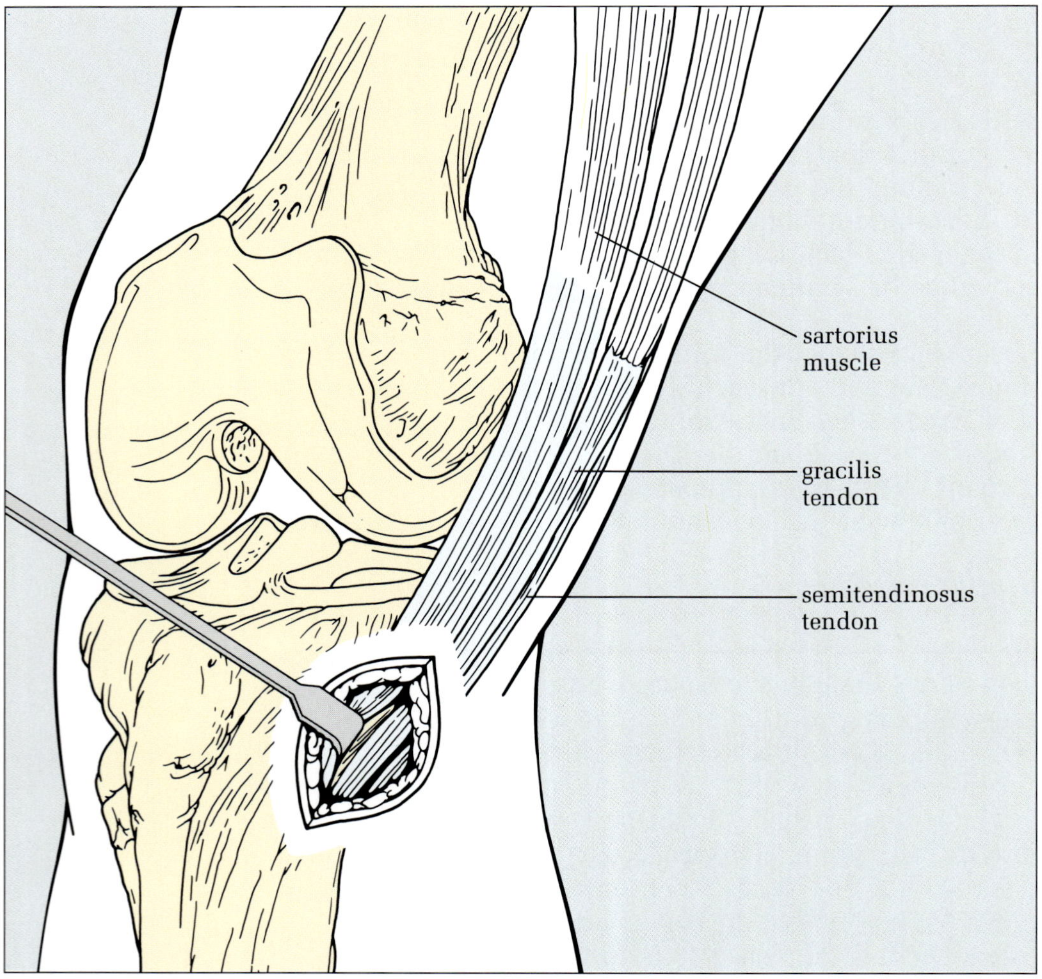

Figure 6.1 Exposure of the semitendinosus and gracilis tendons through an oblique incision over the upper medial tibial metaphysis extending through the sartorius fascia.

medial and lateral compartments should be examined for articular pathology and for meniscal pathology that will require probing and may require examination using a 70° arthroscope through the intercondylar notch. This portion of the examination may be deferred until notchplasty is performed, in which case posterior visualization may be more easily obtained.

The intercondylar notch and cruciate ligaments should be examined and evaluated for the extent of the tear as well as its location and, especially in chronic cases, to determine the amount of narrowing of the intercondylar notch that may have occurred.

Appropriate intraarticular procedures should be performed to correct other pathology, such as resection or repair of meniscus lesions. Notch debridement and notchplasty are routinely carried out laterally and superiorly to expose and define the femoral tunnel location and to prevent graft impingement.

The graft may be harvested before or after the arthroscopic preparation. The tendons are harvested through an oblique skin incision over the upper medial tibial metaphysis. With the knee placed in the figure four position, the semitendinosus tendon is often palpable at the posteromedial border of the upper tibial metaphysis, usually at or just below the level of the tibial tubercle. The tendons are not always easy to identify. The tendons may be exposed by an oblique incision through the sartorius fascia, usually in the direction of the skin incision, and this may be extended proximally or distally (Fig. 6.1). The semitendinosus and gracilis often lie on the deep surface of the sartorius fascia and may be palpated through the fascia or visualized by retracting the fascia. They are then defined, isolated, and retracted with a Penrose drain. The gracilis is the smaller and more proximal of the two tendons. The larger semitendinosus is found more distally.

The tibial attachments of the pes tendons are variable, and these must be defined prior to tendon stripping. Numerous fascial bands often exist. They are found especially between the semitendinosus and the gastrocnemius fascia. In addition, there are often multiple bands of insertion of both the semitendinosus and the gracilis tendon onto the tibial metaphysis. These must be recognized and the aberrant bands isolated and transsected (Fig. 6.2).

Careful digital dissection can confirm that all aberrant and interfering bands that may have prevented proper passage of the tendon stripper have been released for at least 6 cm into the thigh.

Thereafter, a tendon stripper with an open slot is passed about each tendon individually. The stripper should be held at 90° to the tendon as the tendon is placed appropriately into the slot and then the stripper is rotated in line with the direction of the tendon. Traction is exerted on

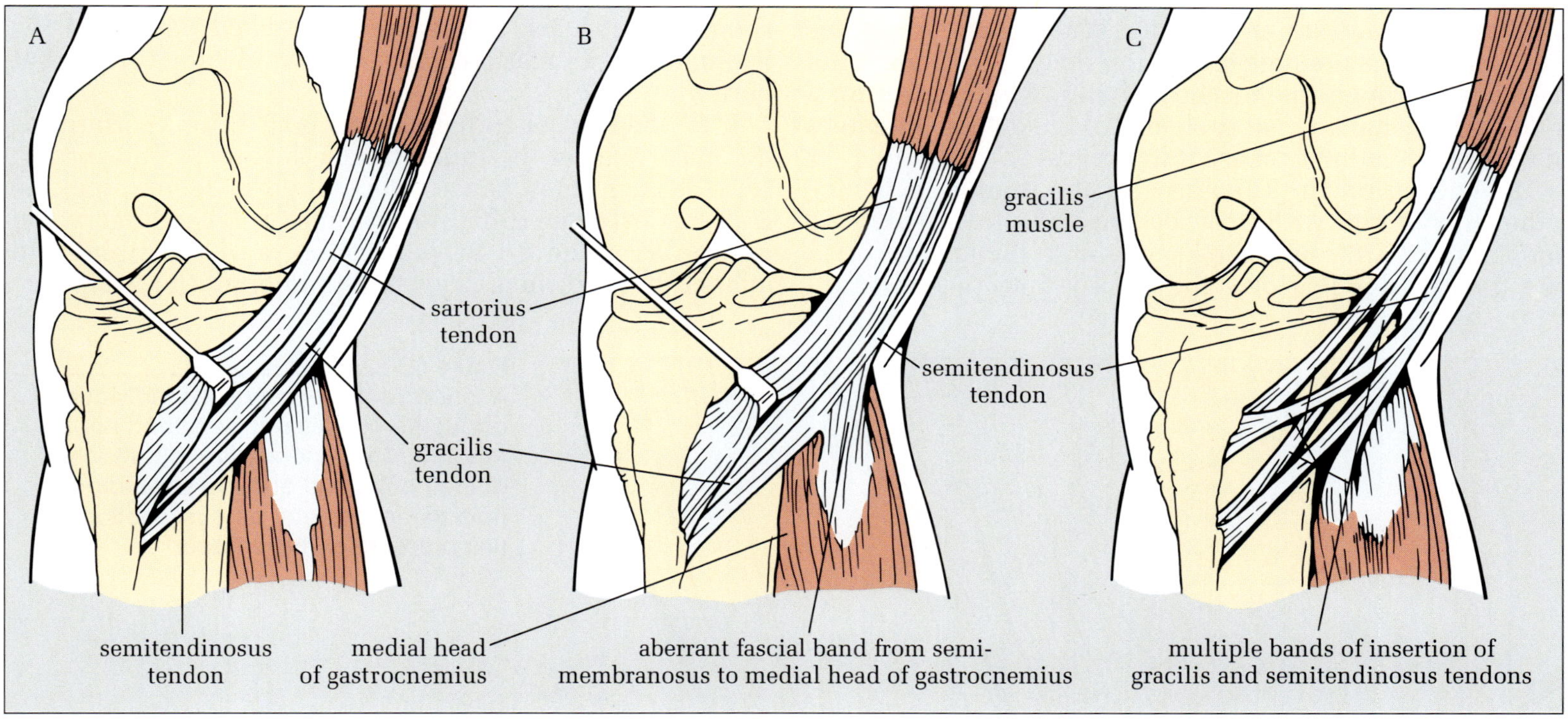

Figure 6.2

(A) Normal attachments of the pes tendinous. (B) Aberrant fascial band attaching the semitendinosus tendon to gastrocnemius fascia. (C) Multiple band of insertion of both the semitendinosus and gracilis tendons to the tibial metaphysis.

each tendon separately with the previously placed Penrose drain or, more ideally, with the index finger of the opposite hand placed around the tendon near its insertion. The tendon is placed under tension by pulling it distally, and the stripper proceeds proximally around the tendon slowly and gently, usually with a slight pronation and supination motion of the wrist (Fig. 6.3). If the tendon has been properly isolated, the stripper will pass easily up to the musculotendinous junction. As the stripper is passed proximally, and tension is exerted on the tendon distally, the tendon will be separated at the musculotendinous junction and delivered into the incision.

The most difficult part of this procedure is proper dissection of the insertion of the tendons and of their fascial bands. If this is not done, the tendon stripper may transect the tendon at the site of the fascial band and, to one's chagrin, deliver a tendon only 5 or 6 cm long. Meticulous care and dissection will prevent this. If, however, one of the tendons (usually the gracilis) is short, the other tendon may have to be doubled over the ligament augmentation device and sutured back upon itself, or a single tendon may have to be used.

When the tendons are obtained and the muscle trimmed from the musculotendinous junction, the ligament augmentation device is attached (Fig. 6.4). To sandwich the device between the tendons, a tension suture is placed in the free end of one tendon, knotted and then passed through the ligament augmentation device to the second tendon, and knotted at the end. When placing sutures through the ligament augmentation device, they must not be placed through the heat-sealed end, which is approximately the distal 1 cm at each end of the device. Puncture of the sealed end may cause it to unravel.

Depending on the thickness of the tendon, a device either 6 or 8 mm wide may be selected. It must be long enough to pass through the knee joint to the lateral cortex and then be doubled over for stapling into place in belt-buckle fashion. For small patients, a 16 cm device is suggested, and for larger patients an 18 cm device is usually sufficient. To determine the length required to affix the composite graft to the lateral femoral cortex, measure a flexible tendon leader passed through the tibial hole intraarticularly and out the femoral hole.

The device should be placed so that at the tibial end its attachment to the graft starts 1 cm from the bony insertion of the graft. Tension on the graft and the device is created by inserting the fingers into the two loops formed in the suture at the free end of the graft, one on either side of the device, and pulling (see Fig. 6.4B). Alternatively, vascular bulldog clamps may be used to hold the device sandwiched between the grafts. This makes it easier to suture but a bit more difficult to apply the proper tension.

The device is sutured between the grafts, starting at the tibial end and proceeding toward the free end. The first four or five nonabsorbable interrupted sutures should be no more than 1 cm apart. Two rows of sutures are placed, one at either edge of the "sandwich." Each suture goes through the gracilis tendon, the device, and then the semitendinosus tendon. The attachment should be strong, and five throws of the suture should be placed.

In the intraarticular portion of the tendon, continuous suture of absorbable or nonabsorbable material may be used at the surgeon's discretion. Again, the sutures should be placed no more than 1 cm apart. The continuous suture should extend toward the free end of the tendons and should be tied just before the heat-sealed portion of the ligament augmentation device to avoid puncturing that portion.

It is often easier to harvest the graft before performing the major part of the intraarticular surgery, because some fluid leakage may cause subcutaneous edema, making graft harvest more difficult. The intraarticular surgery and notchplasty should be performed, and the tibial and femoral holes drilled, prior to formation of the composite

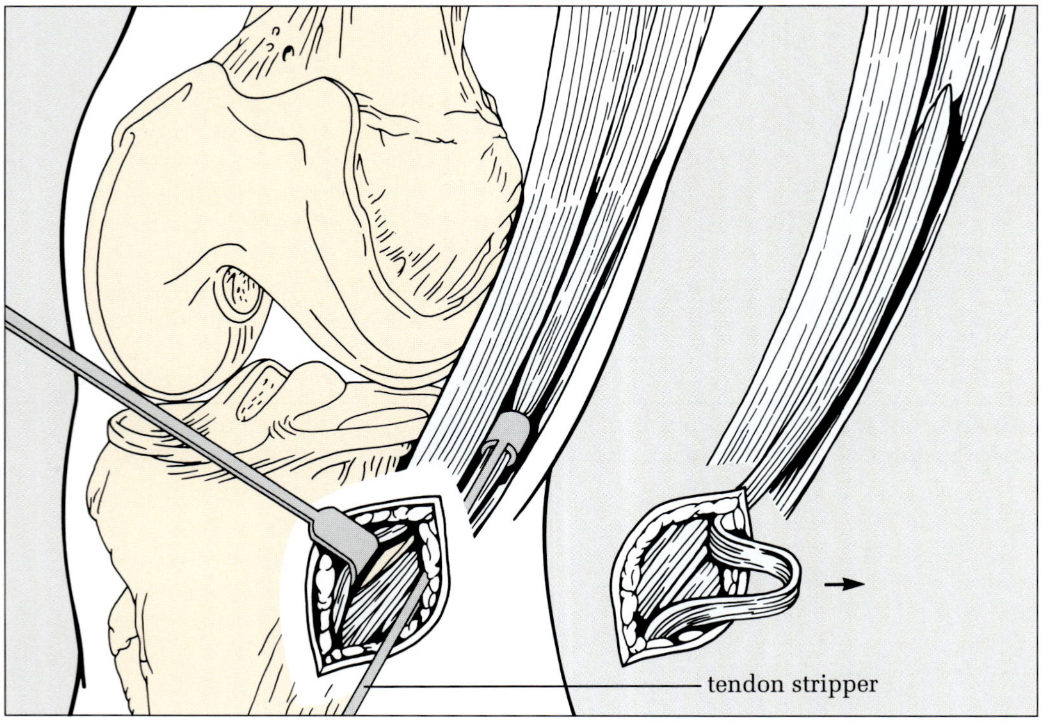

Figure 6.3
A tendon stripper is passed individually about the gracilis and semitendinous tendons. The tendons are left attached at their tibial end and are separated from the musculotendinous junction by firm pressure on the stripper.

graft of the ligament augmentation device. In this way, the length of the ligament augmentation device needed can be measured by the tendon leader.

To prepare the tibial tunnel, a periosteal elevator is used to elevate the remaining insertion of the pes to expose the medial metaphysis at the level of the tibial tubercle.

Intraarticular preparation is similar to that for other types of graft or reconstruction. A tibial drill guide is inserted into the anteromedial portal, the proper point for intraarticular exit of the tibial tunnel selected, and a guidewire placed. Before overdrilling the guidewire, the size of the tunnel is determined by placing the composite graft through a sizer. Usually an 8 mm (with smaller grafts a 7 mm) tunnel will allow passage of the graft. To prevent damage or destruction by the drill, the grafts must be protected with an elevator or osteotome during placement of the guidewire and the drills. After the guidewire has been placed in an appropriate position—I prefer the midpoint of the stump of the anterior cruciate ligament fibers—a cannulated drill is used to make the tibial tunnel.

A plug is placed into the tibial hole to prevent extravasation of intraarticular fluid. The femoral point is then selected and the femoral guide is placed through the same anteromedial portal. A lateral skin incision is made with its distal end at the palpable subcutaneous portion of the lateral femoral condyle and carried proximally through skin and subcutaneous tissues for a distance of about 3 or 4 cm. The fascia lata is split longitudinally. The vastus lateralis may be retracted anteriorly and the lateral femoral cortex exposed subperiosteally.

The femoral guide is then attached to the lateral femoral cortex. The guidewire is drilled from the lateral cortex to the previously determined point on the lateral side of the notch. The appropriate size drill is then used to ream over the guidewire. A flexible leader, which is introduced intraarticularly through the tibial hole and exits from the femoral hole, is used to determine the appropriate length for the ligament augmentation device. It should be at least 2 cm longer than the distance from the medial tibial cortex to the lateral femoral cortex.

The composite graft is then placed into the Chinese finger trap netting at the trailing edge of the leader. A small clamp is passed through the netting at its attachment to the rubber leader. This is then passed out through the hole at the base of the netting. The composite graft is grasped and pulled into the netting as far as possible up to the rubber leader. The graft may be attached to the netting with two figure-eight sutures placed through the graft and around the netting. It is wise to place an additional suture through the flexible leader about 2 cm proximal to its

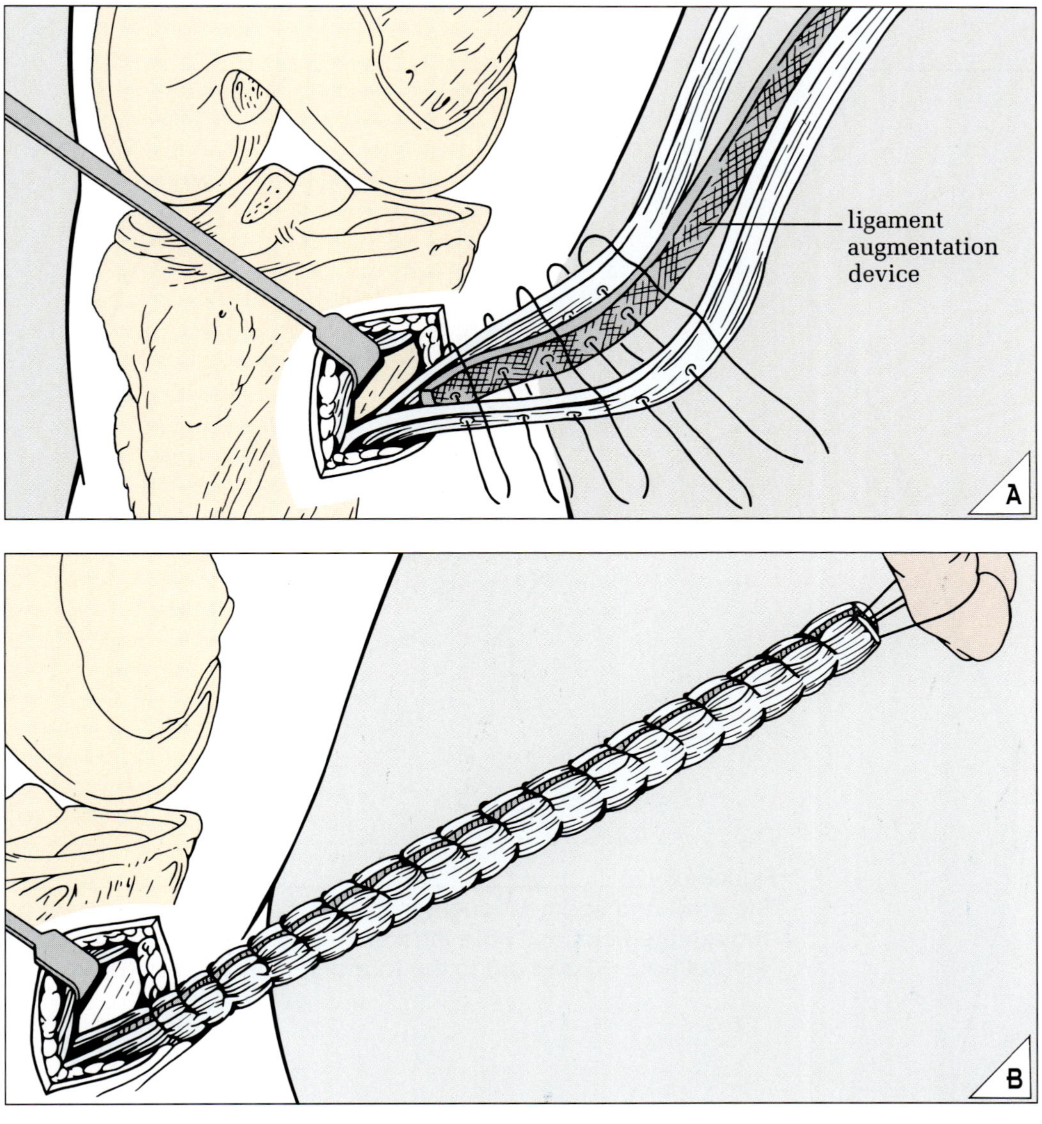

Figure 6.4
The ligament augmentation device is sutured between the two tendons. (A) The initial sutures are interrupted. The intraarticular sutures may be continuous. (B) The tension suture facilitates adjusting the tension of the tendons and the device.

trailing end in order to fix the netting within the leader. Otherwise, strong tension on the leader may pull it away from the netting.

Before placing the graft, it is important that the bony tunnels be well chamfered and smoothed, especially the posterior and lateral edges of the articular end of the tibial tunnel and the anterior and superior edges of the femoral tunnel.

The leader is then placed through the tibial hole, intra-articularly into the joint, and out through the femoral hole under arthroscopic control (Fig. 6.5). If there is any difficulty in running the leader through the femoral hole, a probe may be inserted intraarticularly to move the leader to the proper position. The leader will then exit the femoral hole, or it may be grasped and pulled up from the femoral tunnel, followed by the graft.

The sutures holding the leader to the graft are transected, and the leader is removed. A Kocher clamp is placed longitudinally about the composite graft so that tension may be exerted in the long axis of the femur. A "fish scale" tensiometer scale may be used to apply 20 pounds of longitudinal traction on the graft. Prior to fixation, the graft should be conditioned by fully flexing and fully extending the knee while the graft is under tension. This will remove the "creep" in the graft so that tension may be maintained.

With tension on the graft in the long axis of the femur and with the knee placed at approximately 30° short of full extension and with posterior pressure on the tibial tubercle, the composite graft is attached to the lateral femoral cortex (Fig. 6.6A). I prefer to use two barbed staples in a belt-buckle manner (Fig. 6.6B). The first is placed while tension is applied to the composite graft. The tension is removed, the graft is doubled over the first staple, and a second staple is applied just distal to the first (Fig. 6.7).

The knee is ranged and appropriate stability testing is done. Use of a tourniquet during this procedure may be obviated by the use of an arthroscopic pump for irrigation. The grafts may also be harvested without a tourniquet. The wounds are closed. A Hemovac suction drain is placed through the anteromedial portal into the joint. Dressings are applied. An arthrometer may again be used and its result recorded.

POSTOPERATIVE MANAGEMENT

A CPM machine is placed in the operating room, set initially from 0° to 60°, then increased to 90° over the 48 or 72 hours during which the patient is hospitalized. As soon as comfortable the patient ambulates on crutches. Early motion and early vigorous rehabilitation may be started with this well-fixed composite graft augmented by the ligament augmentation device.

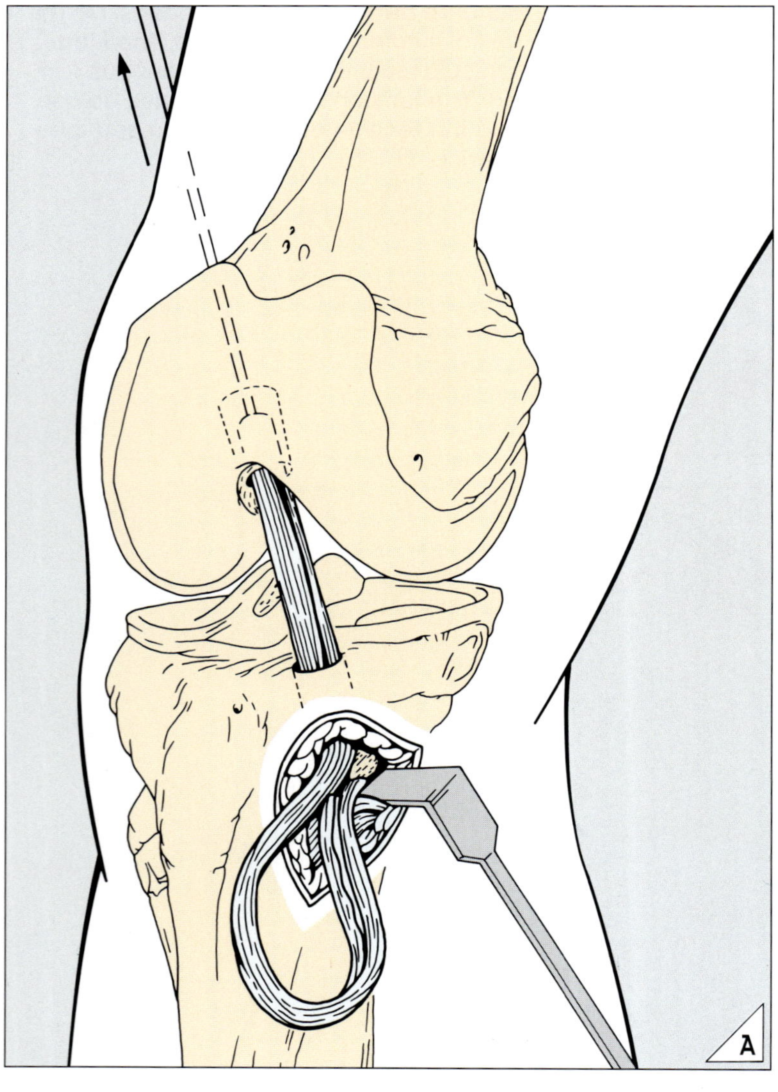

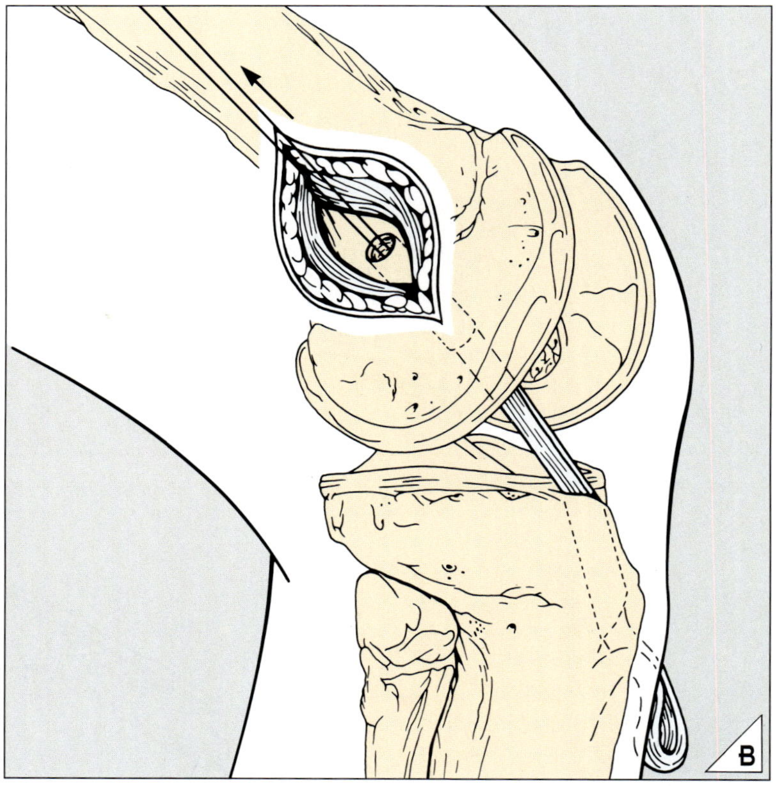

Figure 6.5
The graft and ligament augmentation device are passed through the tibial drill hole intraarticularly to the appropriate femoral hole (A) and out to the lateral femoral cortex (B).

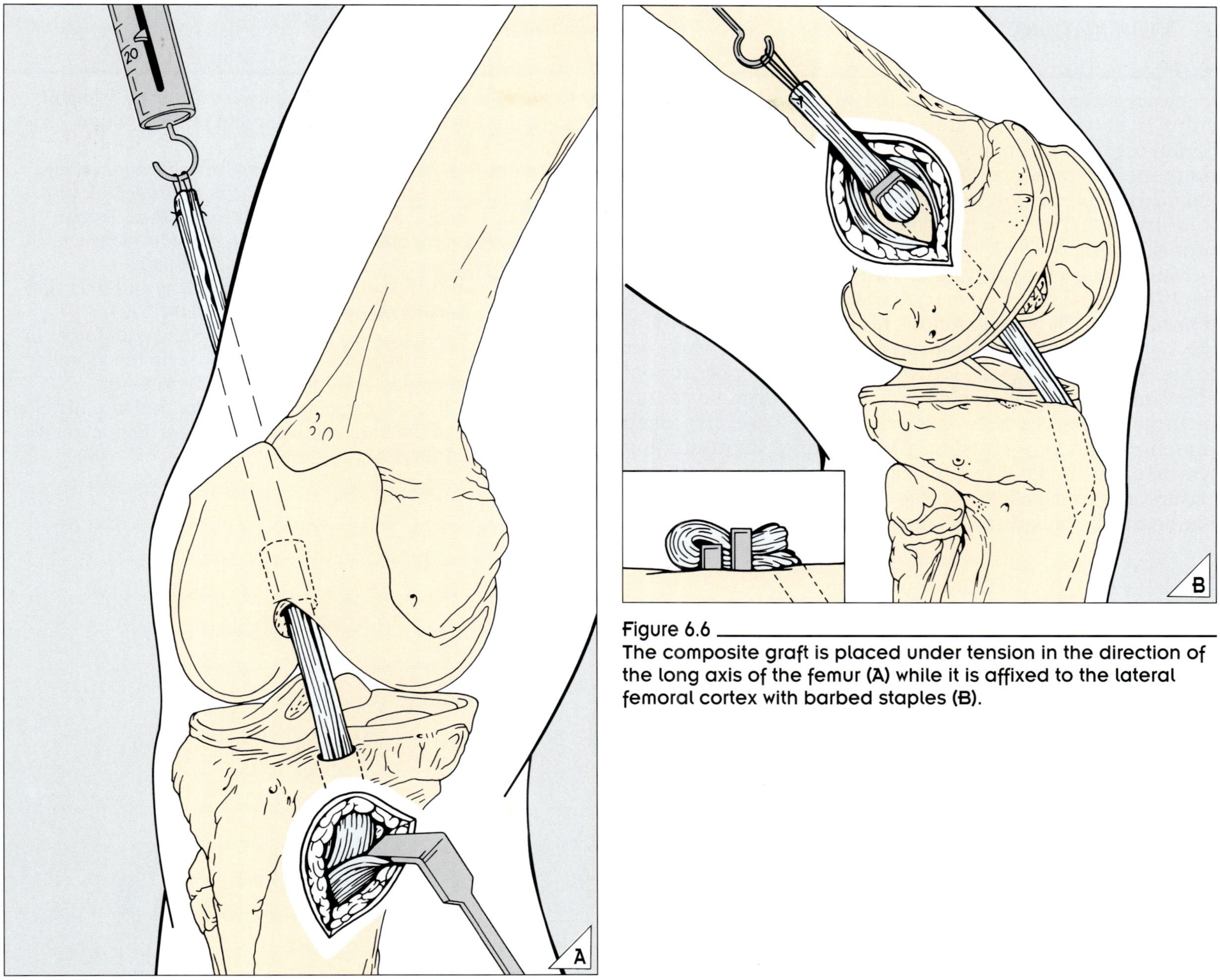

Figure 6.6
The composite graft is placed under tension in the direction of the long axis of the femur (A) while it is affixed to the lateral femoral cortex with barbed staples (B).

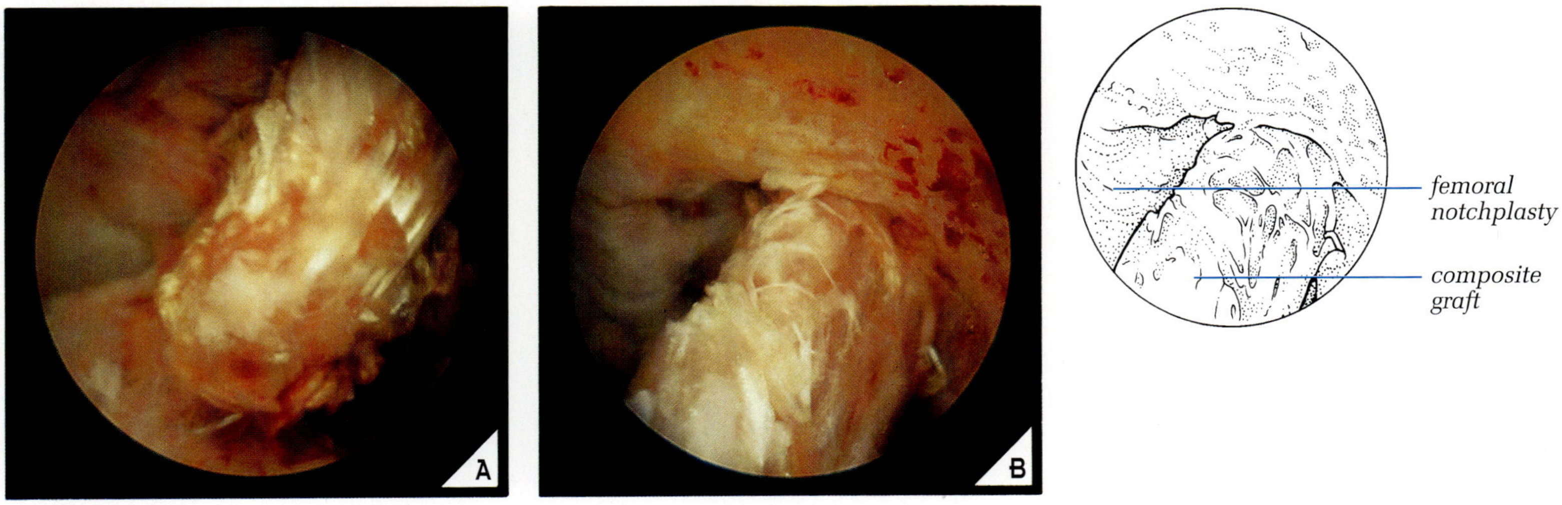

Figure 6.7
(A) Arthroscopic view of the composite graft at its site of exit from the tibial tunnel. (B) Arthroscopic view of graft at its entrance into the femoral tunnel. Note the femoral notchplasty.

COMPLICATIONS AND PITFALLS

In performing this procedure, the main pitfall and difficulty is harvesting the graft. One must be aware of the variations in attachments of the pes tendons to their insertions and the presence of fascial bands that, if recognized, may cause the tendon to be prematurely transected when it is stripped. Thus the graft may be too short to provide a proper length.

Multicenter clinical studies performed for evaluation by the FDA reveal that in over 600 cases, there is a complication rate of 1.7%. In eight cases this resulted in removal of the ligament augmentation device (1.3%). This was due to breakage of the device in two cases (probably because of abrasion from an incomplete notchplasty), fixation failure in three cases, laxity of the graft in one case, one deep infection, and one effusion. Furthermore, manipulation was required in 4.45% of the cases. The need for this procedure should decrease as more vigorous and early rehabilitation results in earlier and more complete joint motion.

REFERENCES

1. Noyes F, et al. Biomechanical analysis of human ligament grafts used in knee ligament repair and reconstruction. *J Bone Joint Surg.* 1984;66A:344–352.
2. Lipscomb AB, Anderson AF. Tears of the anterior cruciate ligament in adolescence. *J Bone Joint Surg.* 1986;68A:19–28.
3. Kennedy J, Roth J, Mendenhal H, Sanford J. Presidential address: intraarticular replacement in the anterior cruciate ligament efficient knee. *Am J Sports Med.* 1980;8:1–8.
4. Lewis JL, Lew ND, Hanley P, et al. Variability and load sharing in ACL repairs. *Trans Orthop Res.* 1988;13:127.
5. Hanley P, Lew ND, Lewis J. Load sharing and graft forces in anterior cruciate ligament reconstruction with the ligament augmentation device. *Am J Sports Med.* 17:414–489.
6. McPherson GK, et al. Experimental, mechanical and histologic evaluation of the Kennedy ligament augmentation device. *Clin Orthop.* 1985;196:186–195.

chapter Seven

ACL Reconstruction Using Fascia Lata Autograft Combined Extraarticular and Intraarticular Arthroscopic Technique

Eugene J. Chandler

Treatment of the symptomatic anterior cruciate ligament deficient knee is an orthopedic challenge. Many surgical operations have been devised. Replacement materials include xenografts, allografts, synthetics, and autografts. The autografts currently being used are the tendons of the semitendinosus, gracilis, patella, and tensor fascia lata.

In the early 1900s Hey Groves described a surgical technique to reconstruct the anterior cruciate ligament of the knee with a 1 1/2-inch strip of the iliotibial band. The iliotibial graft was left attached to the lateral tibial tubercle (Gerdy's) and routed through femoral and tibial osseous tunnels.[1,2] In the 1970s MacIntosh described an anterior cruciate ligament reconstruction of the knee using a 4 cm strip of iliotibial band routed under the lateral collateral ligament and then "over the top" of the lateral femoral condyle through the joint and through a tibial tunnel where the graft was fixated to the bone with a staple. He called this procedure the lateral substitute "over the top" (LSOT).[3] In 1985, Bertoia et al. reported excellent and good results in 31 of 34 (91%) patients using the MacIntosh LSOT operation.[4] In the early 1980s I started using the MacIntosh LSOT operation with equally gratifying results. Gradually, the principles of the MacIntosh LSOT operation were incorporated into an arthroscopic technique.

Arthroscopic reconstruction of the anterior cruciate ligament is becoming the standard of care. Arthroscopy improves visualization of the knee joint and therefore improves the accuracy of the surgical operation. Isometric placement of the graft more closely duplicates normal anterior cruciate ligament function.

INDICATIONS FOR SURGERY

Indications for anterior cruciate ligament reconstruction of the knee are gross anterior lateral rotary instability (i.e., positive lateral pivot shift test[5]), pain, and disability as well as failure to respond to conservative, nonoperative treatment.

The preoperative patient evaluation includes a careful history and physical examination. Stress testing of the knee is done with a KT1000 knee ligament arthrometer (MEDmetric).[6,7] Plain x-rays are obtained in six views—AP, lateral, tunnel, Merchant's, axial views of the patellae,[8] and AP erect views of bilateral knees. Oblique x-ray views are done for recent trauma cases. Magnetic resonance imaging is helpful for planning the surgery. Routine laboratory studies are done within 24 to 48 hours of surgery.

SURGICAL TECHNIQUE

The patient is placed on the operating table in the supine position. General anesthesia is induced. The knee is examined and range of motion and ligament laxity findings are recorded. The leg is elevated and exsanguinated with a 6-inch elastic bandage. A well-padded pneumatic tourniquet is inflated high around the upper thigh to 350 mm Hg. The leg is placed in a circumferential thigh holder, which is sealed off with an impervious U-drape. The foot of the table is lowered. The well leg is wrapped with a 6-inch elastic bandage and placed on a foam rubber splint. The knee, leg, and foot are scrubbed with povidone-iodine soap solution for 8 minutes and then painted with povidone-iodine 10% solution three times. The knee is draped free with impervious arthroscopic drapes.

Diagnostic Arthroscopy

Arthroscopy is carried out through the high infralateral portal with a 4 mm, 30° wide-angled arthroscope under video control in a saline media. The infusion of saline comes through a 5 mm cannula placed in the superome-

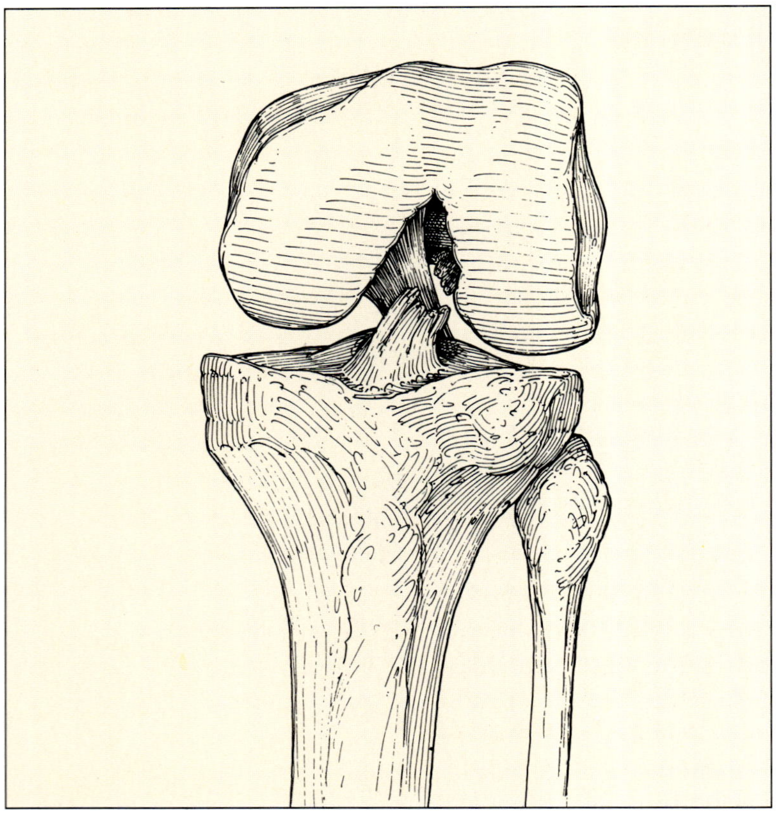

Figure 7.1
Chronic torn anterior cruciate ligament with osteophyte encroachment of the intracondylar notch.

dial portal by gravity feed. Probing is done through an inframedial portal. Patellar tracking is studied through the superomedial portal. If there is significant lateral subluxation of the patella, a lateral release is done at the end of the procedure. The intraarticular pathology is diagnosed precisely.

Surgical Arthroscopy

The intraarticular pathology is corrected by arthroscopic surgical technique. The ligamentum mucosa and the fat pad are debrided to obtain visualization. The anterior cruciate ligament remnants are excised from the femur and the tibia completely in order to determine the anatomic isometric origin and insertion of the anterior cruciate ligament.

Notchplasty

A notchplasty is done using powered instruments. A notchplasty is necessary for adequate visualization of the anatomic isometric origin of the anterior cruciate ligament, adequate room for instrumentation, and obtaining adequate clearance for the graft with knee motion (Figs. 7.1, 7.2).

A dimple is placed at the anatomic isometric origin of the anterior cruciate ligament in the intracondylar notch (Fig. 7.3).[9–13] This dimple is the target for the pointer of the anterior cruciate ligament guide system.

Harvesting the Fascia Lata Graft

A fascia lata autograft left attached to Gerdy's tubercle is harvested. A 10 cm longitudinal skin incision is made centered over the lateral femoral epicondyle. The skin edges are reflected with scissors dissection. The skin is undermined to the midthigh. A fascia lata graft is taken with sharp dissection. The anterior incision is made just posterior to the lateral edge of the patella. The posterior incision is made 5 cm from the anterior incision. This incision is made parallel to the fibers of the iliotibial band. The graft is separated from the underlying vastus lateralis muscle with scissors dissection. A finger is placed under the graft and with proper retraction of the skin edges proximally, the graft is dissected proximal to obtain a 22 cm length of graft from Gerdy's tubercle. The circumferential thigh holder is then released to facilitate harvesting a 22 cm graft. The end of the graft is divided with a general surgeon's gallbladder scissors and the graft

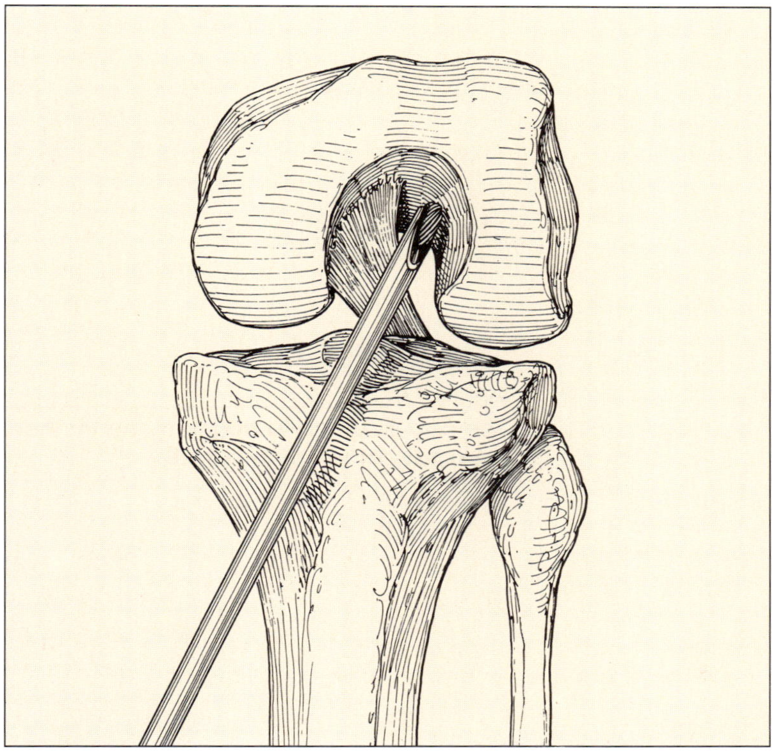

Figure 7.2
Soft tissue debridement and notchplasty.

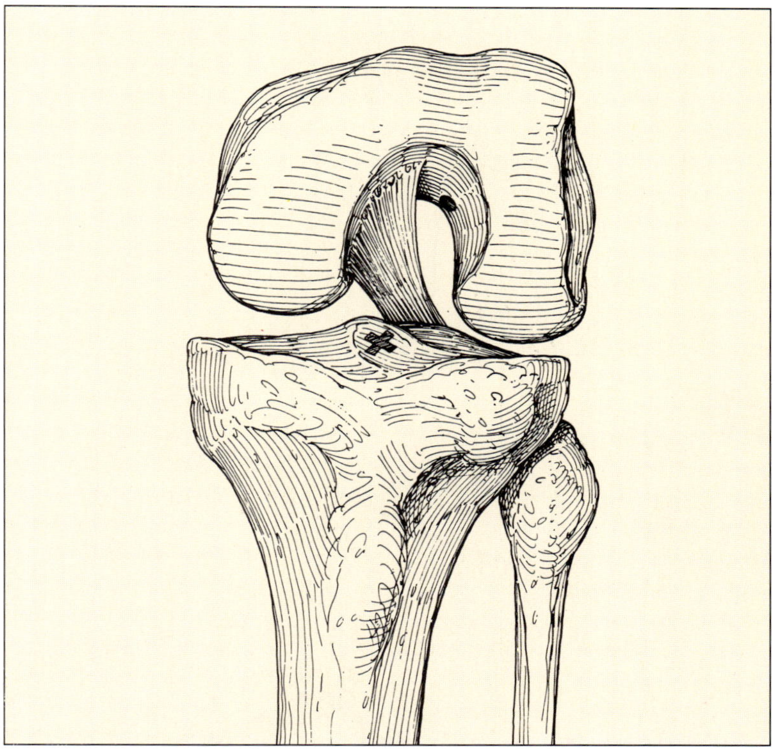

Figure 7.3
A dimple marks the anatomic isometric origin of the anteromedial bundle of the anterior cruciate ligament in the intracondylar notch. The dimple is placed at the superior and posterior edge of the lateral femoral condyle.

is delivered from the wound (Fig. 7.4). A Kocher clamp is then placed on the end of the graft and further dissection is done distally to Gerdy's tubercle. The graft should measure at least 22 cm. The graft is much thicker distally than proximally. To compensate for this fact and to obtain a graft of uniform diameter, a 1 cm strip of fascia lata is split from the graft anteriorly and distally (Fig. 7.5). This flap is then reflected onto the proximal portion of the graft and is incorporated into it with a double running suture of #5 Tycron (Davis & Geck/American Cyanamid). This suture not only strengthens the graft, but compresses it and acts as a leader to pull the graft through the femoral and tibial osseous tunnels (Figs. 7.6, 7.7).

The graft is then sized with an outside diameter gauge

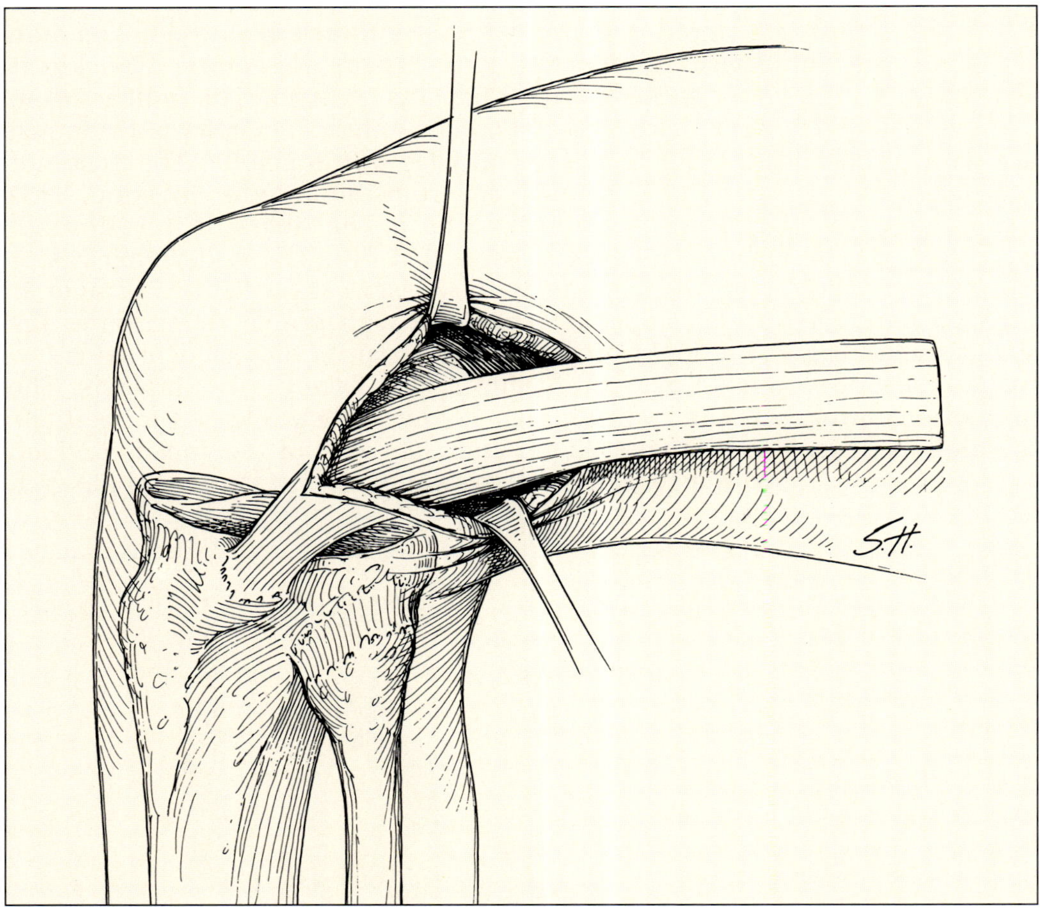

Figure 7.4
A fascia lata graft is harvested—#5 × 22 cm left attached to Gerdy's tubercle.

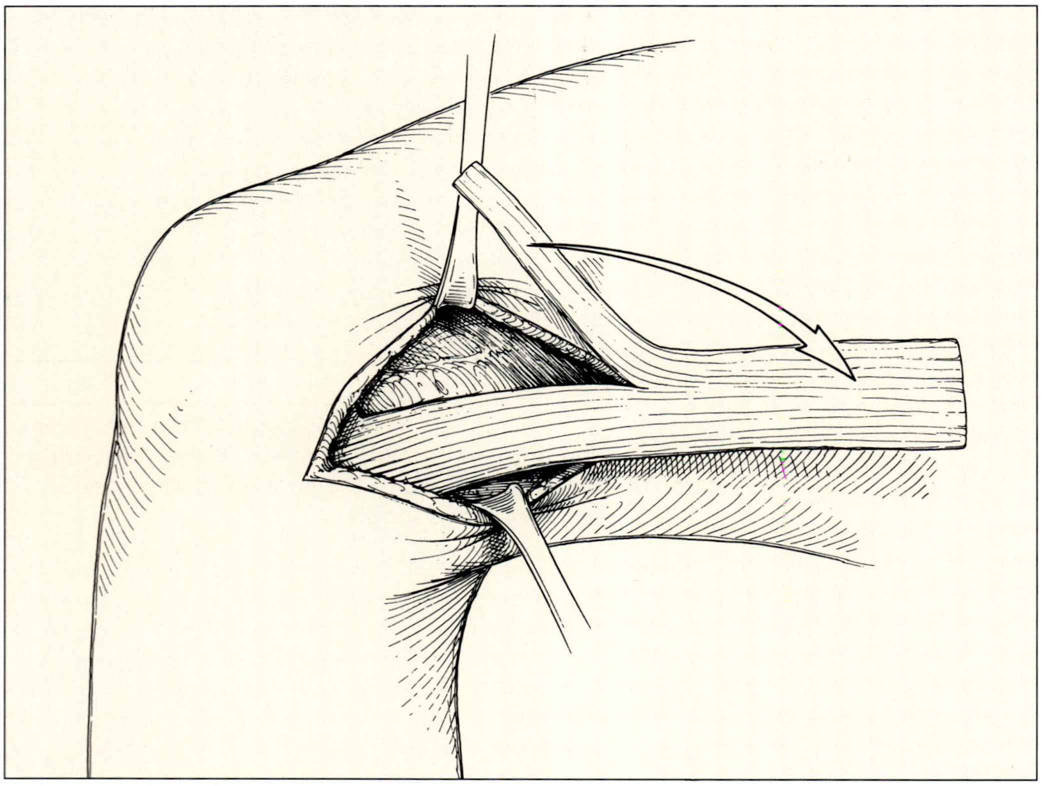

Figure 7.5
The flap is turned to augment the thinner proximal portion of the graft.

in order to select the appropriate drill bits for the femoral and tibial holes. In the average patient the graft size is approximately 10 mm in diameter. If the outside diameter of the graft is not sufficient, the graft may be augmented with a synthetic material (Kennedy LAD, 3M, Orthopaedic Products),[14] however, I have not found this to be necessary.

Tunneling Under the Lateral Collateral Ligament

A tunnel is created under the lateral collateral ligament in order to pass the graft under this ligament. This is the shortest route for the graft and prevents the graft from snapping over the lateral epicondyle with flexion and extension of the knee (see Figs. 7.13, 7.14).

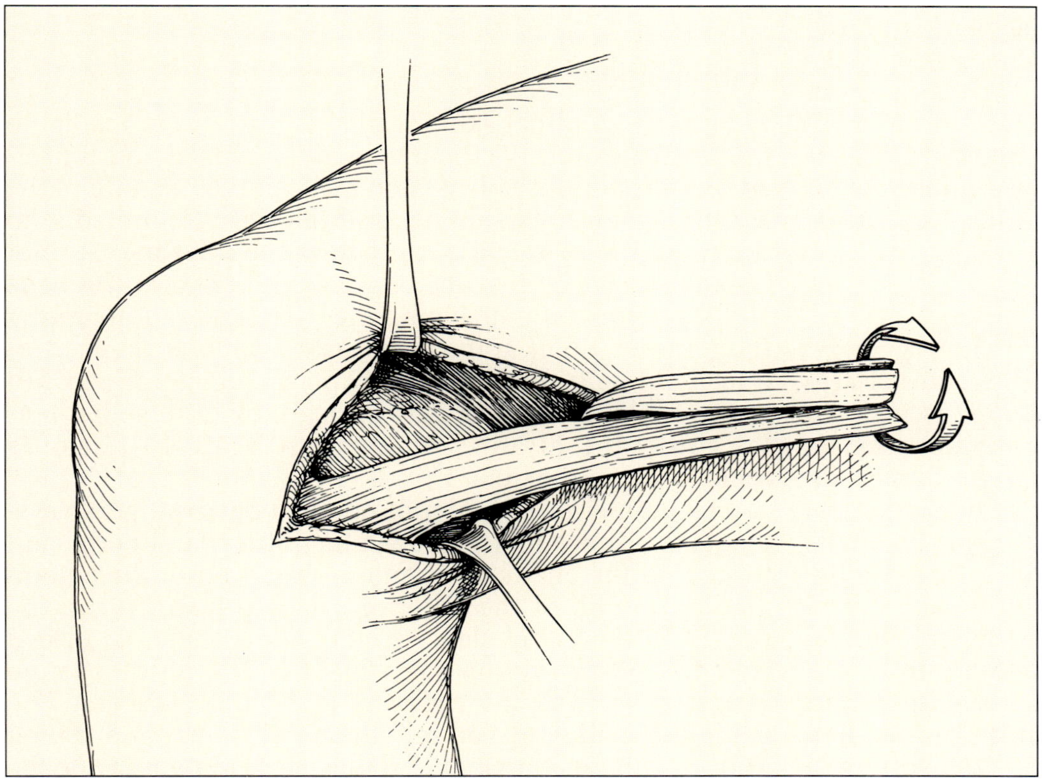

Figure 7.6
Tubing the graft.

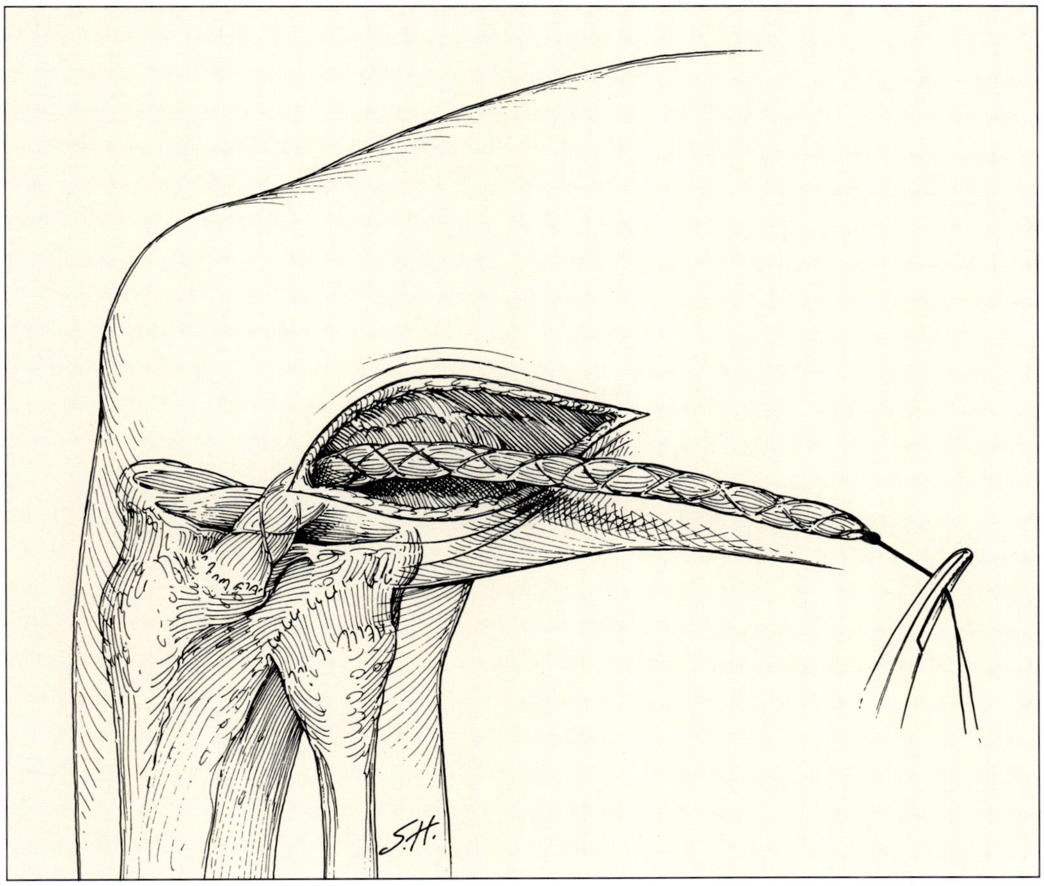

Figure 7.7
The graft is compacted and strengthened with a double running #5 Tycron suture.

Extraarticular Isometry

The extraarticular isometric point on the femur from Gerdy's tubercle is found by placing a 3/32-inch Kirschner wire into Gerdy's tubercle and measuring with an extraarticular isometry gauge while the knee is in full extension and 90° of flexion. This point lies 1 cm proximal to the lateral femoral epicondyle and in line with the posterior aspect of the femur.[15] A periosteal flap is reflected to expose the bone. Another Kirschner wire is placed here and accuracy of the placement is rechecked with the extraarticular isometry gauge (Fig. 7.8). If the location of the femoral pin is isometric, the Kirschner wire is overdrilled with an 8 mm cannulated drill bit. This hole is made 6 to 8 mm deep. This hole serves as a pilot hole for the barrel sleeve of the anterior cruciate ligament guide system. The Kirschner wires are removed.

Femoral Tunnel

The femoral tunnel is made with a Chandler anterior cruciate ligament guide system. The arthroscope is inserted into the inframedial portal. The tip of the anterior cruciate ligament guide system is inserted through the transpatellar portal and placed in the dimple that marks the anatomic origin of the anterior cruciate ligament in the intracondylar notch.[9–13] Holding the anterior cruciate ligament guide system pointer in the dimple, the barrel sleeve is inserted into the pilot hole on the lateral femoral condyle and the guide system is clamped securely. All three wheels of the guide system must be tightened securely to insure its accuracy. The guide pin is then drilled through the barrel sleeve until it hits the pointer of the guide system inside the joint. This can be determined by the vibration of the guide system and also by a few droplets of oil seen as the pin approaches the tip of the guide system pointer seen on the television monitor (Fig. 7.9). The guide system is then removed and the accuracy of the guide pin is confirmed arthroscopically with a hook. The guide pin is then overdrilled with the appropriate sized drill bit corresponding to the outside diameter of the graft. The internal and external holes are chamfered with retrograde and prograde reamers respectively. The hole is then plugged to conserve irrigation liquid.

Tibial Tunnel

A 3 cm longitudinal skin incision is made 2 cm medial to the tibial tubercle. The periosteum is incised and reflected. An 8 mm pilot hole is then made at the junction of the diaphysis and the metaphysis of the tibia 2 cm medial to the tibial tubercle and 3 cm below the jointline. A pilot hole is started by first drilling perpendicular to the bone and then gradually changing the direction and aiming at the anterior tibial spine. The arthroscope is then introduced through the infralateral portal. A motorized full radius resector is introduced through the inframedial portal and residual anterior cruciate ligament tissue is removed from the tibia.

The pointer of the anterior cruciate ligament guide system is then introduced through the inframedial portal and placed on the anatomic isometric insertion of the anteromedial bundle of the anterior cruciate ligament on the tibia.[9–13] The barrel sleeve of the guide system is placed into the pilot hole on the tibia and the guide system clamped securely by tightening all three wheels. The guide pin is then placed into the barrel sleeve and drilled until the tip hits the pointer of the guide system inside the joint. This can be determined by vibration of the guide system and by seeing oil droplets on the video monitor

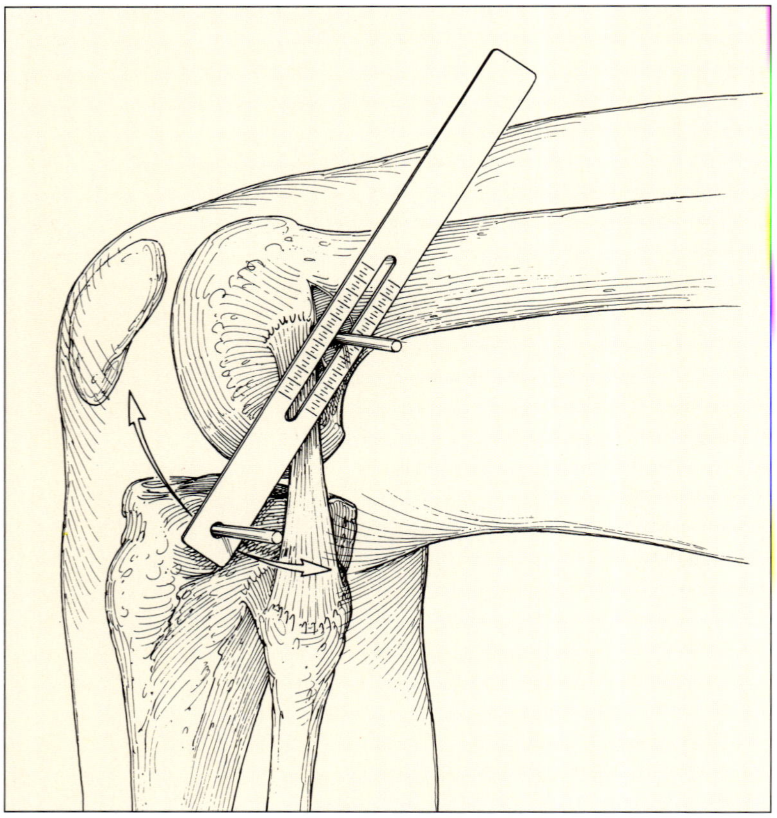

Figure 7.8
Two K-wires and a slotted ruler are used to find the isometric point on the femur from Gerdy's tubercle.

(Fig. 7.10). The guide system is removed. The accuracy of the guide pin is confirmed arthroscopically with a hook probe. The guide pin is overdrilled with a cannulated drill bit of appropriate size of the graft. As the drill bit enters the joint, it frequently creates a bone flap on a tissue hinge. The presence of a bone flap must be ascertained; if one exists, it must be removed because it may block extension of the knee. The internal hole is debrided of soft tissue with a motorized synovial resector. The edges of the internal hole are chamfered with a powered retrograde reamer.

Intraarticular Isometry

Intraarticular isometry is determined with a suture and a spring-loaded strain gauge (Acufex).[10] A #2 braided poly-

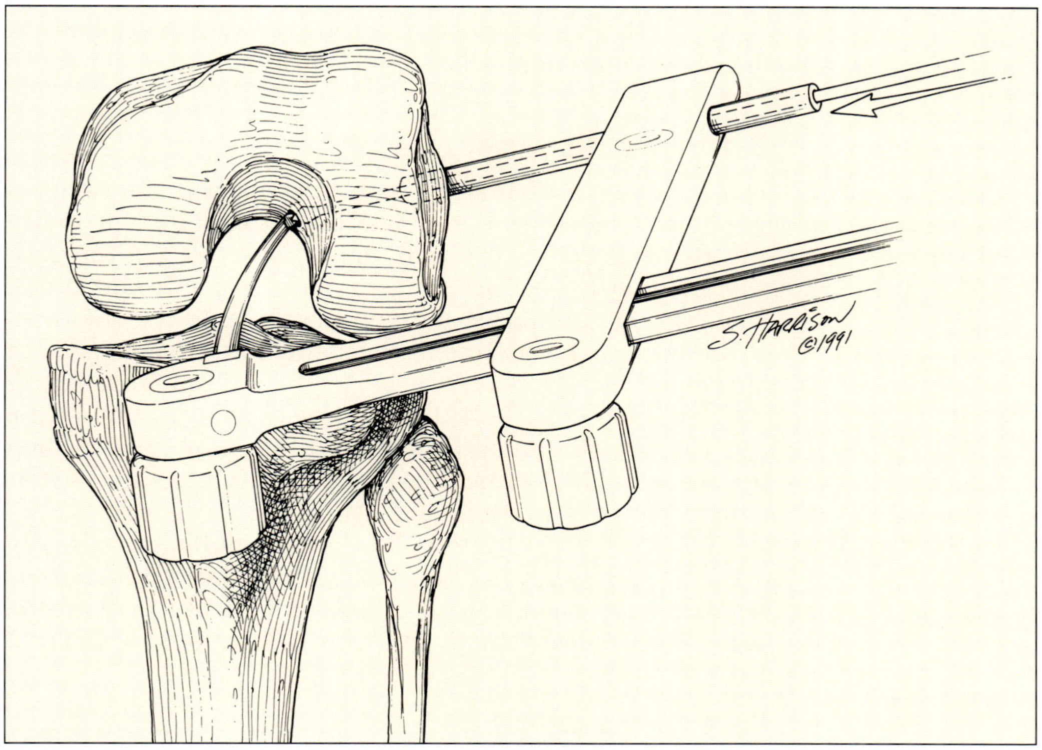

Figure 7.9
The guide pin is drilled from the external isometric point on the femur to the anatomic isometric origin of the anterior cruciate ligament with a Chandler guide system.

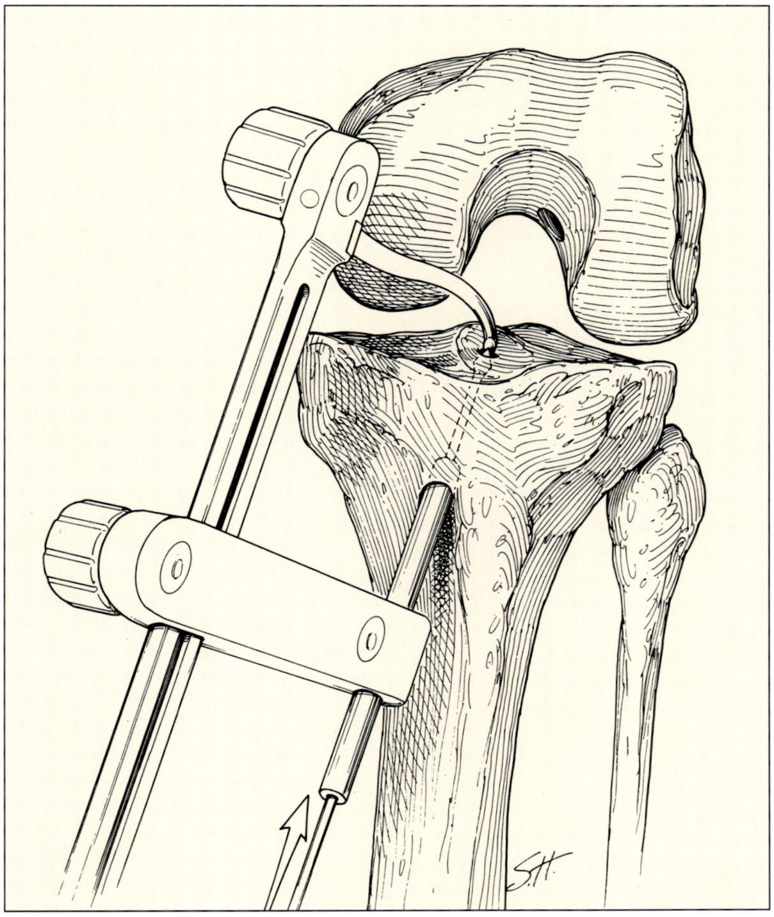

Figure 7.10
The guide pin is drilled from the pilot hole located at the diaphyseal-metaphyseal junction of the tibia to the anteromedial insertion site of the anterior cruciate ligament on the tibia with a Chandler guide system.

ester suture is passed through the femoral tunnel, joint, and tibial tunnel under arthroscopic control. The suture exiting the femoral hole is passed through an adjustable-collared sleeve and tied to a button that acts as a stop. The suture exiting the tibial hole is then passed through an adjustable-collared sleeve and the spring-loaded strain gauge and secured. The knee is manipulated through a range of motion from 0° to 120°. The reading on the strain gauge should be less than 1 mm. The tibial tunnel can be adjusted posteriorly and laterally with a power rasp or reamer to correct isometry of the internal holes to within 1 mm (Fig. 7.11).

Debriding the Osseous Tunnels

The osseous tunnels are debrided and smoothed with a round flexible rasp (Gore). The eyelet on the rasp is tied to the leader suture in the joint and then fed through the osseous tunnels (Fig. 7.12). The rasp is pulled downward with a gentle but firm and continuous motion.

Passing the Graft

The graft is passed under the lateral collateral ligament and drawn tight. The suture in the joint is then tied to the leader suture of the graft. The graft is then fed through the femoral tunnel and simultaneously pulled through the joint and the tibial tunnel with the leader suture. A Kocher clamp is placed on the end of the graft as it exits the tibial tunnel (Fig. 7.13).

Tensioning the Graft

The graft is tensioned with a windlass. The knee is flexed 90° and the tibia is rotated externally to make sure that the tibia is reduced on the femur completely. The Kocher clamp on the end of the graft is used as a windlass to tension the graft. It is very important to note that the graft is being tensioned through both bony tunnels and under the lateral collateral ligament all the way to Gerdy's tubercle. This can best be determined by palpating the graft at Gerdy's tubercle as tension is released and reapplied on the graft with the windlass (Fig. 7.14).

Fixation of the Graft

The graft is fixated to bone with three barbed bone staples (Richards). After the graft has been tensioned properly and the tibia reduced on the femur, one third of the graft is fixated with a barbed stainless steel staple in the lateral femoral condyle tunnel by piercing the anterior one third of the graft with one tine of the staple and then impacting the staple into the bone at a 45° angle with the long axis of the femur (see Fig. 7.14). The extraarticular portion of the graft corrects the lateral pivot shift test. The knee is then positioned at 20° of flexion and the tibia is rotated externally. The graft is tensioned firmly and is fixated with a staple in the tibial tunnel. The graft is pulled proximally over the first staple. The graft is then transfixed with a second staple securing both portions of the graft to the bone in the tibial tunnel. Thus, a "D" ring buckle fixation

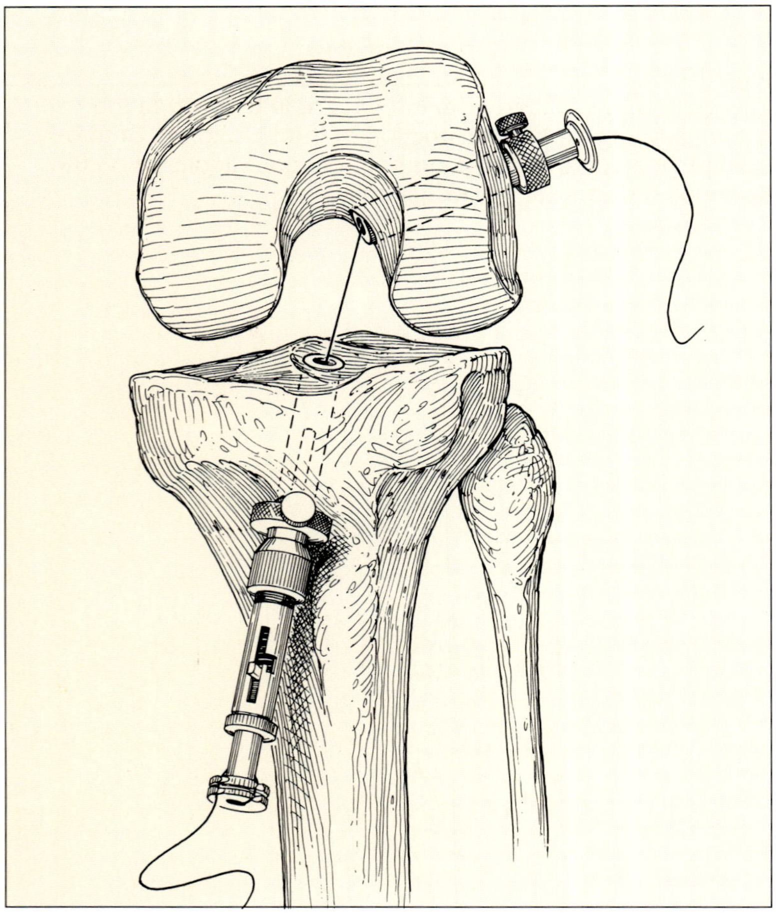

Figure 7.11
The isometry of the internal holes are tested with a suture, two sleeves, and a spring-loaded syringe gauge.

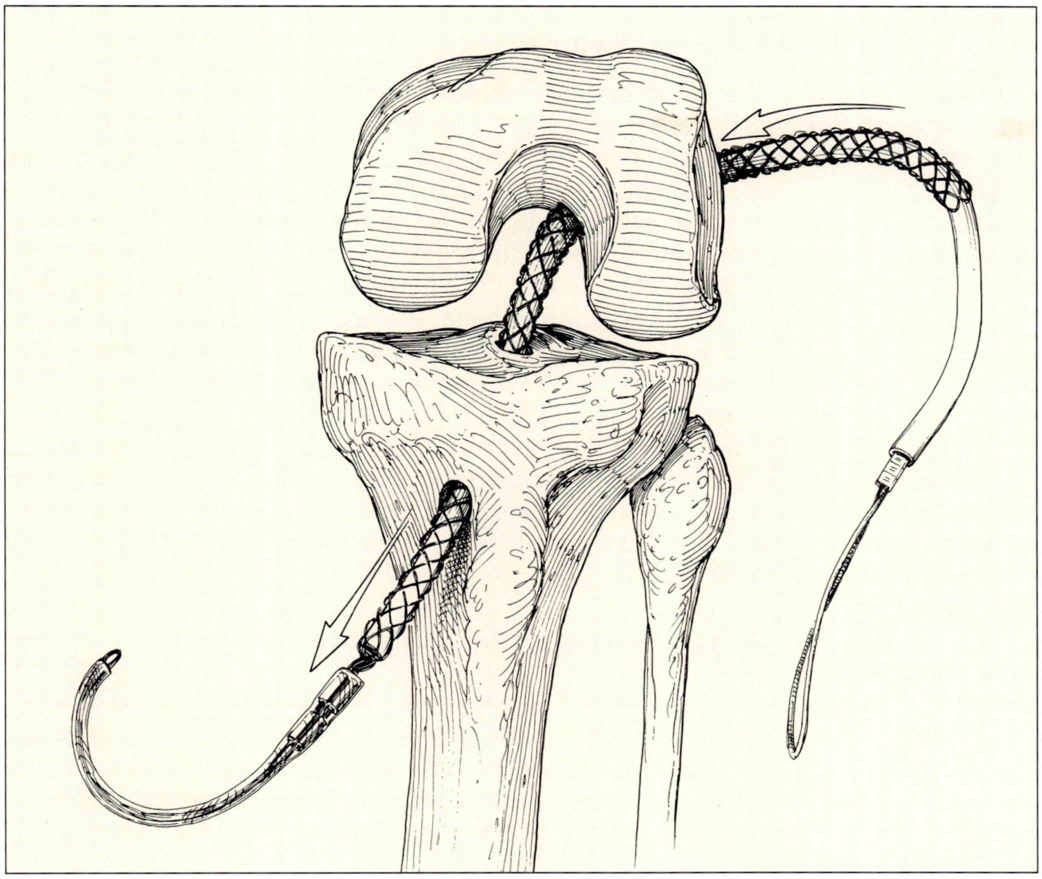

Figure 7.12

The osseous tunnels are debrided and smoothed with a round flexible rasp.

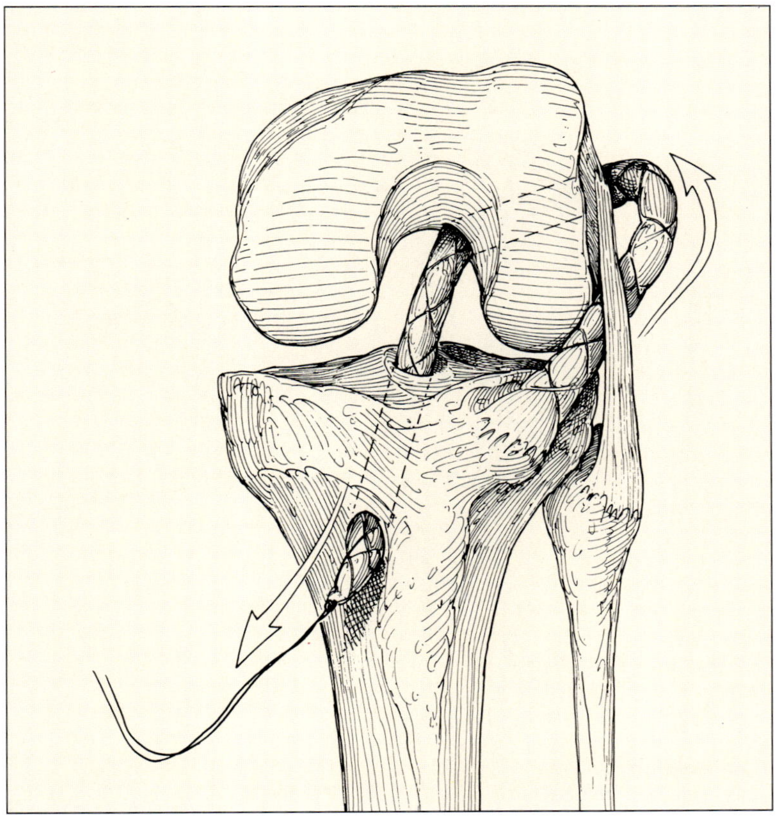

Figure 7.13

The graft is passed under the lateral collateral and through the joint with a suture leader.

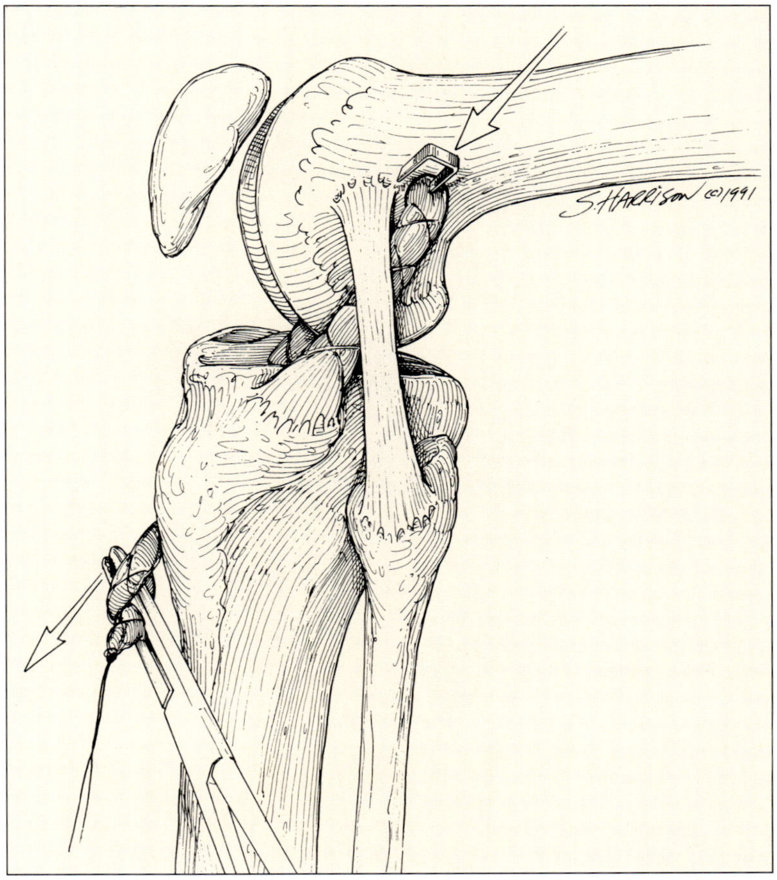

Figure 7.14

A windlass is used to tension the graft. One third of the extra-articular graft is fixated with a staple with the knee at 90° of flexion and the tibia rotated externally.

technique, which fixates the graft to the bone securely, is used. The more the graft pulls the staples into the tunnel, the tighter the fixation becomes; this is similar to a slip knot. The intraarticular portion of the graft corrects the Lachman test (Fig. 7.15). The graft is then studied and tested under direct vision for positioning, lack of pistoning, and adequate clearance in the intracondylar notch by moving the knee through a range of motion from 0° to 120°. Fixation of the graft and stabilization of the knee joint are tested by doing a Lachman test and an anterior drawer test forcibly.

Realignment of the Patella

Lateral subluxation or dislocation of the patella may be present due to the original injury or congenital anomalies. If lateral subluxation of the patella is diagnosed by arthroscopy at the beginning of the procedure, realignment of the patella may be indicated. Realignment of the patella is done by completing the lateral release. This is accomplished by dividing the insertion of the vastus lateralis tendon. If feasible, the vastus lateralis tendon is transferred to the quadriceps tendon and sutured with No. 2 braided polyester sutures in order to preserve power of the vastus lateralis muscle (Fig. 7.16). The lateral geniculate artery is identified and preserved if possible.

Wound Closure

The tourniquet is released and hemostasis is obtained with electrocautery. The fascia lata is reconstituted as much as possible. The posterior remnant of the fascia lata is repaired to the periosteum of the lateral femoral condyle with #2 braided polyester sutures. This repair strengthens the posterolateral corner of the knee to prevent posterolateral rotary instability. The knee is extended fully to make sure these sutures do not untie, break, or pull loose. If they do, they are replaced under corrected tension (Fig. 7.17). The wounds are closed in layers with sutures. One medium-sized suction catheter drain is placed in the lateral wound and brought out through a separate stab wound in the skin. Another suction catheter drain is placed in the joint through the superomedial portal. A bulky compression dressing is applied with extra thick padding over the lateral thigh—the graft donor site.

Postoperative Management

Following surgery the patient is taken to the postanesthesia care unit where the operative limb is placed in a CPM machine. Prophylactic antibiotics (Cefazolin), which were started by the anesthesiologist just prior to surgery, are

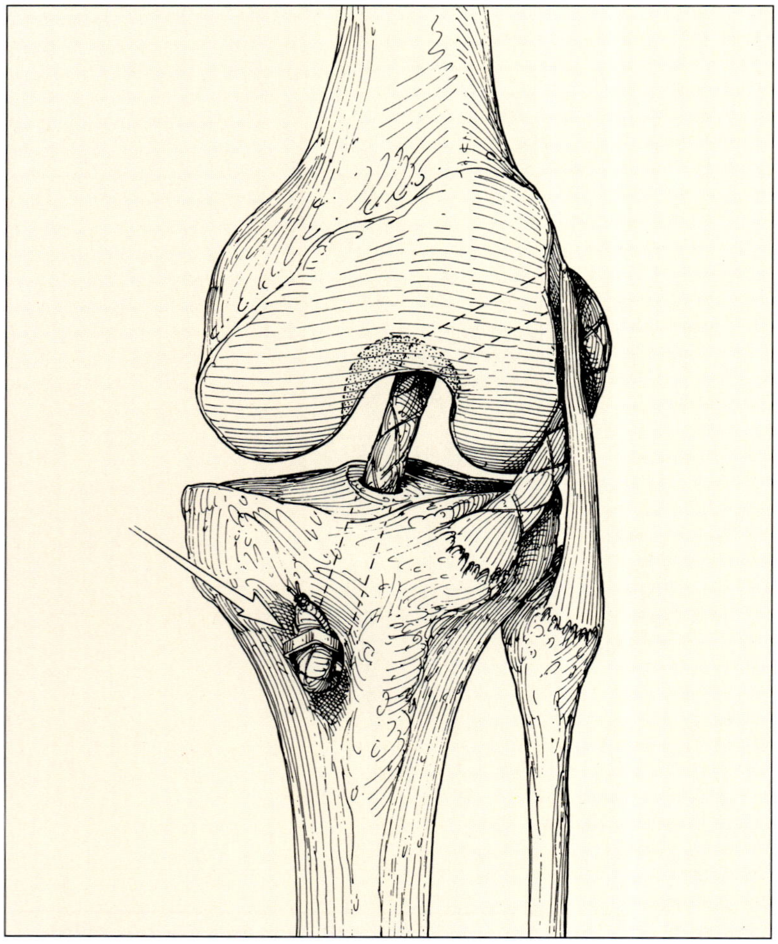

Figure 7.15
The graft is fixed to the tibia with a double staple. The "D" ring buckle technique is used with the knee in 20° of flexion.

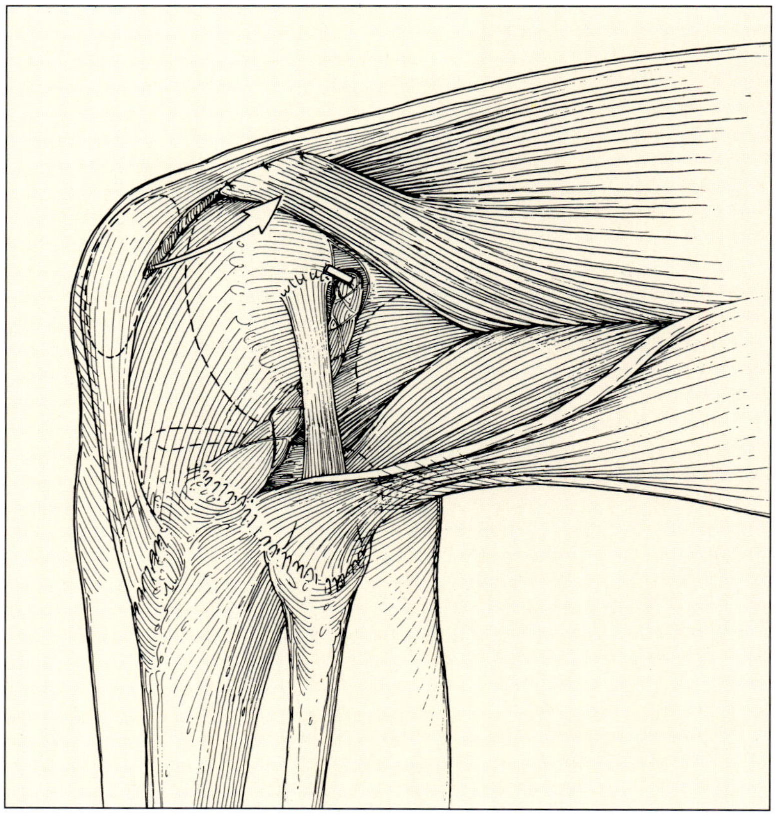

Figure 7.16
The vastus lateralis tendon is released and transfered from the patella to the quadriceps tendon to correct lateral patellar subluxation.

continued intravenously for 24 to 48 hours. The CPM is set at 0° to 60° motion and flexion is increased 10° twice daily to 110° as tolerated. The wound drains are removed at 24 to 48 hours.

On the first postoperative day, physical therapy is started. The patient is instructed in knee rehabilitation exercise program and crutch ambulation full weight bearing as tolerated. No casts or braces are necessary for most patients. Patients at risk are fitted with a removable rigid splint to assist with ambulation and maintain full extension. Patients with a torn medial collateral ligament are fitted with a removable double caliper knee hinged brace (Bledsoe) with 0° and 90° stops. The patient is instructed in active and passive range of motion exercises as well as gravity-assisted passive knee extension and flexion exercises. Gravity-assisted knee extension exercises are in the prone position on the table with knees and legs hanging off the end of the table. Heel heights are checked and if not equal, passive manipulation and/or ankle weights are used to achieve and maintain full knee extension. Gravity-assisted knee flexion exercises are done with the patient in the supine position. The patient grasps both thighs with the hands and pulls the knees toward the chest. Ankle weights can be added to achieve flexion to at least 120°. The patient is discharged from the hospital on the second or third postoperative day.

The patient is seen in the office on the fourth to seventh postoperative day. Wound care is done. X-rays are taken in AP and lateral views to check the position of the osseous tunnels and the staples (Fig. 7.18). A bulky compression dressing with extra padding over the graft donor site is continued for 7 to 10 days. If active range of motion

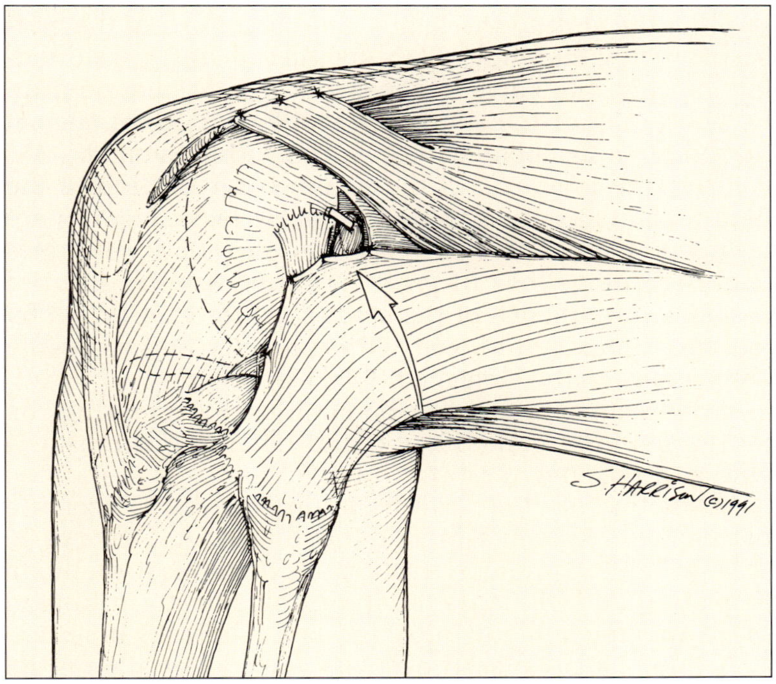

Figure 7.17
The posterior fascia lata to the periosteum on the lateral femoral condyle is repaired.

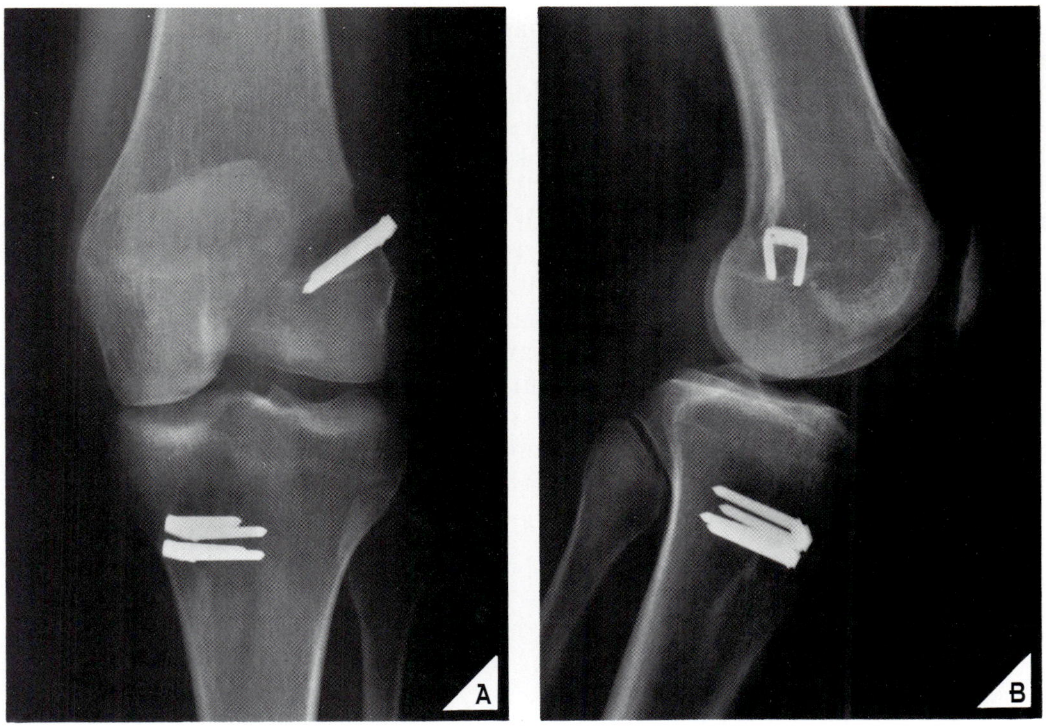

Figure 7.18
Postoperative AP (A) and lateral (B) x-rays of the left knee demonstrate the osseous tunnels in the proximal tibia and the distal femur as well as one staple in the lateral femoral condyle laterally and two staples in the proximal tibia anteromedially in ideal position.

is less than 5° to 90° or if the patient is unable to maintain full passive extension, outpatient physical therapy is instituted 3 to 5 times weekly. Crutches are discarded only when the patient is walking normally—usually in 1 to 3 weeks. Progressive resistant exercises are instituted.

Patients are seen at weekly and then monthly intervals to check their progress. They are reinstructed in their home exercise program repeatedly. Most patients are able to rehabilitate their knee in 3 to 6 months. Full rehabilitation of the knee means a full painless range of motion, good stability, no thigh atrophy, and at least 85% power and strength by isokinetic muscle testing (Cybex/Lumex). When patients reach this level of rehabilitation, they are released for most activities including recreational sports. Collision sports are not recommended for 1 year.

Patients with special interests in high demand activities or competitive sports should be referred to a certified athletic trainer (ATC) for further strengthening, conditioning, and training. Patients who intend to participate in collision sports should be fitted with a custom made knee brace (Orthotech). Patients are seen at 6- to 12-month intervals indefinitely for periodic medical maintenance and KT1000 testing.

Complications and Pitfalls

Some of the pitfalls encountered in this surgical procedure are:

- Poor tissue quality
- Nonisometric osseous tunnel placement
- Wound hematoma
- Graft fixation technical problems
- Cosmetic deformities
- Slip and fall accidents.

Poor tissue quality is frequently found in patients with hypermobile joints and hyperelastic tissue. The iliotibial band may be underdeveloped and/or the fascia lata may be very thin. In these cases it may be prudent to switch to another source of graft material or augment the fascia lata autograft. The fascia lata autograft can be augmented with autogenous semitendonosus and/or gracilis tendon(s) or synthetic materials such as polypropylene braid or dacron. The selected material is used as the core in the tubed composite graft.

The most serious intraoperative problem is the nonisometric placement of the graft on the femur. This mistake can be avoided by doing an adequate notchplasty. You must be able to visualize the intracondylar notch all the way to the back of the joint. You should see the "black hole" and see and feel the "over the top position" on the lateral femoral condyle with a hook probe to make sure you are seeing the anatomical origin of the anterior medial bundle of the anterior cruciate ligament. When the site is confirmed precisely, a dimple is placed in the bone with a power burr at the 1 o'clock position in a left knee and at the 11 o'clock position in a right knee. This dimple serves as a visual landmark for easy arthroscopic identification when positioning the pointer of the femoral guide system. If the femoral osseous tunnel is placed too far anteriorly, the tunnel should be bone grafted and redrilled. If the femoral tunnel cannot be placed in the proper position, the graft can be routed over the top of the lateral femoral condyle as a salvage procedure. Nonisometric placement of the tibial tunnel can be avoided by placing the guide pin slightly anterior and medial to the isometric center of the anterior cruciate ligament (i.e., the anterior medial bundle insertion site). If the tibial hole is not isometric, the hole can be adjusted posteriorly and laterally by ovaling the hole with a power reamer or rasp. Conversely, if the hole is placed too far posteriorly and laterally, the hole has to be bone grafted and redrilled to correct isometry.

Graft fixation problems can be avoided if strict attention is given to specific details of the technique. When stapling the graft to the femur, only one third of the graft is covered by the staple. Stapling the full graft risks dividing the graft into halves if the staple is impacted too firmly. Loosening of the staples is avoided by using special barbed bone ligament staples and inserting them at a 45° angle to the long axis of the femur. Graft fixation to the tibia with dual staples using the buckle technique has not been a problem. There have been no cases of tibial staples backing out or loss of graft fixation. Among thinner patients, prominence of the staples can be minimized by making the exit hole oval with a reamer and recessing both staples in the elongated tibial exit hole.

Wound hematomas can be avoided by releasing the tourniquet after graft fixation and obtaining hemostasis with electrocautery prior to wound closure.

Cosmetic deformity can be minimized by 1) accurate placement of skin incisions so that they do not have to be enlarged and 2) proper retraction of skin edges to facilitate exposure, and meticulous wound closure to minimize scar formation and bulging of the vastus lateralis muscle.

A thick pad is placed over the graft donor site on the lateral thigh and incorporated into the compression dressing. This pad is maintained over the lateral thigh for 7 to 10 days to minimize bulging of the vastus lateralis muscle. Patients should be forewarned of the cosmetic residuals prior to surgery so they are not surprised later.

The most serious complication following this surgery is due to slip and fall accidents. Patients should be warned of the hazards with crutch ambulation. They should wear sturdy shoes and avoid wet, slippery, and unstable surfaces in and out of the house. They should be cautioned about showers, bathtubs, and swimming pools. They should avoid unpaved surfaces and uneven terrain. Prophylactic bracing may be prudent for the less agile or high risk patients.

There have been no functional deficits of the lateral side of the knee from using the iliotibial band in performing this operation.

REFERENCES

1. Hey Groves EW. Operation for repair of the crucial ligaments. *Lancet.* 1917;2:674.
2. Hey Groves EW. The crucial ligaments of the knee joint: their function, rupture, and the operative treatment of same. *Br J Surg.* 1920;7:505–515.
3. MacIntosh DL, Darby TA. Lateral substitution reconstruction. In the proceedings of the Canadian Orthopaedic Association. *J Bone Joint Surg.* 1976;58B:142.
4. Bertoia JT, Urovitz EP, Richards RR, Gross AE. Anterior cruciate reconstruction using the MacIntosh lateral-substitution over-the-top repair. *J Bone Joint Surg.* 1985;67A:1183–1188.
5. Galway HR, MacIntosh DL. The lateral pivot shift: a symptom and sign of anterior cruciate ligament insufficiency. *Clin Ortho Related Res.* 1980;147:45–50.
6. Bach JR, Bach BR, Warren RF, Flynn WM, Kroll M, Wickiewicz TL. Arthrometric evaluation of knees that have a torn anterior cruciate ligament. *J Bone Joint Surg.* 1990;72A:1299–1306.
7. Daniel DM, Malcom LL, Losse G, Stone ML, Sachs R, Burks R. Instrumented measurement of anterior laxity of the knee. *J Bone Joint Surg.* 1985;67A:720–726.
8. Merchant A, Mercer RL, Jacobsen RH, Kool CR. Roentgenographic analysis of patellofemoral congruence. *J Bone Joint Surg.* 1974;56A:1391–1396.
9. Clancy WG Jr, Ray JM. Anterior cruciate ligament autografts. In: Jackson DW, Drez D Jr, eds. *The Anterior Cruciate Deficient Knee. New Concepts In Ligament Repair.* St. Louis, Mo: CV Mosby; 1987:193–210.
10. Graf B. Isometric placement of substitutes for the anterior cruciate ligament. In: Jackson DW, Drez D Jr, eds. *The Anterior Cruciate Deficient Knee. New Concepts In Ligament Repair.* St. Louis, Mo: CV Mosby; 1987:102–113.
11. Norwood LA, Cross MJ. Anterior cruciate ligament functional anatomy of its bundles in rotatory stabilities. *Am J Sports Med.* 1979;7:23.
12. Sapega AA, Moyer RA, Schneck C, Komalahiranya N. Testing for isometry during reconstruction of the anterior cruciate ligament. *J Bone Joint Surg.* 1990;72A:259–267.
13. Sidles JA, Larson RV, Garbini JL, Downey DJ, Matsen RA III. Ligament length relationships in the moving knee. *J Orthop Res.* 1988;6:593–610.
14. Roth JH, Kennedy JC, Lockstadt H, McCallum CL, Cunning LA. Polypropylene braid augmented and nonaugmented intraarticular anterior cruciate ligament reconstruction. *Am J Sports Med.* 1985;13:321–336.
15. Krackow KA, Brooks RL. Optimization of the knee ligament position for lateral extraarticular reconstruction. *Am J Sports Med.* 1983;11:293–302.

chapter Eight

Anterior Cruciate Ligament Reconstruction Using Fresh Frozen Patellar Tendon Allografts

Freddie H. Fu
Eric J. Olson

Compared with autogenous reconstruction, allograft reconstruction of the knee offers a number of advantages in the treatment of symptomatic anterior cruciate ligament deficiency: The use of allografts means that no autogenous tissue is sacrificed; allograft tissue is available if an autograft has failed; allograft reconstruction requires a smaller incision than autograft reconstruction; and by sparing the patellar tendon and extensor mechanisms, allograft reconstruction causes less extensor mechanism morbidity.[1–3]

A further advance in allograft reconstruction has been made at our center. A quadriceps sparing procedure, also known as the "one-shot" technique, allows the entire anterior cruciate ligament reconstruction to be performed through a single 2 to 3 cm medial tibial incision. No incision is made on the distal lateral thigh. By avoiding a separate approach to the distal lateral quadriceps, operative time is reduced. Additionally, four patients who have had one knee reconstructed with the traditional rear-entry guide technique and the other reconstructed using the quadriceps-sparing reconstruction, report that the knee that underwent the "one-shot" reconstruction felt "normal" in 2 months compared to 4 months for the opposite knee.

OBTAINING ALLOGRAFTS

Patients who undergo anterior cruciate ligament reconstruction with allografts need to be fully informed about the relative risks and benefits of this procedure. The possible transmission of the human immunodeficiency virus (HIV) and other infections must be discussed so the patients feel comfortable with their decision to use autograft or allograft tissue.

Surgeons need to be careful about where they obtain their allografts. Tissue banks that adhere to the standards of the American Association of Tissue Banks (AATB)[4] will provide higher quality grafts than "in-house" banks. American Association tissue banks carefully screen potential donors to minimize the chance of procuring tissue from a donor in the "window period," the time between their exposure to HIV and disclosure of the HIV infection by antibody or antigen testing. Current antigen testing becomes positive in approximately 2 weeks. Third generation HIV antibody tests have the potential to reduce this window to less than 2 weeks.

At our center, we avoid using ethylene oxide sterilized allografts for several reasons. First, Jackson et al.[5] and Roberts et al.[6] have reported cyst formation around bone tunnels into which ethylene oxide allografts have been placed. Investigators have also reported effusions, an "applesauce reaction," and graft dissolution following reconstruction with ethylene oxide-treated allografts.[7] Additionally, in our own laboratory, Silvaggio demonstrated that wear particles generated from ethylene oxide-treated allografts induce significantly increased levels of interleukin-I from synovial cells than do wear particles from fresh frozen allografts.[8] This data supports the notion that ethylene oxide may induce inflammation in the synovial lining of the knee. This inflamed synovium produces cytokines that may cause graft deterioration and subsequent cyst formation in the bone surrounding the allograft's bone plugs.

Fresh frozen allografts are preferred over fresh grafts for several reasons. Freezing decreases the graft immunogenicity[9] by causing the lysis of the "passenger leukocytes,"[10] which are the principle cellular features responsible for allograft immunogenicity. Additionally, freezing grafts is necessary to allow adequate time for completion of screening tests that insure graft safety.

Grafts may be radiated to further minimize the risk of viral transmission. While doses of 15 to 25 kGy are employed, some investigations suggest that this dosage does not eliminate the risk of HIV transmission.[11,12] Furthermore, there are several disadvantages to radiating anterior cruciate ligament allografts. Studies have demonstrated that the collagen crimping pattern is altered and the collagen cross-linking is lost after allografts have been exposed to radiation.[13,14] These changes may alter the graft's biomechanical properties.[15,16] The tissue bank from which we currently obtain allografts radiates the tissue with between 15 and 20 kGy due to recent reports of HIV transmission following allograft use.

SURGICAL TECHNIQUE

After satisfactory general anesthesia the patient is placed supine on the operating table. The well leg is placed in a padded, elevated leg holder with the hip and knee flexed 90° and secured with an ace bandage. Elevating and abducting the well leg minimizes blood pooling in this leg during surgery and provides improved access to the operative extremity. The operative leg is placed in a leg holder. A tourniquet is placed inside the leg holder and positioned so that approximately 20 cm of the distal thigh are exposed below the lower edge of the tourniquet and leg holder. The infragluteal crease is positioned so it is just above the edge of the operative table. The limb is exsanguinated with an Esmarch bandage, and the tourniquet is inflated to between 250 and 300 mm Hg (Fig. 8.1).

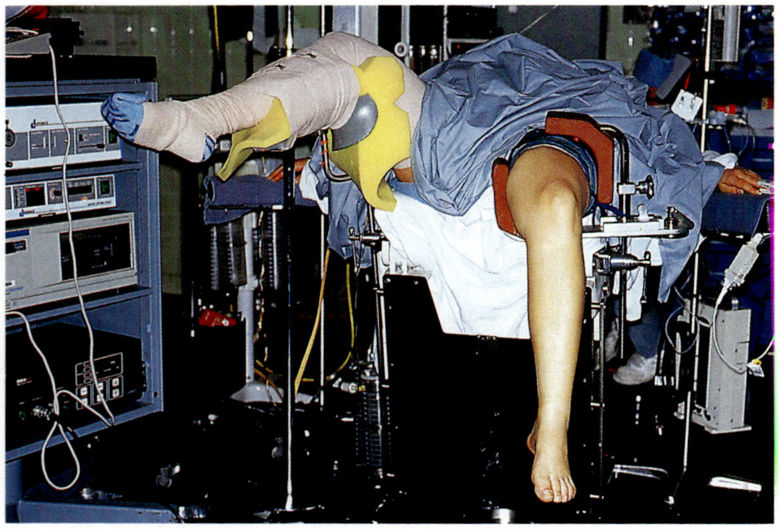

Figure 8.1
Patient positioned on operating table with well leg elevated in a leg holder and the operative leg positioned in a tourniquet-enclosing leg holder.

Portal Placement

A superior medial inflow portal is made posterior to the vastus medialis obliquus but anterior to the intermuscular septum. This must be of adequate diameter to permit good inflow. A lateral parapatellar viewing portal is made just adjacent to the patellar tendon. A medial parapatellar operative portal is made in the soft spot just adjacent to the tendon. Placing the portal in this location rather than further medial gives better access to the medial wall of the lateral femoral condyle posteriorly during notch preparation (Fig. 8.2).

Clearing Soft Tissue Debris

After the arthroscope has been placed, attention is immediately turned to clearing any excessive soft tissue in the anterior aspect of the knee. This is necessary to obtain an unobstructed view of the intercondylar notch. It allows rapid meniscal diagnosis and minimizes the time spent orienting and positioning instruments inside the knee. Moreover, this soft tissue clearance will eventually need to be performed for anterior cruciate ligament tunnel placement and reconstruction. A slow cutting speed with the full radius resector (for example, 800 to 1,000 rpm) using a 5.5 mm full radius resector works well for this portion of the procedure.

Meniscal Procedures

We address any meniscal pathology first, performing a partial meniscectomy if necessary or, if healing is possible, a meniscal repair. If a meniscal repair is performed, sutures are placed, but the knots are not tied until after anterior cruciate ligament reconstruction fixation is in place. This prevents undue intraoperative shear placed on the repair and minimizes the risk of disrupting the meniscal repair while completing the anterior cruciate ligament reconstruction.

Notchplasty

The torn anterior cruciate ligament fibers are completely removed. A large basket forceps or pituitary grasper used in a twisting motion helps speed the debridement process

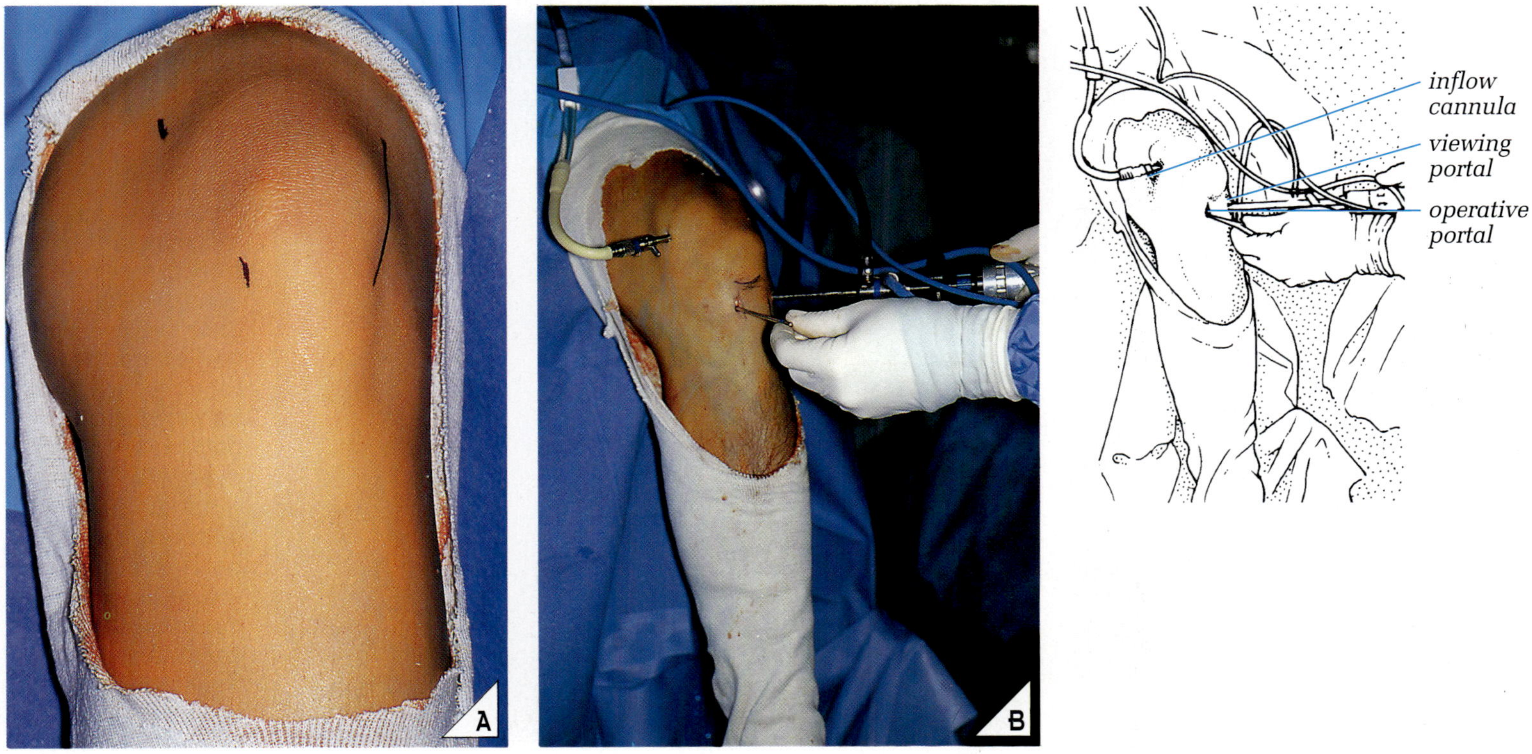

Figure 8.2
(A, B) Instruments placed in the arthroscopic portals of the knee: viewing portal, operative portal, inflow portal.

(Fig. 8.3). At times a small stump of tissue is left on the tibial insertion to help orient placement of the tibial tunnel. Approximately 3 to 4 mm of bone are typically removed from the medial wall of the lateral femoral condyle. When learning to perform this procedure, it may help to mark the amount of bone to be taken with an arthroscopic osteotome. With experience, the amount of bone to be removed will be apparent from inspecting the intercondylar notch directly. Several tips are helpful in performing a good notchplasty:

- First, it is important to remove more bone anteriorly and almost none posteriorly in the notch. This "trumpeting" of the bone resection prevents excessive lateralization of the femoral anterior cruciate ligament origin point, and it removes the bone anteriorly and superiorly where impingement typically occurs.
- Second, at some point during notchplasty, it is important to flex the knee greater than 90° to allow improved access to the inferior posterior aspect of the medial wall of the lateral femoral condyle. A ridge of bone may be inadvertently left in this region if the knee is not adequately flexed. Because this ridge of bone rests against the tibial plateau, some surgeons avoid resecting it because they fear causing injury to the tibial articular cartilage. However, if this ridge remains, it may saw against the anterior cruciate ligament reconstruction and cause graft failure in extreme knee flexion.
- Third, we have found that bone may be resected with a 5.5 mm full radius resector run at maximum speed or with a burr. We found that after initial bone removal, running the burr backwards allows greater control and prevents gouging of cancellous bone of the lateral femoral condyle. This is useful for smoothing the notchplasty surfaces (Fig. 8.4).

Tibial Tunnel Placement

The goal of tibial tunnel placement is to create a tunnel that allows access to the starting point of the femoral tunnel and yields a graft with satisfactory isometricity. No allograft or autograft anterior cruciate ligament reconstruction is truly "isometric". However, in terminal extension a graft should tighten no more than 3 mm for the reconstruction to remain appropriately tensioned in the range of motion in which the pivot shift phenomenon typically occurs—which is 15° to 20° of flexion. A graft that becomes lax in terminal extension is unacceptable. The graft should also be placed in a position that will minimize impingement and risk to surrounding structures.

We have found in a cadaveric anatomical study that measuring the distance between the apex of the tibial tubercle and the medial aspect of the tibia, then selecting a point halfway in between, results in a consistently good tibial tunnel starting point. In an average-sized individual, this will be 3 to 4 cm medial from the apex of the tibial

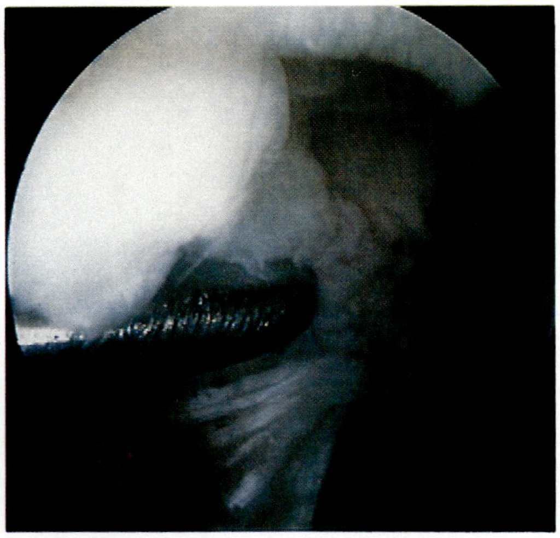

Figure 8.3
Intraarticular view of a pituitary grasper or large basket forceps debriding the stump of a torn anterior cruciate ligament.

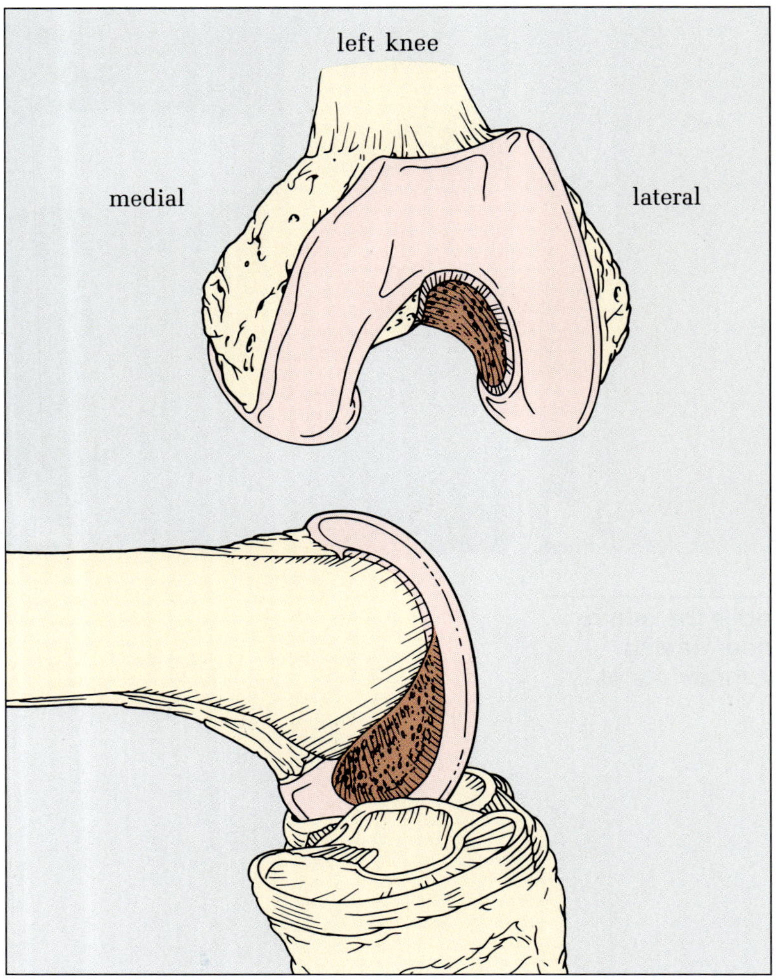

Figure 8.4
Intraarticular notch after completed notchplasty—anterior view (top) and lateral view (bottom, depicted with medial half half of femur removed). Three to 4 mm of bone was removed from the anterior portion of the medial wall of the lateral femoral condyle, tapering the notchplasty in order to take less bone posteriorly.

tubercle (Fig. 8.5). We use an Acufex or Concept tibial tunnel guide, positioning its intraarticular portion through the medial parapatellar portal so that the tip is in the midportion of the tibial anterior cruciate ligament stump. Extending the knee at this point will help to show that the tip of the tibial guide is "captured" within the anterior portion of the intracondylar notch.

The surgeon should position the external portion of the tibial tunnel guide against the proximal medial tibia at the previously determined starting point. If the extraarticular starting point is too lateral, i.e., too close to the tibial tubercle, the resulting tibial tunnel will have several problems. A K-wire placed through a lateral tunnel will tend to skive off the medial wall of the lateral femoral condyle and fall toward the posterior aspect of the intercondylar notch. Curetting a depression in the femoral wall allows the K-wire to be captured.

A femoral tunnel drilled over a K-wire placed too parallel to the medial wall of the lateral femoral condyle results in a shallow angle between the lateral aspect of the notch and the allograft, predisposing the reconstruction to impingement.

Additionally, if the tibial tunnel starting point is too close to the tibial tubercle, the femoral tunnel created through it will be too parallel to the femur. When a Beeth needle, used to draw the allograft into the knee, is passed through such a tunnel, the needle tends to emerge too proximal from the lateral thigh. The needle may be difficult to retrieve distal to the tourniquet and leg holder.

Starting the tibial tunnel too medially, however, causes graft impingement against the lateral edge of the medial femoral condyle and makes it difficult to reach adequately into the posterior aspect of the intracondylar notch.

The proximal-to-distal starting point is determined by the tibial tunnel guide. Once the tip of the tibial tunnel guide has been positioned against the tibial plateau, the external portion of the guide is applied against the anteromedial tibia. The tibial tunnel guide measures the tunnel's length. The tunnel should be 35 to 45 mm long to permit interference screw fixation of the allograft. Dropping the starting point distally helps prevent a short, shallow tunnel. A satisfactory tunnel usually results if the surgeon initiates the tunnel at the level of the tibial tubercle and drills the tunnel at a 45° angle as seen from a lateral projection (Fig. 8.6).

A 2 to 3 cm incision is created, extending just proximal to the starting point marked on the skin. The tibial drill guide is securely positioned against the periosteum and the position is rechecked. A K-wire is advanced through the tibial drill guide until it emerges through the tibial plateau. The position is rechecked. Extending the knee allows the surgeon to verify "capture" of the tibial insertion of the anterior cruciate ligament reconstruction within the femur's anterior intracondylar notch. If unsatisfactory, the guide wire is removed and redrilled until an acceptable position is achieved. The tibial tunnel is then created by overdrilling the K-wire with a cannulated 10 mm drill. Care must be taken not to plunge when breaking through the tibial plateau. Inadvertent posterior cruciate ligament injury can result from careless drilling.

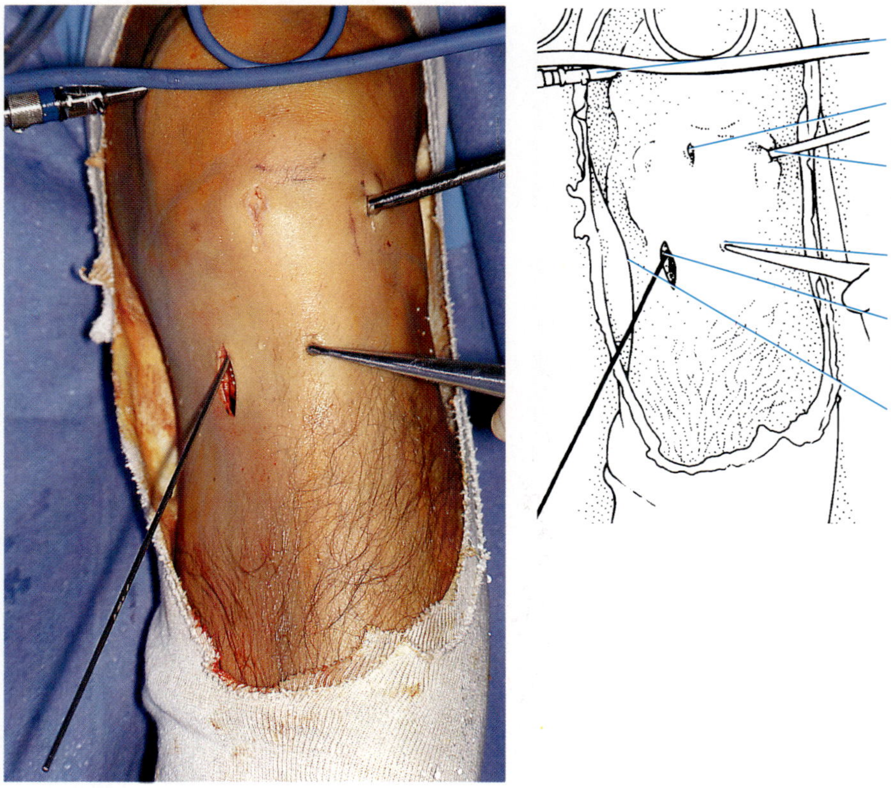

Figure 8.5
Tibial tunnel starting point incisor approximately 3 cm medial to the medial aspect of the tibial tubercle, i.e., halfway between the apex of the tibial tubercle and the most medial portion of the tibia.

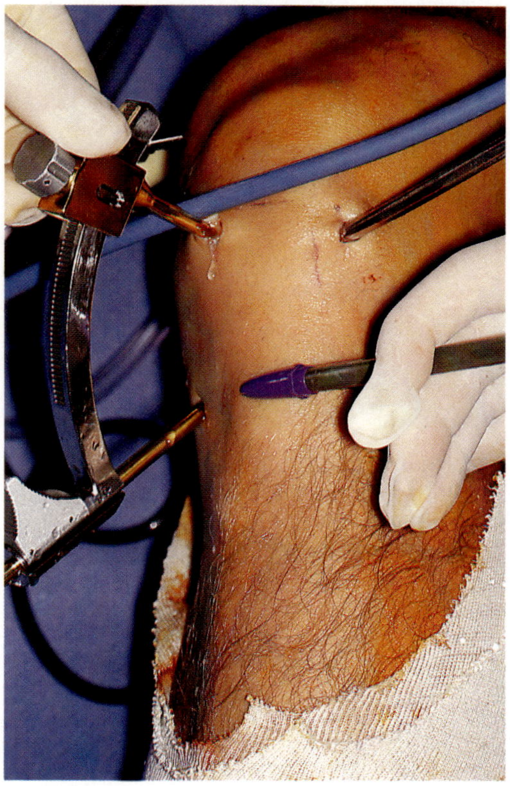

Figure 8.6
Tibial tunnel guide in place on the tibia shows the length of the tunnel (35 to 45 mm), the angle of the tunnel (45°), and the guide secured where the incision will be made.

Chamfering the Tibial Tunnel

The rasps and full radius resector smooth and chamfer the edges of the tibial tunnel, particularly posteriorly and laterally on the tibial plateau. The femoral tunnel guidewire can reach the posterior medial aspect of the lateral femoral condyle more easily if the surgeon removes bone from the posterior and lateral aspects of the tibial tunnel. This also minimizes the risk of graft failure due to abrasion against a sharp bone edge.

Selecting the Femoral Tunnel Starting Point

Choosing the appropriate femoral tunnel starting point is critical for operative success. Correct placement will allow the femoral tunnel to be drilled through the tibial tunnel, precluding the need for a distal lateral thigh incision. The femoral tunnel should not be started too posteriorly, which could result in a posterior "blowout" fracture of the lateral femoral condyle. This prevents satisfactory interference screw fixation of the femoral bone block. To assist selection of the femoral tunnel starting point, mentally divide the femoral intercondylar notch into a clock face. Nine o'clock and 3 o'clock are the left and right edges of the notch, while 12 o'clock is the roof. For right knee reconstruction, the 10 o'clock position is used. For left knees, the 2 o'clock position is used. Studies by Hefzy and others[17] have shown the relatively isometric region of the femoral condyle lies more anteriorly as one moves down from the roof of the intracondylar notch. Therefore, selecting a starting point in these regions minimizes the risk of a blowout fracture, and is also more kinematically sound. Once the medial lateral starting point has been selected, the anteroposterior starting point is determined.

It is critical that the posterior edge of the femoral condyle be cleared of soft tissue so the surgeon can be certain that the posterior cortex within the intercondylar notch is adequately visualized. Once this posterior edge of the femoral condyle has been well exposed, a point 5 to 10 mm anterior to the edge is selected for the femoral tunnel starting point.

The starting point is marked with a curette placed through the medial parapatellar portal. Creating a concavity in the medial wall of the lateral femoral condyle facilitates placement of the femoral tunnel guidewire. If no depression is made, the guidewire may skive off the condyle and move posteriorly or become engaged in a location not selected by the surgeon (Fig. 8.7).

The surgeon must insure that the knee is flexed 90° before placing the femoral tunnel guidewire through the tibial tunnel and up into the lateral femoral condyle. Extending the knee to "help" the guidewire reach a posterior point on the femur increases the risk of a femoral blowout fracture. Rather than extending the knee to get the guidewire posterior, additional bone should be resected from the posterior aspect of the tibial tunnel where it emerges through the tibial plateau.

Once the tip of the guidewire has been passed through the tibial tunnel and is engaged into the lateral femoral

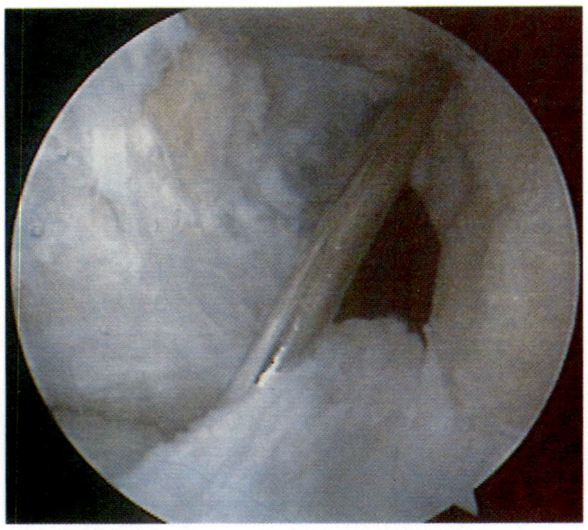

Figure 8.7
K-wire positioned in curetted concavity along the medial wall of the lateral femoral chondyle. Note the appropriate femoral tunnel starting point.

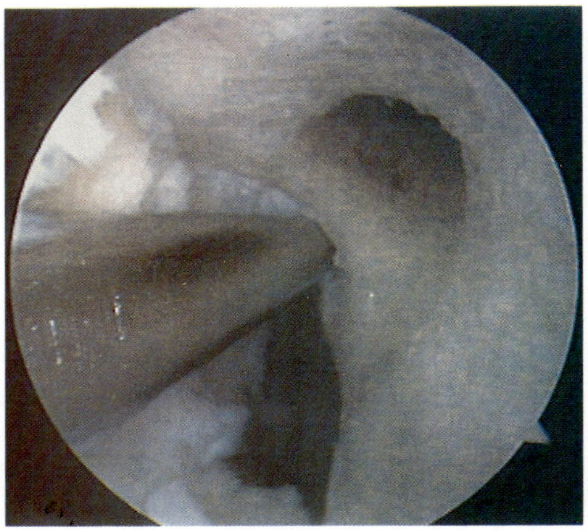

Figure 8.8
A well chamfered femoral bone tunnel, minimizing risk of graft abrasion and failure.

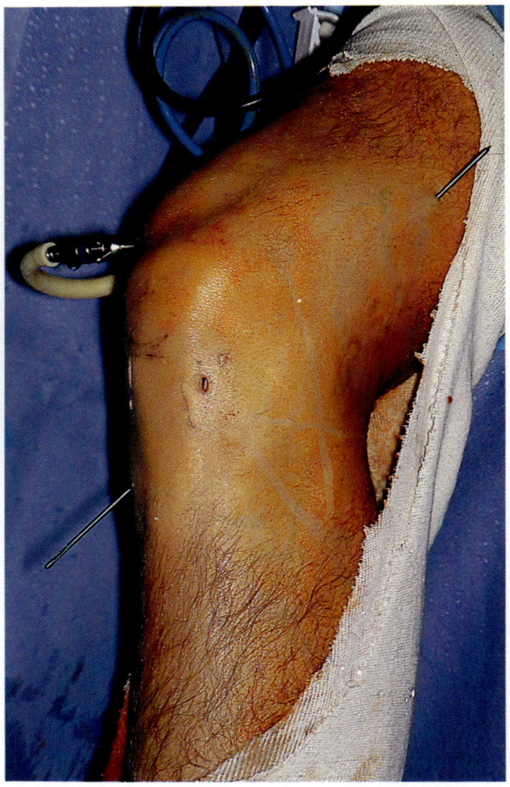

Figure 8.9
Beeth needle in place through the knee, ready to accept allograft sutures through the eye of the needle. Note where the Beeth needle emerges from lateral thigh.

condyle, it is hammered 1 to 2 cm into the femur. At this point the knee must not be flexed or extended, which would bend the guidewire. A 10 mm endoscopic drill is then placed over the femoral guidewire and manually advanced through the tibial tunnel, through the knee (taking care not to damage the posterior cruciate ligament), then engaged against the medial wall of the lateral femoral condyle. A power drill advances the endoscopic bit into the lateral femoral condyle to a depth of approximately 35 mm. We have found the lateral cortex of the lateral femoral condyle is typically 40 to 45 mm from the femoral tunnel starting point. Plunging through this cortex with the endoscopic drill risks injuring the superior lateral geniculate artery, particularly if the selected femoral starting point is too posterior.

Once the endoscopic drill and the K-wire are removed, the surgeon should see an intact cylinder of bone in the lateral femoral condyle with no compromise of bone along the posterior aspect of the tunnel. The anterior edge of the tunnel should then be chamfered and smoothed with the rasps and the full radius resector (Fig. 8.8). The rasps and the full radius resector may then be used to make a slot in the anterior edge of the tunnel to facilitate positioning the interference screw fixation later. The femoral cortex is perforated with a long 1/4 inch drill passed through the tibial tunnel and then the femoral tunnel. This perforation eases passage of the Beeth needle (a long K-wire with an eye at one end), and the knots of the sutures that draw the allograft into the knee. A Beeth needle is advanced through the knee from the tibia, through the femoral tunnel, until the tip emerges through the skin in the distal lateral thigh. The eye of the Beeth needle should remain accessible just outside the tibial tunnel (Fig. 8.9).

Allograft Preparation

The thawed allograft should be rinsed in two baths of saline, which are not heated above 40° C because the allograft's collagen can be denatured. Instead, saline 37° to 38° C should be used. If the saline feels too warm for bathing, the graft should not be put in it. The allograft should be inspected to determine the region with optimal preservation of tendon bone insertion. The graft is then shaped with oscillating saws and rongeurs so that it can easily be passed through a 10 mm-sizing guide (Figs. 8.10, 8.11). The fiber insertion into the bone blocks must be optimally preserved. In shaping the allograft, the surgeon must balance the need for ease of graft passage with the need to fill the tunnel with the graft's bone plugs. Good bone plug fit will facilitate union between the allograft and the surrounding host bone cylinder. We typically make bone plugs 25 mm in length. Each bone block is perforated with a hand drill, then a #5 Tycron suture is passed through the block. The leading edge of the femoral bone block is "bulleted" to ease passage through the knee.

Passage of the Graft Into the Knee

The femoral bone block suture is tied to the Beeth needle, which is drawn through the knee pulling the Tycron suture out through the distal lateral thigh. The surgeon should insure that the knot passes out through the skin before the allograft is advanced into the knee. This eliminates the potential for failure of the suture knot as the allograft is being drawn into the knee. Allograft passage is facilitated by grasping the Tycron suture with a Kocher clamp.

After the graft has been drawn into the knee, the

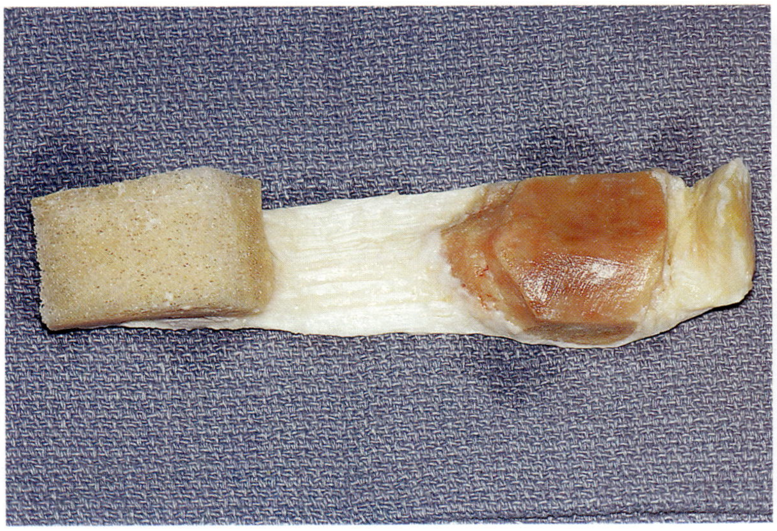

Figure 8.10
Bone-patellar tendon-bone allograft prior to shaping and preparation. It is critical to maintain the tendon bone attachments during graft preparation.

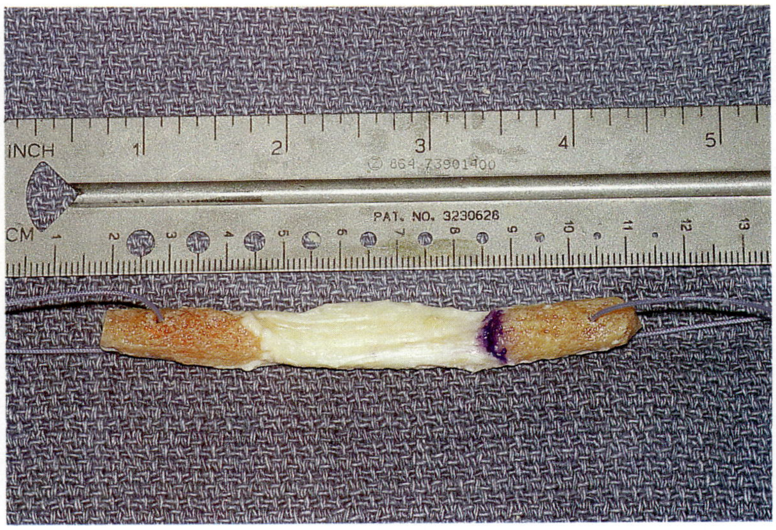

Figure 8.11
Bone-patellar tendon-bone allograft after shaping to pass through a 10 mm tunnel. Note the suture placement in bone block.

femoral bone block should be positioned so that the graft's fibers are posterior. Conversely, the portion of the bone block without fiber attachment should be anterior. This minimizes the risk of graft fiber damage during interference screw placement. Once the graft is drawn into the knee, a flexible guidewire for the interference screw is placed through the medial parapatellar portal. This flexible wire is positioned between the femoral bone block and its surrounding femoral tunnel. If the femoral bone block is left a little "proud" by not fully pulling the block into the femoral tunnel, the tip of the flexible guidewire can be positioned between the bone plug and the femoral tunnel (Fig. 8.12), then drawn up into this interface by fully seating the femoral bone plug into the femoral tunnel (Fig. 8.13). This helps make the access of the interference screw parallel with that of the bone block.

The knee should then be fully flexed. A Kirowsaca or other interference screw is advanced over the flexible guidewire and screwed into the interval between the bone block and surrounding tunnel (Fig. 8.14). The flexible guidewire is removed and the femur's Tycron suture is removed.

Fixation of the Tibial Bone Block

The tibial bone block is drawn distally as the knee is cycled approximately 20 times through flexion and extension. The change of graft length with terminal extension should be recorded by the surgeon. It should be less than 3 mm. If 20 mm or more of the tibial bone block remains inside the tibial tunnel, the bone block is fixed with an interference screw. The knee is flexed approximately 20° and approximately 20 pounds of tension are applied to the tibial bone block. An interference screw is placed between the tibial bone block and the surrounding tibia, taking care not to cut the sutures with the screw, which would result in inadequate graft tensioning.

If, however, less than 15 to 20 mm of bone remain in the tibial tunnel, satisfactory interference screw fixation cannot be achieved. Instead, the tibial incision is lengthened distally several centimeters. The tibial periosteum is elevated for 2 to 3 cm directly distal to the tibial tunnel. A 10 mm trough is created in the tibia just distal to the tunnel. The graft is then tensioned and one or two Richard's bone staples are used to fix the graft into the trough (Fig. 8.15). Sutures are removed from the tibial bone block, and the wounds are closed in the usual fashion.

Conclusion

Quadriceps-sparing anterior cruciate ligament reconstruction with fresh frozen patellar tendon allografts provides an attractive alternative to traditional central third anterior cruciate ligament reconstruction. It provides patients with improved cosmesis, avoids iatrogenic injury to their patellar extensor mechanism, and prevents direct injury to their quadriceps musculature.

At our center, we have performed approximately 450 allograft anterior cruciate ligament reconstructions over the past 6 years. We have had no cases of rejection or adverse clinical responses due to the allograft tissue. While technically demanding, particularly with regard to tibial tunnel placement for optimal "one-shot" femoral tunnel creation, the technique described in this chapter provides surgeons with a desirable method for reconstruction of symptomatic anterior cruciate ligament deficient knees.

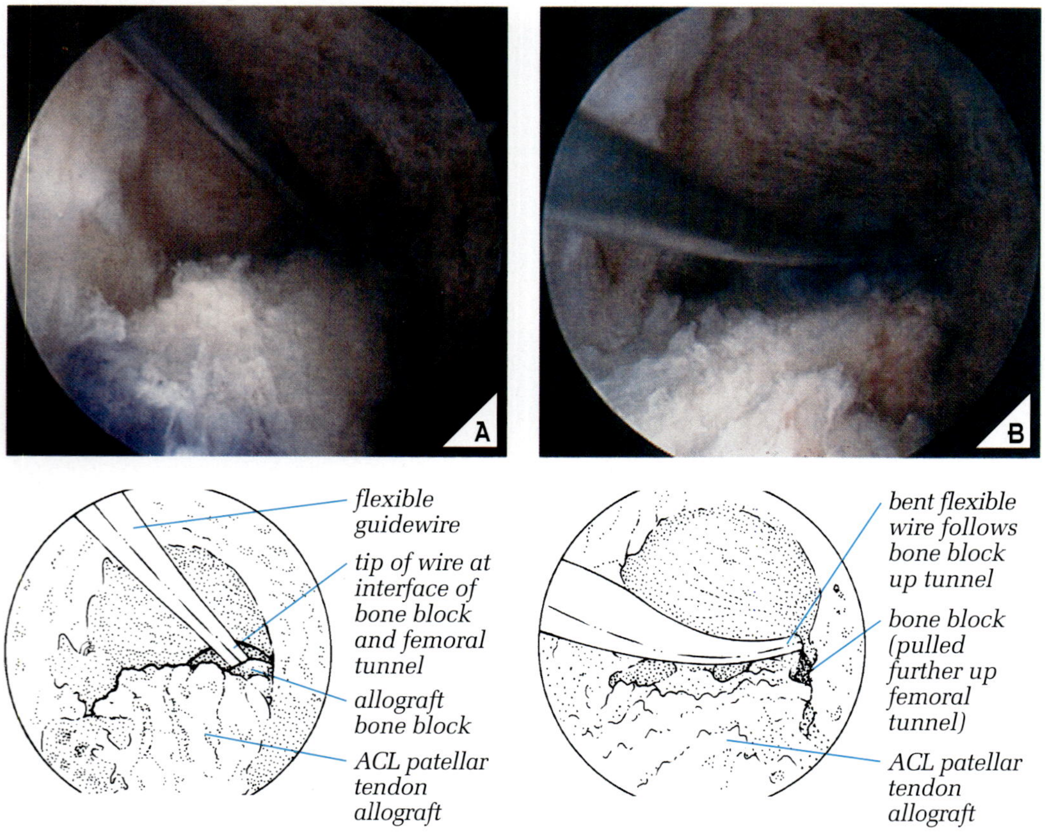

Figure 8.12
(A) Femoral bone block/femoral tunnel interface. The femoral bone plug is a little "proud," and the flexible wire is resting at the junction between the tunnel and the bone plug. (B) The bone plug is pulled up into the femoral tunnel and the flexible wire is drawn into the gap between the bone plug and femoral tunnel, which facilitates placing the interference screw parallel to the femoral bone block.

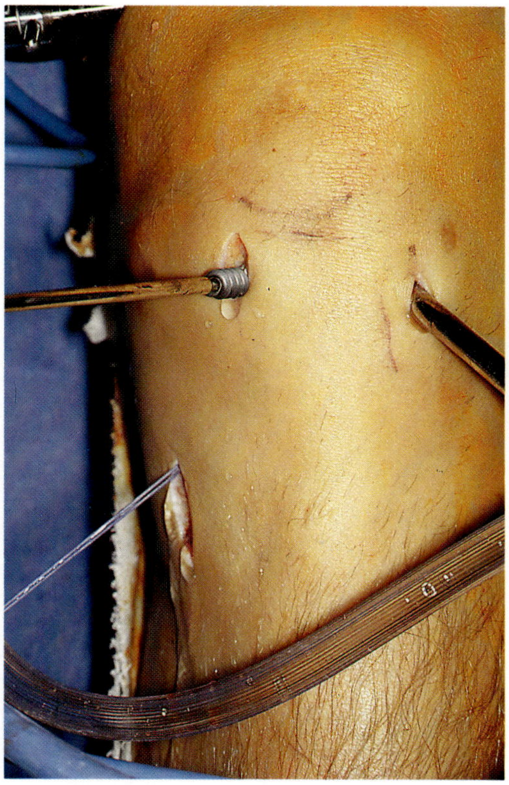

Figure 8.13
The interference screw is introduced into the knee over the flexible guidewire.

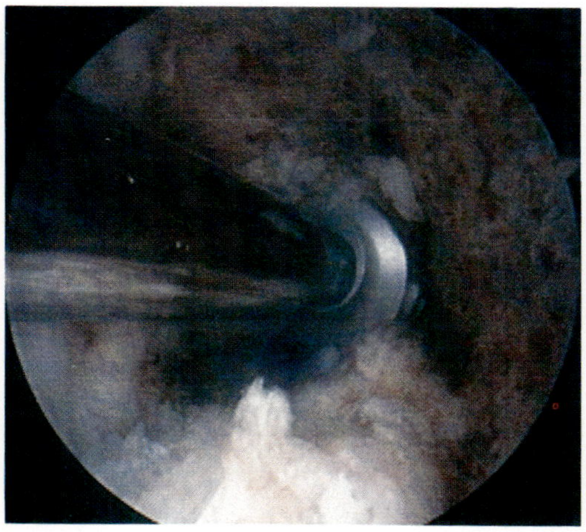

Figure 8.14
The interference screw is introduced between the femoral bone block and the femoral tunnel.

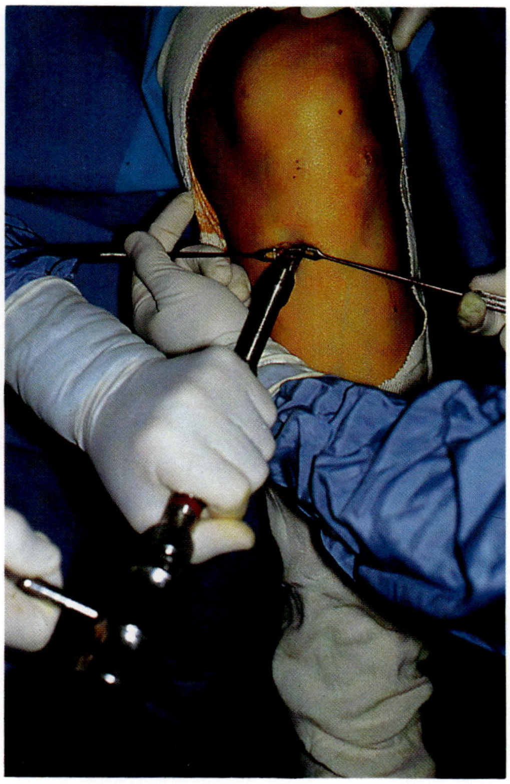

Figure 8.15
Tibial bone block fixation with two Richard's staples.

REFERENCES

1. Bonamo JJ, Krinick RM, Sporn A. Rupture of the patellar ligament after use of its central third for anterior cruciate reconstruction. report of two cases. *J Bone Joint Surg.* 1984; 66A:1294–1297.
2. DeLee JC, Craviotto DF. Rupture of the quadriceps tendon after central third patellar tendon anterior cruciate ligament reconstruction. *Am J Sports Med.* 1991;19:415–416.
3. McCarroll JR. Fracture of the patella during a golf swing following a reconstruction of the anterior cruciate ligament. a case report. *Am J Sports Med.* 1983;11:26–27.
4. American Association of Tissue Banks. *Standards for Tissue Banking.* Arlington, Va: American Association of Tissue Banks; 1984.
5. Jackson DW, Windler GE, Simon TM. Intraarticular reaction associated with the use of freeze-dried, ethylene oxide sterilized bone-patellar tendon-bone allografts in the reconstruction of the anterior cruciate ligament. *Am J Sports Med.* 1990;18:1–11.
6. Roberts TS, Drez D, McCarthy W, Paine R. Anterior cruciate ligament reconstruction using freeze-dried, ethylene oxide-sterilized, bone-patellar tendon allografts. two year results in thirty-six patients. *Am J Sports Med.* 1991;19:35–41.
7. Paulos LE, Rosenberg TD, Gurley WD. Anterior cruciate ligament allografts. In: Friedman MJ, Ferkel RD, eds. *Prosthetic Ligament Reconstruction of the Knee.* Philadelphia, Pa: WB Saunders Co; 1988:186–192.
8. Silvaggio VJ, Fu FH, Georgescu HI, Evans CH. The induction of IL-1 by freeze dried ethylene oxide treated bone-patellar tendon-bone allograft wear particles: an *in vitro* study. *Trans Orth Res Soc.* 1991;16:207.
9. Bos GD, Goldberg VM, Gordon NH, et al. The long-term fate of fresh and frozen orthotopic bone allografts in genetically defined rats. *Clin Orthop.* 1985;197:245–254.
10. Czitrom AA, Axelrod T, Fernandes B. Antigen presenting cells and bone allotransplantation. *Clin Orthop.* 1985; 197:27–31.
11. Conway B, Tomford WW, Hirsch MS, Schooley RT, Mankin HJ. Effects of gamma irradiation of HIV-1 in a bone allograft model. *Trans Orth Res Soc.* 1990;15:225.
12. Withrow SJ, Oulton SA, Suto TL, et al. Evaluation of the antiretroviral effect of various methods of sterilizing/preserving corticocancellous bone. *Trans Orth Res Soc.* 1990;15:226.
13. Haut RC, Powlison AC. Order of irradiation and lypophilization on the strength of patellar tendon allografts. *Trans Orth Res Soc.* 1989;14:514.
14. Haut RC, Powlison AC. The effects of test environment and cyclic stretching on the failure properties of human patellar tendons. *J Orthop Res Soc.* 1990;8:532–540.
15. Gibbons MJ, Butler DL, Grood ED, et al. Dose dependent effects of gamma radiation on the material properties of frozen bone-patellar tendon-bone. *Trans Orth Res Soc.* 1989;14:513.
16. France EP, Paulos LE, Rosenberg TD, Harner CD. The biomechanics of anterior cruciate allografts. In: Friedman MJ, Ferkel RD, eds. *Prosthetic Ligament Reconstruction of the Knee.* Philadelphia, Pa: WB Saunders Co; 1988:180–185.
17. Hefzy MS, Grood ES, Noyes FR. Factors affecting the region of most isometric femoral attachments, II: the anterior cruciate ligament. *Am J Sports Med.* 1989;17:208–216.

chapter Nine

Arthroscopic Technique for Anterior Cruciate Reconstruction Using an Artificial Ligament

James A. Hill

Many prosthetic anterior cruciate ligament devices have been tried. The Gore-Tex prosthesis is intended as a permanent implant for correction of anterior cruciate ligament instability. Approval by the FDA was given in 1986 for its commercial use in patients who had undergone previous failed intraarticular reconstructions. This multifilamentous prosthesis is made of expanded polytetrafluorethylene (PTFE). It is constructed of a single continuous fiber of PTFE, which is arranged in bundles that are braided with an eyelet at each end to provide secure internal fixation with a screw (Fig. 9.1). The Gore-Tex prosthesis can be implanted by an arthroscopic technique.

Surgical Technique

Initially, a thorough joint evaluation is performed to document associated intraarticular pathology (e.g., articular surface damage) and to treat lesions such as meniscal tears and loose bodies. Once the joint has been evaluated, attention is directed to the intracondylar notch, where a large shaver removes synovium and a portion of the fat pad to aid visualization. A large burr is then used to resect the lateral and superior portion of the notch to prevent impingement on the prosthesis (Fig. 9.2).

After the notchplasty has been performed a 5 cm longitudinal incision is made 1 cm medial to the patellar tendon, beginning 3 cm below the medial tibial plateau. A 2.4 mm (3/32 inch) Kirschner wire is then drilled, beginning 2 to 3 cm distal to the tibial rim and 1 cm medial to the patellar tendon. Under arthroscopic visualization, this wire should exit on the tibial plateau at the center of the normal insertion of the anterior cruciate ligament (Fig. 9.3). A drill guide may facilitate proper placement. To double check the correct position of the K-wire, the wire should be pointed directly at the posterior aspect of the intercondylar notch just medial to the lateral femoral condyle with the knee in full extension (Fig. 9.4).

The K-wire is then overdrilled with a 7.9 mm (5/16 inch) cannulated drill bit (Fig. 9.5). At the time of drilling, the tip of the intraarticular guide pin is covered with a small curette to prevent the guide pin from being inadvertently driven across the joint and puncturing the articular surface or the posterior capsular area. The edge of the tibia drill hole is then smoothed and chamfered with a smoother, rasp, or burr (Fig. 9.6). This is extremely important because passing the prosthesis over sharp bone edges will damage the prosthesis and lead to failure.

Attention is then directed to the femur, where a 7 cm lateral suprapatellar incision is made to expose the femur proximal to the lateral femoral epicondyle. The fascia lata is incised parallel to its fibers. The lateral femoral shaft and popliteal space are approached with blunt dissection. A 2.4 mm (3/32 inch) K-wire is used to make the femoral tunnel, beginning on the lateral surface of the femur anterior and approximately 4 to 5 cm proximal to the lateral epicondyle. The K-wire is angled posteriorly, distally,

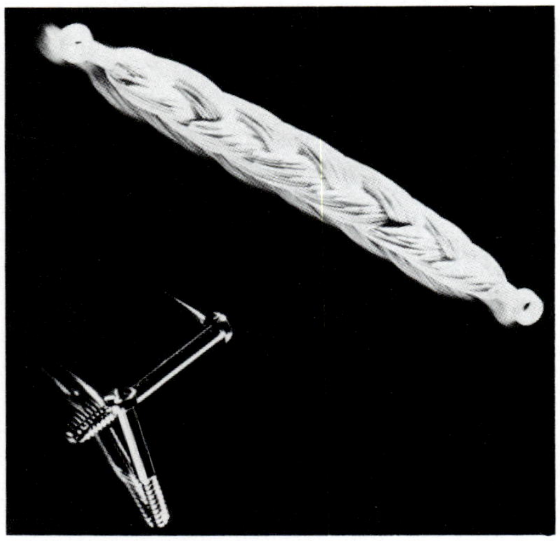

Figure 9.1
Gore-Tex prosthetic ligament.

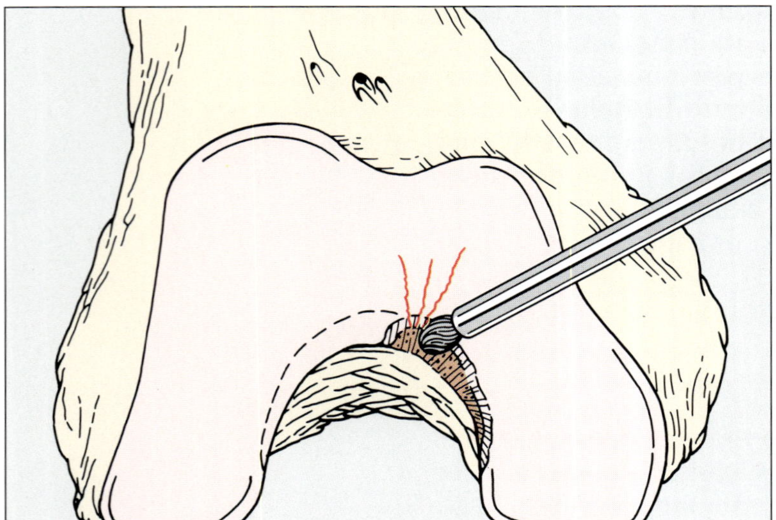

Figure 9.2
Intracondylar notchplasty of the superior and lateral portions to prevent impingement.

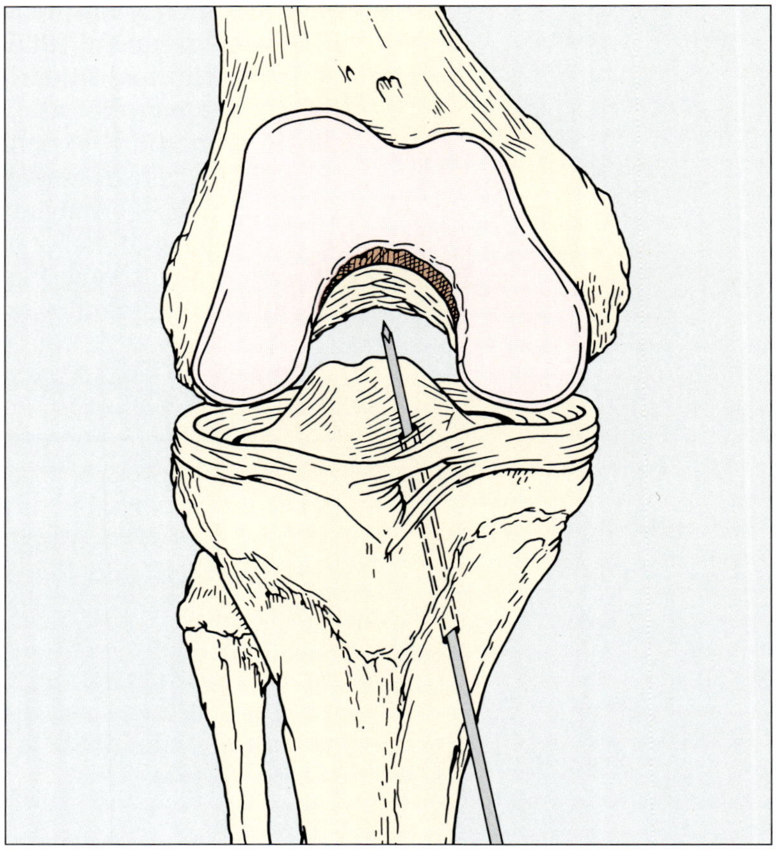

Figure 9.3
Tibial K-wire.

and medially to exit on the popliteal surface of the distal femur. The exit site should be extracapsular, approximately 1 to 2 cm proximal to the capsular attachment at the intercondylar ridge and approximately 1 cm lateral to the midline of the intercondylar notch (Fig. 9.7). Care should be taken to insure that no soft tissue is near the exit hole because of the close proximity of neurovascular structures. A drill guide may facilitate proper placement. The tunnel must be drilled distally, posteriorly, medially, and inferiorly to avoid a transverse placement from the lateral femoral surface to the popliteal fossa. A transverse placement of the femoral tunnel will place greater stress on the

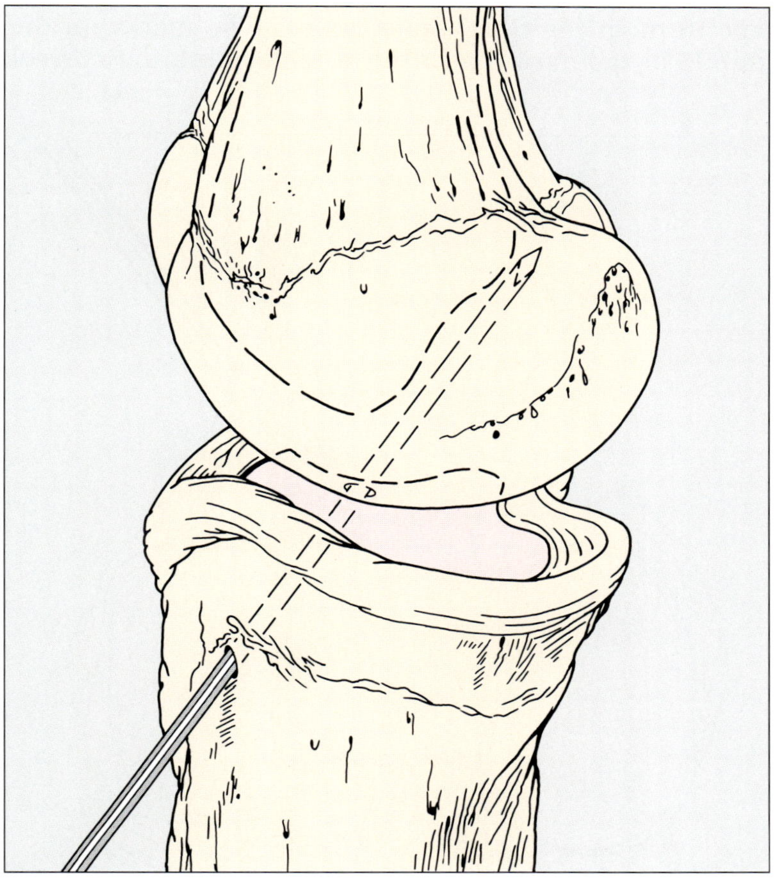

Figure 9.4
Proper placement of the tibial guide pin.

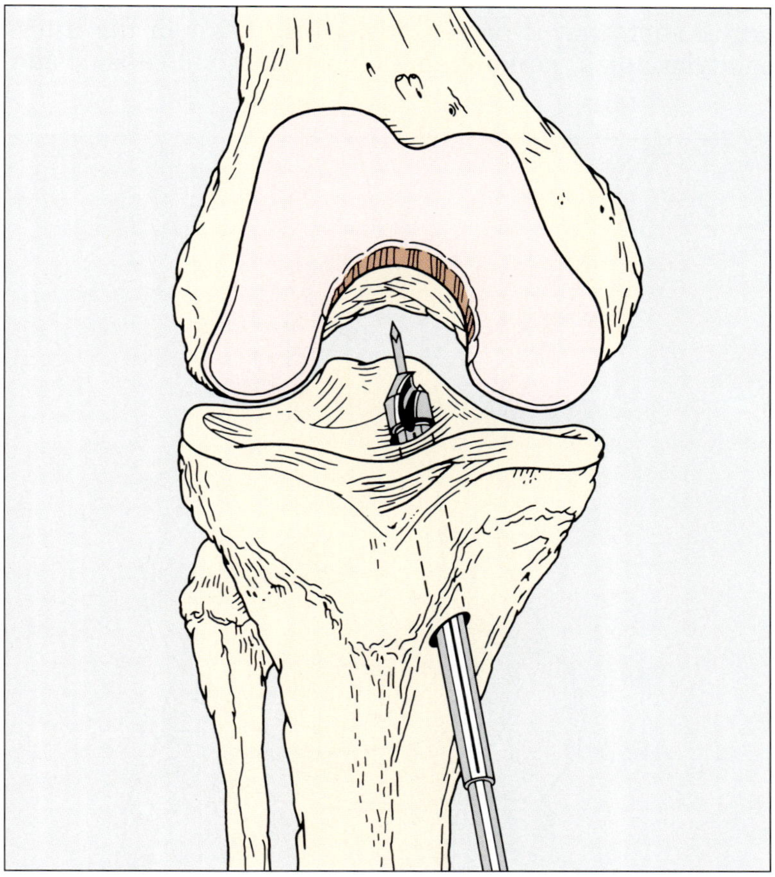

Figure 9.5
Overdrilling of the tibial guide pin with a cannulated drill bit.

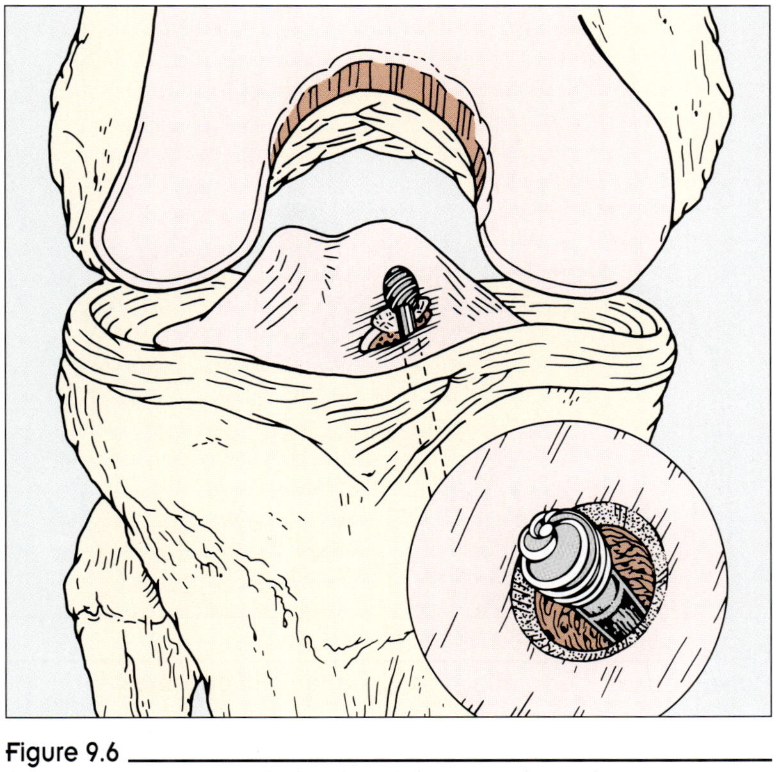

Figure 9.6
Smoothing and chamfering the tibial bone tunnel.

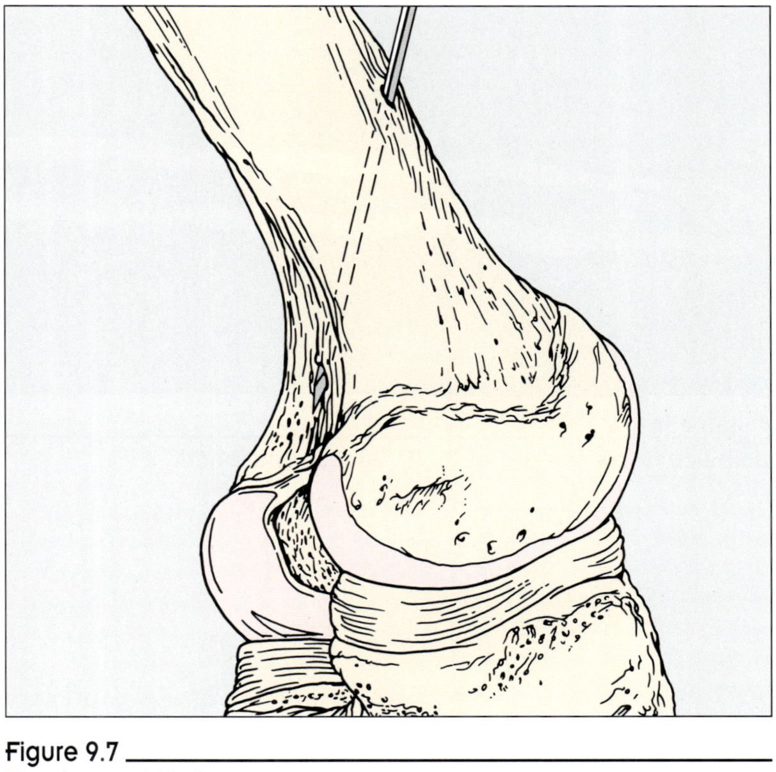

Figure 9.7
The femoral K-wire.

prosthesis, which could result in failure. Next, the K-wire is overdrilled with a 7.9 mm (5/16 inch) cannulated drill bit (Fig. 9.8). The femoral drill hole is then smoothed and chamfered with a smoother, rasp, or burr (Fig. 9.9).

After the bony tunnels have been prepared, 100 cm umbilical tape is folded in half and marked with a surgical marking pen at 16, 18, 20, 22, and 24 cm (Fig. 9.10). A large, curved passer is then directed through an anterior portal such that it passes posteriorly through the intercondylar notch, perforating the posterior joint capsule and exiting the lateral popliteal space (Fig. 9.11). The joint capsule must be perforated at its femoral attachment directly inferior to the posterior femoral bone tunnel exit. Soft tissue beneath the prosthesis should be avoided because it may lead to future laxity. The looped end of the umbilical tape is then passed through the femoral bone tunnel, and the curved passer is used to bring the tape into the joint. Once in the joint, a gripper is used to pull the tape through the tibial bone tunnel. The marks on the umbilical tape are then used to determine the correct

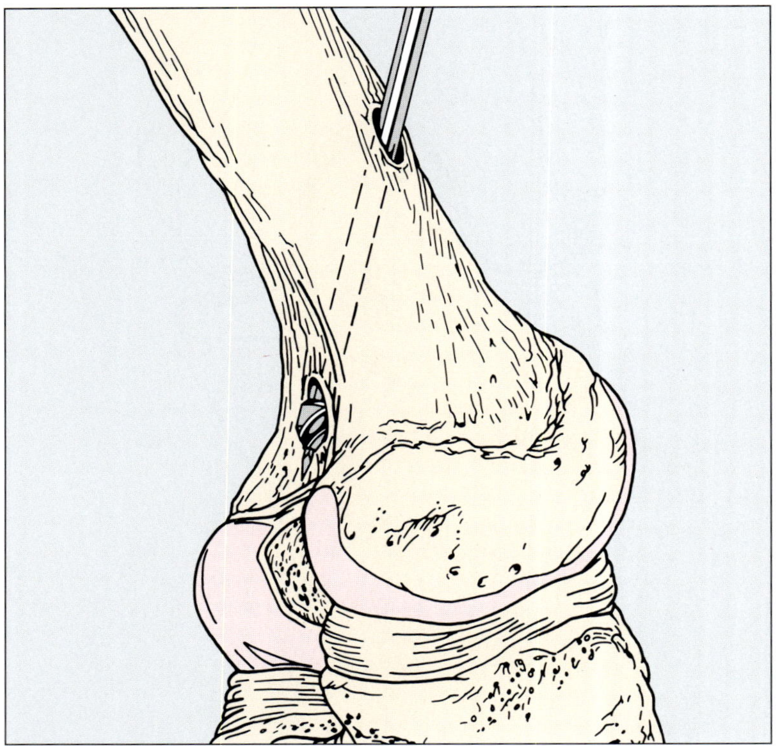

Figure 9.8
Overdrilling of the femoral guide pin with a cannulated drill bit.

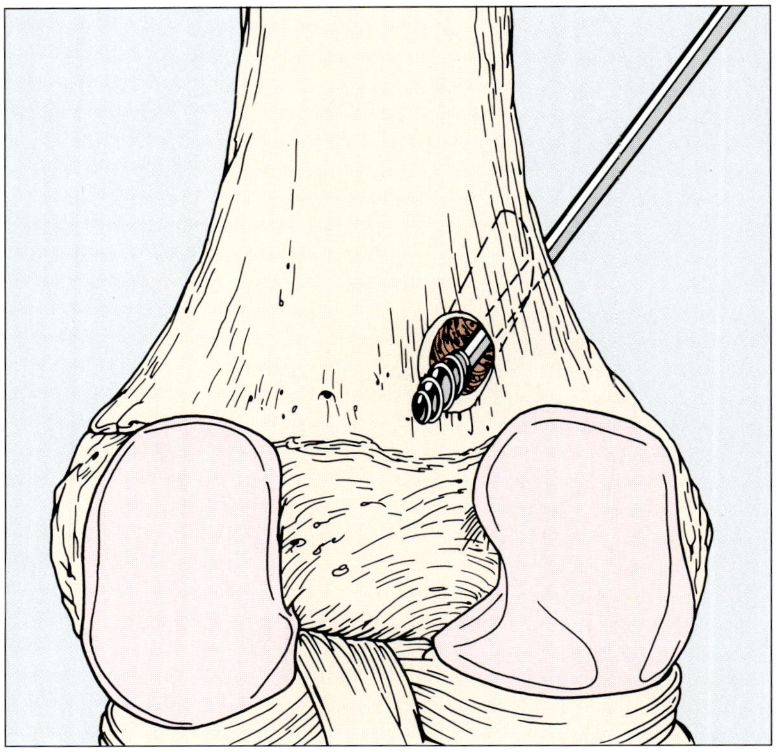

Figure 9.9
Smoothing and chamfering the femoral bone tunnel.

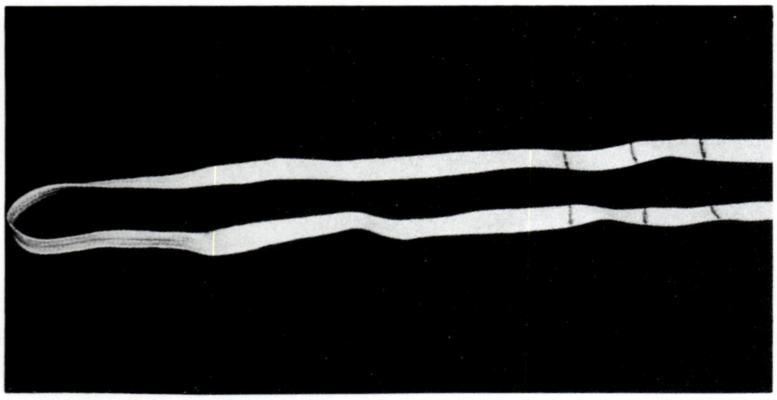

Figure 9.10
Umbilical tape marked at 16, 18, 20, 22, and 24 cm.

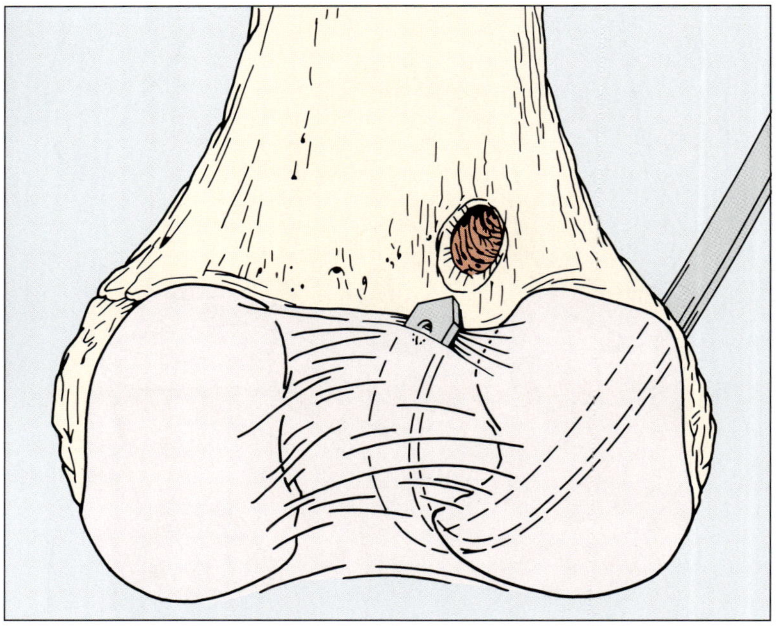

Figure 9.11
Curved passer perforating the posterior joint capsule.

length of the prosthesis to be used. The marked, looped end is positioned about 2 cm distal to the edge of the exit hole on the medial tibial crest. The other end is pulled taut. Then a mark is selected (16, 18, 20, 22, or 24 cm) that is at least 2 cm or more from the proximal edge of the exit hole on the lateral femoral cortex. This insures proper prosthesis length. It is always better to select a prosthesis that is longer than the measurement rather than shorter. The looped end of the umbilical tape is passed through the prosthesis eyelet, and the entire prosthesis is passed through the looped end of the umbilical tape, which locks it on (Fig. 9.12). Gentle tension is then applied to tape as the prosthesis is carefully pulled into position (Fig. 9.13). To facilitate placement, the prosthesis is pulled through in stages. First, the prosthesis is passed through the tibial hole, across the joint space, through the posterior joint capsule, and laterally into the popliteal space. At this point, the prosthesis is slid back and forth several times to confirm that it does not bind or catch anywhere. The prosthesis is then directed into the femoral hole and pulled into its final position (Fig. 9.14). Once the prosthesis is in position, it is again important to slide it back and forth several times to help redistribute the braid and to make certain there is no excessive laxity in the system. The prosthesis is then adjusted so that an equal length of the ligament extends out of each bone tunnel and each eyelet is at least 2.0 cm from the edges of the bone tunnels.

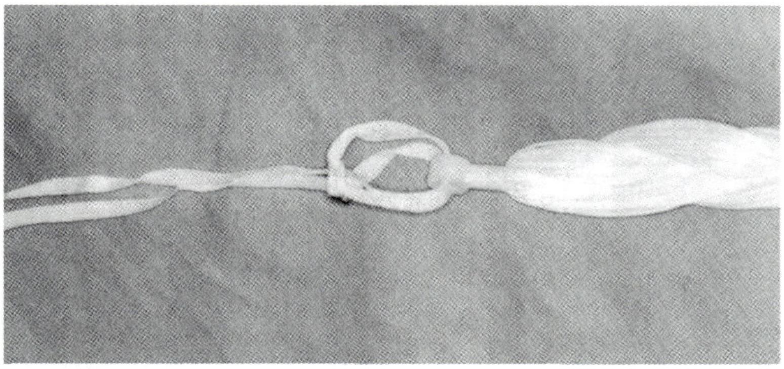

Figure 9.12
Gore-Tex ligament looped over the umbilical tape.

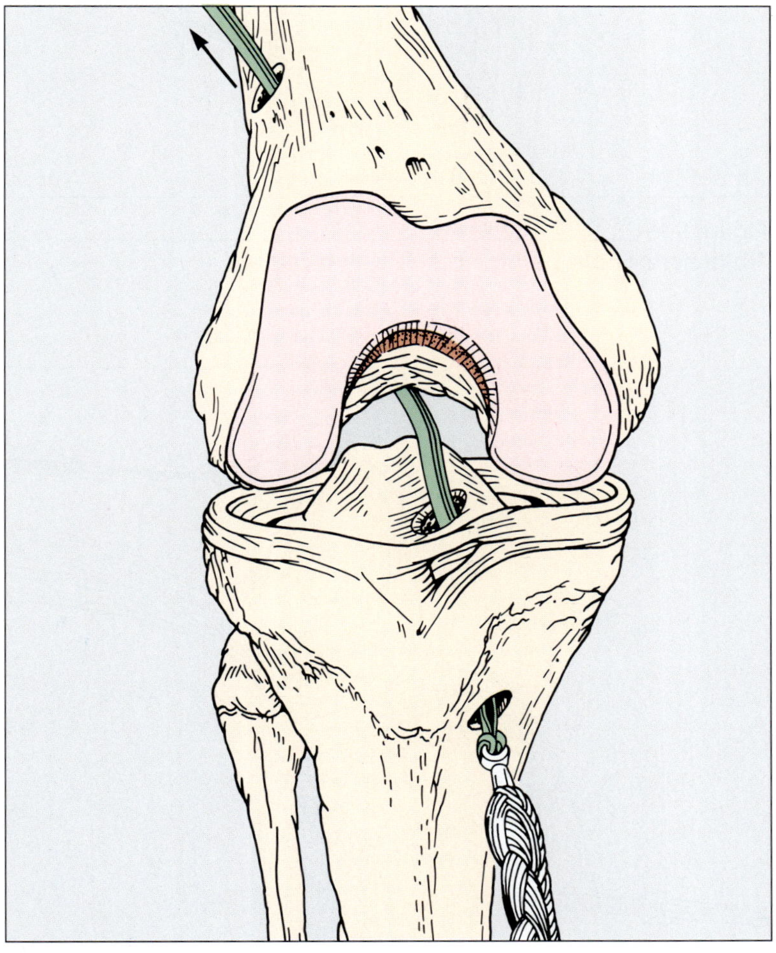

Figure 9.13
Gore-Tex ligament pulled into place.

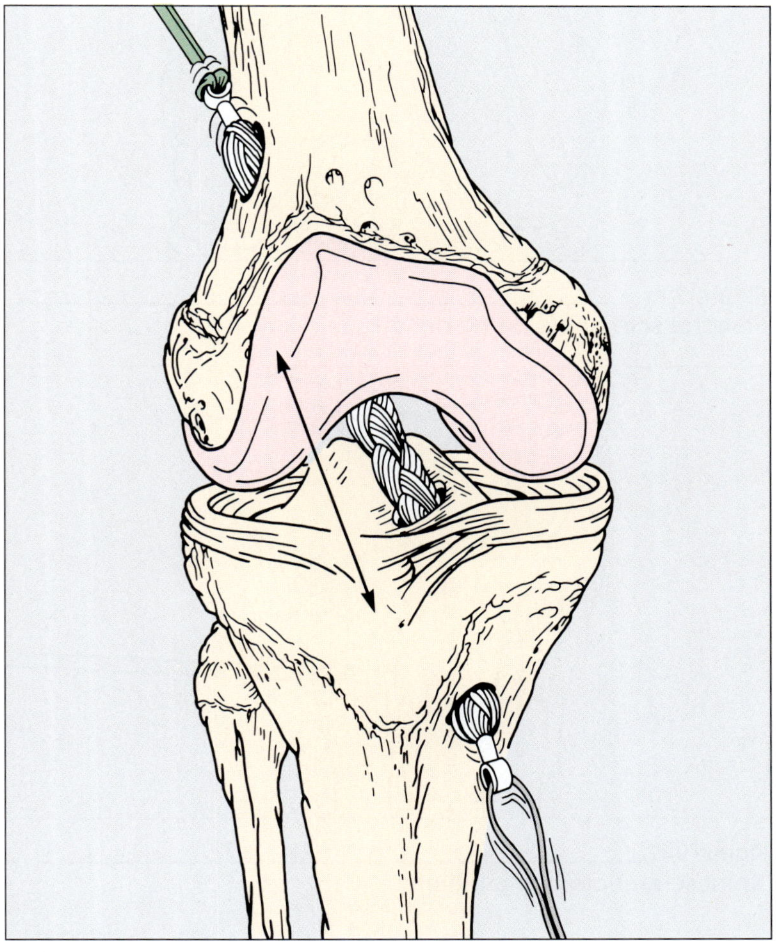

Figure 9.14
Gore-Tex ligament in final position.

The femoral end of the prosthesis is attached first. A punch is used to set the drill site on the femur. The screw hole is drilled with a 3.2-mm (1/8 inch) drill bit (Fig. 9.15). The drill bit should completely penetrate the opposite cortex. A depth gauge is used to determine the length of the hole and 3 mm are added to the depth measurement to account for the thickness of the eyelet. The screw hole is then tapped with a 4.5 mm A-O bone tap. A specially designed bone screw is inserted through the eyelet and tightened until the eyelet begins to bulge.

Attention is next directed to the tibial end of the prosthesis. The tibial eyelet is engaged with the bone punch and the prosthesis is pulled tight. One person holds the punch with firm tension while a second person takes the leg through a full range of motion 20 times. After this has been completed, the knee is placed in 20° of flexion and a posterior force of at least 20 pounds is applied to the proximal tibia. The tibial screw site is then selected with the punch (Fig. 9.16). A 3.2 mm (1/8 inch) drill bit is used to drill through the tibial punch mark, piercing both cortices (Fig. 9.17). A depth gauge is used to determine the length of the tibial screw, with 3 mm again being added to allow for the thickness of the eyelet. The screw hole is then tapped with a 4.5 mm A-O bone tap. Before insertion of the screw, the knee is flexed to 90° (Fig. 9.18). This position provides laxity in the prosthesis while the screw is being inserted, thereby facilitating placement of the screw and reducing the potential for damage to the eyelet or the screw.

After the prosthesis has been inserted it is important to take the knee through a full range of motion to make sure that it is not inhibited (Figs. 9.19). In addition, stability should be tested, keeping in mind that because of the nonisometric over-the-top position of the prosthesis there will always be some laxity in flexion, although this should be minimal. Finally, the prosthesis should again

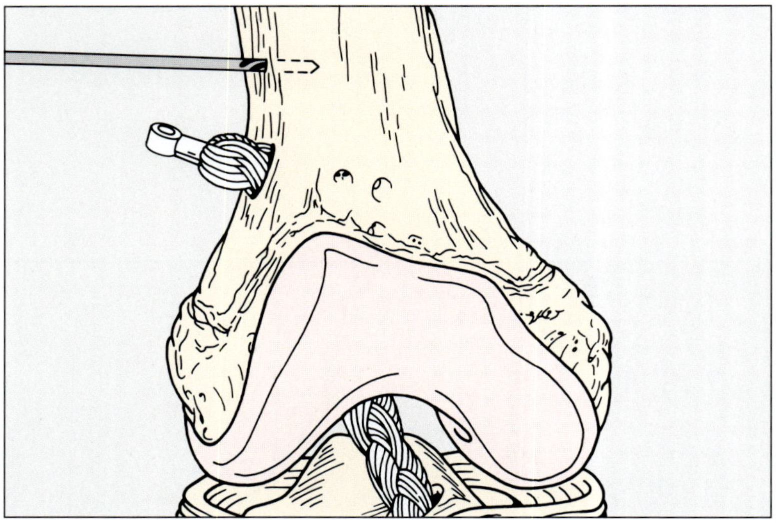

Figure 9.15
Femoral screw hole being drilled.

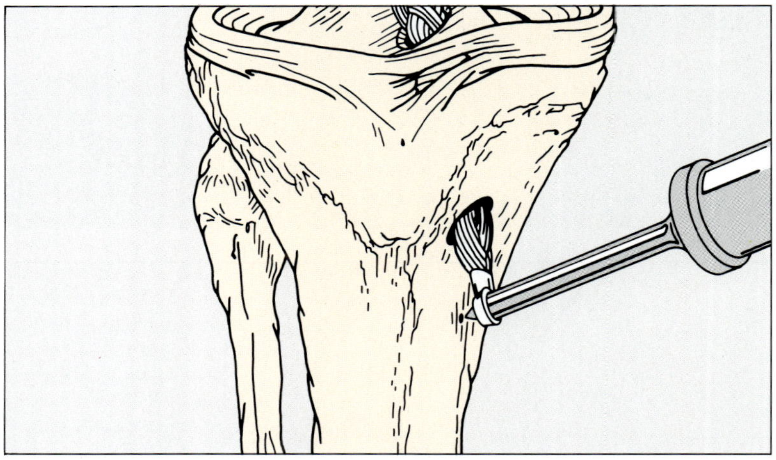

Figure 9.16
Tibial screw hole being marked with a punch.

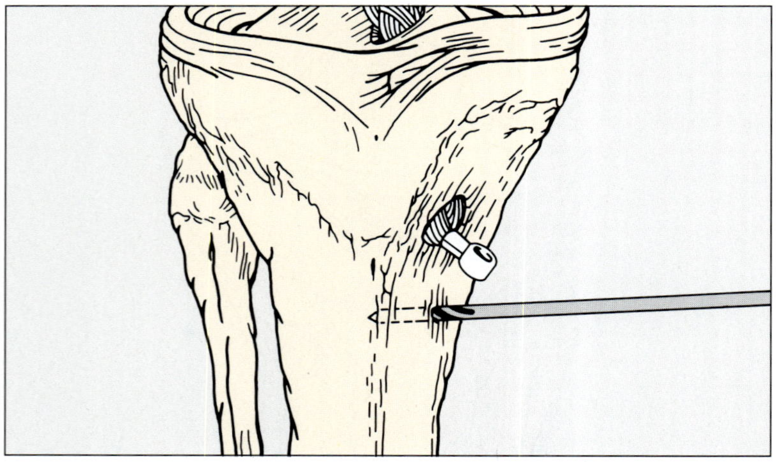

Figure 9.17
Tibial screw hole being drilled.

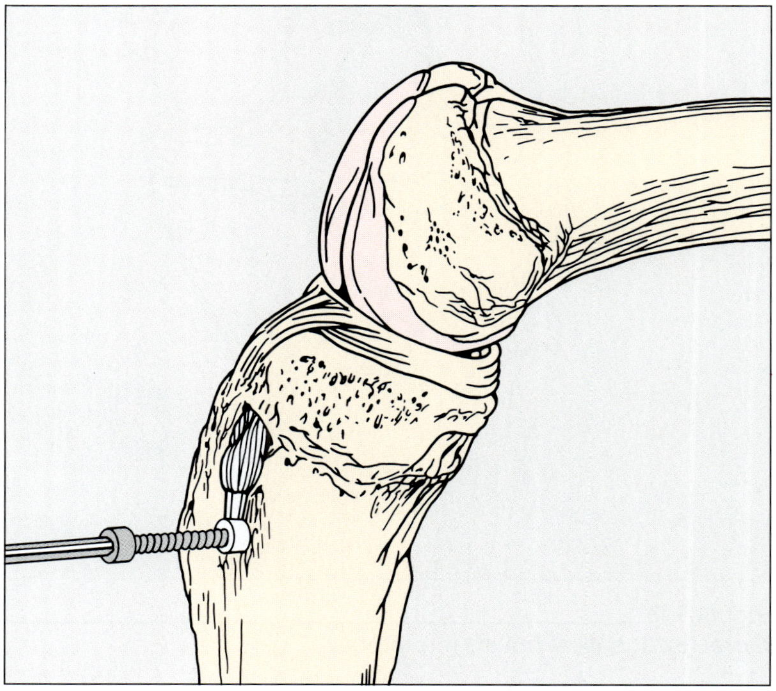

Figure 9.18
Insertion of the tibial screw.

be visualized arthroscopically, going through a range of motion to make sure that the notch is not impinging on the prosthesis (Fig. 9.20). The wounds are then closed in a standard fashion.

Postoperative Management

Postoperatively, patients are placed in a continuous passive motion machine. Active and passive range of motion exercises are started immediately. The patient is also started on straight leg raises, quadriceps sets, and ankle pumping exercises. Initially, the patient is allowed full weight-bearing with crutches and a splint with knee hinges. Resistance exercises are added as tolerated. Biking and swimming are started as soon as the wound has healed. Sporting activities are started after 3 months, if the patient has achieved adequate rehabilitation.

Complications and Pitfalls

Infrequent complications associated with the Gore-Tex prosthesis are effusions, rupture, loosening, and infection. Effusions in one series occurred in 34% of patients[1] and were often associated with partial rupture of the prosthesis. Rupture of the prosthesis increases with time and occurs primarily at the posterior notch on the femoral side. Loosening can also occur and increases with time. As with any implanted prosthesis, infection is a concern

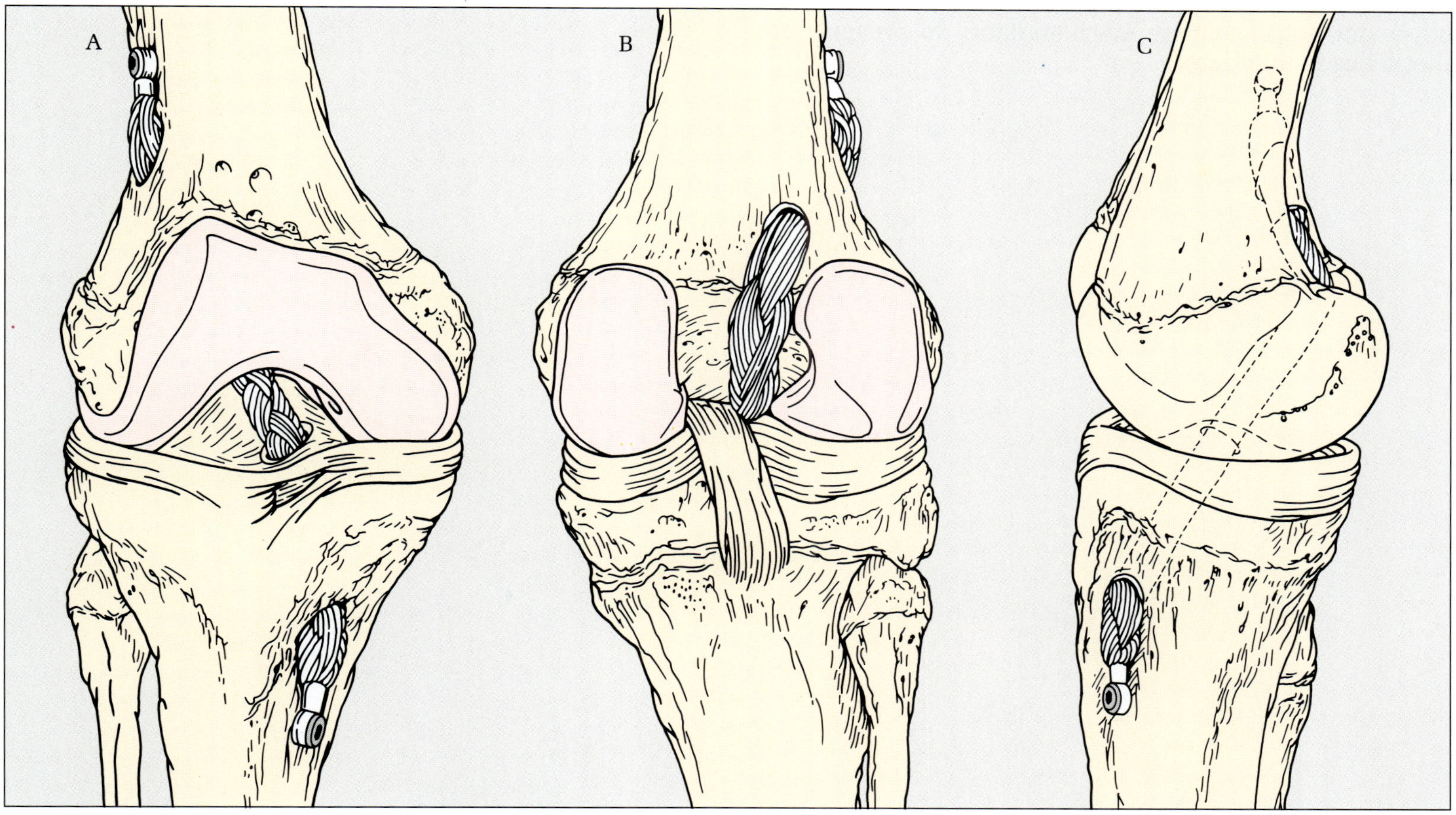

Figures 9.19
Anterior (A), posterior (B), and lateral (C) views of the Gore-Tex ligament after insertion.

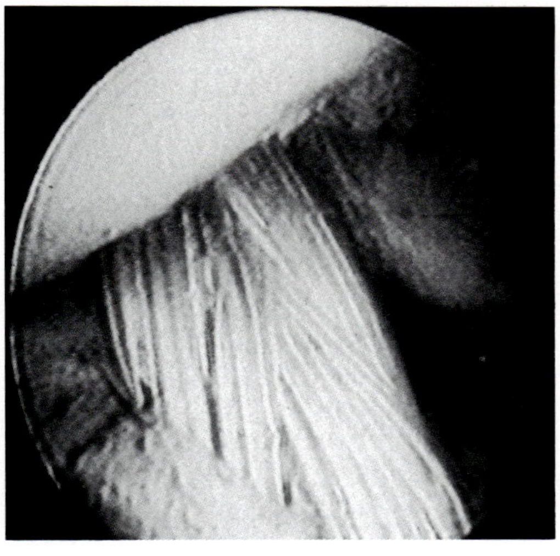

Figure 9.20
Arthroscopic view of the Gore-Tex ligament.

and has been reported in different series to occur in a range of 1.3% to 2.7%.[1,2] It should always be remembered that the prosthesis is a nonorganic substance and carries a risk of late infection. Prophylactic antibiotics should be given to any patient in whom there is a risk of seeding the joint with bacteria.

CONCLUSION

The Gore-Tex prosthetic ligament insertion for anterior cruciate ligament instability is a salvage procedure to be used in patients for whom the more conventional anterior ligament reconstructive procedures are not appropriate. Attention to detail in implanting the device, with proper chamfering of the bone tunnels to avoid sharp bony impingement areas and notchplasty to prevent any sharp edges and impingement, are mandatory to prevent prosthetic ligament failure.

REFERENCES

1. Grewe SR, Paulos LE. Prosthetic replacement of the anterior cruciate ligament with expanded polytetrafluoroethylene. In: Tullos HS, ed. *Instructional Course Lectures.* Park Ridge, Ill: American Academy of Orthopaedic Surgery; 1991:60:213–217.
2. Collins HR. US experience with Gore-Tex reconstruction of the anterior cruciate ligament In: Friedman MJ, Ferkel RD, eds. *Prosthetic Ligament Reconstruction of the Knee.* Philadelphia, Pa: WB Saunders Co; 1988:156–164.

chapter Ten

Arthroscopically Assisted Posterior Cruciate Ligament Reconstruction Using Allograft Tendon

Mehrdad M. Malek
Gregory C. Fanelli

Arthroscopically assisted posterior cruciate ligament reconstruction is a technically demanding procedure that should be performed in the proper setting by only the experienced arthroscopic knee surgeon. It requires a meticulous approach, with strict attention to detail, to insure proper tunnel and graft placement and prevent neurovascular complications.[1–7]

Our technique for arthroscopically assisted posterior cruciate ligament reconstruction using an Achilles tendon allograft will be presented. This technique is also applicable to other graft sources; although their mode of fixation varies.

Preoperative Preparation

Preoperative planning begins with a physical examination to determine the severity of tibial dropback as demonstrated by the posterior drawer test and measurement of the tibial step offs. It is very important at this time to document the presence of posterolateral, posteromedial, or anterior cruciate ligament insufficiency, since all aspects of a combined instability pattern must be addressed for posterior cruciate ligament reconstruction to be successful.

A KT1000 knee arthrometer is used to compare pre- and postoperative tibial excursion. Strength is evaluated using isokinetic measurements, and a knee rating form is used to quantitate knee function.

Surgical Technique

The patient is positioned supine on the operating table. The surgical leg is placed in a leg holder, lateral post, or left completely free, depending on the surgeon's preference (Fig. 10.1A). A less restricted surgical leg allows the surgeon more flexibility during the procedure. The well leg may be held in a support or rested flat on the operating room table (Fig. 10.1B). The video cabinet is placed at the side of the operating room table opposite the surgeon. It is important to have an experienced orthopedic operating team to expedite the procedure and to keep the tourniquet time under 90 minutes.

Joint Preparation

Diagnostic arthroscopy is performed in the usual manner with correction of other pathology as needed. The notchplasty consists of soft tissue debridement, usually with no bone resection necessary in posterior cruciate ligament reconstruction. Motorized synovial resectors and hand tools are used to debride the posterior cruciate ligament stump.

Specially curved rasps, curettes, and knives are used to elevate the capsule from the posterior proximal tibia (Figs. 10.2–10.4). During the entire operation, the arthroscope is

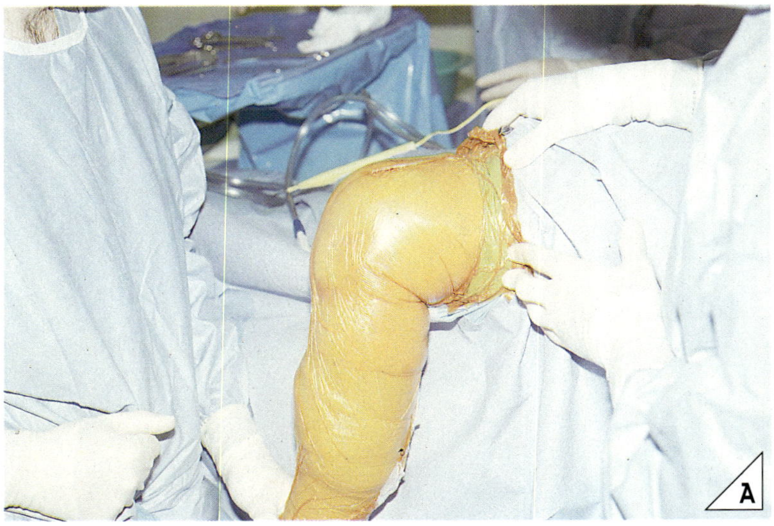

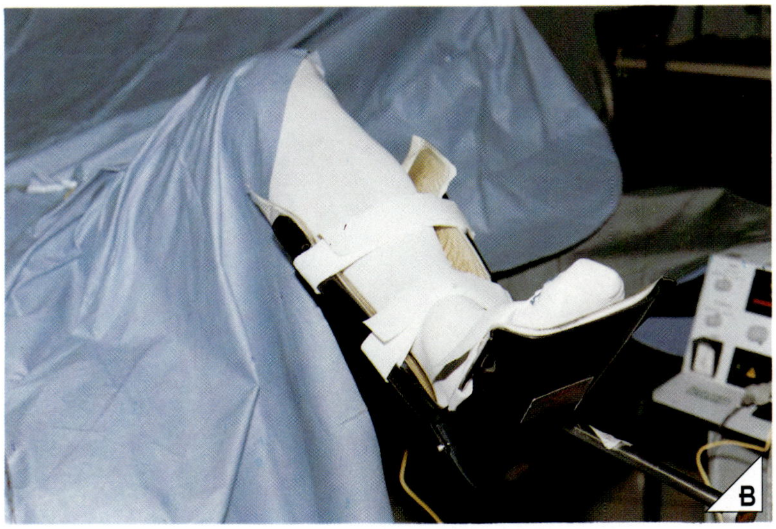

Figure 10.1
The patient is positioned supine on the operating table. (A) The surgical leg is placed in a leg holder, padded properly, and draped away from the surgical field. (B) The other leg is draped free and is in a 90° position.

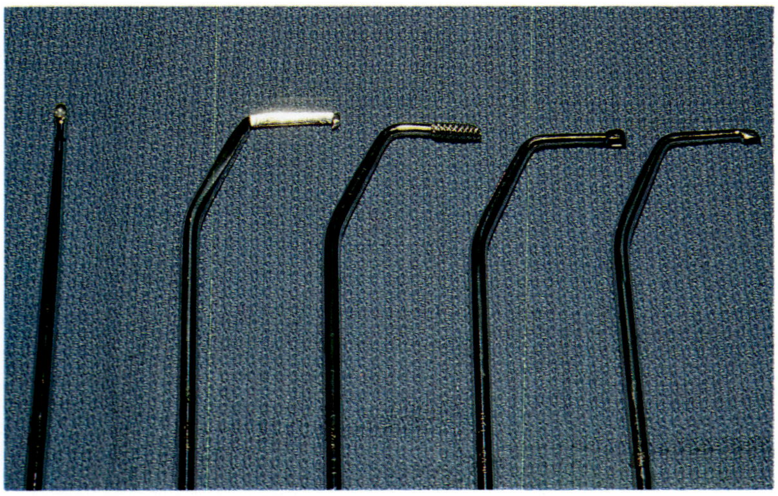

Figure 10.2
The curved rasps and curettes used for arthroscopically aided posterior cruciate ligament reconstruction (Acufex Microsurgical).

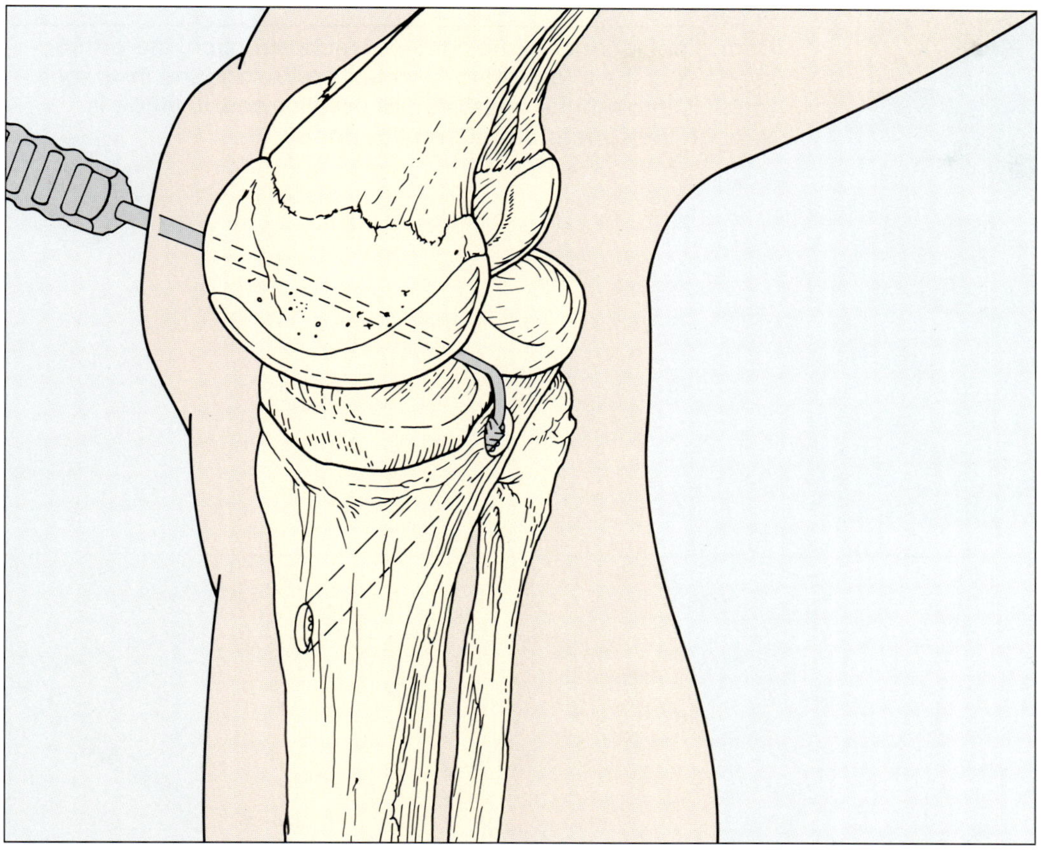

Figure 10.3

The curved posterior cruciate rasps are used to elevate the capsule where the tibial tunnel will be placed. Note the position of the tunnel and the distance from the articular surface.

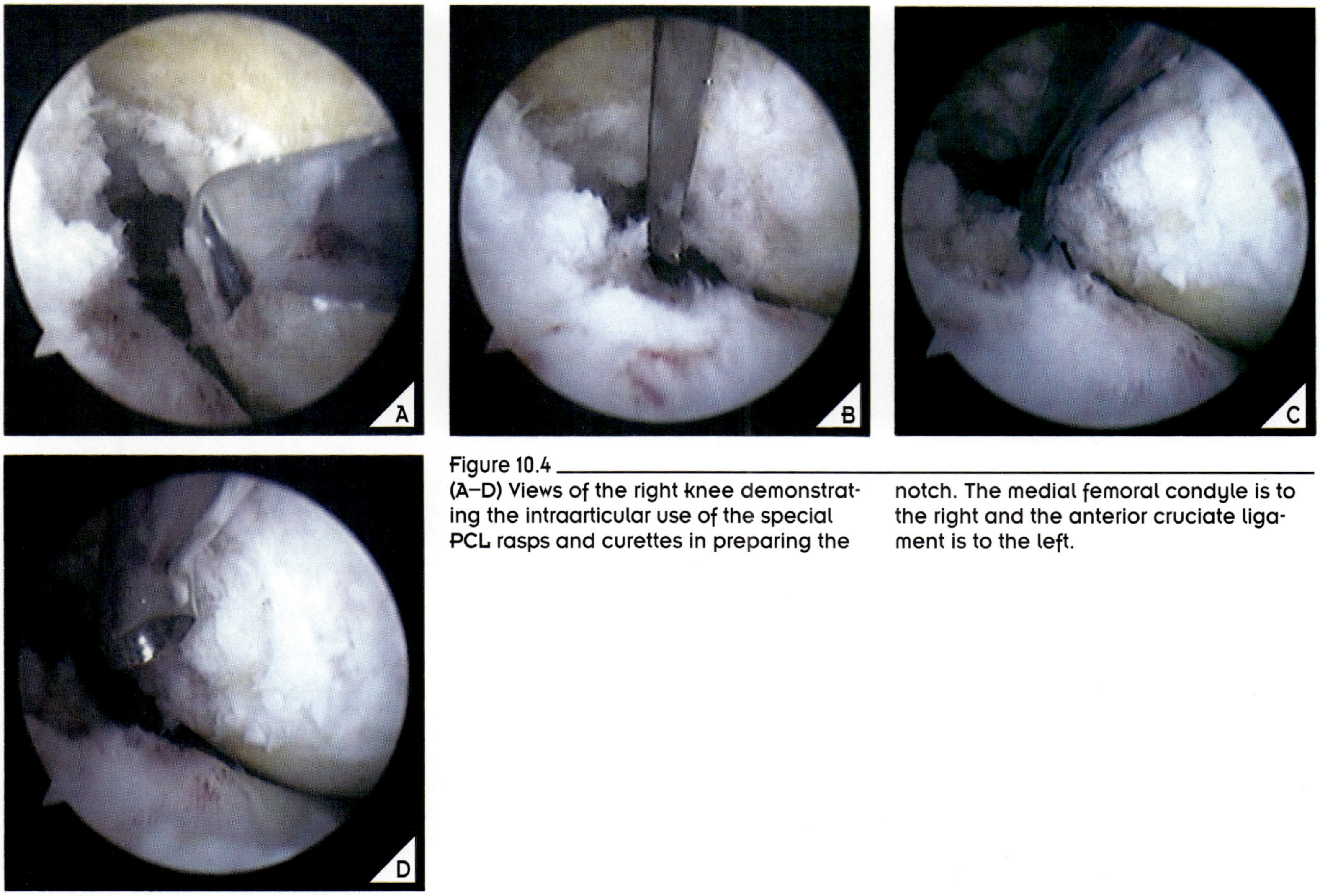

Figure 10.4

(A–D) Views of the right knee demonstrating the intraarticular use of the special PCL rasps and curettes in preparing the notch. The medial femoral condyle is to the right and the anterior cruciate ligament is to the left.

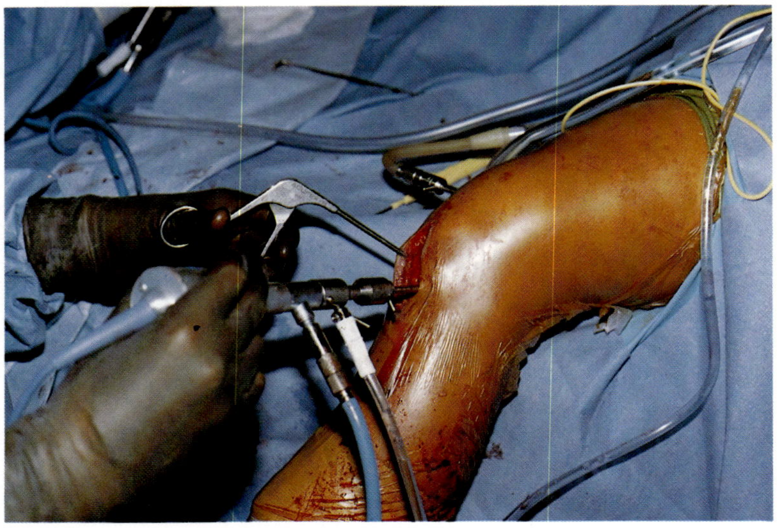

Figure 10.5
During posterior cruciate ligament reconstruction, the arthroscope is in the inferolateral patellar portal, and the instrumentation is through the inferomedial patellar portal. Inflow is through the superolateral patellar portal.

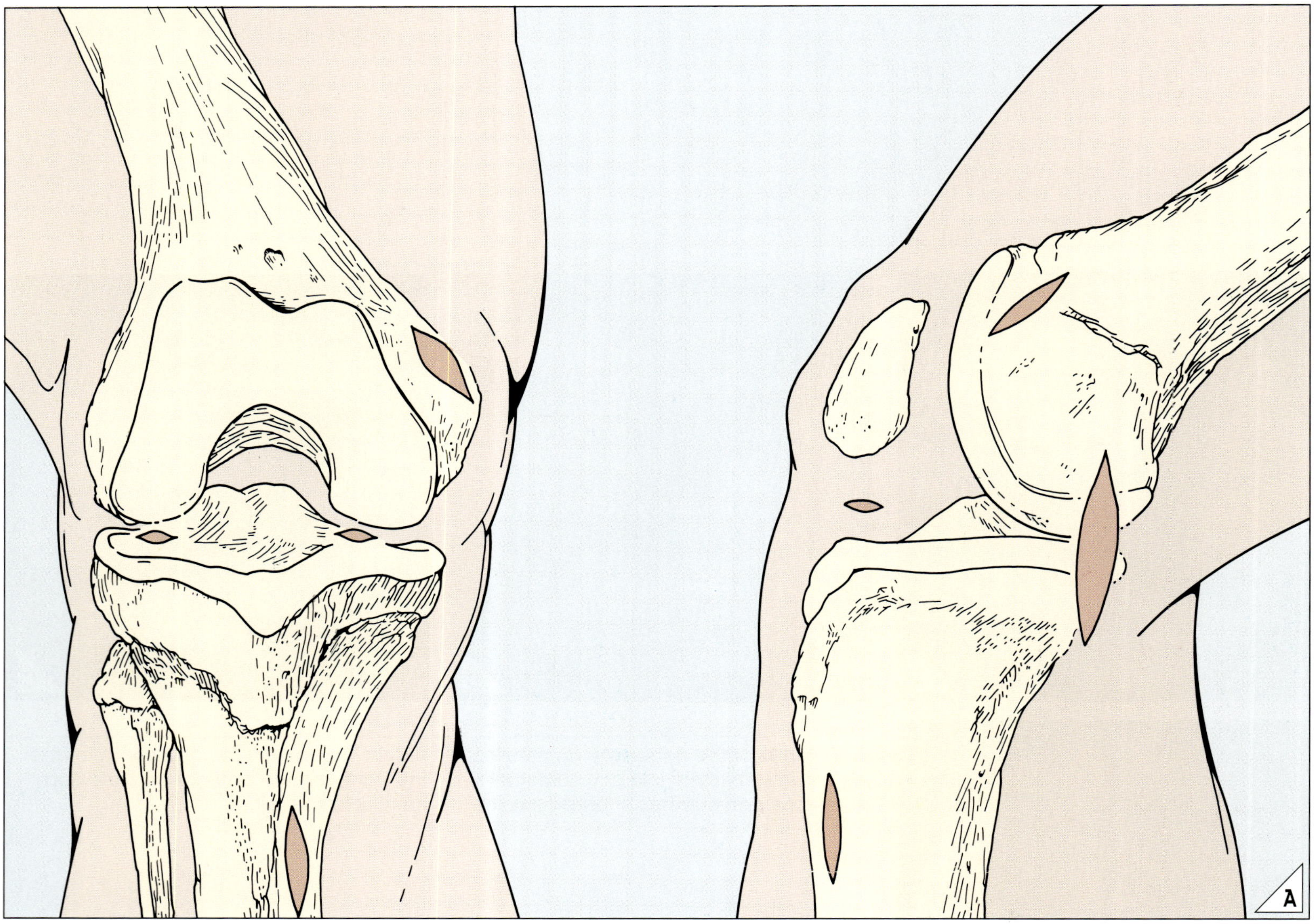

Figure 10.6
(A) Incision about the knee. Note the 3 cm posteromedial incision and the 3 cm anteromedial incision. The posteromedial incision is for the surgeon's finger to identify and protect the neurovascular structures. The anteromedial incision, located 1 to 2 cm below the tibial tubercle, is for entrance of the tibial guidewire and tunnel placement. By using a C-arm and 70° scope, the posteromedial incision may be eliminated. However, this incision is recommended for protection of the neurovascular structures and proper placement of the tibial guidewire. (continued on next page)

in the inferolateral patellar portal and the instrumentation is through the inferomedial patellar portal. Inflow is through the superolateral patellar portal (Fig. 10.5). We do not use a pump.

Tibial Tunnel Preparation

After the notch is prepared, the surgeon assumes the seated position with the patient's knee flexed 90° and the foot resting in the surgeon's lap. A small, 3 cm posteromedial incision is made and an interval developed between the medial head of the gastrocnemius tendon and the posterior capsule (Fig. 10.6). During tibial reaming and drilling procedures the surgeon's finger is kept in this interval to protect the neurovascular structures—a very important safety measure.

A 3 cm incision is then made on the anteromedial aspect of the proximal tibia, beginning at the tibial tubercle and extending distally (see Fig. 10.6). The tibial posterior cruciate ligament drill guide (Acufex Microsurgical) is positioned so that the 3/32 inch guidewire enters the anteromedial proximal tibial 1 to 2 cm below the tibial tubercle (Fig. 10.7). The guidewire exits posteriorly in the posterior cruciate ligament fossa of the posterior proximal tibia. The appropriate size reamer is used to create the tibial tunnel. The surgeon's gloved finger should be placed

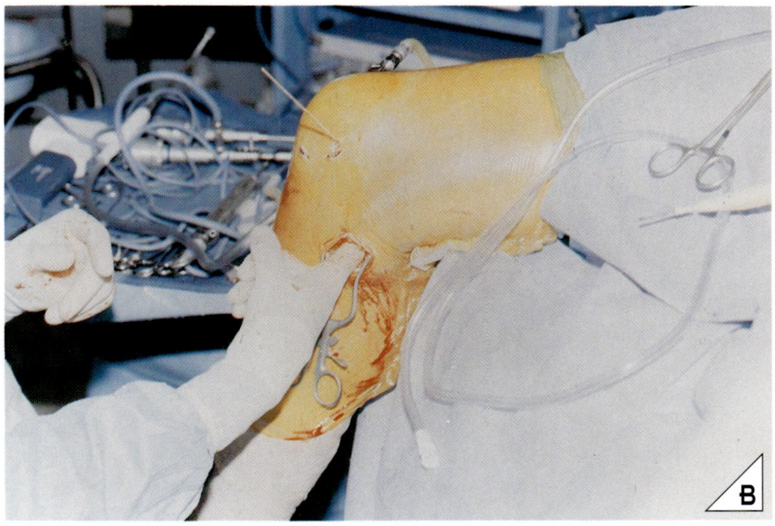

Figure 10.6 (continued)
(B) Note the 3 cm posteromedial incision and the surgeon's finger placement.

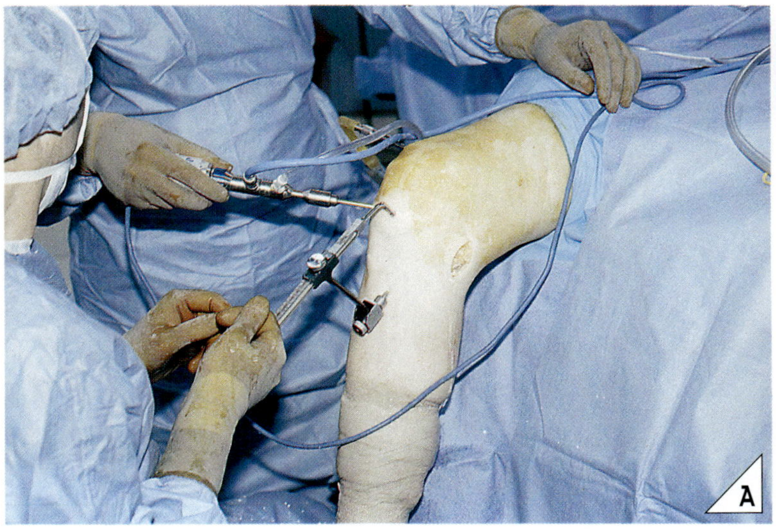

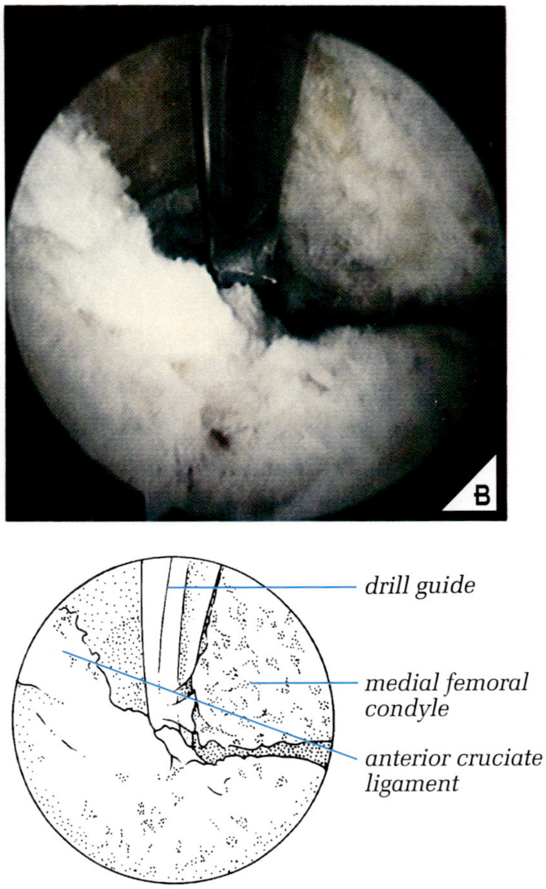

Figure 10.7
Correct drill guide position for making the tibial tunnel. The drill guide is placed through the anteroinferior medial patellar portal of the right foot and positioned in the intercondylar notch. (A) The guide is positioned so the 3/32 inch guidewire enters the anteromedial proximal tibia 1 to 2 cm below the tibial tubercle. (B) The intraarticular position of the posterior cruciate ligament tibial drill guide.

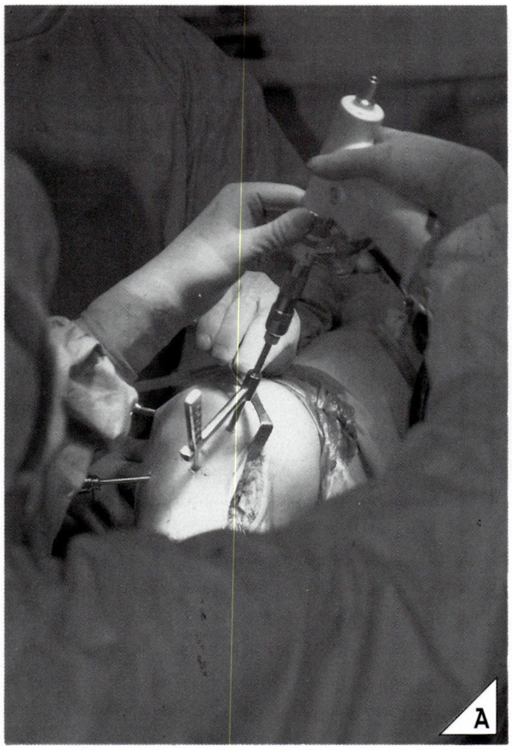

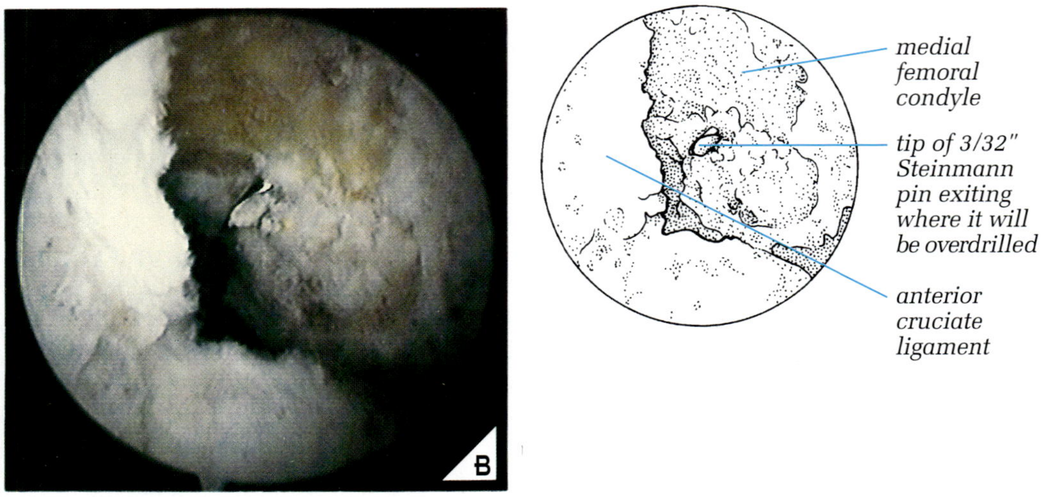

Figure 10.8

External position of the femoral drill guide on the right knee (Acufex Microsurgical). (A) The additional medial incision in this particular case was for reconstruction of the medial and posteromedial structures. (B) The guidewire exits through the center of the stump of the posterior cruciate ligament in the intercondylar notch of the right knee.

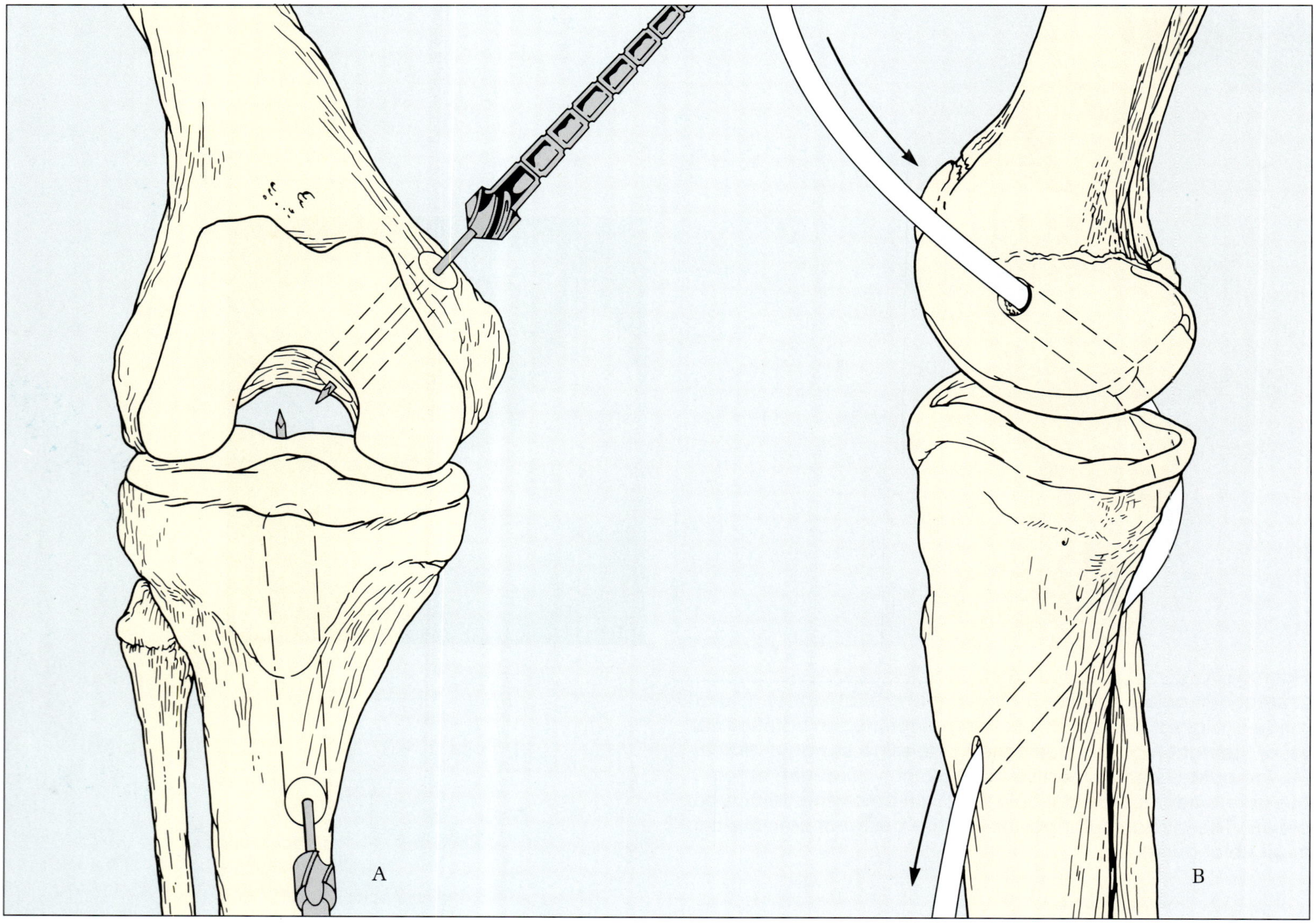

Figure 10.9

The tibial and femoral tunnels (A) are reamed to the appropriate size using cannulated reamers over the guidewires. (B) The Gore-Tex smoother (W.L. Gore) passes through the femoral tunnel, the joint, and the tibial tunnel to smooth the tunnel edges as well as aid in passing the graft through the joint.

between the posterior capsule and the neurovascular structures to protect the neurovascular structures during the drilling procedures. The tibial tunnel is now complete.

Preparation of the Femur

The femoral guide is positioned so the guidewire enters the medial cortex of the medial femoral condyle midway between the medial epicondyle and the medial femoral condylar articular surface, in line with the upper one third of the patella when the knee is flexed 90° as described by Paulos (Fig. 10.8).[7] The guidewire enters through the center of the femoral posterior cruciate ligament stump, which minimizes tunnel divergence. The appropriate size reamer is used to create the femoral tunnel.

When the tibial and femoral tunnels are complete, a Gore-Tex smoother (W.L. Gore) is passed through the femoral tunnel, through the joint, and through the tibial tunnel (Figs. 10.9, 10.10). With the knee at 0°, 30°, 60°, 90°, and 120° of flexion, the tunnel edges are rasped and chamfered using the Gore-Tex smoother. The smoother is then used to pull the graft into position.

Graft Preparation

We routinely prepare the allograft Achilles tendon prior to bringing the patient into the operating room (Fig. 10.11A). The allograft, which must be no less than 21 cm long, is formed into a tube using #0 absorbable suture. The circumference of the tubed graft determines the diameter of

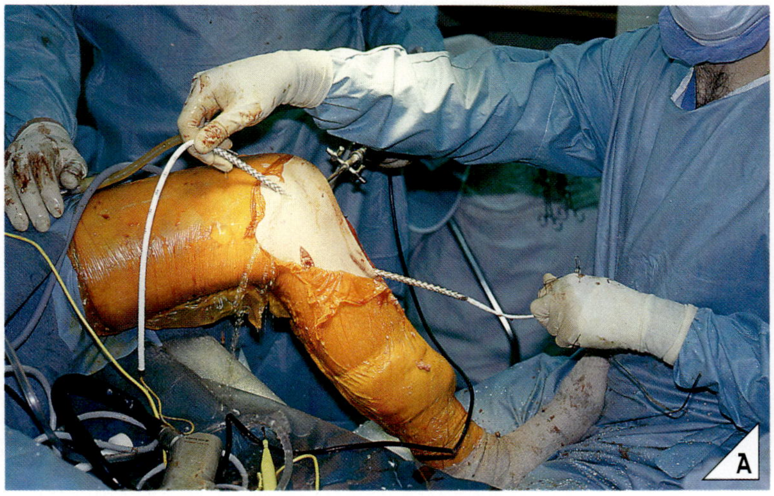

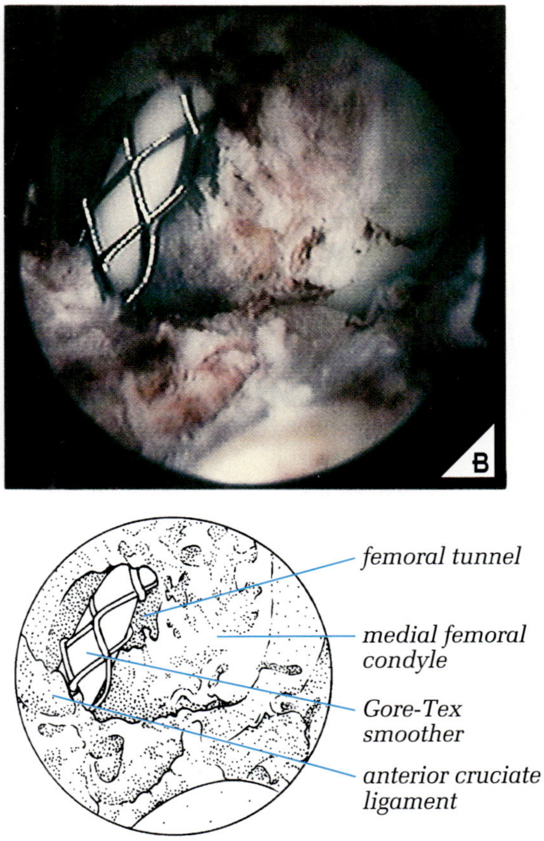

Figure 10.10
(A) The Gore-Tex smoother passes through the femoral tunnel into the joint, exits the tibial tunnel, and is moved back and forth to smooth the tunnel edges. (B) Internal view from the inferolateral portal of the Gore-Tex smoother as it exits the femoral tunnel and enters the area behind the tibial plateau and then the tibial tunnel of the right knee.

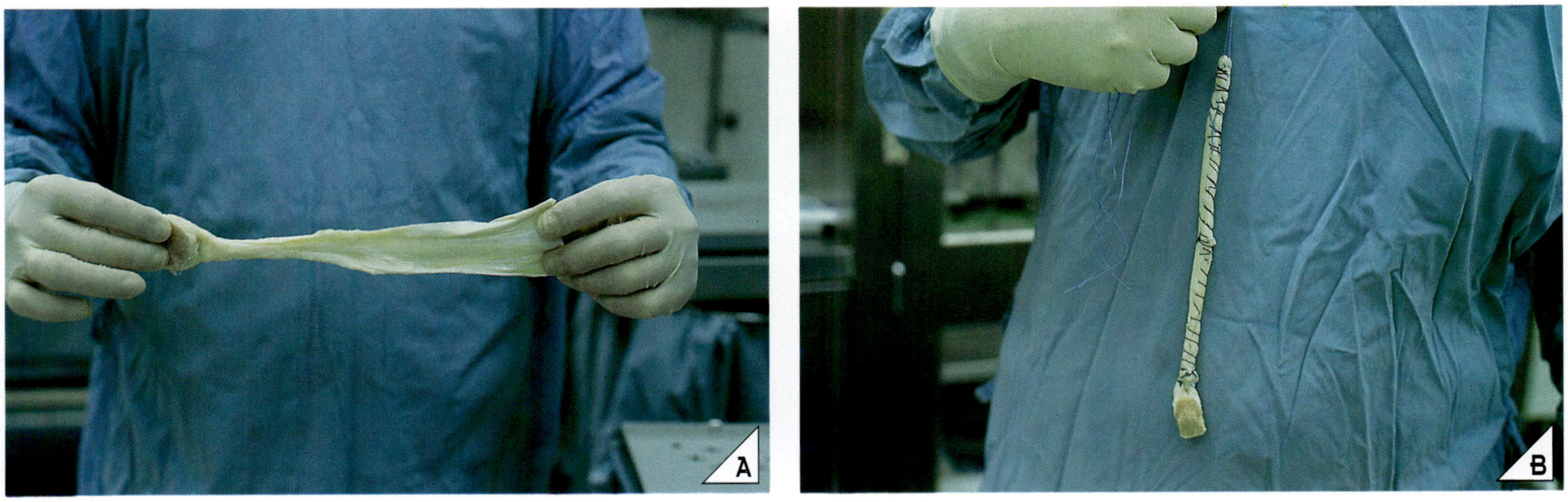

Figure 10.11
(A) The Achilles tendon allograft prior to preparation for insertion into the knee. (B) The prepared Achilles tendon allograft with a tendinous portion is shaped into a tube using sutures on a noncutting needle. The bone plug is contoured into a wedge for press or interference fit.

the tibial and femoral tunnels, which is most often 12 mm. The calcaneous bone block is contoured into a wedge shape for press or interference fit fixation in the femoral tunnel (Fig. 10.11B). After completion of graft preparation, the patient is brought into the operating room.

Graft Passage and Fixation

The traction sutures on the Achilles tendon allograft are tied to the Gore-Tex smoother. The graft is pulled first through the femoral tunnel, then through the joint into the tibial tunnel, and out to the anteromedial aspect of the proximal tibia (Fig. 10.12). The contoured calcaneous bone plug is tapped into the femoral tunnel and held in place by a press fit or an interference fit screw (Fig. 10.13). The graft is viewed arthroscopically as the knee is placed through a range of motion. The knee should be adjusted to 0° to 20° of flexion, and a firm anterior drawer force should be applied to the proximal tibia. This will reduce the posterior tibial subluxation and create tension on the graft. The Achilles tendon allograft is then secured to the tibia using a bicortical screw with a spiked washer (Figs. 10.14, 10.15).

The knee is placed through a full range of motion. The posterior drawer should be eliminated and the tibial step off should be equal to that of the normal knee. If postero-

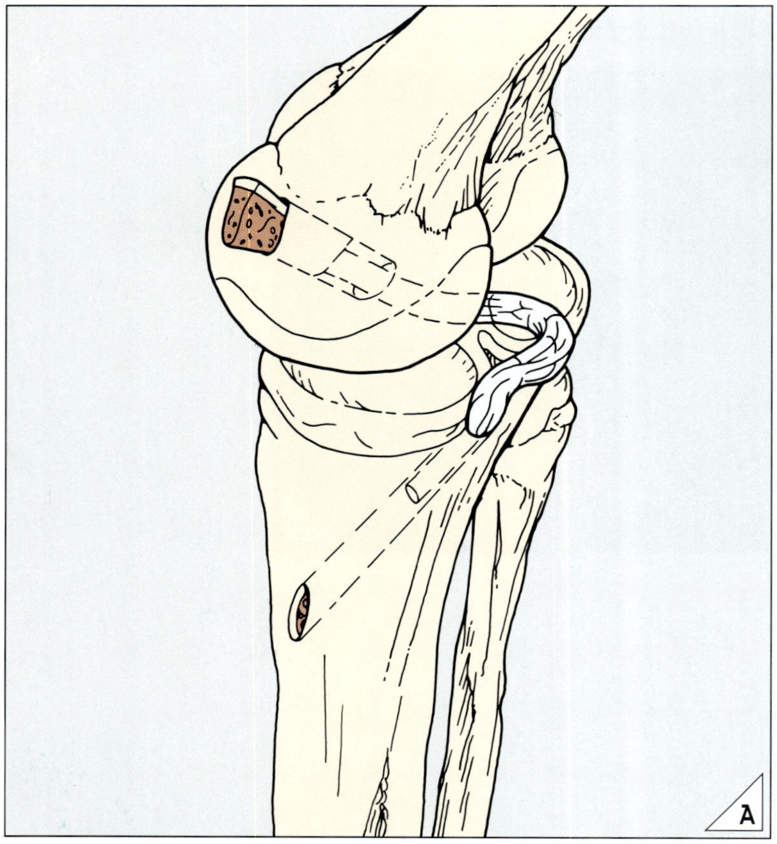

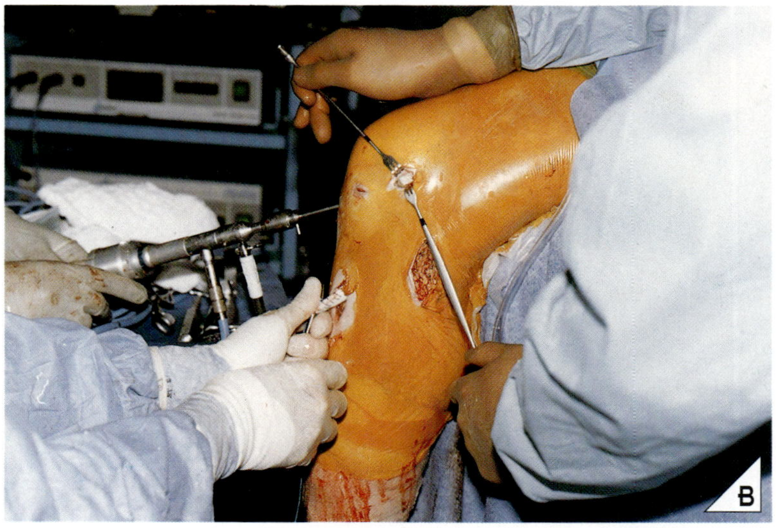

Figure 10.12
The Achilles tendon allograft being pulled into position in the tunnel. (A) The allograft is pulled into the femoral tunnel first, then through the joint and, finally, through the tibial tunnel. (B) Intraoperative photo of the Achilles tendon allograft being pulled into the femoral tunnel and (C) intraarticular positioning of the Achilles tendon allograft during posterior cruciate ligament reconstruction.

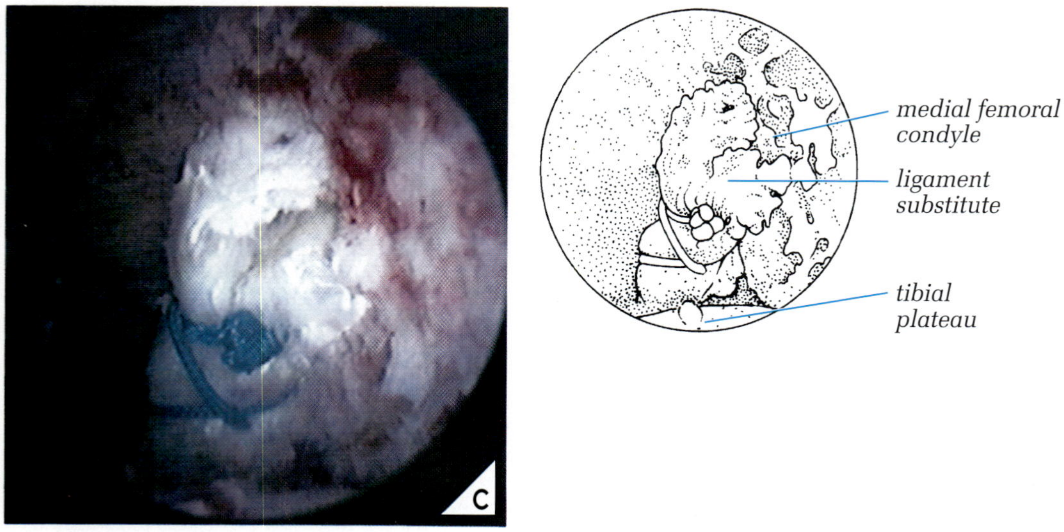

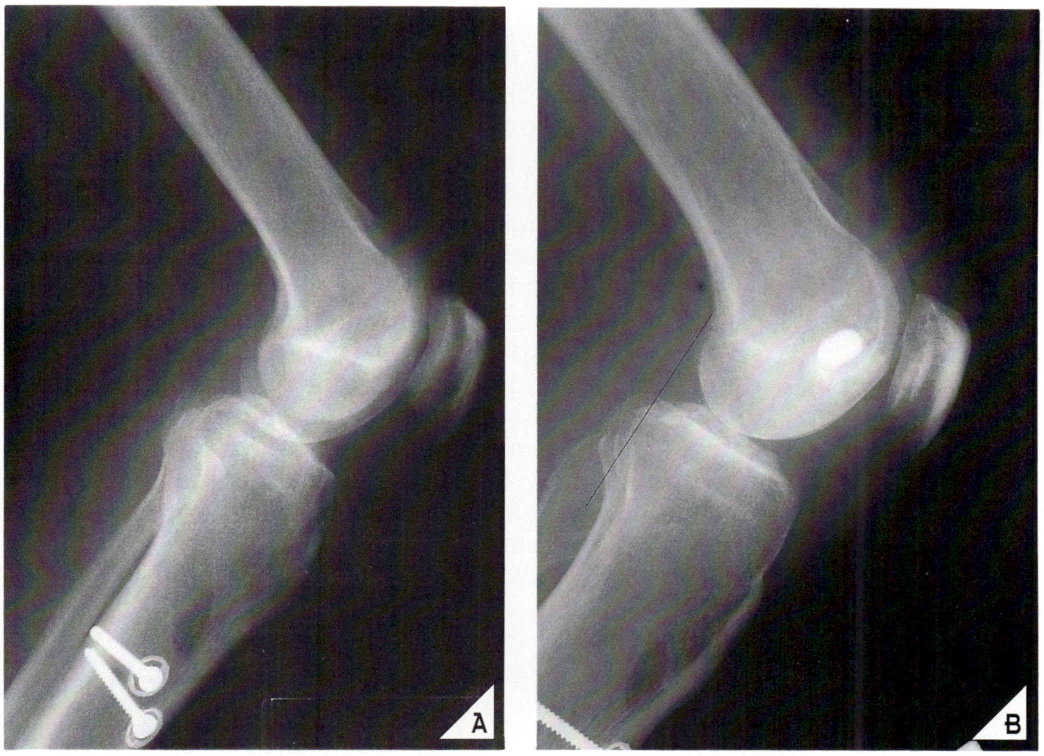

Figure 10.13
(A) Fixation of the femoral tunnel with the press fit technique. (B) Femoral fixation with the interference fit fixation technique.

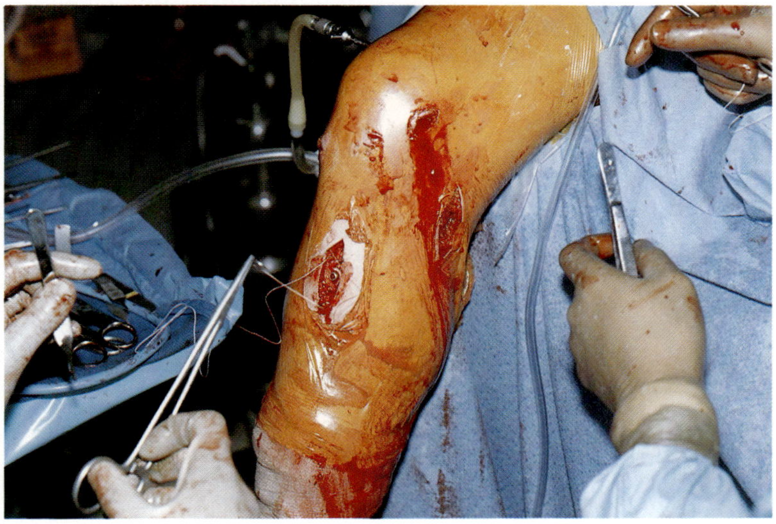

Figure 10.14
The distal end of the allograft has been tensioned and fixed to the proximal tibia with screw and washer. The tourniquet has been deflated and incisions are being closed.

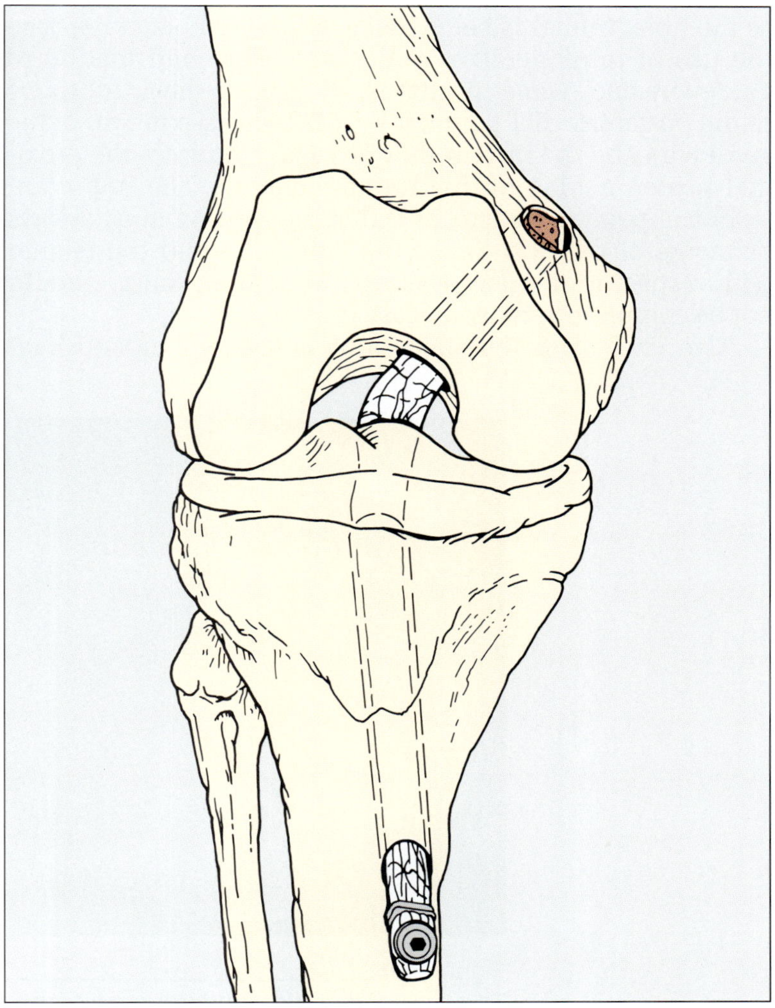

Figure 10.15
Fixation of the Achilles tendon allograft in the femoral tunnel and on the anteromedial aspect of the proximal tibia.

lateral or posteromedial insufficiency coexists with posterior cruciate ligament insufficiency, these must be corrected before final tensioning and tibial fixation of the Achilles tendon allograft. Failure to do so will result in graft laxity.

Closure

The tourniquet is deflated, hemostasis obtained, and the wound closed in layers. Sterile dressing is applied and the patient is placed in a postoperative rehabilitation brace locked in full extension. Rehabilitation proceeds as per our postoperative guidelines (Fig. 10.16).

Technical Considerations

When performing posterior cruciate ligament surgery, the potential for damage to the neurovascular structures must always be kept in mind. We emphasize the use of a small posteromedial incision so that the surgeon's gloved finger can be passed through the posterior capsule and in front of the neurovascular structures. This allows the surgeon to palpate the tip of the guidewire and also the tip of the reamer as the tibial tunnel is being made. Other authors emphasize the use of intraoperative radiographs for confirmation of guidewire and reamer positions. By placing the arthroscope in the posteromedial portal, it is possible to see the tip of the guidewire and the drill as they are emerging from the proximal posterior tibia during tunnel creation. The important technical point to remember is that the surgeon must always be aware of the position of the guidewire and the reamer with respect to the neurovascular structures. Safety should not be compromised in any case (Fig. 10.17).

Also critical to the success of posterior cruciate ligament reconstruction, as with anterior cruciate ligament, is tunnel placement. It is important that the femoral guidewire exit through the center of the stump of the femoral insertion of the posterior cruciate ligament so the subsequent tunnel will be in an anatomic position. It is extremely important that the tip of the guidewire exit through the apex of the posterior tibial ridge so that after the tunnel is reamed, the posterior cruciate ligament substitute will pass through a tunnel in the posterior cruciate ligament fossa, thus giving anatomic position to the graft.

Passage of the posterior cruciate ligament can sometimes be a frustrating experience for a surgeon performing this procedure for the first time. It is absolutely essential that the posterior capsule be elevated from the tibial ridge and approximately 1 cm below the tibial ridge. This facilitates graft passage after the creation of the tibial tunnel since capsular tissues will not interfere with the passage of the guidewire, the Gore-Tex smoother, and the posterior cruciate ligament substitute graft.

Finally, it is essential to achieve secure fixation of the femoral and tibial ends of the Achilles tendon allograft or the patellar tendon graft. We have found that putting the knee through approximately 20 cycles of full range of motion flexion and extension removes most of the laxity from the ligament substitute. The knee is then placed in approximately 20° of flexion with a firm anterior drawer force applied to the proximal posterior tibia. This reduces the posterior tibial subluxation. The graft, previously secured with internal fixation or wedge fit on the femoral side, is now secured with internal fixation on the proximal tibia. This allows for consistent tension and fixation of the allograft or autograft tissue.

Preparation of this manuscript was supported in part by a grant from the National Knee Research and Education Foundation.

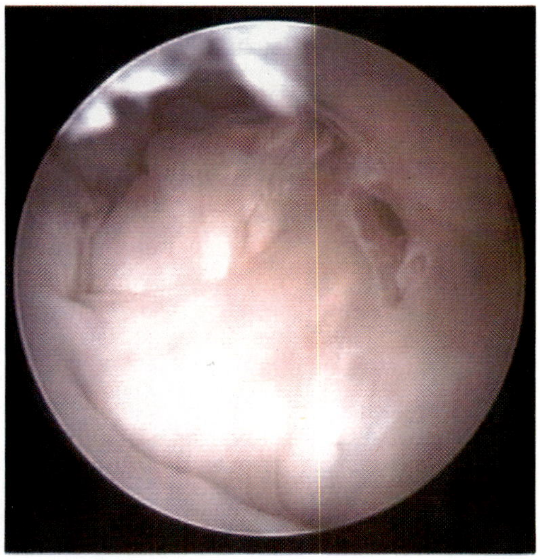

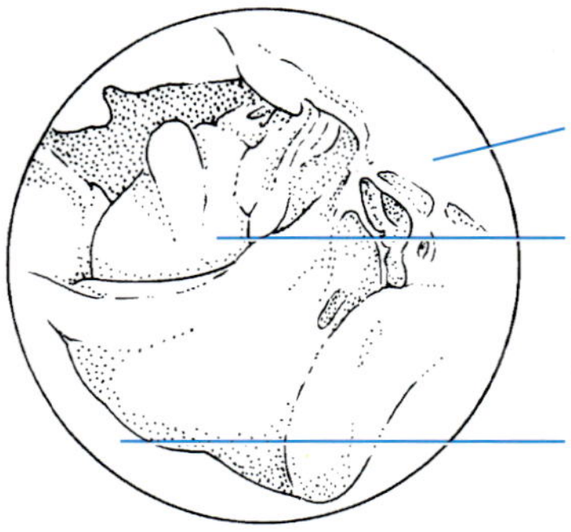

Figure 10.16
This view of the intercondylar area of the right knee shows the appearance of a well-positioned and synovialized posterior cruciate ligament allograft 6 months postoperatively. The allograft is at the center of the medial femoral condyle to the right and the anterior cruciate ligament is to the left.

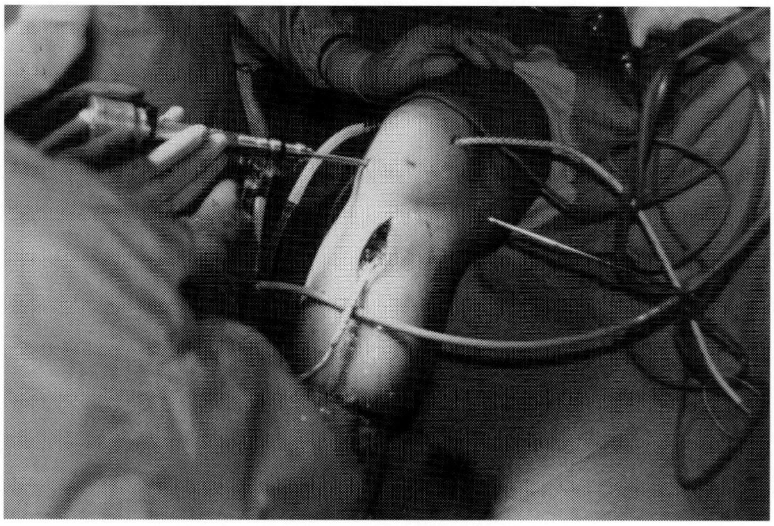

Figure 10.17

Switching stick shows position of posteromedial arthroscopic portal for visualization of the proximal tibia during tunnel creation.

REFERENCES

1. Clancy WG. Repair and reconstruction of the posterior cruciate ligament. In: Chapman MW, ed. *Operative Orthopaedics.* Philadelphia, Pa: JB Lippincott; 1988.
2. Daniel DM, Stone ML, Barnett P, Sachs R. Use of the quadriceps active test to diagnose posterior cruciate ligament disruption and measure posterior laxity of the knee. *J Bone Joint Surg.* 1988;70A:386–391.
3. Daniel D, Akeson W, O'Connor J: *Knee Ligaments: Function, Injury, and Repair.* New York, NY: Raven Press; 1990.
4. Fanelli GC. Three zone concept of arthroscopic PCL evaluation. Presented at the Cherry Blossom Seminar; McLean, Va; March, 1991.
5. Parolie JM, Bergfeld JA. Long-term results of nonoperative treatment of isolated posterior cruciate ligament injuries in the athlete. *Am J Sports Med.* 1986;14:35–38.
6. Paulos L. *Arthroscopically Assisted Posterior Cruciate Ligament Reconstruction Using Precision Drill Guides.* Mansfield, Mass: Acufex Microsurgical Inc; 1986.
7. Stanish WO, Rubinovich M, Armason T, et al. Posterior cruciate ligament tears in wrestlers. *Can J Applied Sports Sci.* 1986;4:173–177.

Section Two

The Shoulder

chapter

Eleven

Arthroscopy of the Shoulder: Basic Techniques

J. Serge Parisien

The arthroscope is a useful tool for the evaluation and management of various pathologic shoulder conditions. Diagnostic procedures are easy and usually require two portals, one anterior and one posterior. Surgical procedures are technically more demanding, and successful results depend on the surgeon's accurate knowledge of portal anatomy, meticulous techniques, and proper choice of patients.[1–12]

Positioning of the Patient

Lateral Decubitus Position

The patient can be placed in the lateral recumbent position with the affected side up. If arthroscopic surgery is contemplated, the shoulder is placed in traction with the arm in a position between 30° to 70° of abduction and 10° to 15° of forward flexion (Fig. 11.1). The patient can be tilted backward approximately 15° to 20° from the vertical to accommodate for the anterior slope of the glenoid. When arthroscopic acromioplasty is performed, it may be necessary to decrease the amount of abduction so as not to close the subacromial space.

Sitting Position

Because of concern about the possible compromise of neurovascular status associated with traction, the sitting position for shoulder arthroscopy is being used more frequently. A standard operating table is used and the patient can be adjusted to a semisitting or a sitting position. If the superior quarter panel of the table can be removed and replaced by a neurosurgical head holder, the patient is moved upward to clear the scapula from the superior edge of the table. Otherwise, the patient is moved to the edge of the operating table with the shoulder tilted forward by means of a bolster placed beneath the scapula. Recently, Chandler[13] advocated the use of modular shoulder cutouts and a narrowed head piece on a standard surgical operating table, in order to gain better access to the posterior aspect of the shoulder (Fig. 11.2). With a semisitting or sitting position, traction need not be applied to the shoulder, and there is no need to reposition the patient or to redrape and reprepare the surgical field for an open procedure. To prevent external rotation of the lower extremities and any abnormal compression of the peroneal nerve at the fibula head, the feet and ankles are held together with adhesive tape.

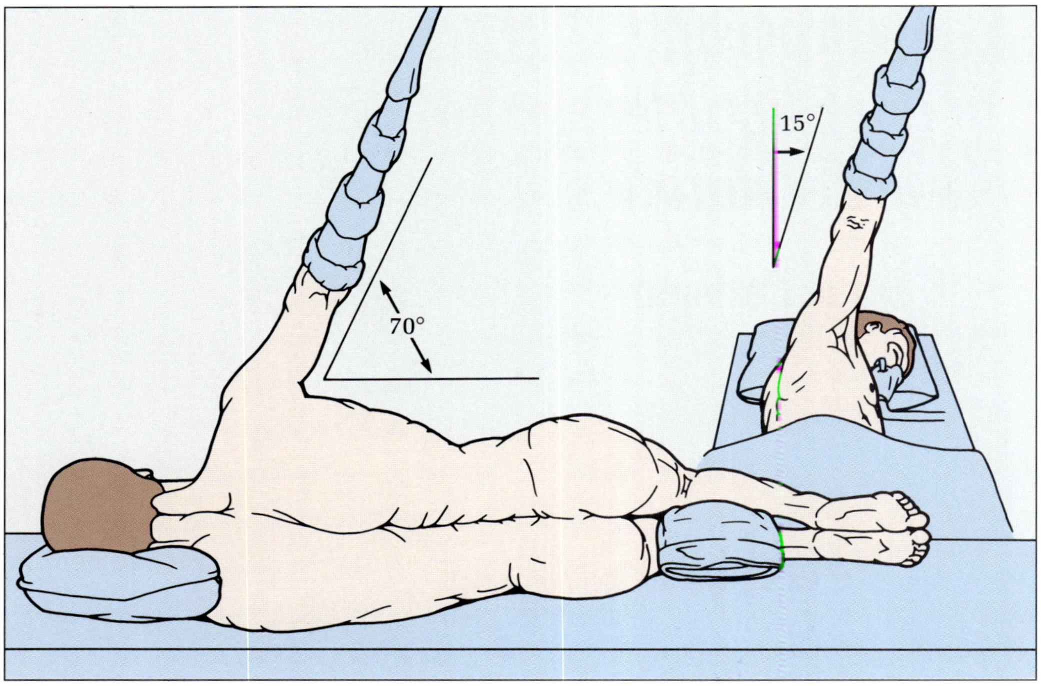

Figure 11.1
Patient in the lateral decubitus position.

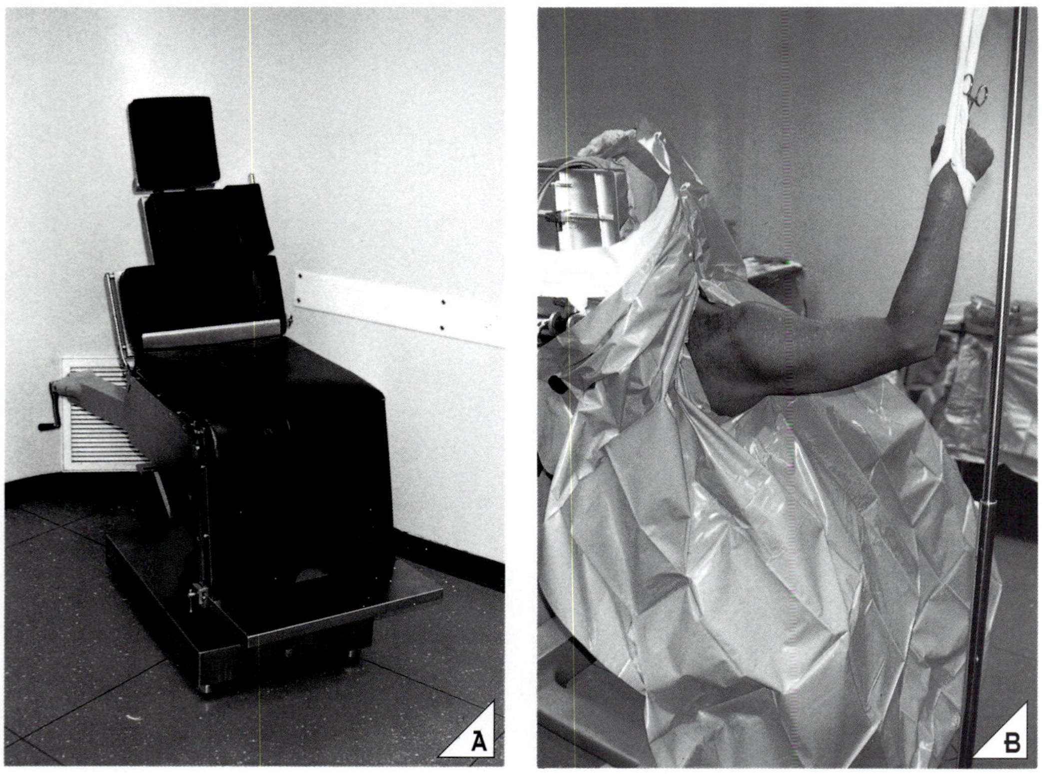

Figure 11.2
(A) Operating table modified with modular cutouts for access to the posterior aspect of the shoulder. (Courtesy of Eugene Chandler MD, Scottsdale, Arizona) (B) Patient in the sitting position with modular shoulder cutouts and a narrowed headpiece.

PORTAL ANATOMY

At the beginning of the procedure a marking pen is used to outline the bony anatomic landmarks about the shoulder, mainly the coracoid process, the acromioclavicular joint, the anterior, lateral, and posterior borders of the acromion, and the spine of the scapula. Various neurovascular structures are at risk posteriorly, laterally, superiorly, and anteriorly when the three main shoulder portals are developed.

Posterior Portal

The posterior portal is located approximately 2 cm inferior and 1 cm medial to the posterolateral corner of the acromion. The arthroscope pierces the skin and subcutaneous tissue, the posterior third of the deltoid muscle, the infraspinatus muscle or the interval between the infraspinatus and teres minor muscles, and finally the joint capsule. At this level the posterior portal avoids violating the quadrangular and triangular spaces of the posterior aspect of the shoulder, located approximately 6 cm below the acromion, and the sites of the posterior humeral circumflex artery and axillary nerve and scapular circumflex artery, respectively (Fig. 11.3).

Anterior Portal

The anterior portal is located lateral to the tip of the coracoid process, inferior to the anterolateral corner of the acromion. This portal pierces the skin, subcutaneous tissue, the anterior third of the deltoid muscle, and finally the joint capsule. The musculocutaneous nerve, which is at risk with this portal, is located approximately 3 cm inferior and

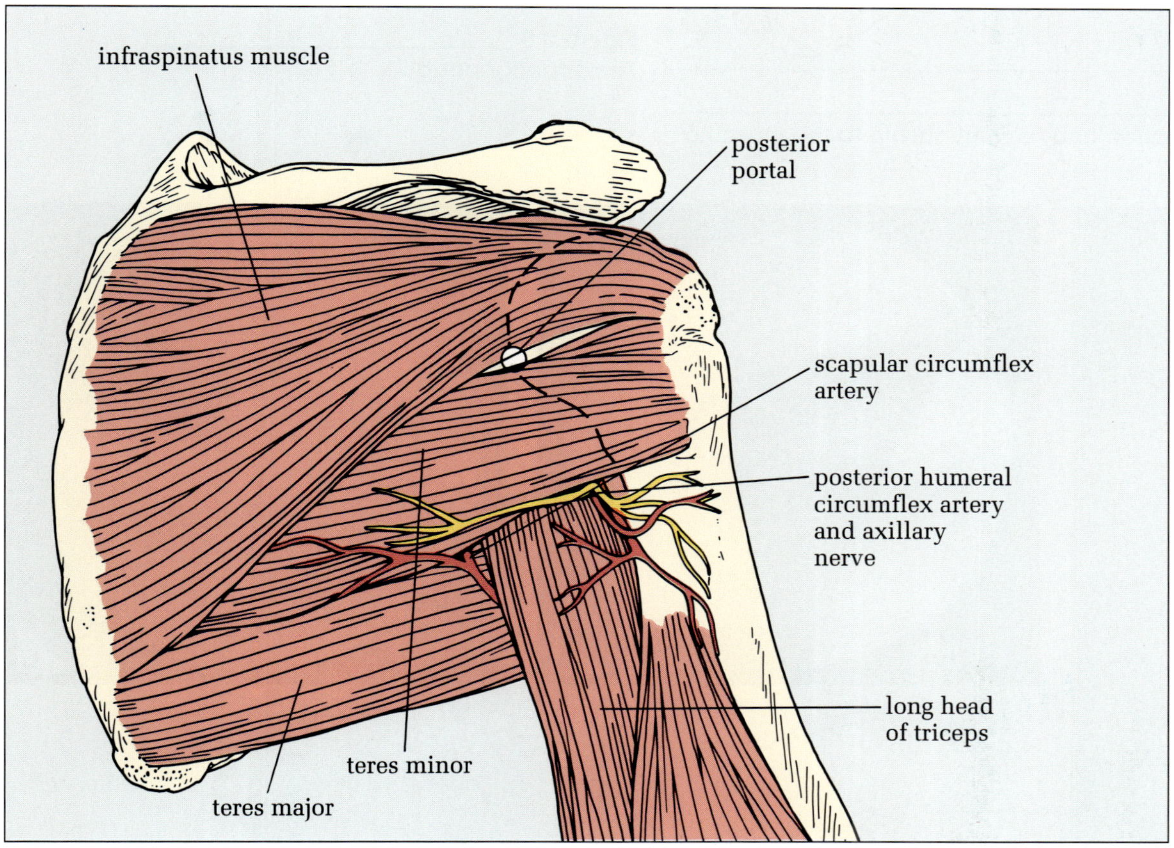

Figure 11.3 The posterior portal location and its relationship to the neurovascular structures.

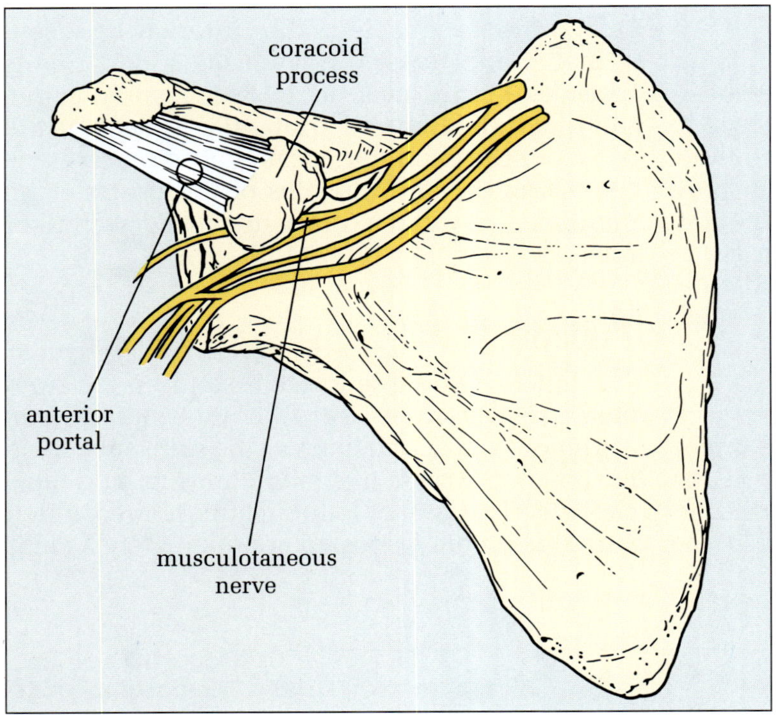

Figure 11.4
The anterior portal location and its relationship to the musculocutaneous nerve.

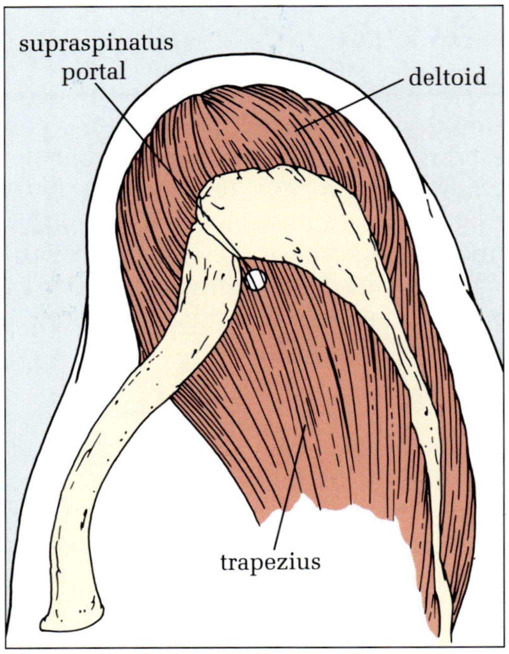

Figure 11.5
The superior portal.

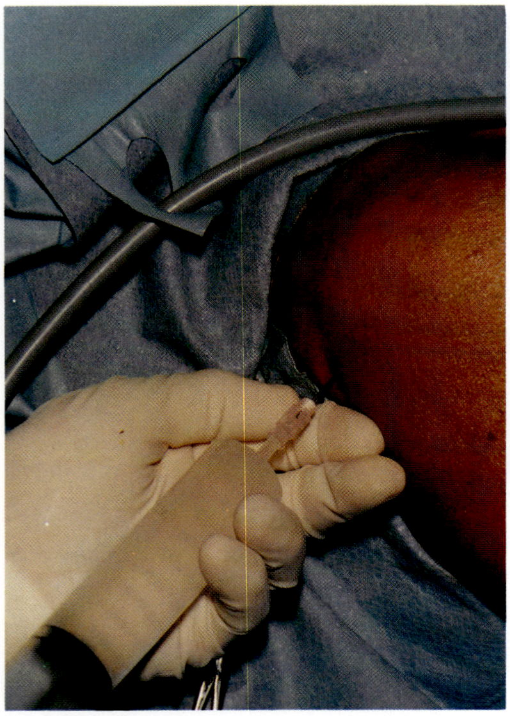

Figure 11.6
Spinal needle attached to syringe filled with normal saline to inflate the joint cavity.

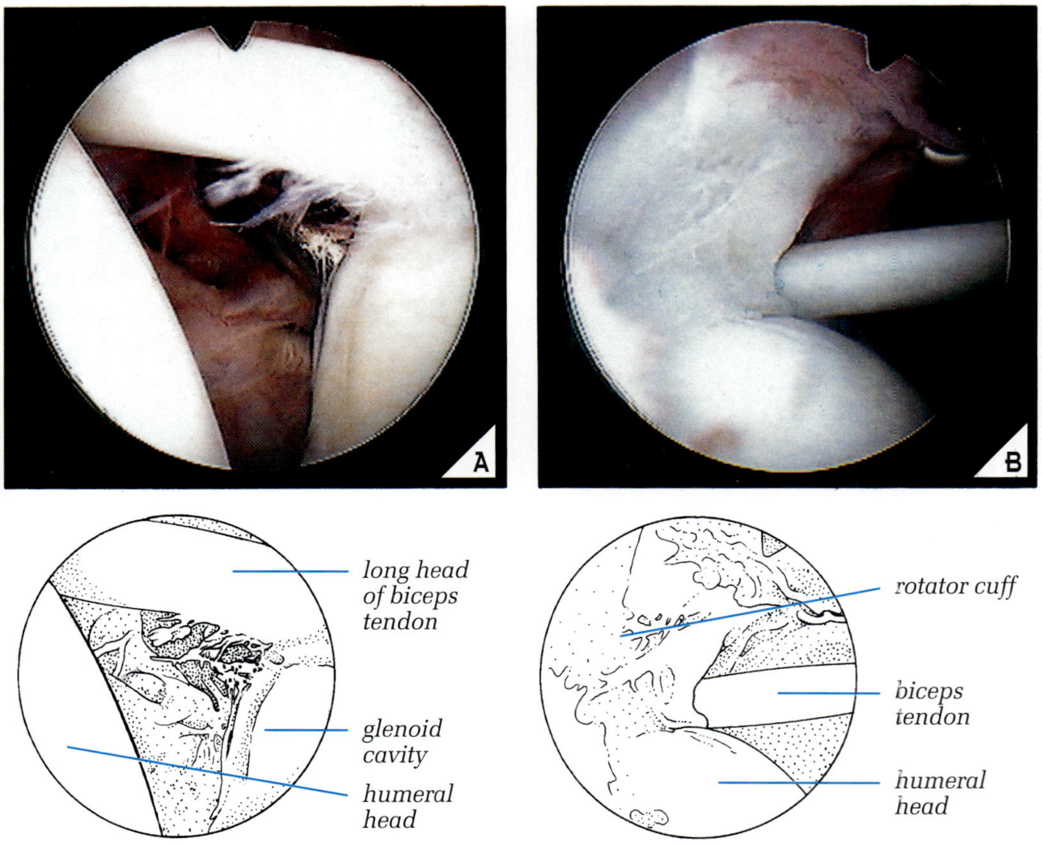

Figure 11.7
(A) Visualization of the long head of the biceps tendon in the left shoulder, with the patient in the sitting position.
(B) Biceps tendon exiting under transverse ligament.

medial to the coracoid process (Fig. 11.4). This portal can be developed by inserting a spinal needle into the intraarticular triangle described by Matthews,[8] formed by the biceps tendon, the glenoid labrum, and the humeral head. This anterior portal can also be developed by placing a long rod (Wissenger rod) from the posterior portal through the arthroscope cannula, against the anterior capsule in the intraarticular triangle. Another cannula placed over the protruding rod anteriorly enters the joint to establish the portal. An accessory anterior portal can be used and should be located adjacent and lateral to the coracoid process.

Superior Portal

The superior portal is located in the supraspinatus fossa and is limited anteriorly by the posterior aspect of the clavicle, laterally by the medial border of the acromion, and posteriorly by the spine of the scapula. The arthroscope pierces the skin, subcutaneous tissue, the trapezius muscle medial to the acromion, and the supraspinatus muscle, avoiding its tendinous portion. The suprascapular artery and nerve are approximately 2.5 cm medial to the portal. When this portal is used, care should be taken to avoid the area adjacent to the suprascapular notch, thus avoiding injury to the suprascapular artery and nerve (Fig. 11.5).

Surgical Technique

At the posterior portal located approximately 2 cm inferior and 1 cm medial to the posterolateral tip of the acromion, a spinal needle is introduced into the shoulder joint and 40 to 70 mL of normal saline is used to inflate the joint cavity (Fig. 11.6). The needle is removed after the saline is seen to flow out freely, and the skin is punctured with a #11 scalpel. The smooth obdurator of a 4 mm arthroscope, aimed at the coracoid process, is inserted into the joint. As the posterior capsule is felt, penetration of the joint is followed by escape of the fluid medium from the cannula. The arthroscope attached to the video camera is then introduced into the joint. For diagnostic examination, a Veres needle is placed via the anterior portal between the coracoid process and acromion. Its entry can be confirmed by direct vision. With the overhead irrigation fluid connected to the scope, a flow is established to keep the joint capsule clear of blood and articular debris.

The first intraarticular landmark to be identified is the long head of the biceps tendon (Fig. 11.7A). The tendon, which is round in cross section, appears to arise from the labrum and crosses the humeral head to exit anteriorly under the transverse humeral ligament (Fig. 11.7B). Then the intraarticular part of the subscapularis tendon is seen in a synovial recess between the superior and middle glenohumeral ligaments. These two ligaments form the superior and inferior margins of the entrance of the subscapularis recess. The inferior glenohumeral ligament, the most important of the glenohumeral ligaments, can then be visualized. Its superior band, placed beneath the middle glenohumeral ligament, seems to originate from the anterior labrum (Fig. 11.8). The scope is withdrawn gently so that the inferior recess of the joint can be seen. By rotating the scope, the posterior aspect of the humeral head,

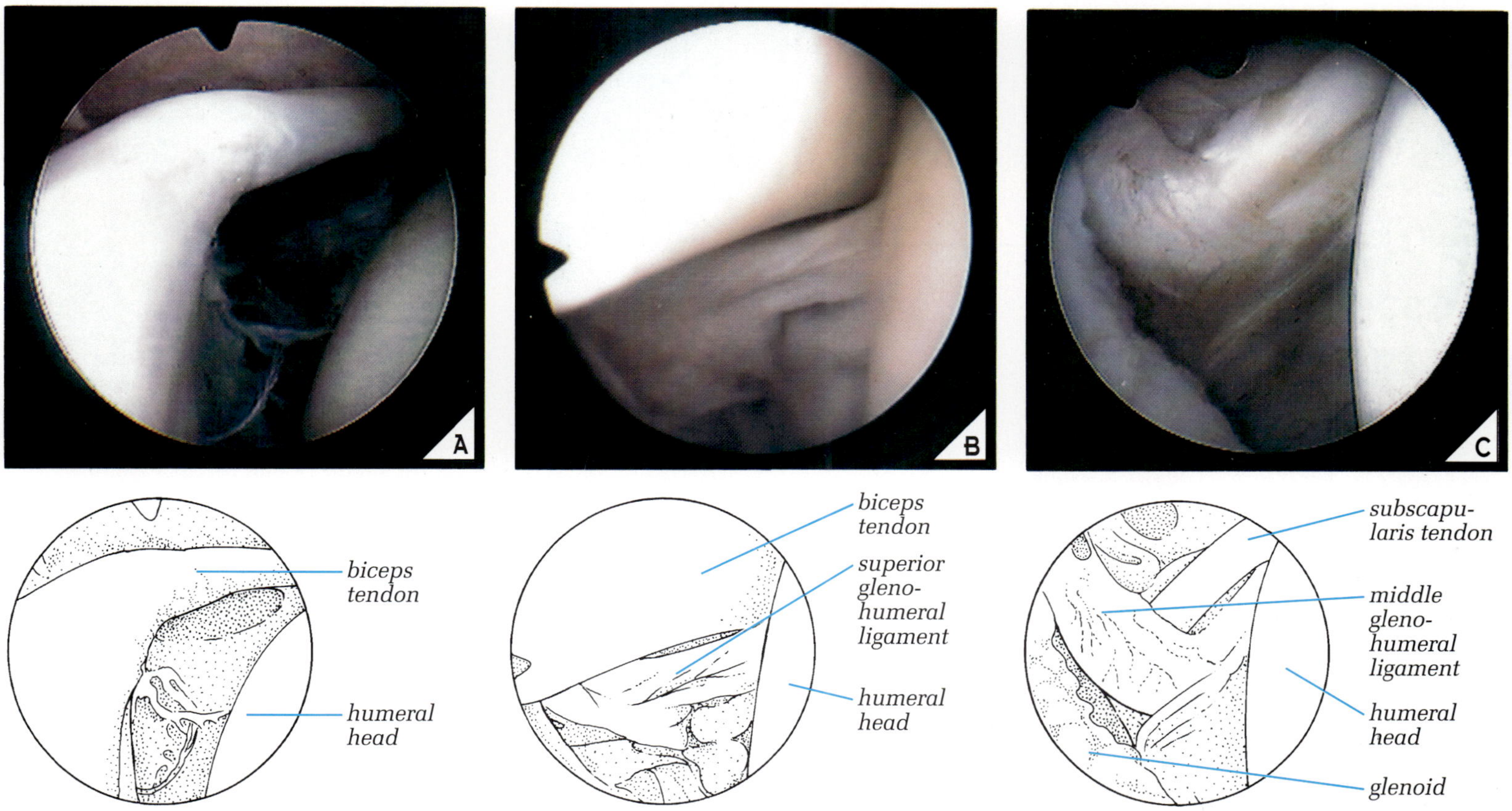

Figure 11.8

Visualization of the right shoulder showing the origin of the long head of the biceps tendon (A), the superior glenohumeral ligament (B), the middle glenohumeral ligament with subscapularis tendon (C), the inferior glenohumeral ligament (D, E), and the inferior synovial recess (F). The patient is in the sitting position.) (continued on next page) the posterior glenoid and labrum, and the posterior synovial recess can be visualized.

An area of bare bone with multiple fenestrations is normally found at the posterolateral aspect of the humeral head between the capsular insertion and the articular lining of the head. It should not be confused with a pathologic Hill–Sachs lesion, which is usually secondary to glenohumeral instability (Figs. 11.9, 11.10). The examination then proceeds to the superior aspect of the joint to inspect the rotator cuff. The supraspinatus tendon will be seen superior to the biceps tendon, followed by the infraspinatus and teres minor tendons more superiorly and posteriorly. Abduction of the shoulder will improve visualization of the superior humeral attachment of the cuff. To facilitate a thorough examination of the joint, a probe is introduced through the anterior portal previously described.

Diagnostic Arthroscopy

Diagnostic arthroscopy of the shoulder is valuable in suspected tears of the rotator cuff (Fig. 11.11) when the patient is allergic to contrast material. In suspected cases

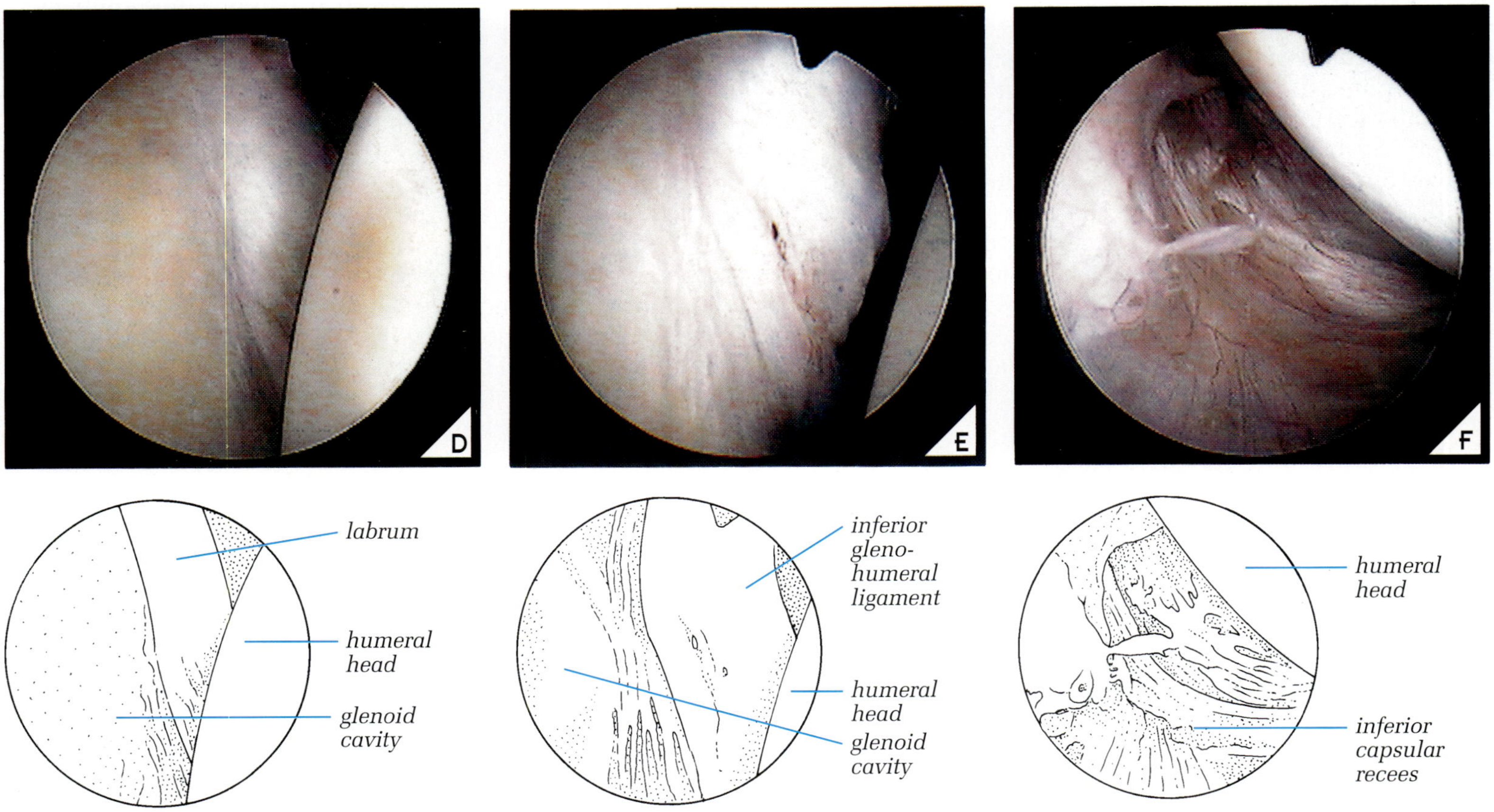

Figure 11.8 (continued)

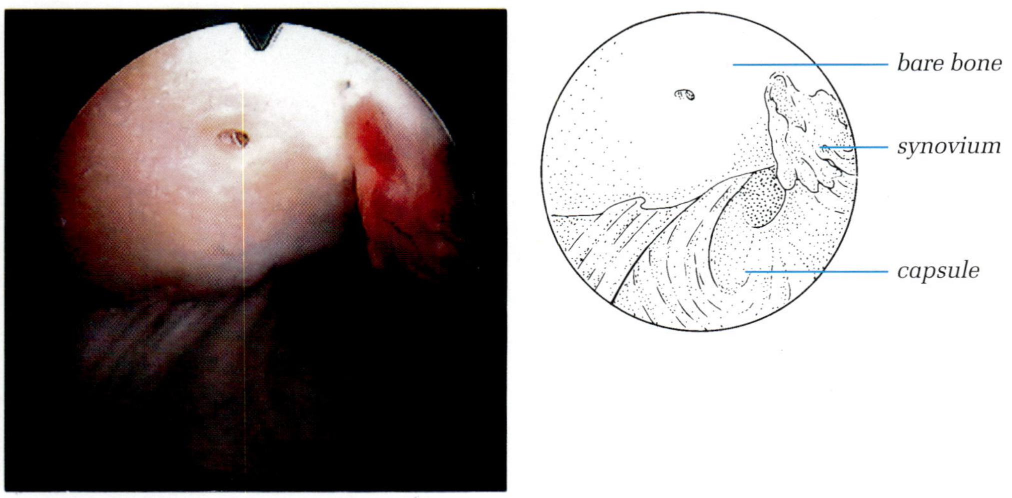

Figure 11.9
An area of bare bone at the posterolateral aspect of the humeral head left shoulder. The head is on the left. The patient is in the sitting position

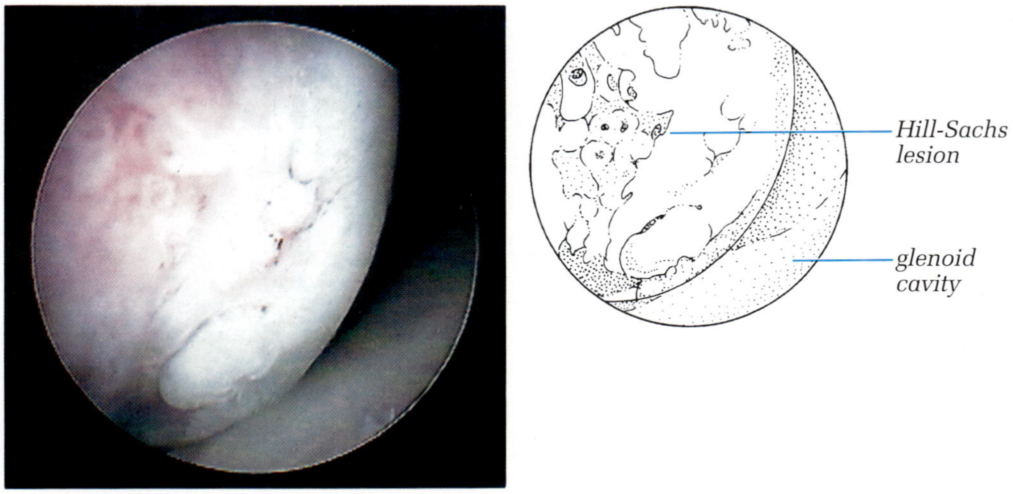

Figure 11.10
A true Hill-Sachs lesion of the left shoulder. The humeral head is on the left. The patient is in the sitting position.

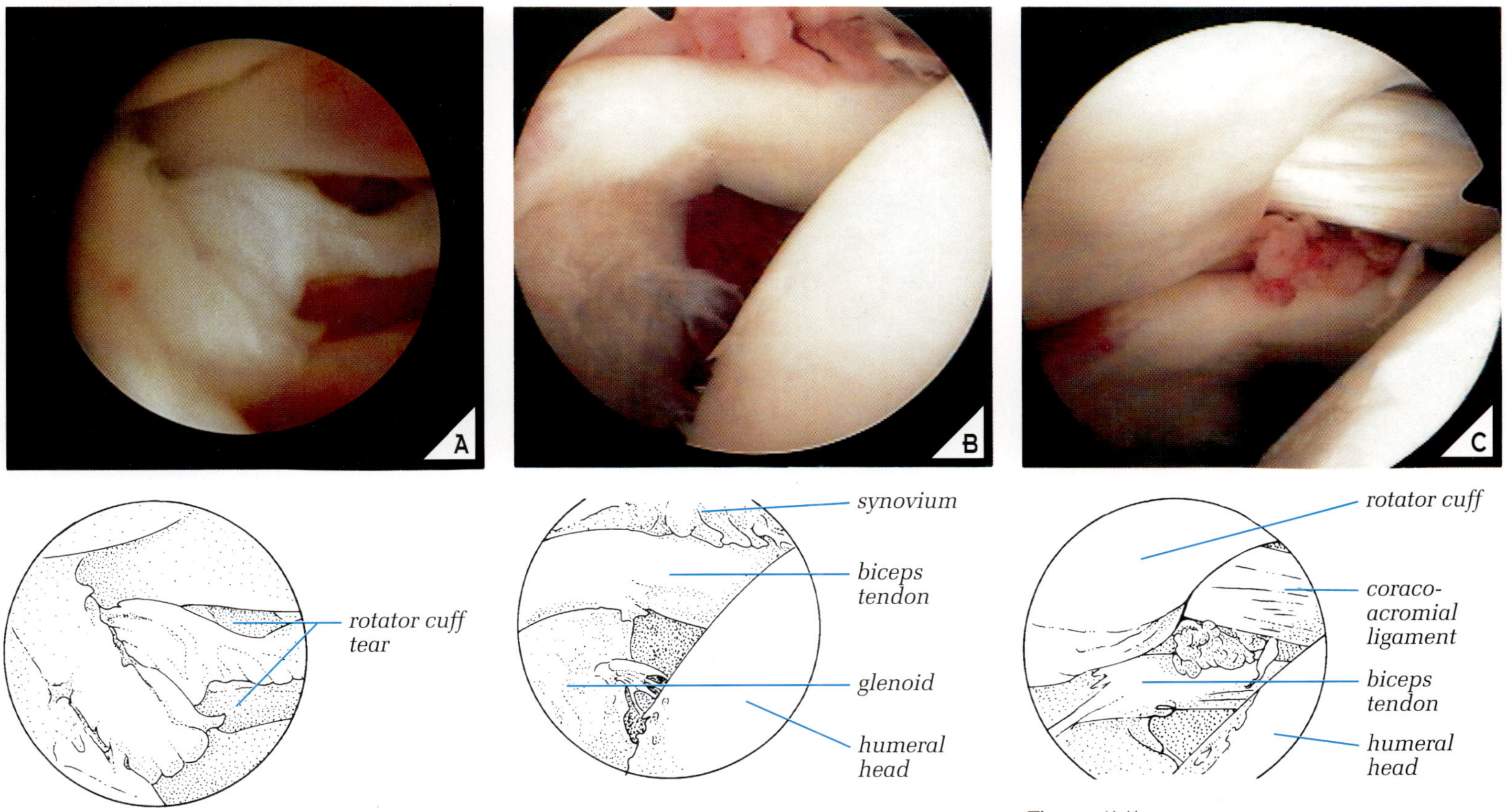

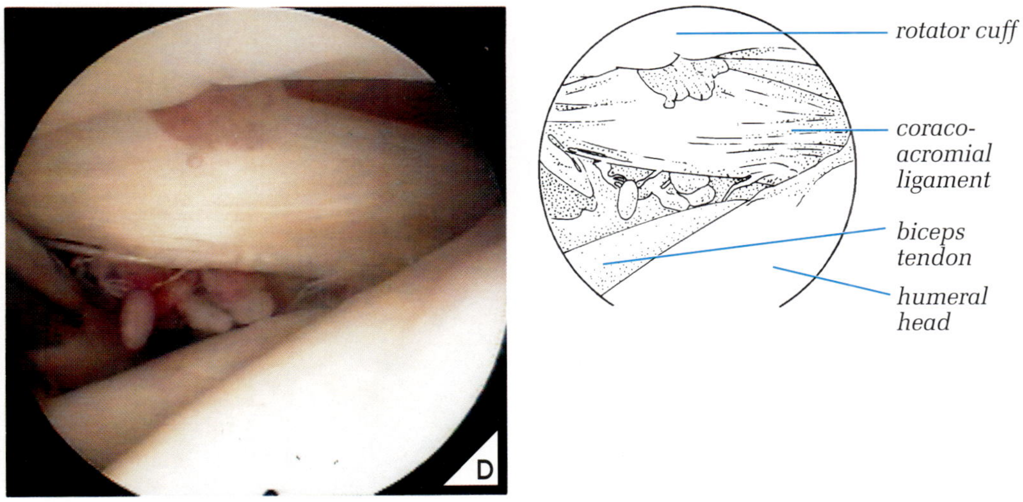

Figure 11.11
(A) Rotator cuff tear. (B) The insertion of the biceps tendon. (C, D) Steps in the visualization of a large rotator cuff of the right shoulder, with the coracoacromial ligament seen through the tear.

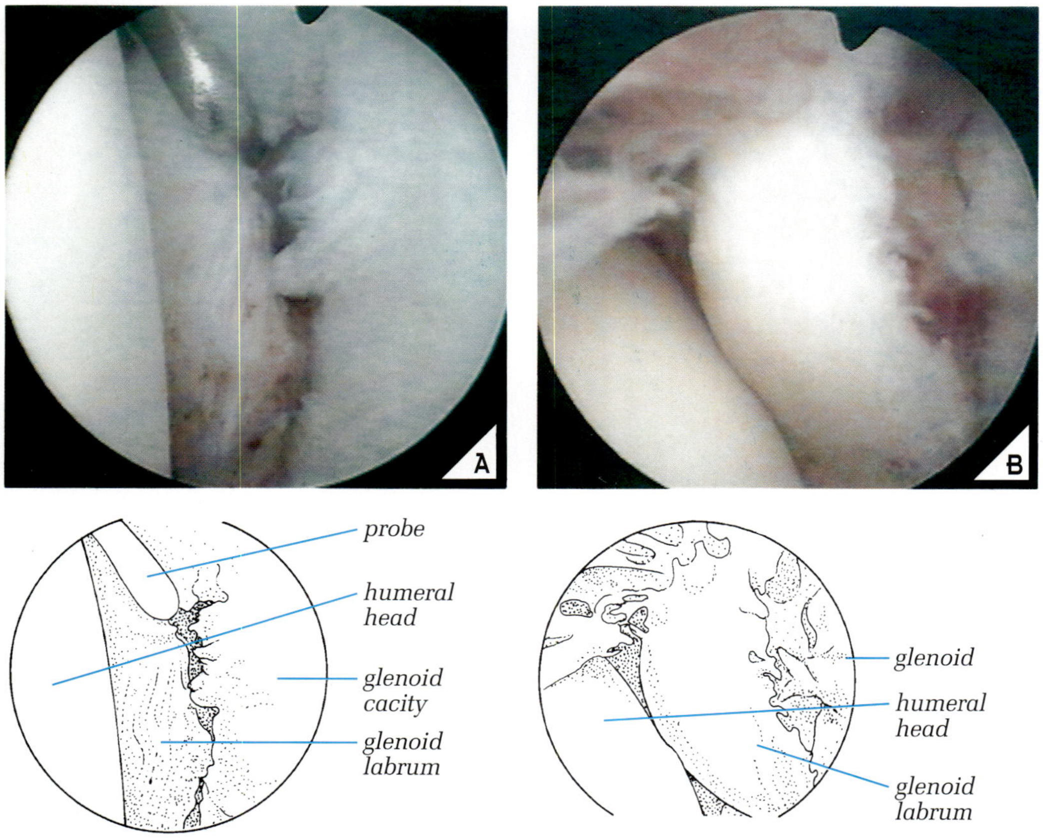

Figure 11.12

(A, B) Examples of anterior labrum detachment of the left shoulder. The patient is in the sitting position.

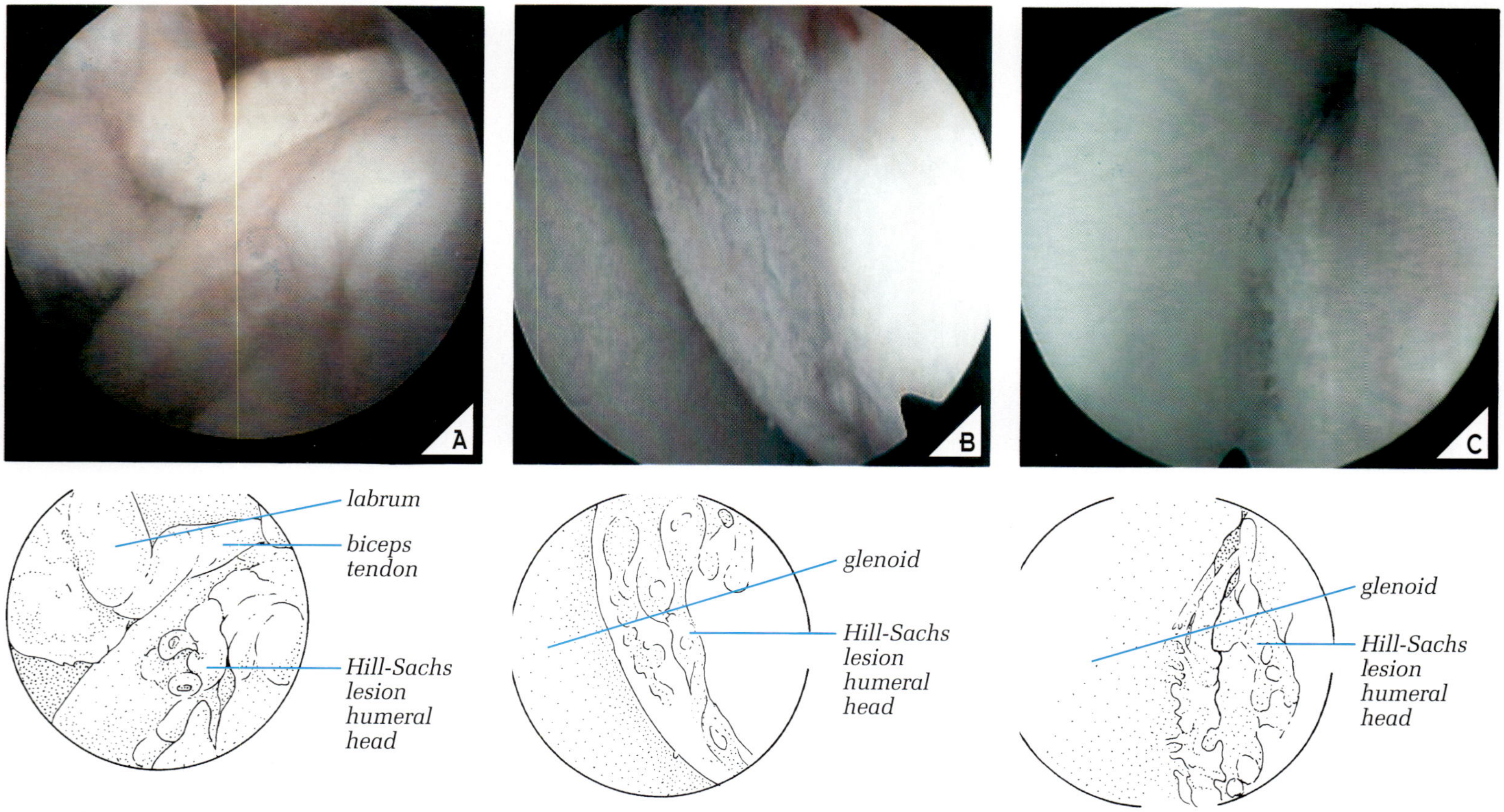

Figure 11.13

(A) Instability of the right shoulder with tear and detachment of the labrum and a Hill-Sachs lesion. The posterior aspect of the head is on the right. (B, C) Hill-Sachs lesion of the right shoulder. The patient is in the sitting position.

of shoulder instability it may be necessary to combine an examination under anesthesia with diagnostic exploration of the joint. Some pathologic findings such as labral tears, damage to the inferior glenohumeral ligament, Bankart lesion, Hill–Sachs lesion, or the presence of a loose body may confirm a diagnosis of shoulder instability (Figs. 11.12–11.14). In a young, athletic individual with atypical pain in the shoulder, arthroscopy can help assess the joint to rule out labral tears, loose bodies, or early degenerative changes. When an open or closed subacromial decompression is performed, diagnostic arthroscopy of the glenohumeral joint is recommended to rule out or to treat any associated intraarticular pathology.[4,5,7,9,10,14–17]

Surgical Arthroscopy

Operative arthroscopy of the shoulder is indicated for treatment of any loose body or osteochondral lesions of

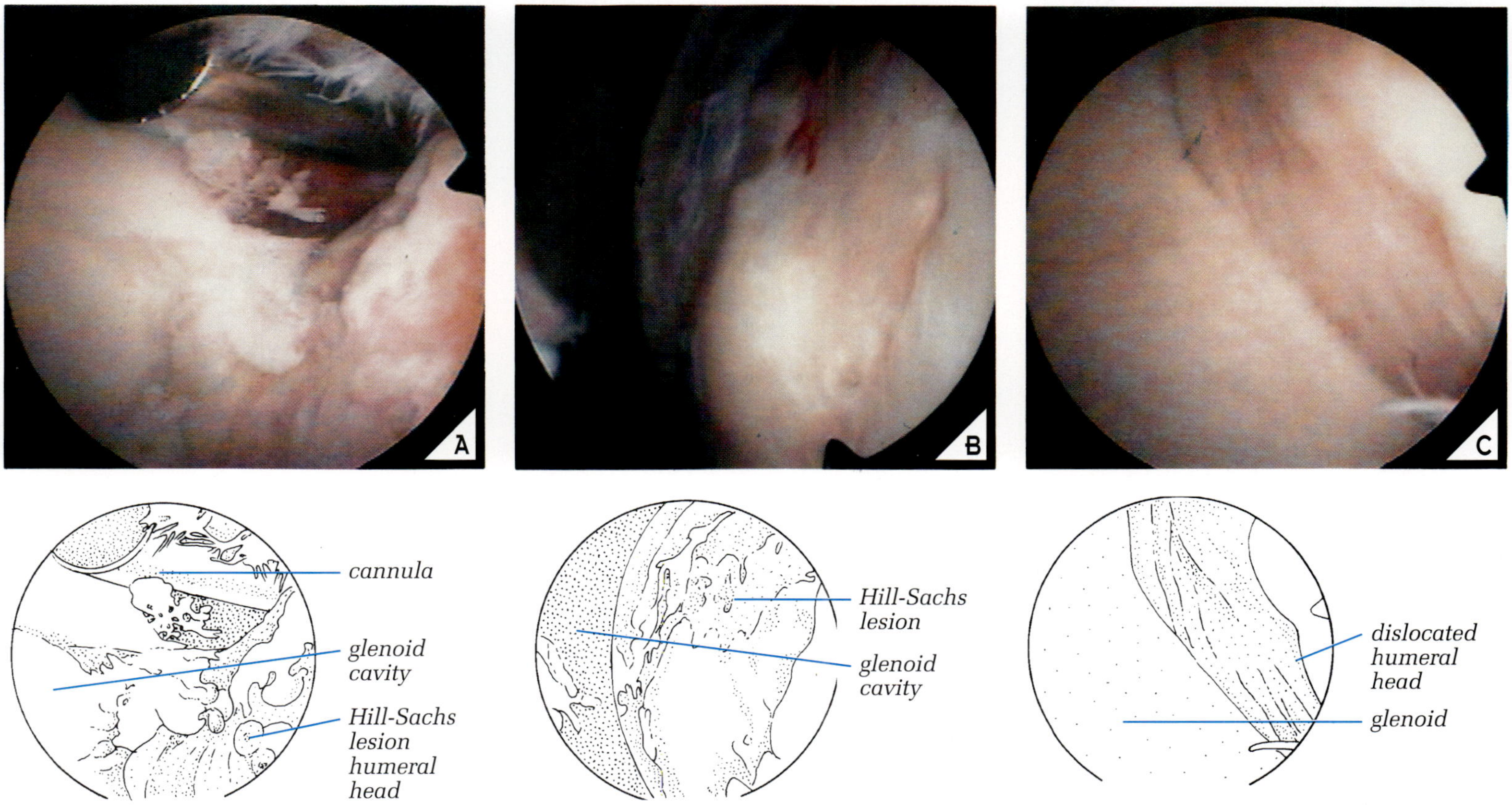

Figure 11.14
Instability of right shoulder with posterolateral defect (A, B) and anteroinferior dislocation (C). The patient is in the sitting position.

the glenohumeral joint (Fig. 11.15). Synovial disorders (rheumatoid arthritis, pigmented villonodular synovitis, synovial osteochondromatosis, pyarthrosis) can be managed arthroscopically using the above-mentioned arthroscopic portals (Figs. 11.16–11.18). Isolated lesions of the biceps tendon can be managed if the proximal part of the tendon is impinging in the joint. Partial thickness tear of the rotator cuff can be debrided, sometimes in combination with subacromial decompression. Some large deposits of calcific tendinitis, not amenable to the needle aspiration technique, can be debrided arthroscopically, using subacromial portals as described in Chapter 15. Arthroscopic surgery can also be very helpful in tears of the labrum not associated with instability of the shoulder.

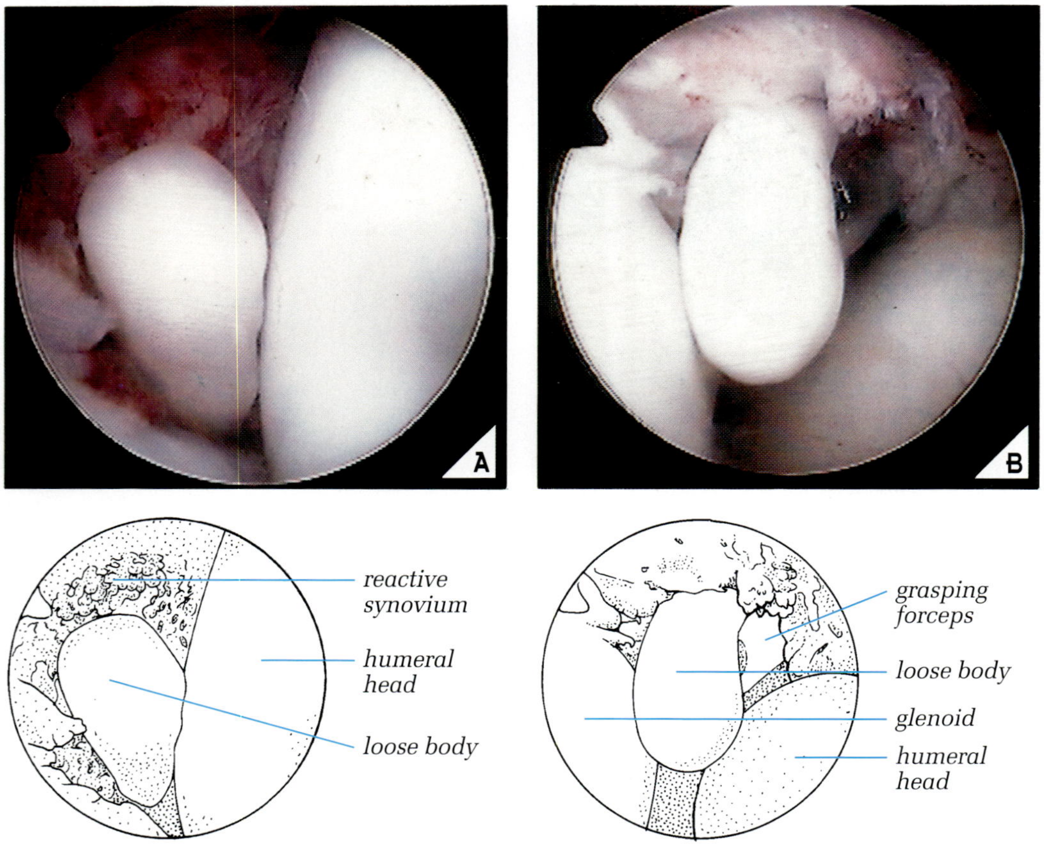

Figure 11.15
A loose body of the right shoulder before (A) and after (B) excision.

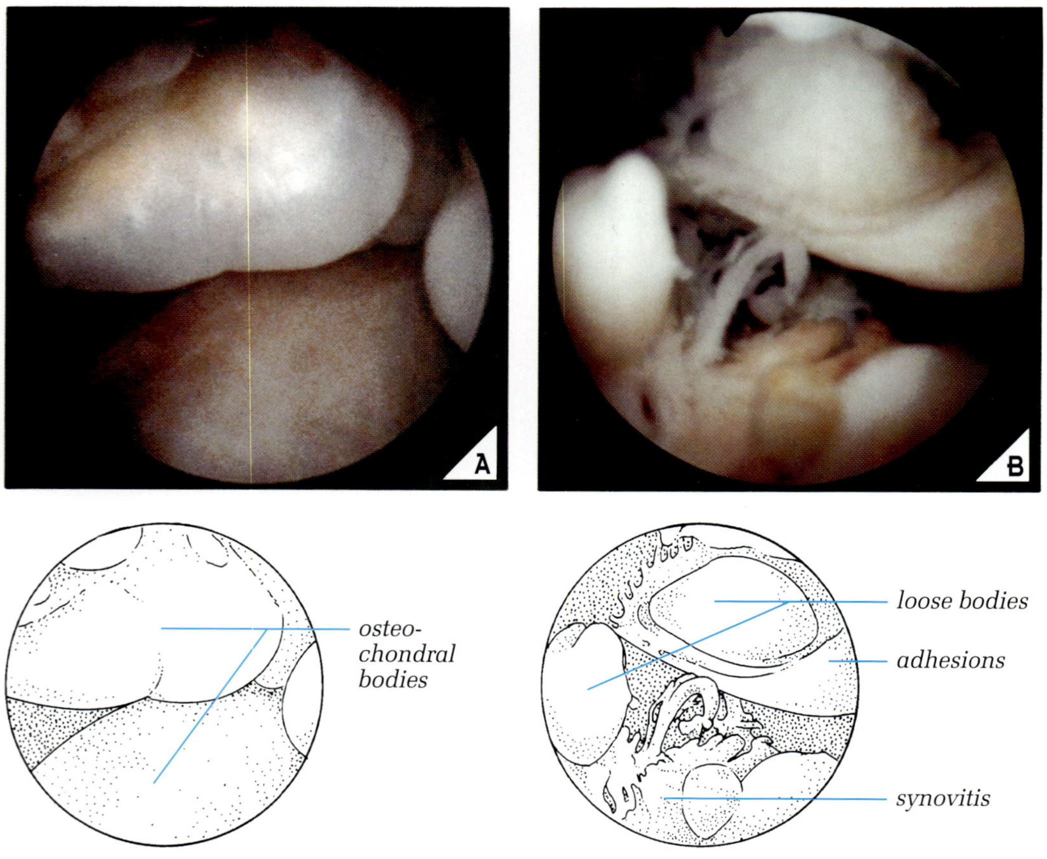

Figure 11.16
(A) Loose bodies of the shoulder in synovial osteochondromatosis. (B) Loose bodies, hypertrophic synovium, and adhesions in posttraumatic arthritis of shoulder. **(continued on next page)**

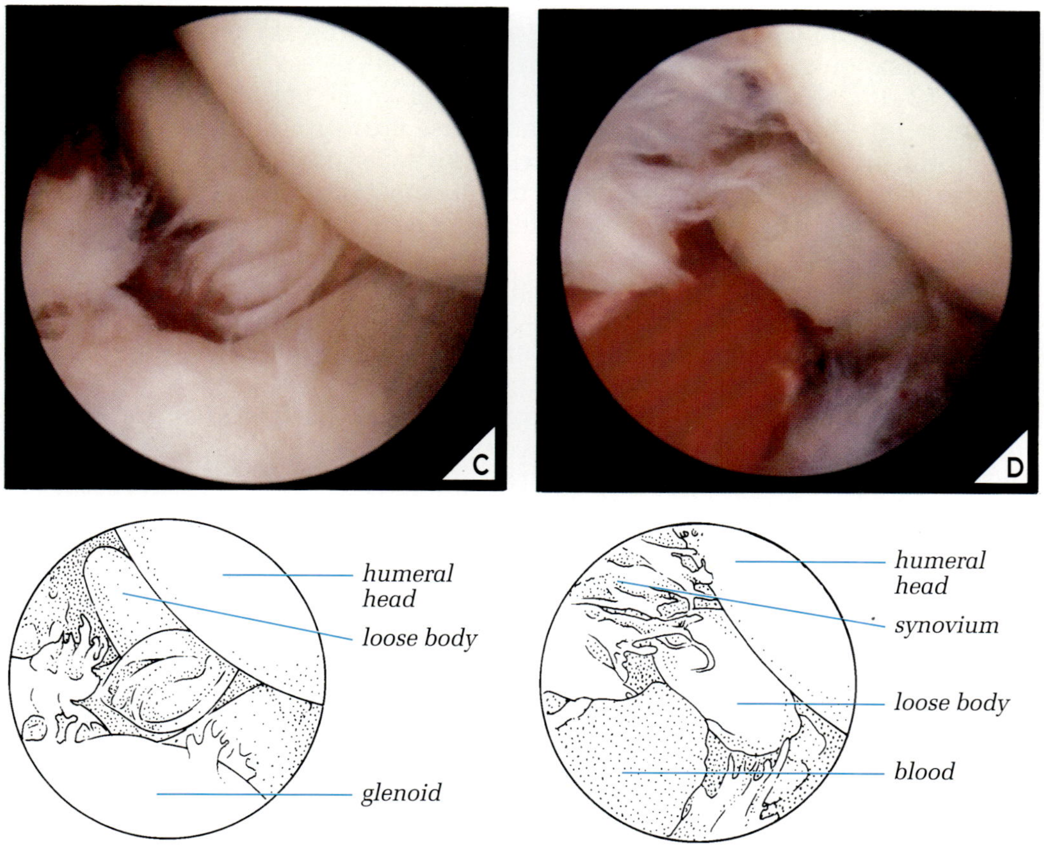

Figure 11.16 (continued)
(C, D) Loose body in subscapularis recess of the right shoulder. The patient was placed in lateral decubitis position.

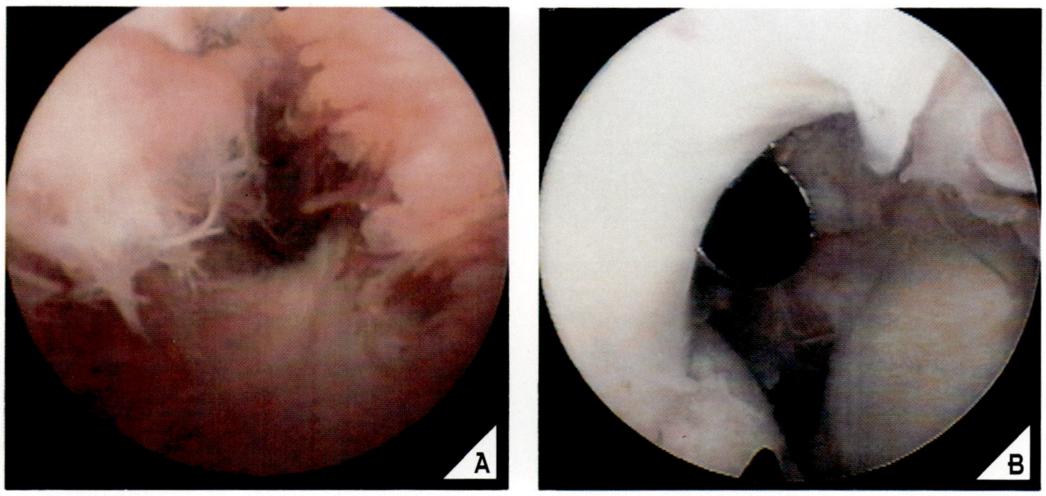

Figure 11.17
(A, B) Synovitis of the left shoulder before and after arthroscopic debridement.

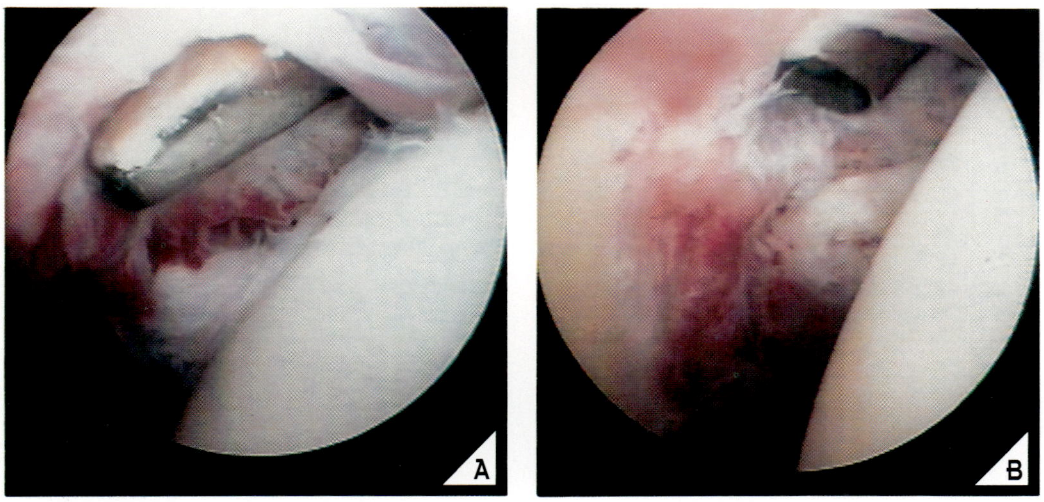

Figure 11.18
(A, B) Steps of excision of localized synovial lesion of the right shoulder. The patient is in the sitting position.

Isolated flap tears and bucket-handle tears of the labrum with "clicking" or locking of the shoulder will respond very well to arthroscopic debridement (Figs. 11.19–11.21). In addition, arthroscopic debridement may be helpful in some selected cases of degenerative arthritis of the shoulder when the rotator cuff shows no evidence of tear or degeneration.

Complications and Pitfalls

The posterior portal is the most commonly used portal in arthroscopy of the shoulder. If it is placed correctly, the surgeon will avoid the neurovascular structures at risk with this approach. If the scope is placed too medially, damage can be inflicted to the suprascapular nerve, artery, or vein. If the portal is placed too distally, the posterior humeral circumflex artery, axillary nerve, and scapular circumflex artery will be injured. When the posterior labrum and posterior synovial recess are visualized with this portal, the surgeon must take care that manipulation of the scope does not cause it to slip from the joint.

When the anterior portal is used, it must be kept in mind that inferior to the coracoid process lie the divisions of the brachial plexus. The musculocutaneous nerve is particularly at risk, since it is located approximately 3 cm inferior and medial to the coracoid process. The intraarticular triangle, as described by Matthews, is a safe area through which to enter the joint anteriorly while viewing from the posterior portal.

When the superior portal is used, the suprascapular nerve, artery, and vein are at risk, since the suprascapular notch is medial to this portal.

Excessive strain on the brachial plexus can be avoided by using approximately 10 to 15 pounds of traction when the patient is placed in the lateral decubitus position.

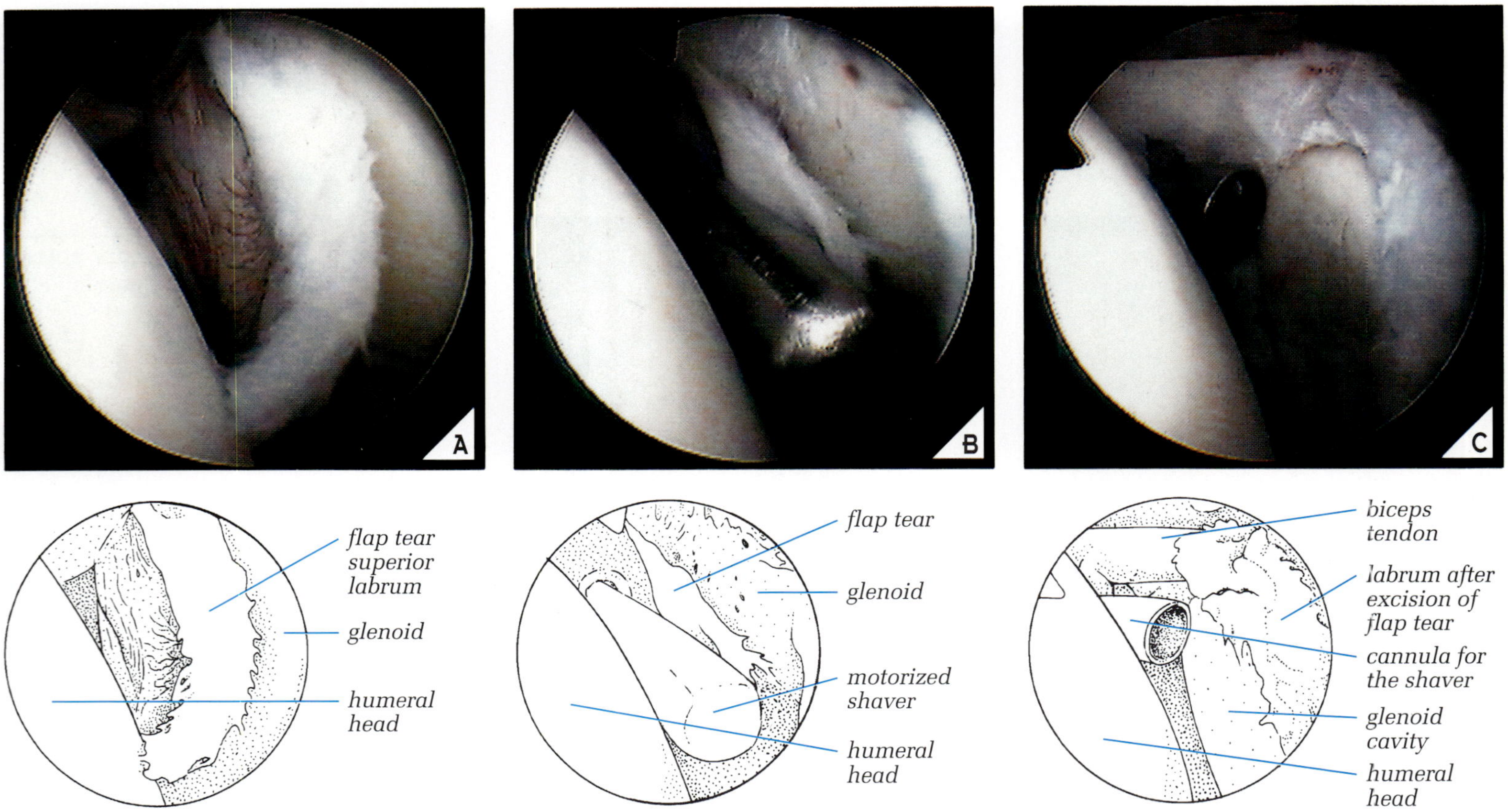

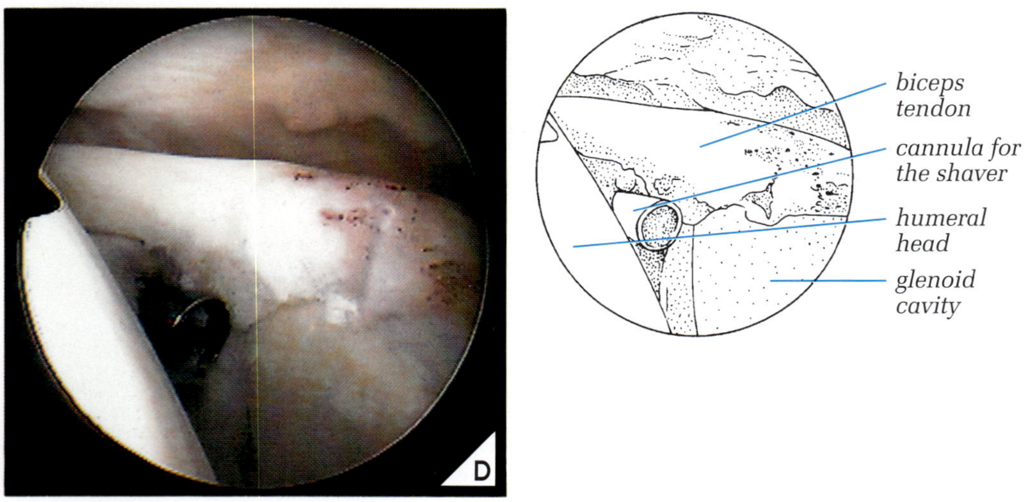

Figure 11.19
(A–D) Steps of excision of a flap tear of the superior labrum of the left shoulder. The patient is in the sitting position.

Although Fu[5,17] has shown experimentally that the best position for traction is 45° of forward flexion with 90° of abduction, many surgeons use abduction ranging from 45° or 60° to 70° and 15° of forward flexion. Pitman,[14] using somatosensory evoked potentials during shoulder arthroscopy, found that neuropraxia is probably secondary to a combination of factors such as position of the arm, the amount of traction, and intraarticular distention.

Fluid extravasation can be avoided when it is secondary to excessive pressure of the irrigation fluid and a lengthy procedure. It is sometimes related to a large tear of the rotator cuff or a loose biceps tendon sheath. In most situations, the soft tissue swelling will resorb in a matter of hours.

When the superior portal is used, damage to the tendinous portion of the supraspinatus muscle[18] can be avoided, according to Baker,[11] by keeping the shoulder in a position of no more than 45° of abduction with no forward flexion.

Elderly patients, placed in sitting position, may develop *hypotension*.[19] This can be prevented by applying compression leg stockings on the lower extremities to minimize pooling of blood in the lower extremities or using an interscalene regional block.

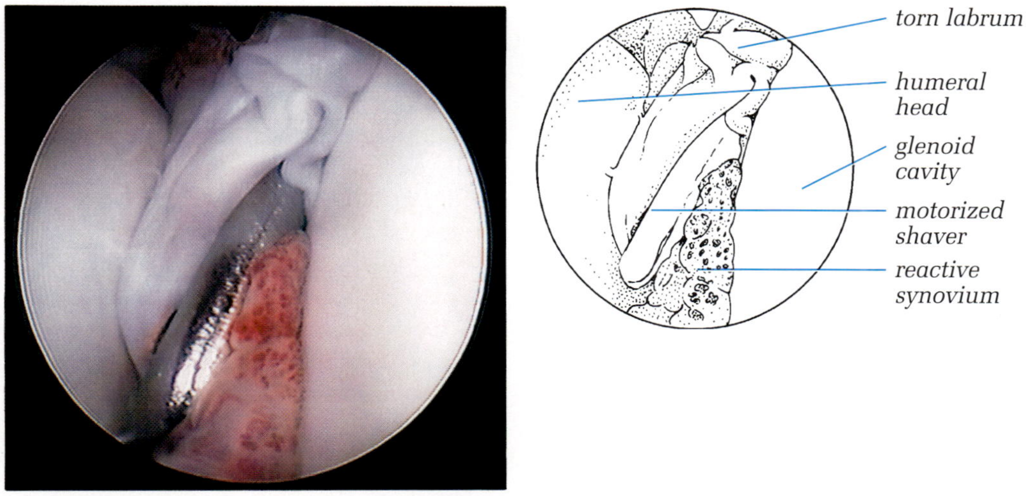

Figure 11.20 Arthroscopic excision of a bucket-handle tear of the labrum of the left shoulder using a motorized shaver.

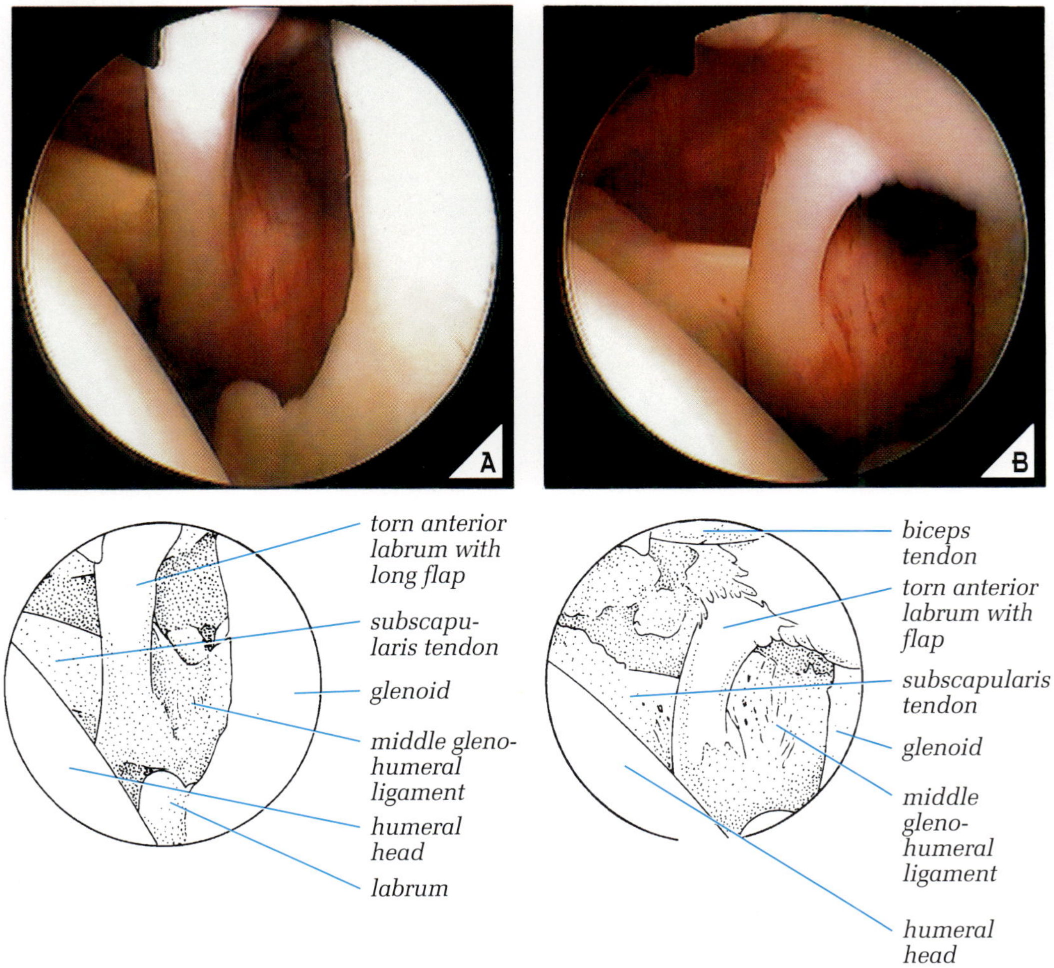

Figure 11.21 (A, B) Isolated tear of the anterior labrum of the left shoulder. The distal part of the flap is attached to the middle glenohumeral ligament in front of the subscapularis tendon.

REFERENCES

1. Andrews JR, Carson WG, Ortega K. Arthroscopy of the shoulder: technique and normal anatomy. *Am J Sports Med.* 1984;12:1–7.
2. Blachut PA, Day B. Arthroscopic anatomy of the shoulder. *Arthroscopy.* 1989;5:1–10.
3. Bryant WJ, Schauder K, Tullos HS. The axillary nerve and its relationship to common sports medicine shoulder procedures. *Am J Sports Med.* 1986;14: 113–116.
4. Caspari RB. Shoulder arthroscopy—a review of the present state of the art. *Contemp Orthop.* 1982;5:523–530.
5. Fu FM, Klein AH. Shoulder arthroscopy, complications and pitfalls. *Techniques in Orthopaedics.* 1988;3:27–32.
6. Gross RM, Fitzgibbon TC. Shoulder arthroscopy, a modified approach. *Arthroscopy.* 1985;1:152–159.
7. Johnson LL. Arthroscopy of the shoulder. *Orthop Clin North Am.* 1980;11:197–204.
8. Matthews LS, Zarins B, Michael RH, Helfet DL. Anterior portal selection for shoulder arthroscopy. *Arthroscopy.* 1985;1:33–39.
9. Ogilvie-Harris DJ, Wholey AM. Arthroscopic surgery of the shoulder: a general appraisal. *J Bone Joint Surg.* 1986; 68B:201–207.
10. Parisien JS. Shoulder arthroscopy technique and indications. *Bull Hosp Jt Dis Orthop Inst.* 1983;43:56–69.
11. Souryal TO, Baker CL. Anatomy of the supraclavicular fossa portal in shoulder arthroscopy. *Arthroscopy.* 1990;6:297–300.
12. Wolf EM. Anterior portals in shoulder arthroscopy. *Arthroscopy.* 1989;5:201–208.
13. Chandler E. Shoulder arthroscopy with the patient in the sitting position. *Contemp Orthop.* 1992;24:191–195.
14. Pitman MI, Nainzadeh N, Ergas E, Springer S. The use of somatosensory evoked potentials for detection of neuropraxia during shoulder arthroscopy. *Arthroscopy.* 1988;4:250–255.
15. Skyhar MJ, Altchek DW, Waren RF, et al. Shoulder arthroscopy with the patient in the beach chair position. *Arthroscopy.* 1988;4:256–259.
16. Snyder SJ, Karzel RP, Del Pizzo W, et al. SLAP lesions of the shoulder. *Arthroscopy.* 1990;6:274–279.
17. Klein AH, France JC, Mutschler TA, Fu FH. Measurement of brachial plexus strain in arthroscopy of the shoulder. *Arthroscopy.* 1987;3:45–52.
18. Norwood LA, Fowler HL. Rotator cuff tears, a shoulder arthroscopy complication. *Am J Sports Med.* 1989;17:837–841.
19. Martin JT. The head elevated position. In: *Positioning in Anesthesia and Surgery.* Philadelphia, Pa: WB Saunders Co: 1987:44–79.

chapter Twelve

Arthroscopic Suture Capsulorrhaphy for Anterior Shoulder Instability

Donald J. Rose

Arthroscopic stabilization procedures for anterior shoulder instability offer several possible advantages over open techniques, including reduced postoperative morbidity and hospitalization time, decreased loss of range of motion, improved assessment and treatment of associated intraarticular pathology,[1–3] and improved cosmesis. However, arthroscopic techniques using metal staples or other metal devices have led to a significant incidence of hardware complications, including loosening, migration, and breakage of hardware[4]; soft tissue tearing, irritation, or erosion[5]; humeral head impingement[4–6]; and secondary procedures for removal of hardware.[5,7,8]

The following technique of arthroscopic suture capsulorrhaphy selectively repairs the Bankart lesion and excessive anteroinferior capsular laxity found in anterior shoulder instability. The advantages of an arthroscopic procedure are maintained, while many of the potential complications of capsulorrhaphy with arthroscopic staples or other hardware are avoided. The procedure is indicated for nonhabitual anterior or anteroinferior shoulder luxators.

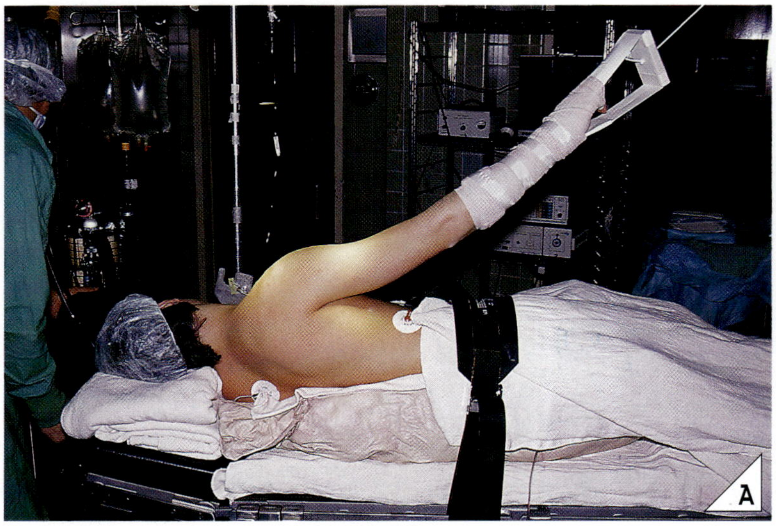

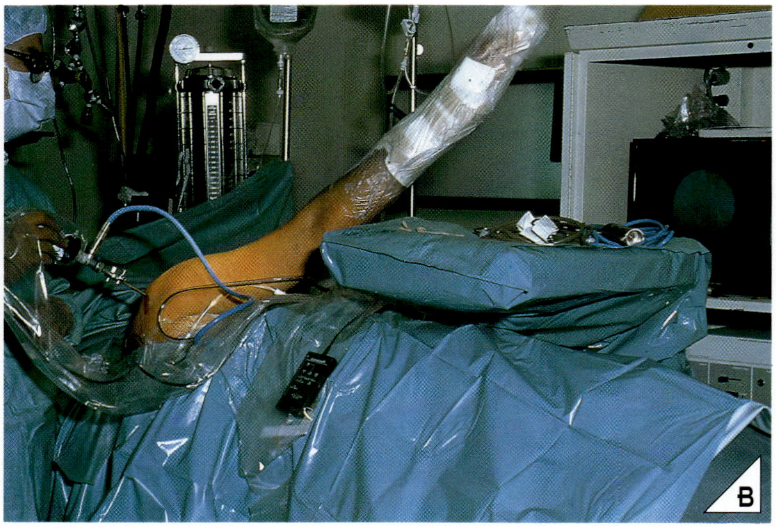

Figure 12.1
(A) Patient in the lateral decubitus position with operative shoulder suspended. (B) The arthroscope is inserted via posterior portal.

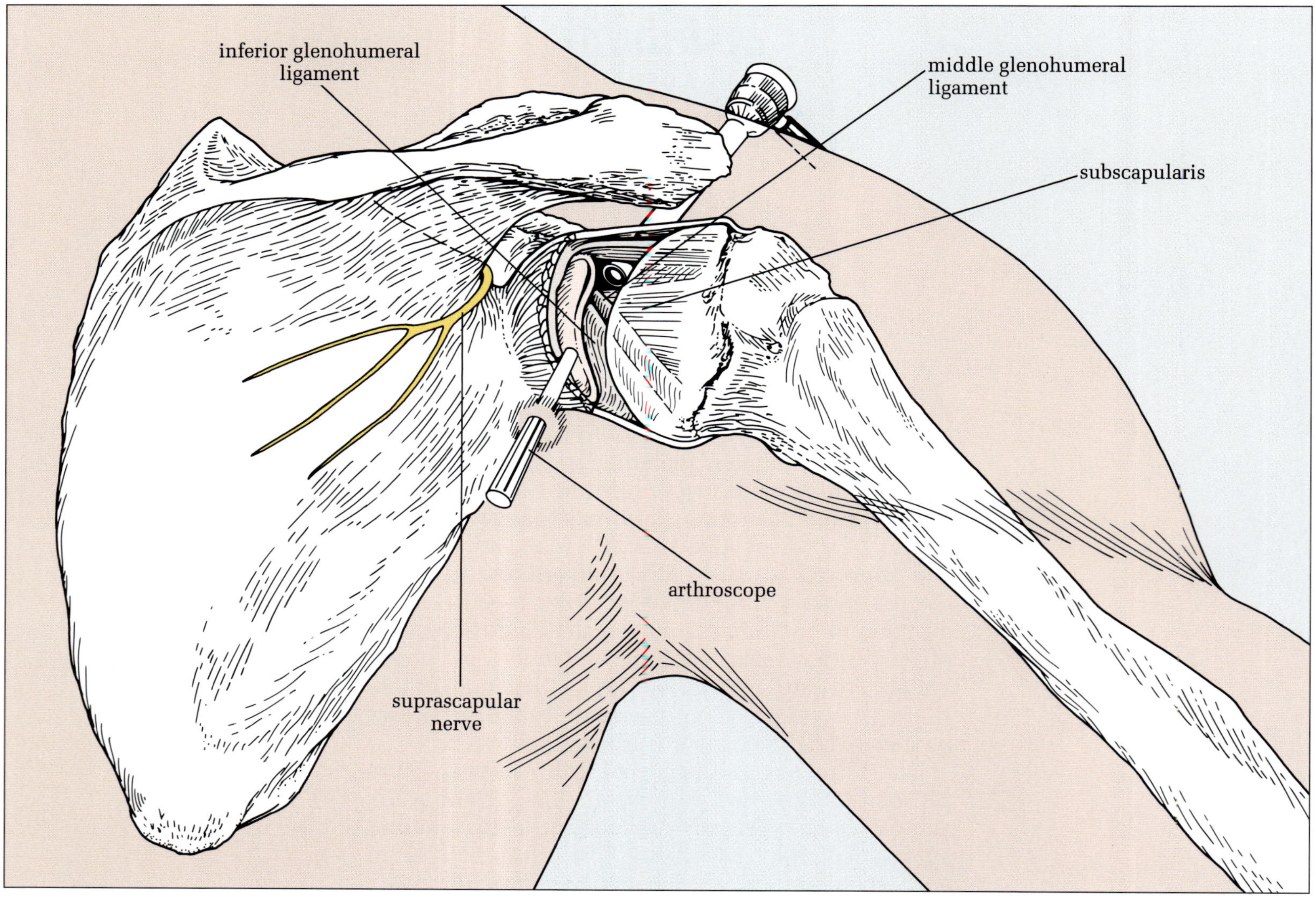

Figure 12.2
Posterior view of the pertinent arthroscopic anatomy of the right shoulder.

SURGICAL TECHNIQUE

Following induction of general endotracheal anesthesia, both shoulders are examined. The patient is placed in a lateral decubitus position with the operative shoulder suspended overhead in approximately 40° of abduction and 20° of flexion (Fig. 12.1). The scapular blade is left exposed during prepping and draping.

Arthroscopic Evaluation

The arthroscope is inserted through a standard posterior arthroscopic portal with normal saline inflow established through the arthroscopic cannula. Using a Wissinger rod placed through the arthroscopic cannula, a disposable cannula with a 7 mm inner diameter is inserted with the aid of a cannulated obturator through the triangular space bordered by the anterior glenoid rim, the superior edge of the subscapularis tendon, and the biceps tendon (Fig. 12.2). The 7 mm cannula may be sutured to the skin anteriorly during the procedure to prevent inadvertent withdrawal. Outflow is established through the cannula's accessory portal, and all subsequent instrumentation is passed through the cannula. An arthroscopic examination of the shoulder is then performed. The presence of a detached anterior glenohumeral ligament–labral complex (Bankart lesion) is confirmed (Fig. 12.3). The quality of tissues, degree of separation, and amount of anterior and/or inferior capsular laxity is thoroughly assessed. All associated intraarticular pathology (e.g., chondral damage, labral tears, loose bodies, hypertrophic synovitis) is evaluated and treated.

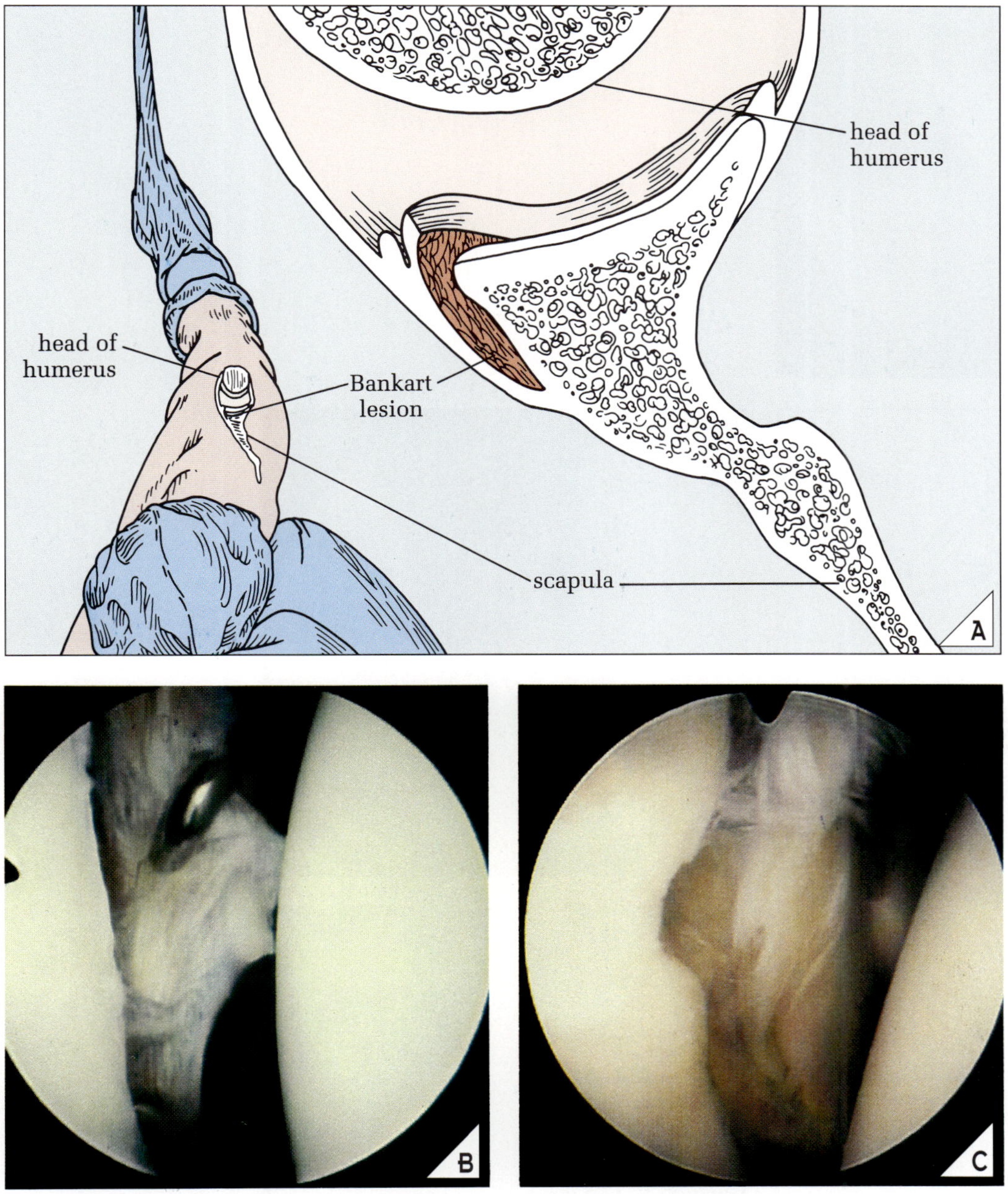

Figure 12.3
(A) Horizontal cross section of the glenoid demonstrating a Bankart lesion.
(B, C) Posterior views of the Bankart lesion.

Preparation of Anterior Glenoid Neck

A motorized shaver or rasp is placed through the anterior cannula and soft tissue removed from the anterior surface of the glenoid neck in the region of the Bankart lesion (Fig. 12.4). An abrader is then used to decorticate the anterior glenoid neck (Fig. 12.5).

Capsular Shift

A superior shift of the inferior glenohumeral ligament is then performed as required. A shoulder stitcher is used to pass multiple #0 or #1 monofilament nonabsorbable, or absorbable if desired, sutures through the superior band of the inferior glenohumeral ligament. The suture end exiting from the tip of the suture passer is retrieved using a suture snare or small grasper (Fig. 12.6) and brought out through the anterior cannula (Fig. 12.7). Both ends of each suture are tagged until later in the procedure.

Repair of Bankart Lesion

Repair of the Bankart lesion, using horizontal mattress sutures, is then performed. The sharp end of a suture pin is passed via the anterior cannula through the detached glenohumeral ligament–labral complex (Fig. 12.8). The

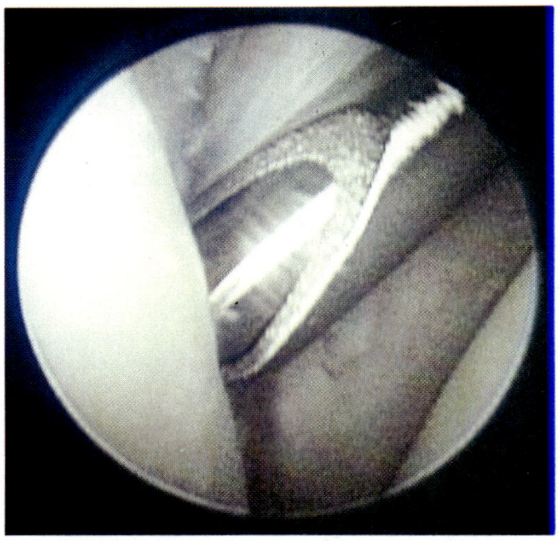

Figure 12.4
Soft tissue from the anterior surface of the glenoid neck region of the Bankart lesion is removed with a motorized shaver.

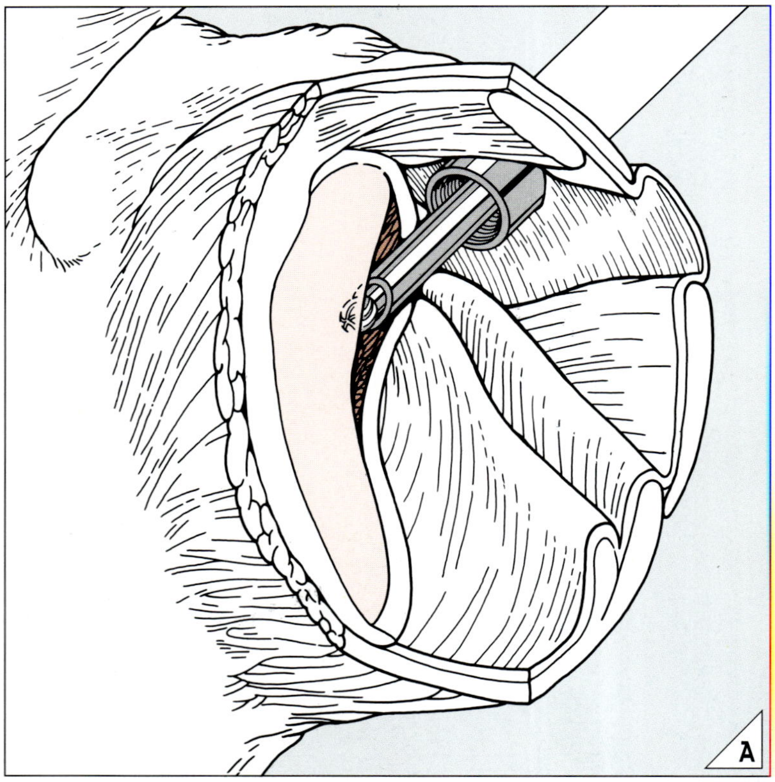

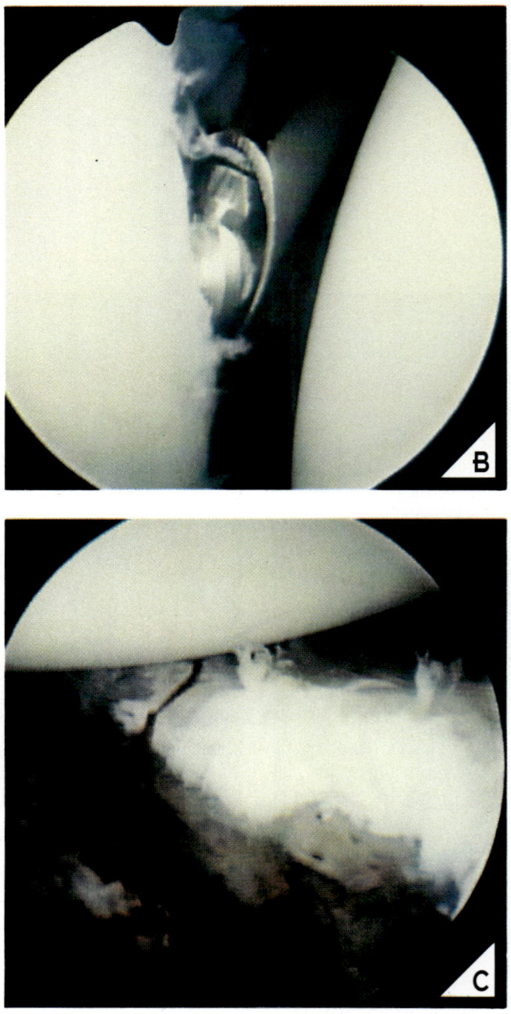

Figure 12.5
(A, B) Motorized abrader decorticating the anterior glenoid neck region. (C) View of the anterior glenoid neck from the anterior portal following decortication.

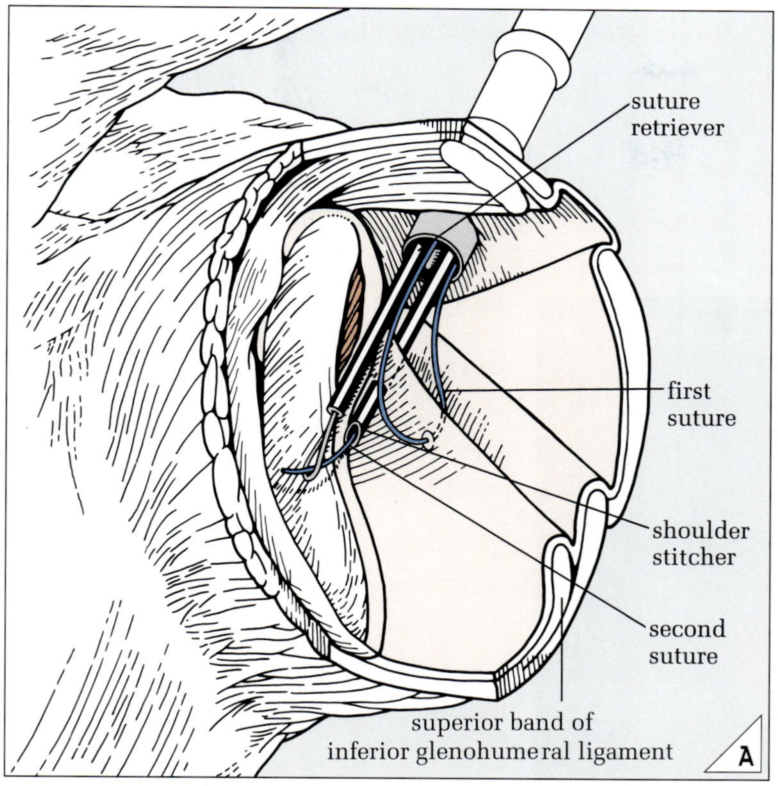

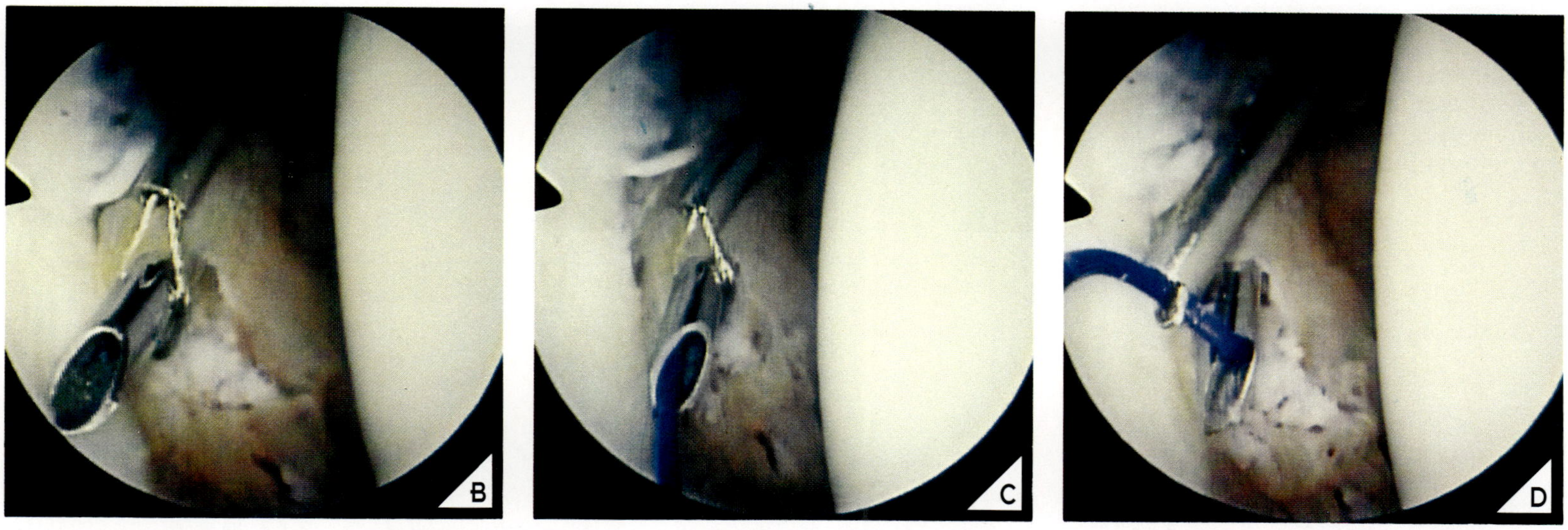

Figure 12.6

Schematic illustration (A) and arthroscopic views (B–D) of a shoulder stitcher passing the suture through the superior band of the inferior glenohumeral ligament to be retrieved by a suture snare.

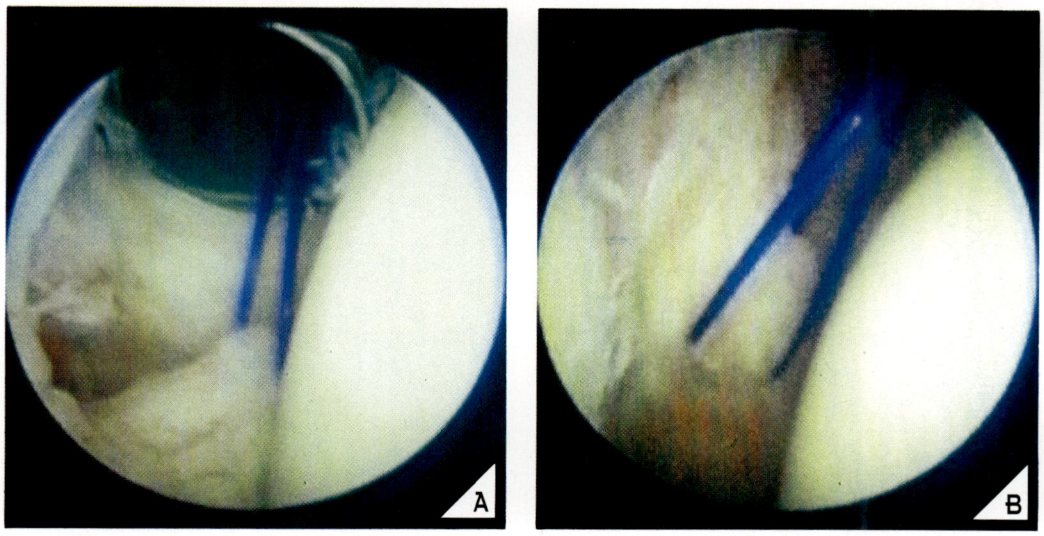

Figure 12.7

Single (A) and then double (B) sutures passed through the superior portion of the glenohumeral ligament.

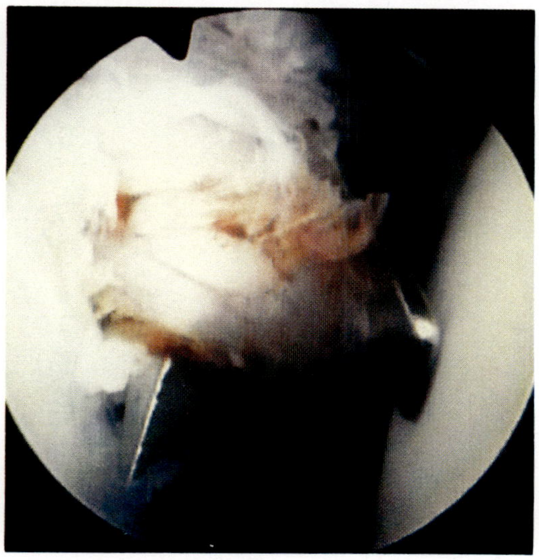

Figure 12.8

The suture pin is passed through the detached glenohumeral ligament–labral complex.

suture pin cannula portion of the shoulder guide system is placed over the suture pin, with its flange on the anterior edge of the glenoid articular surface (Fig. 12.9), to permit accurate placement and to prevent inadvertent medial migration of the suture pin. The tip of the suture pin may be gently tapped into the abraded bone surface of the anterior glenoid neck.

The assembled shoulder guide is used to direct pin exit posteriorly toward a point approximately 4 to 5 cm inferior to the scapular spine and less than 15° medial to the articular surface of the glenoid (Fig. 12.10). The pin is drilled posteriorly through the glenoid neck and out through a small skin incision (Fig. 12.11). The shoulder guide, including the suture pin cannula, is removed. One

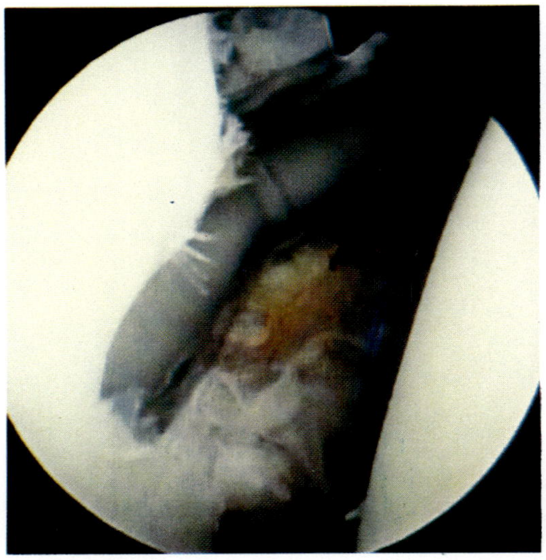

Figure 12.9

Glenohumeral ligament–labral complex is advanced to the anterior edge of the glenoid using the flange of the suture pin cannula for placement.

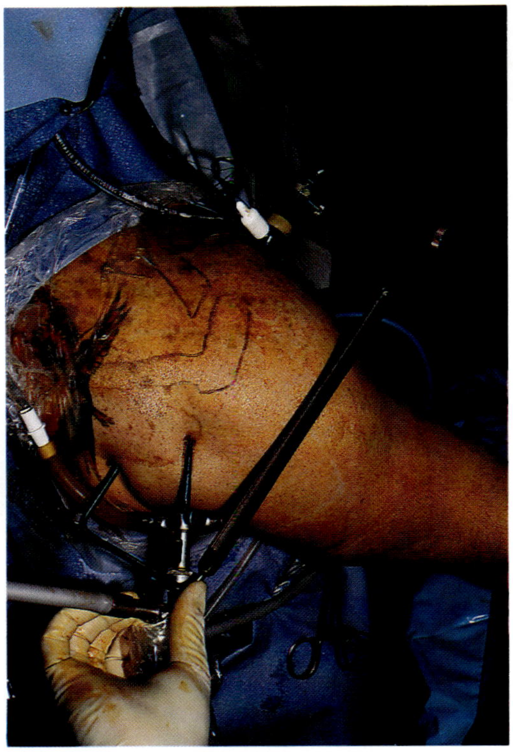

Figure 12.10

The shoulder guide is used to direct the exit of the suture pin posteriorly.

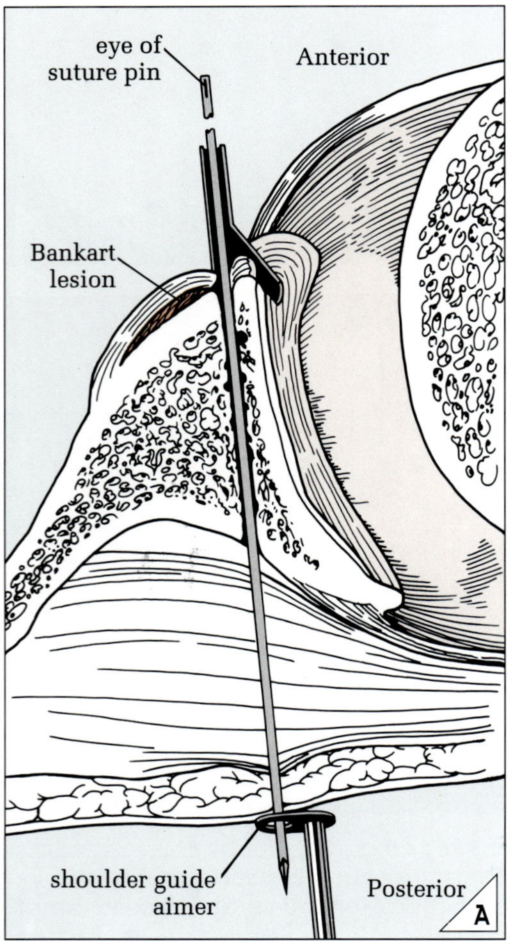

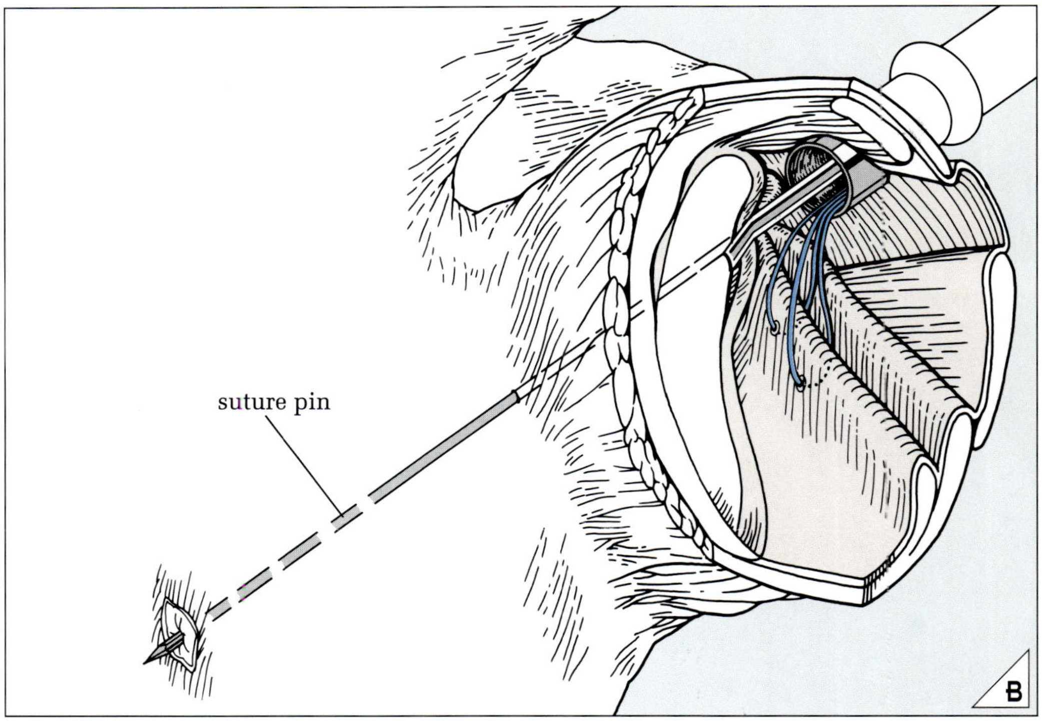

Figure 12.11

(A, B) The suture pin is drilled posteriorly through the glenoid neck and out through a small skin incision.

end of a #1 or #2 braided nonabsorbable suture is placed through the hole in the trailing end of the suture pin, which is advanced with pliers. Using the guide system, a second suture pin is placed in a similar fashion, with its posterior exit directed toward the first pin exit point (Fig. 12.12). Use of the guide system minimizes the risk of damage to the supracapsular nerve by accurately directing the suture pins and minimizing capture of soft tissue between the two pins. Maintaining the first pin within the glenoid neck while the second pin is drilled prevents inadvertent cutting of the sutures by the second pin. Soft tissue is retracted from between the two suture pins posteriorly prior to exit of the second pin through the soft tissue. This allows for later tying of the sutures down to the bone with minimal capture of soft tissue structures posteriorly. The other end of the braided suture is passed through the eye of the second suture pin anteriorly and both pins, together with the ends of the sutures, are brought out posteriorly (Fig. 12.13). The multiple monofilament sutures placed earlier in the inferior glenohumeral ligament are also passed posteriorly via one or both of the suture pins.

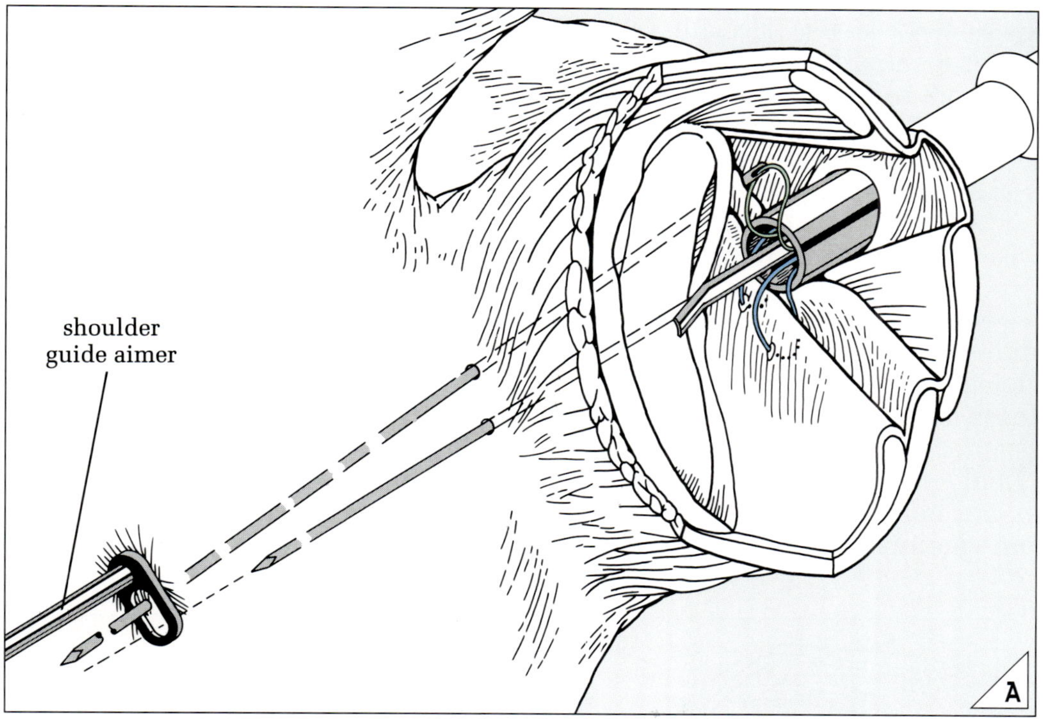

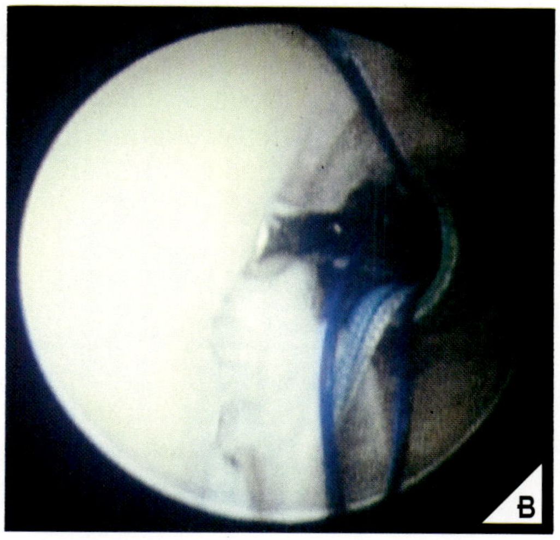

Figure 12.12
(A, B) The second suture pin being drilled through the glenoid neck using the shoulder guide to converge the pins posteriorly.

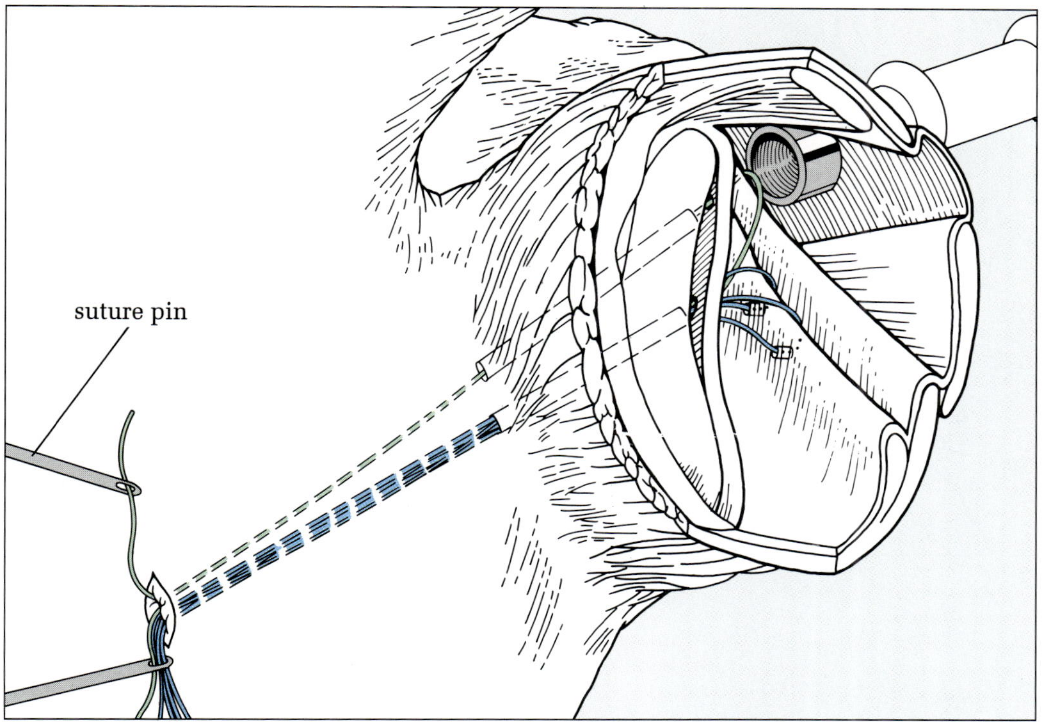

Figure 12.13
Suture pins are brought out posteriorly together with the ends of the sutures.

After traction is removed and the upper extremity internally rotated, tension is placed on the suture ends posteriorly. The sutures are tied to themselves over the posterior cortex of the scapular neck, thus repairing the Bankart lesion and superiorly shifting the inferior glenohumeral ligament (Fig. 12.14).

After the reconstruction is evaluated arthroscopically, all instruments are removed from the shoulder. The shoulder is thoroughly irrigated, all incisions are closed, and a sterile compression dressing is applied.

Postoperative Management

Postoperatively, the patient is maintained in a shoulder immobilizer for 3 to 4 weeks, after which progressive range-of-motion and strengthening exercises are begun. Throwing and overhead sports are restricted for approximately 4 months. Contact sports are allowed at 6 months.

Complications and Pitfalls

Arthroscopic suture stabilization procedures are technically demanding, and not without their potential complications and and pitfalls. Being aware of these can shorten the learning curve.

The use of suture pins may lead to inadvertent pin migration. The newer, less flexible pins are helpful in avoiding this problem, as is the suture pin cannula. The cannula decreases the working length of the pin, while the flange on the cannula prevents medial migration of the pin prior to entry into the bone anteriorly.

The suprascapular nerve is at risk as the suture pins exit the scapular neck posteriorly, although this complication has not been reported. By using a guide to direct pin exit posteriorly towards the "safe zone"[9] the likelihood of damage to the nerve can be significantly decreased, although not eliminated.

Careful dissection through the infraspinatus muscle and tying the sutures down to the bone avoids entrapping the large muscle belly, especially if nonabsorbable sutures are preferred. Absorbable sutures tied over infraspinatus fascia have not been noted to have adverse consequences, however, by those surgeons who have routinely used that technique.[10]

Inappropriately medializing the repaired tissue anteriorly can result in a lack of restoration of the "buttress." The use of a flanged pin cannula avoids this medialization by placing the suture pin entrance, and thus the soft tissue repair, at the rim of the glenoid.

Appropriate restoration of the inferior glenohumeral ligament tension by superior shift is important to the success of the procedure. Lack of proper capsular tension may result in either recurrent instability[11] or restriction of full shoulder motion. Arthroscopic evaluation of this tension requires experience. More of a shift is usually required in the presence of an inferior component to the shoulder luxation, or when the patient has generalized ligamentous laxity (for example, hyperextensible elbows).

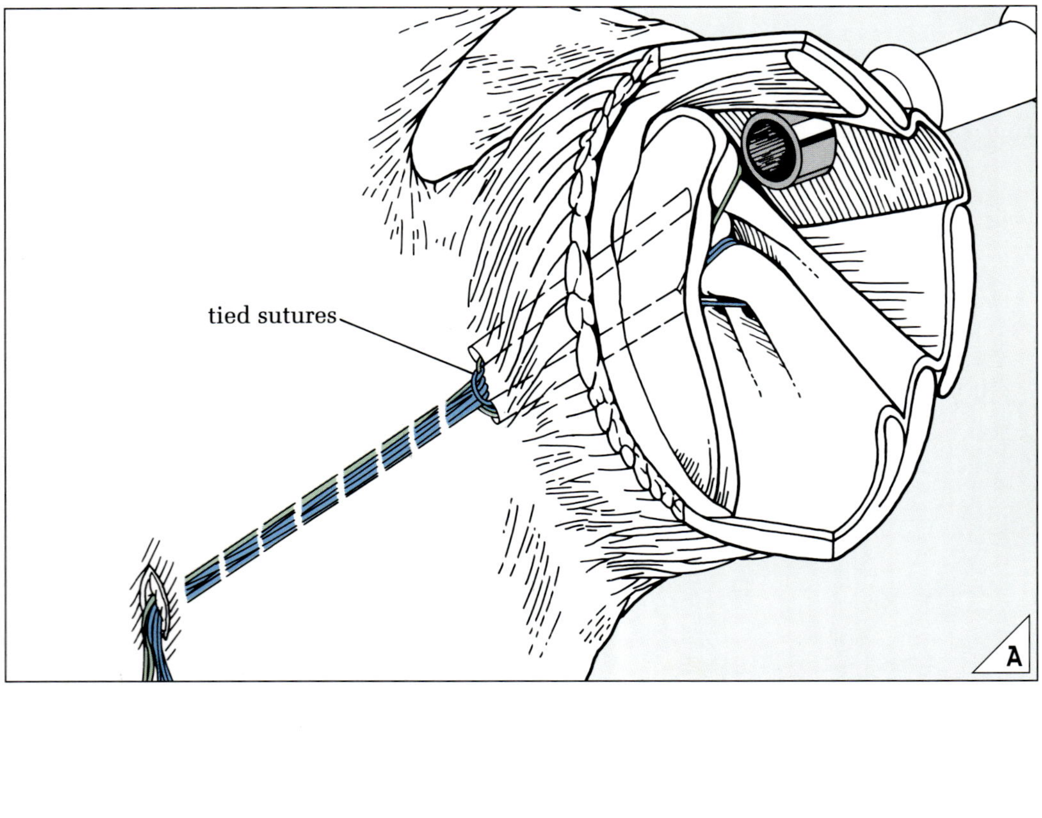

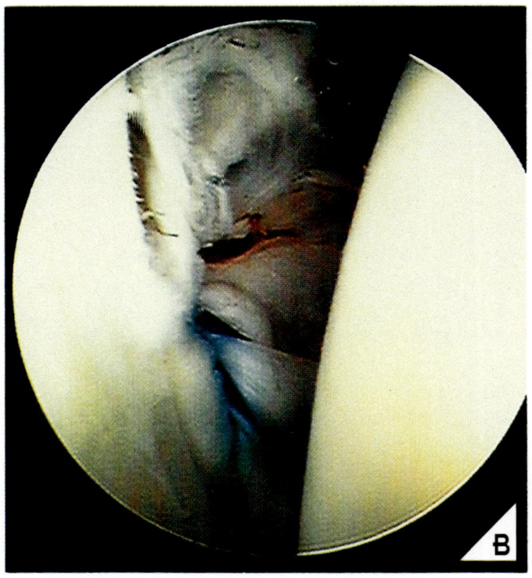

Figure 12.14
(A, B) Completed Bankart lesion repair and superior shift of the inferior glenohumeral ligament.

REFERENCES

1. Johnson LL. The shoulder joint: an arthroscopic perspective of anatomy and pathology. *Clin Orthop.* 1987;223:113–125.
2. McGlynn FJ, Caspari RB. Arthroscopic findings in the subluxating shoulder. *Clin Orthop.* 1984;183:173–178.
3. Ellman H. Shoulder arthroscopy: current indications and techniques. *Orthopaedics.* 1988;2:45–51.
4. Small NC. Complications in arthroscopy: the knee and other joints. *Arthroscopy.* 1986;2:253–258.
5. Mathews LS, Vetter WL, Oneida SJ. Arthroscopic staple capsulorrhaphy for recurrent anterior shoulder instability. *Arthroscopy.* 1988;4:106–111.
6. Small MC. Complications in arthroscopic surgery performed by experienced arthroscopists. *Arthroscopy.* 1988;4:215–221.
7. Kareney MF, Wilson FD. Arthroscopic staple capsulorrhaphy for recurrent shoulder instability. Presented at the Fourth Open Meeting of the American Shoulder and Elbow Surgeons; Atlanta, Ga; February, 1988.
8. Johnson LL. *Arthroscopic Surgery: Principles and Practice,* 3rd ed. St. Louis, Mo: CV Mosby Co;1986.
9. Bigliani LU, Dalsey RM, McCann PD, et al. An anatomical study of the suprascapular nerve. *Arthroscopy.* 1990;4: 301–305.
10. Morgan CD. Arthroscopic transglenoid Bankart suture repair. *Operative Tech Orthop.* 1991;1:171–179.
11. Wolin PA. Arthroscopic glenoid suture repair. Presented at the Annual Meeting of the AAOS; New Orleans, La; February, 1990.

chapter Thirteen

Arthroscopic Capsulolabral Repair Using Suture Anchors

Eugene M. Wolf

In an effort to treat recurrent anterior shoulder instability, orthopedic surgeons have devised more than 150 different operations designed to prevent recurrent anterior subluxation or dislocation. Theories regarding the etiology of recurrent anterior instability of the shoulder have evolved considerably over recent years. They initially centered around three concepts: 1) a labral avulsion popularized by Bankart,[1] 2) muscular insufficiencies described by Symeonides,[2] Magnuson and Stack,[3] and dePalma,[4] and 3) bone abnormalities of the glenoid or humeral head.[5,6]

The Bankart lesion has received the most attention and is the most significant of the lesions responsible for anterior instability. The basic open Bankart repair became a standard of care in dealing with cases of recurrent anterior dislocations.

Many studies have documented the functional significance of the anteroinferior capsular labral structures in maintaining stability of the glenohumeral joint throughout ranges of motion.[1,7–10] These studies emphasize the importance of the inferior glenohumeral ligament–labrum complex in providing a stabilizing force, especially with increasing abduction.

OPEN PROCEDURES

The majority of orthopedic surgeons use an open procedure for surgical treatment of the unstable shoulder, with numerous techniques proposed by many surgeons. Studies have shown significant variation in intraoperative pathologic findings and long-term results, depending on the procedure employed. The Bristow-Latarjet, Bankart, Putti-Platt, and Magnuson-Stack procedures have become the most popular methods for treating recurrent anterior instability of the shoulder in the United States. There appears to be a regional preference for each specific approach.

Although there have been several modifications of the Bristow procedure, the recurrence rate in two large series has been between 8.5% and 13%.[11,12] Other problems with this repair are limitations in external rotation, muscle weakness, and the development of severe glenohumeral arthritis.[11] The Putti-Platt procedure has a reported recurrence rate ranging from 0% to 12.5%, and a recent study by Hawkins also reported that glenohumeral osteoarthritis can develop as a late complication in patients treated with this procedure.[13,14] The functional results of the Magnuson-Stack procedure have been less satisfactory, a common complaint being loss of external rotation and therefore limitations in returning to overhead activities.

The standard open Bankart procedure restores stability by suturing the lateral capsular flap created anterior to the glenoid rim. The medial capsular flap and labrum are then tied over the lateral flap but are not reattached directly to the glenoid rim. The procedure has a failure rate of between 2% and 10%, depending on the series reviewed.[15] The standard Bankart repair popularized by Rowe is technically difficult, especially with respect to dissection of the subscapularis tendon and muscle from the capsule and the creation of suture holes in the anterior glenoid rim that are necessary to complete the repair. These holes pass from the scapular neck side of the rim up through the subchondral bone and the articular cartilage of the anterior glenoid. Several approaches have been developed to accomplish this invariably awkward step. Towel clips, curved awls, angled drills, and, more recently, the Midas Rex,[15] have all been used to make these holes. In an attempt to simplify this step of the Bankart repair, a suture anchor (Mitek) was designed to enable the lateral capsular border sutures to be securely fixed to the anterior glenoid edge with minimal difficulty.

The suture anchor consists of a titanium body and a nitenol arc with a memory property that allows insertion through a small drill hole, thereby simplifying the open technique. A stepped drill, drill guide, and an insertion device allow accurate and predictable placement of sutures and anchors. Bench studies performed on cadaver scapulae have compared the pull-out strength of the suture anchor to that of a plain suture placed through a curved suture hole, with satisfying results. With a #2 polyester suture, the suture anchor was found to be slightly weaker than the suture alone (82.5N versus 135N). However, the suture anchor was strong enough to provide a safe margin in reattaching the capsular complex to the anterior glenoid rim.[16] A review of 17 patients with more than 1 year of follow up (out of a total of 32 patients) who had been treated with an open Bankart repair using suture anchors revealed one dislocation, which occurred in a football player 1 year postoperatively during an arm tackle.[17] Recently, a second-generation suture anchor has been developed that employs a double-armed device, with fixation even stronger than the original anchor (Fig. 13.1). Testing of the newer anchor with #2 polyester suture revealed a strength almost comparable to that of the suture alone (90.1N versus 98.4N), confirming the suitability of a suture anchor in securing soft tissue to bone.[18]

ARTHROSCOPIC PROCEDURES

Our ability to diagnose and treat recurrent anterior instability of the shoulder has been advanced by a number of different diagnostic means, including open exploration, arthrography, postarthrogram CT scans, arthroscopy, and, more recently, MRI scans. Current trends in the diagnosis of shoulder pathology lean towards noninvasive techniques such as MRI; however, the arthroscope has emerged as the most effective and accurate means of identifying the intraarticular pathology in the unstable shoulder.

We have a better and more precise understanding of the normal and pathologic anatomy of the glenohumeral ligament–labrum complex. Three specific lesions of this complex can be identified in anterior instability: avulsion of the glenohumeral ligament–labral complex from the glenoid rim; in-substance tears; and avulsion of the complex from the humerus.

Rowe found the avulsion of the glenohumeral ligament–labral complex to be present in 85% of his cases and believed diffuse capsular laxity to be the causative factor in the remaining 15%, but the difficult sharp surgical dissection of the subscapularis tendon and muscle from the capsular complex would render the identification of lesions other than the classic Bankart extremely difficult. Appreciation of these other lesions is important to the design of surgical approaches and, ultimately, in improving long-term results. I reviewed 64 consecutive cases of anterior instability and found 47 patients (73.5%) with glenoid avulsions of the ligament complex, 11 patients (17.2%) with diffuse capsular laxity, and 6 patients (9.3%) with humeral avulsions of the glenohumeral ligament.

As arthroscopic skills have improved, various devices and techniques have been developed in an effort to restore shoulder stability while avoiding the morbidity and the long-term complications of open procedures.

Initial efforts at arthroscopic stabilization involved the use of a staple similar to the device used by du Toit. However, the results were discouraging, with one study reporting a 16% incidence of redislocation or subluxation, and only 67% of patients achieved a good or excellent result in another study.[19,20] The complications of staple capsulorrhaphy have included loosening, migration, breakage, improper positioning, and cutting through the anterior capsule, all of which can lead to pain, recurrent instability, or arthrosis.[21] Other devices have been used, such as cannulated screws with ligament washers[22] and removable metal rivets.[23] More recently, efforts have been directed towards arthroscopic reconstruction of the detached inferior glenohumeral ligament–labrum complex, with several approaches demonstrating the potential to restore the integrity of the capsular/labral structures.

A technique of arthroscopic Bankart suture repair has been successfully employed by Morgan and Bodenstab, with preliminary results showing no recurrent instability and no complications.[24] More recent data in a greatly expanded series have revealed a 5.2% rate of traumatic redislocation, with seven of eight recurrences in collision athletes.[25]

Morgan has used a transglenoid suture technique that requires drilling suture pins through the scapular neck and out the back of the shoulder. The sutures are tied over fascia and muscle where they exit posteriorly. This procedure has been performed only when a clear cut Bankart lesion was arthroscopically identified. The transglenoid techniques risk injury to the suprascapular nerve, and tying the suture over muscle and fascia that is often distended with extravasated fluid is less than reassuring.

We have attempted to restore the anatomic integrity of the inferior glenohumeral ligament–labral complex through an arthroscopic capsulolabral repair using an arthroscopic suture delivery device, the suture hook (Concept Surgical), and a Mitek G II suture anchor. Using an arthroscopic approach with twin anterior portals, we have been able to place suture anchors in the anterior glenoid and suture the inferior ligament–labrum complex back to its normal anatomic position. This technique addresses the issue of labral detachment as well as the often associated capsular laxity. With this arthroscopic technique, we have eliminated the limitations of, objections to, and potential complications of the transglenoid approach using suture pins.

PATIENT SELECTION

A careful preoperative assessment of the patient must be made to clarify the direction and degree of instability. The patient with radiographic evidence of recurrent anterior dislocation or with clinical evidence of recurrent subluxation is ideal for this procedure. An effort to document the direction and degree of instability should be made through the patient's history and physical examination.

SURGICAL TECHNIQUE

Shoulder arthroscopy is carried out with the patient on a beanbag in the lateral decubitus position because this provides optimal exposure for instrument placement while allowing for distraction and internal rotation of the glenohumeral joint. The technique involves modifying previously described patient positioning and portals, to facilitate the insertion of suture anchors.[26] The operating table is positioned to provide 180° of access to the shoulder, placing the anesthesiologist at the level of the patient's abdomen (Figs. 13.2, 13.3). The twin traction set up is

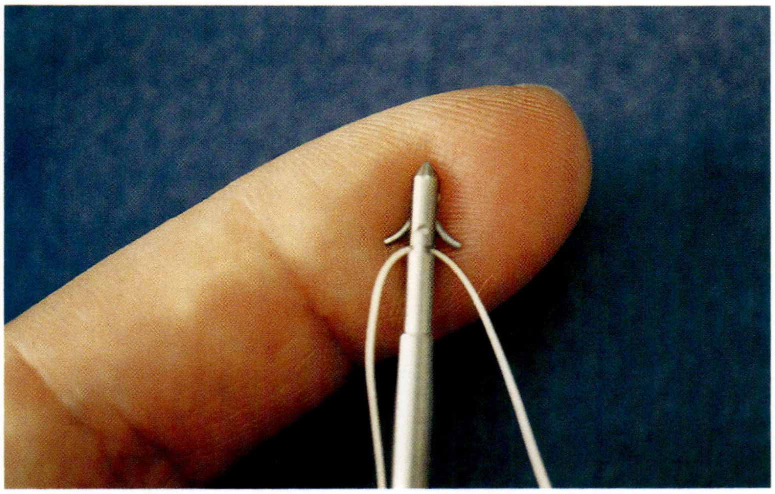

Figure 13.1
The Mitek Generation II anchor.

essential to stabilize and distract the shoulder in a slightly abducted and internally rotated position. The internal rotation helps to relax the anterior capsule and increases the working space anteriorly. During the procedure, the position of the shoulder can be altered as necessary by modification of the weights and the angles of the traction devices. This procedure cannot be performed in the beach chair position.

Examination Under Anesthesia

Once the patient is under anesthesia, intubated, and positioned, the shoulder is examined to assess the direction and degree of instability (Fig. 13.4). The examination must be performed in a systematic fashion. It must be accurate, reproducible, and capable of detecting all types and degrees of instability. Examination under anesthesia is critical because the findings will be used, in conjunction with arthroscopic findings, to decide on the surgical approach. To insure accuracy, the examination must be done bilaterally, in both lateral decubitus positions, with abduction to 90°, axial compression of the humeral head on the glenoid surface, and stabilization of the scapula.

All the above steps of the examination under anesthesia are essential to properly assess shoulder instability. In some respects this examination is similar to Barlow's test in the congenital hip, in which the pelvis is stabilized and the hip dislocated. It is also analogous to the Lachman's test in that to appreciate the anterior translation of the

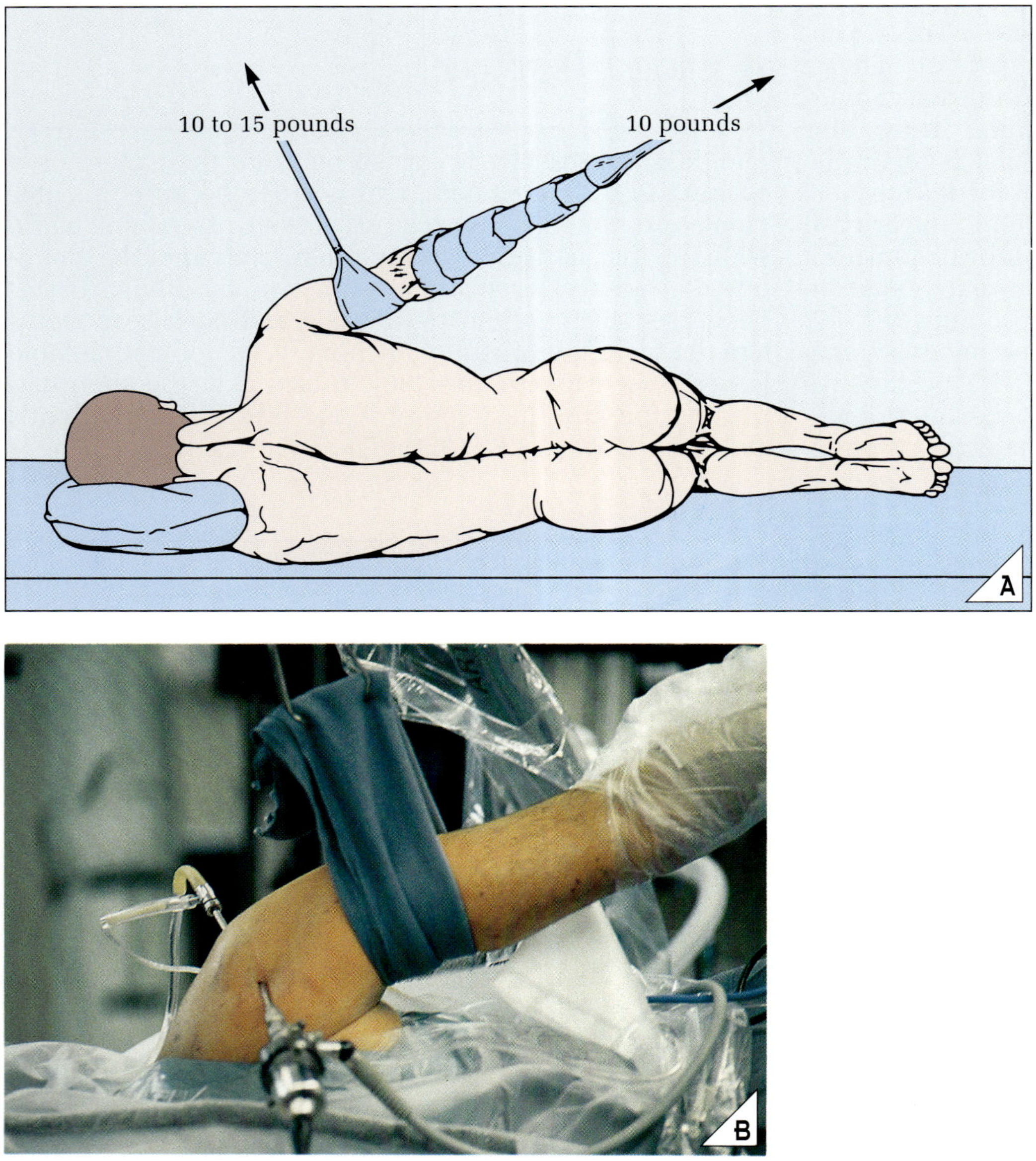

Figure 13.2
Patient set up and positioning with twin traction units, allowing for adjustments during the procedure. After prep and draping, the arm is adducted and the underarm traction sling is applied. Ten to 15 pounds are used for this underarm sling, depending on the size of the patient, and 10 pounds are used distally (A). Operative view (B).

tibia on the femur, the femur must be stabilized when anterior force is applied to the posterior aspect of the tibia. To appreciate the instability or lack thereof in the glenohumeral joint, the scapula must be stabilized and the humerus abducted to 90°. Turkel[8] demonstrated that the main stabilizing structure with respect to anterior instability is the inferior glenohumeral ligament and that this structure functions maximally at 90° of abduction.

With compression of the humeral head on the glenoid, one can clearly appreciate when the convexity of the humeral head goes over and beyond the glenoid rim in any direction. Once this information is obtained, the sur-

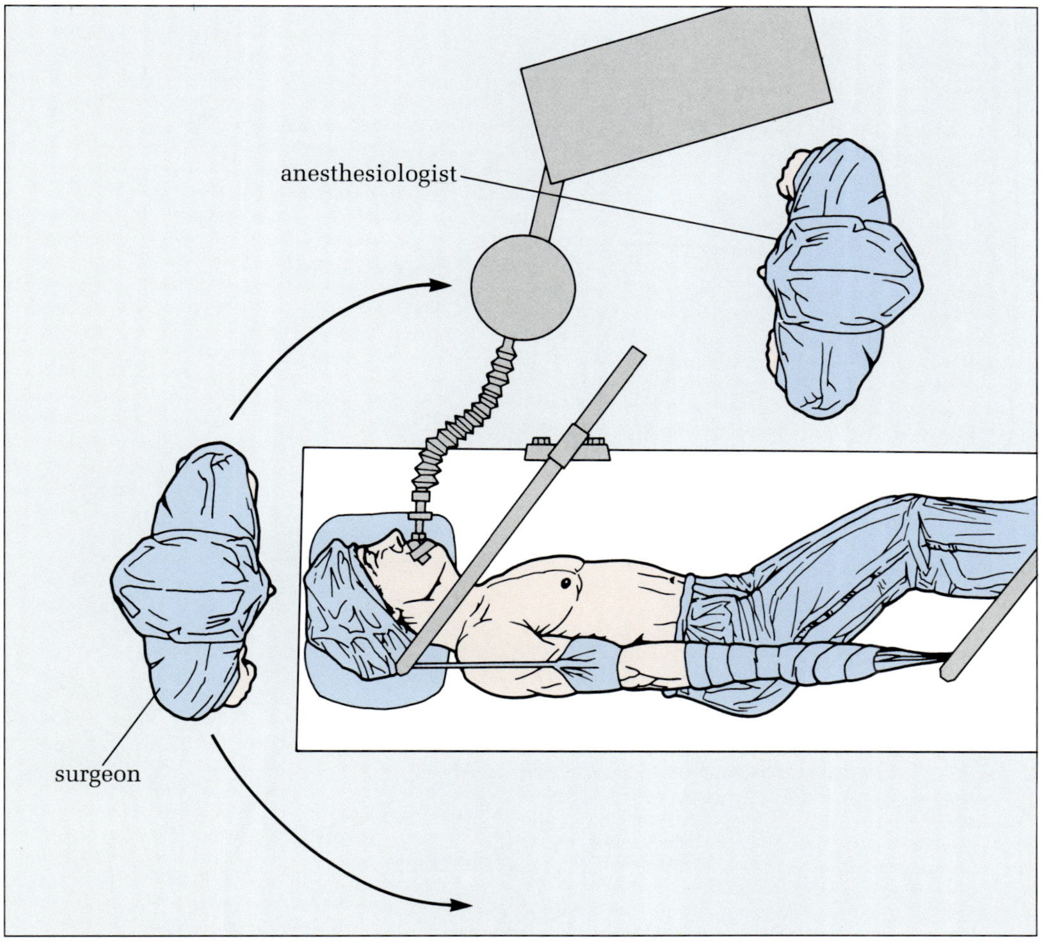

Figure 13.3

The table is rotated 120° so that anesthesia is out of the way. This allows 180° of access to the shoulder.

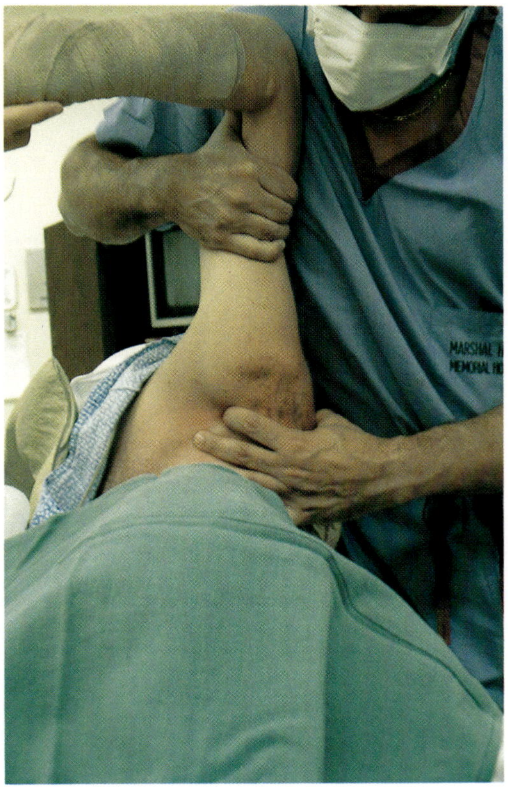

Figure 13.4

The examination under anesthesia must be bilateral, in the lateral decubitus position, with 90° of abduction and external rotation, axial compression of the humeral head on the glenoid, and stabilization of the scapula.

geon should proceed with the arthroscopic examination. The surgical approach is determined by the results of the EUA and the arthroscopic findings. An arthroscopic anterior capsulolabral reconstruction is undertaken only in the presence of anterior instability.

Portals

There are two anterior portals—anterosuperior and anteroinferior—and two posterior portals—posterosuperior and posteroinferior (Fig. 13.5).

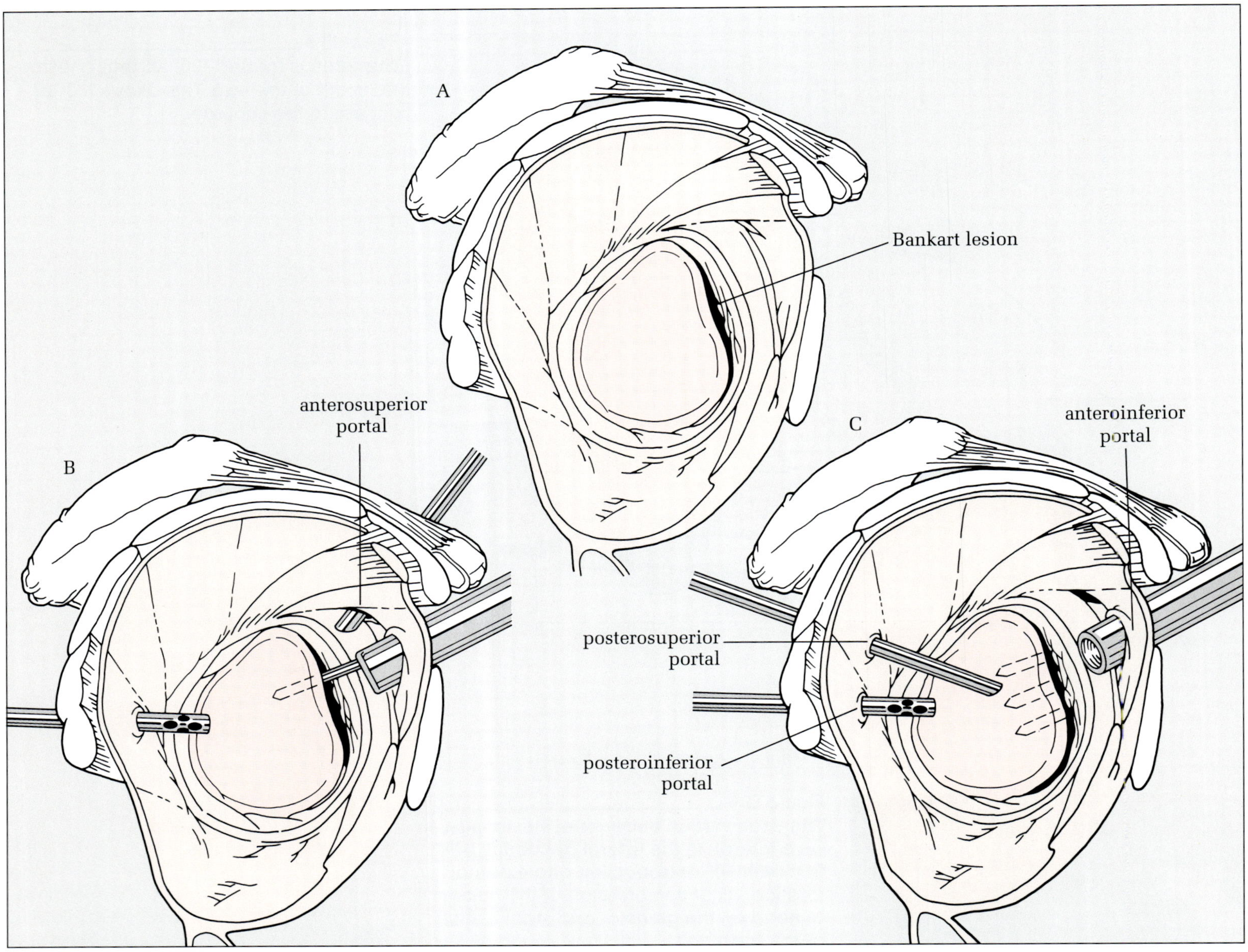

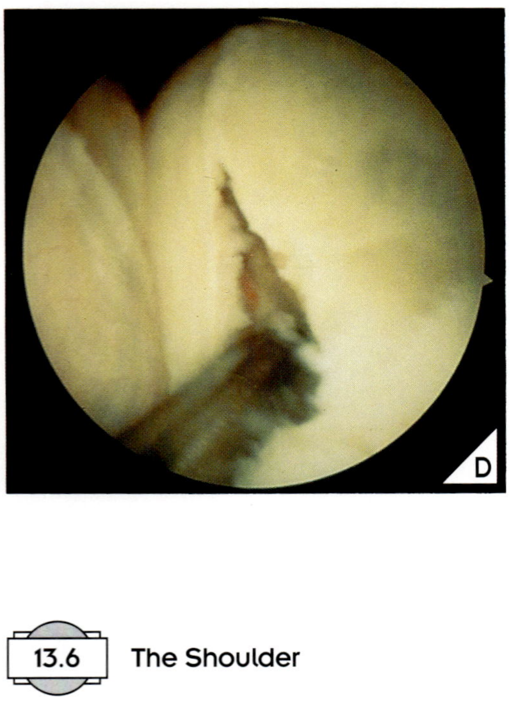

Figure 13.5

(A) The Bankart lesion among otherwise normal intraarticular shoulder anatomy. (B) This working configuration uses two anterior portals. The arthroscope is in the anterosuperior portal and the large Concept cannula is in the anteroinferior portal. A drill bit is making the drill holes in the glenoid rim. The transduction outflow cannula is in the posteroinferior portal. (C) After preparation and drilling of the glenoid rim, it is often advantageous to switch to a 70° scope in a posterosuperior portal. (D) Arthroscopic view from the anterosuperior portal.

After marking the surface landmarks, particularly the posterior lateral edge of the acromion and the coracoid, the posterior superior portal is created at the posterior bone margin of the acromion at the level of the joint line. This joint line is easily palpated with the patient in traction, by rotating the arm while pressure of the thumb allows palpation of the posterior level of the glenohumeral joint. The arthroscope cannula with a blunt obturator is inserted and passed through the deltoid and infraspinatus muscle bellies to palpate the bone contours of the humeral head and the posterior superior rim of the glenoid. One should not fill the joint cavity with saline, which, in fact, might preclude an adequate assessment of the anatomy with the blunt obturator in the arthroscope sheath. There are no sharp trocars on a shoulder arthroscopy set. Once the interval between the humeral head and glenoid is palpated, the blunt trocar is easily popped through the thin posterosuperior capsule and enters the joint. The arthroscopic cannula, with its blunt trocar, is advanced anteriorly to palpate the coracoid, which lies within the safe triangle created by the superior edge of the subscapularis, the inferior border of the biceps tendon, and the anterosuperior edge of the glenoid. Once the coracoid is palpated, the blunt tip is allowed to slip off the inferior edge of the coracoid, is advanced through the capsule and the deltoid, and tents the skin just inferior and lateral to the coracoid tip. A #15 blade is used to open the anteroinferior portal. A cannula is then retrograded back into the joint, where it is held for entry of a shaver, burr, and other instrumentation used during the course of the procedure.

A posteroinferior portal, created 3 cm distal to the posterosuperior portal, is used to place the combination cannula of a 3M arthroscopy pump (3M), which is essential for maintaining distention and flow in the shoulder joint during the procedure.

An anterosuperior portal is then created with an inside-out technique. This is done by palpating the inferior border of the coracoacromial ligament in the rotator cuff interval with the blunt obturator in the scope sheath. When the coracoacromial ligament is located, the sheath and obturator are popped through the rotator cuff interval, and a cannula is retrograded back into the joint. This anterior portal is used to better visualize the intraarticular pathology in the anteroinferior aspect of the shoulder and to directly visualize the abrasion of the glenoid rim and scapular neck.

One must be familiar with the use of switching sticks and frequent changes in instrument and scope configurations. Visualization of the suturing process may be excellent with the scope in the anterosuperior portal, but as sutures are placed from inferior to superior it may be preferable to switch to a 70° scope in the posterosuperior portal to gain better visualization (see Fig. 13.5B, C)

Preparation of the fibroblastic bed by debridement and abrasion of the anterior rim of the glenoid and scapula neck is accomplished with the scope in the anterosuperior portal and the burr in the anteroinferior portal.

In summary, there are two posterior portals—the posterosuperior portal at the posterior border of the acromion at the level of the joint line and the posteroinferior portal at the level of the joint line, 3 cm distal to the posterosuperior portal. There are two anterior portals—the anterosuperior portal, which is used for visualization, and the anteroinferior portal, which allows introduction of the suture and anchor instrumentation.

Arthroscopic Examination

The arthroscopic capsulolabral repair using suture anchors often requires all four portals, which can be created as described above. For surgeons performing this procedure for the first time, even those experienced in arthroscopy, I recommend that the procedure begin with the creation of the commonly used portals familiar to most surgeons—the anterosuperior portal and the posteroinferior portal. As described above, the anterosuperior portal is slightly more anterior and superior than is generally used in shoulder arthroscopy. The posteroinferior portal is 3 cm from the inferior border of the acromion. Therefore, it is slightly more distal than the "soft spot" most commonly used. The surgeon enters the joint with the arthroscope via the posteroinferior portal, distends the joint, and visualizes the area of the anterosuperior portal, with the spinal needle coming in the region of the most superior part of the rotator cuff interval. This allows establishment of flow and arthroscopic evaluation of the joint to begin. This procedure, performed with the standard 30° scope from the posteroinferior portal, usually allows identification of a classic Bankart lesion. A 70° scope further facilitates the inspection from the posterior portal. The surgeon can visualize from the posterior portal and use the anterior cannula to probe the ligament–labrum complex.

The arthroscopic examination is not complete until the structures are visualized from the anterosuperior portal. A 30° scope is used for this purpose. With switching sticks, the outflow cannula is placed in the posteroinferior portal and the arthroscope in the anterosuperior portal. This permits the best possible evaluation of the anteroinferior structures.

If the patient has already had an examination that clearly demonstrated anteroinferior instability and significant pathology of the glenohumeral ligament–labrum complex has been noted arthroscopically, the anteroinferior portal can be created.

It is critical to maintain these portals at all times with a cannula in place. Threaded cannulas that are screwed into the soft tissues over a switching stick are key elements in preventing portal loss and soft tissue extravasation. Extravasation will be minimized if this is done carefully, and the portals are always maintained with cannulas within them. This careful technique, plus use of a pump to control intraarticular pressure and distention while maintaining flow, will minimize extravasation and will result in remarkably little soft tissue distention when the procedures are completed.

Anteroinferior Portal

The key to obtaining access to the anteroinferior aspect of the glenoid, where the pathology usually exists in recurrent anterior dislocations or subluxation, is the anteroinferior portal. The anteroinferior portal is created with the blunt obturator in the arthroscope sheath. After entering the joint through the posteroinferior portal, the tip of the coracoid should be identified by palpation with the blunt obturator. The sheathed obturator is advanced until it slips off the inferior border of the coracoid tip and is pushed out through the capsule at the angle created by the lateral border of the conjoined tendon and the superior border of the subscapularis tendon. An incision in this area must be made very carefully because of the proximity of the cephalic vein. It is important to retrograde a cannula of choice back into the joint over the tip of the scope sheath and obturator, insuring that both tips are within the joint before allowing contact of the cannula and release of the obturator.

Preparation of the Anterior Glenoid Rim and Scapular Neck

After the portals have been created, the surgeon should prepare the anterior glenoid rim and scapular neck for the creation of the fibroblastic bed and the drill holes. The arthroscope is positioned in the anterosuperior portal to best visualize the anterior glenoid rim and scapula neck. The detached labrum is visualized, and an aggressive full-radius resector is used in the anteroinferior portal with minimal suction to clear the field. Viable tissues of the inferior glenohumeral ligament–labrum complex needed for repair should not be suctioned into the full-radius resector. An aggressive full-radius resector allows excellent dissection along the scapula neck and glenoid rim to prepare the Bankart lesion (see Fig. 13.5D). This allows advancement and retensioning of the ligament–labrum complex. Once the soft tissue has been removed from the scapula neck, a motorized burr decorticates the glenoid rim and scapula neck to bleeding bone.

Creating Drill Holes

At this point, it is necessary to switch cannulas in the anteroinferior portal and to place an 8.5 mm threaded arthroscopic cannula that can accommodate the drill guide, the drill bits, suture hook, and anchors.

Once the threaded cannula is inserted, the Mitek drill guide and drill are inserted. Three widely spaced drill holes are made along the anterior glenoid rim. One drill hole is created as inferiorly as possible on the glenoid rim and another as far superiorly as possible within the lesion on the glenoid rim. The third hole is created between the two previously drilled holes.

It is important to check the direction of the drill bit and drill guide. The bit must be angled at approximately 15° to 20° to the plane of the glenoid surface—going under the glenoid surface. It is critical that the holes are made at the anterior-most border of the cartilaginous surface and not medial on the scapular neck. This enables the inferior glenohumeral ligament–labrum complex to be brought up onto the glenoid rim, recreating a labral buttress anteriorly and increasing the depth of the glenoid.

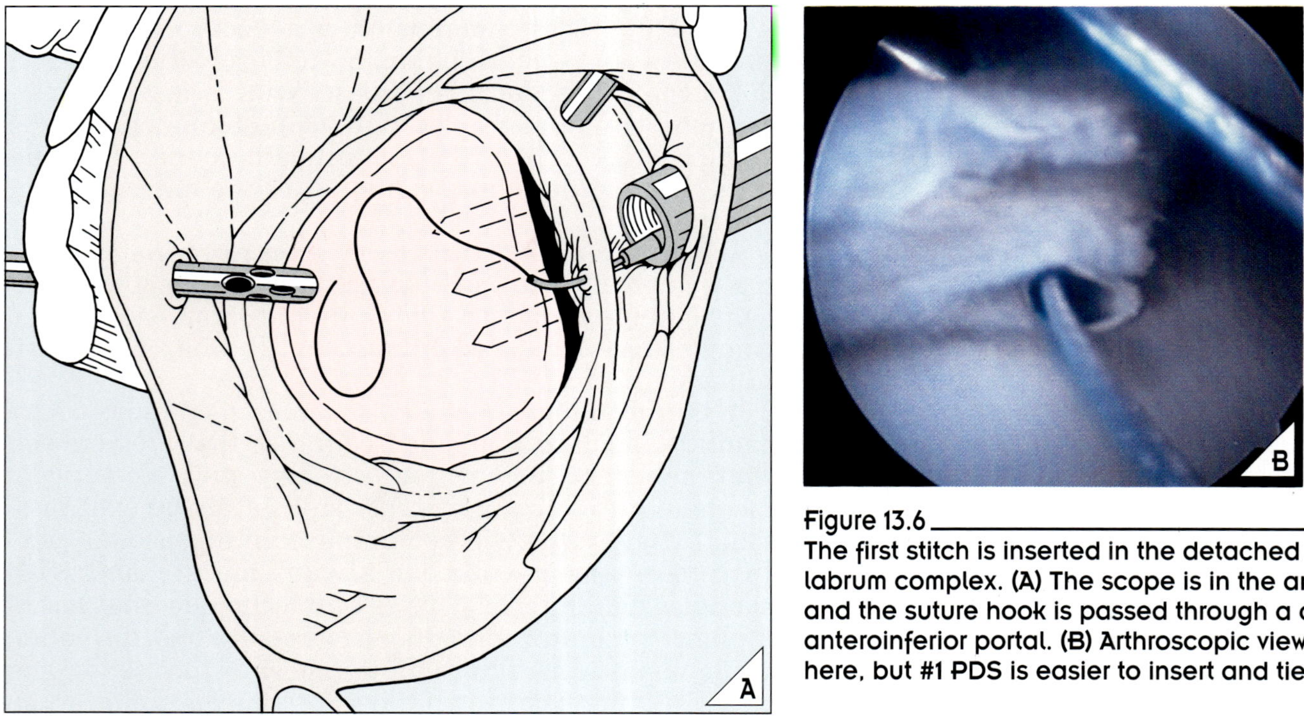

Figure 13.6

The first stitch is inserted in the detached inferior ligament–labrum complex. (A) The scope is in the anterosuperior portal and the suture hook is passed through a cannula in the anteroinferior portal. (B) Arthroscopic view. #0 Tycron is pictured here, but #1 PDS is easier to insert and tie.

Insertion of the Suture and Anchors

Still viewing through the anterosuperior portal with the 8.5 mm cannula in the anteroinferior portal, a suture hook is placed through the most inferior portion of the detached glenohumeral ligament–labrum complex (Fig. 13.6). In cases where there is a very cleanly detached ligament–labrum complex, it is sufficient to have the scope in the anterosuperior portal and the cannula in the anteroinferior portal. There are occasions when the ligament–labrum complex has healed to the scapular neck a medial and inferior position. An arthroscope periosteal elevator is an essential tool in this situation. Vigorous dissection along the scapular neck with the elevator in the anteroinferior portal will often bring up a surprisingly intact labrum and attached ligaments that can be restored to the glenoid rim. An appropriate suture hook is passed through the ligament–labrum complex once it is mobilized.

The suture hook will feed a #1 PDS suture into the joint a sufficient distance so that the hook can be withdrawn, leaving the suture through the detached ligament–labrum complex. A suture grasper is then inserted to pull out the "inside limb" of the inserted suture and create a loop going down through the cannula, through the ligament, and back out the cannula.

An anchor is secured to the inserter and fixed with a stitch of #0 Dexon tied over the handle of the inserter. This prevents loss of the anchor within the joint. The mounted suture anchor is slid down the "inside limb" of the suture—the end of the suture that came through the avulsed surface to be applied to the glenoid rim. It passes down through the cannula and slides over the suture to enter the first drill hole (Figs. 13.7A, B).

The anchor is then inserted into the first drill hole and the security suture, used to maintain the anchor secure on the inserter, is cut. The inserter is withdrawn, thus leaving a loop of suture going down through the cannula, through the detached ligament–labrum complex, into the drill hole, through the base of the anchor, back out the drill hole, and out the cannula (Fig. 13.7C).

The Generation 2 Mitek anchor allows the suture to slide within the anchor and within its drill hole. The loop is closed, using a slip knot that is tied outside of the cannula, tightened outside the cannula, and slid down the

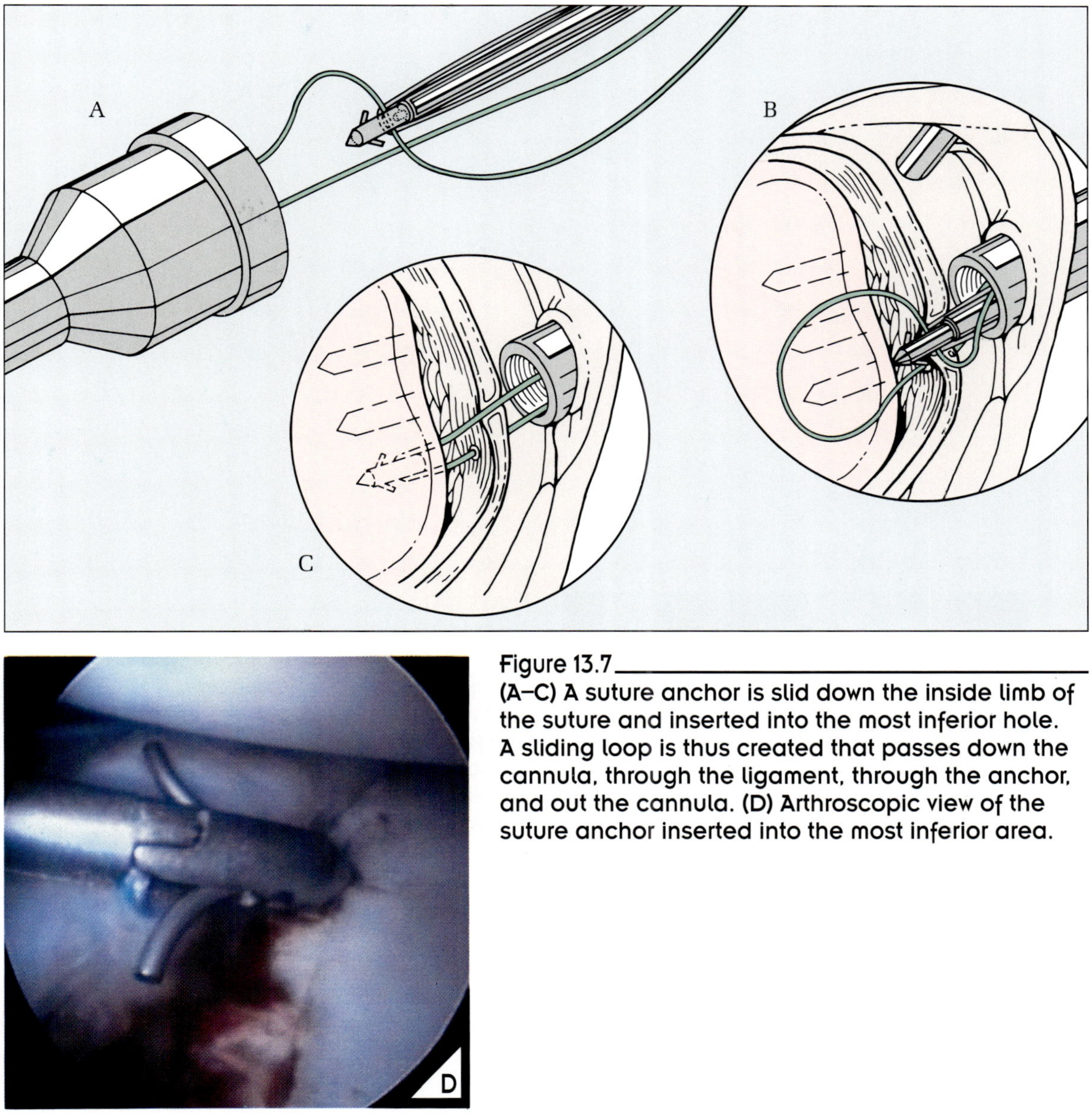

Figure 13.7
(A–C) A suture anchor is slid down the inside limb of the suture and inserted into the most inferior hole. A sliding loop is thus created that passes down the cannula, through the ligament, through the anchor, and out the cannula. (D) Arthroscopic view of the suture anchor inserted into the most inferior area.

cannula, tightening the loop and approximating the ligament–labrum complex (Fig. 13.8).

In general, three anchors and sutures are inserted, but two may be sufficient in some cases. The more proximal anchor and suture can be inserted with the scope in a posterior portal. This avoids crowding in the anterior aspect of the joint and, with a 70° scope, permits visualization of the drill holes and allows the insertion of suture and anchor.

Before the wound is closed, the shoulder is injected with 20 mL of 0.25% bupivacaine with epinephrine. Once the repair is complete (Fig. 13.9), all arthroscopic equipment is withdrawn and the portals are closed with simple nylon sutures. A compressive dressing and immobilizer are applied.

Postoperative Management

The immobilizer is worn continuously, except during bathing and pendulum and pulley exercises, for 3 weeks, then only at night for 3 additional weeks. Patients are advised that after 24 hours the dressing may be replaced by Band-Aids. The sutures are removed in 5 days.

At 6 weeks the patients are advanced to an aggressive phase of therapy, with a full range of active and resistive motion exercises. A home therapy program suffices in the majority of cases. Rarely does a patient require a formal physical therapy program. Only the most apprehensive and pain-intolerant patients have difficulty regaining motion, and most have full motion at 12 weeks.

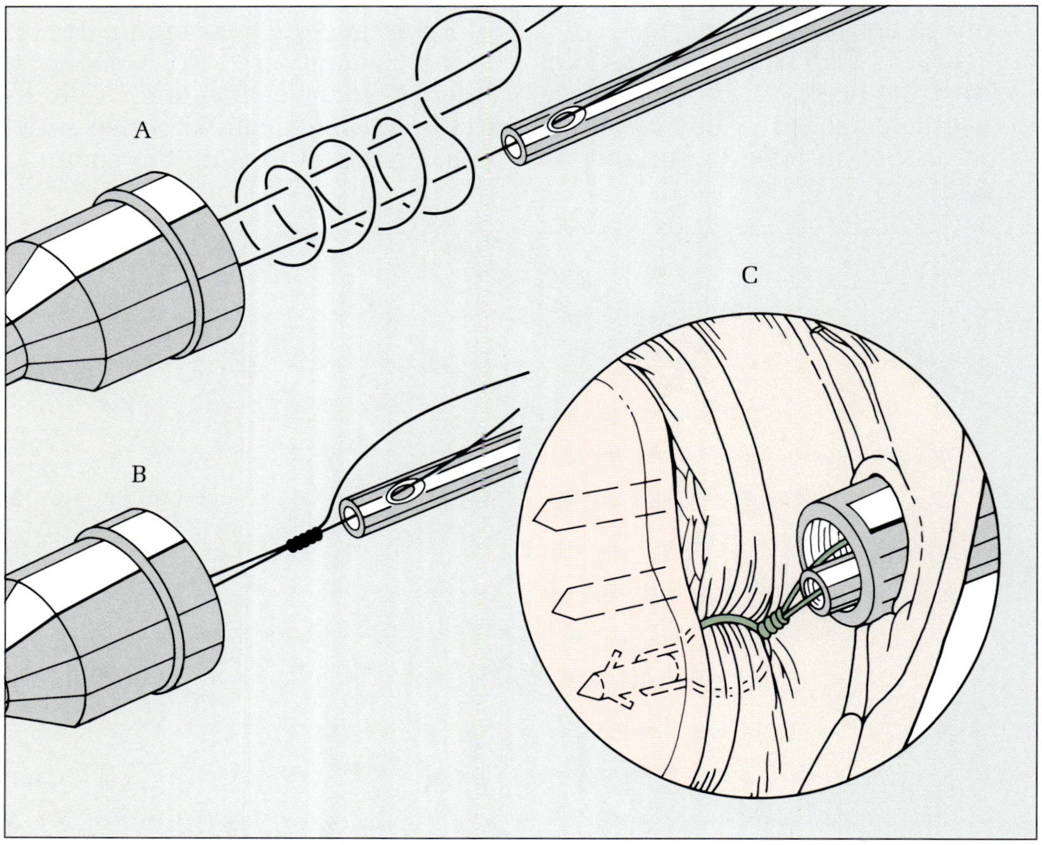

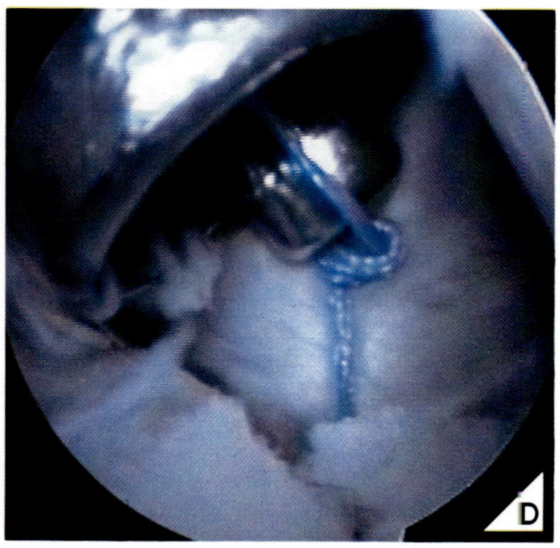

Figure 13.8

A common fishing knot (A) is made and slid down the cannula with a knot pusher (B), thereby tightening a noose created around the ligament–labrum complex and reapproximating it to the glenoid (C). (D) Arthroscopic view showing the noose being tightened. #0 Tycron is shown here but #1 PDS is recommended.

RESULTS

This procedure has been performed in more than 40 patients since September 1989. There have been no complications and only two recurrences in 44 patients followed 1 to 3 years. The follow up is short and the results will have to be assessed in several years. However, this arthroscopic capsulolabral repair does restore the inferior glenohumeral ligament–labrum complex as anatomically as possible, without either the morbidity of an arthrotomy or the major modifications of joint mechanics inherent in most open procedures.

This technique also allows for a degree of capsular plication when there is capsular laxity. The suture hook can pass not only through the labrum but also through a selected amount of capsule beyond the labrum. With capsular plication, as well as with labral advancement, patients experience an immediate sensation of stability as soon as they begin their rehabilitation.

CONCLUSION

As with many arthroscopic techniques and shoulder surgery, this procedure is extremely demanding and should be performed only by surgeons who possess superior arthroscopic skills. Even the most skilled surgeons will encounter a difficult learning curve.

The technique described here continues to evolve but the basic principles remain the same.

As orthopedic surgeons, we have the benefit (or the curse) of many methods with which we can treat the multitude of problems that may need to be addressed in caring for a patient with a disorder of the musculoskeletal system. Throughout modern times, surgeons have attempted to develop techniques that offer the highest chance of success with the lowest possibility of complication or failure. Our experience in treating shoulder pathology has been aided by the advent of arthroscopic techniques, which allow better visualization of the anatomic structures associated with the various problems that involve the shoulder. At the same time, we have refined our skills and have devised new instruments and techniques that permit surgical repair of injured shoulder tissues. As with most areas of orthopedic surgery, the physician must have a broad knowledge base for proper decision making when the care of an orthopedic problem is planned. Here we have presented a different arthroscopic approach to the diagnosis and treatment of anterior shoulder instability. These techniques are in various stages of development, and the ultimate success of any technique will have to stand the test of time.

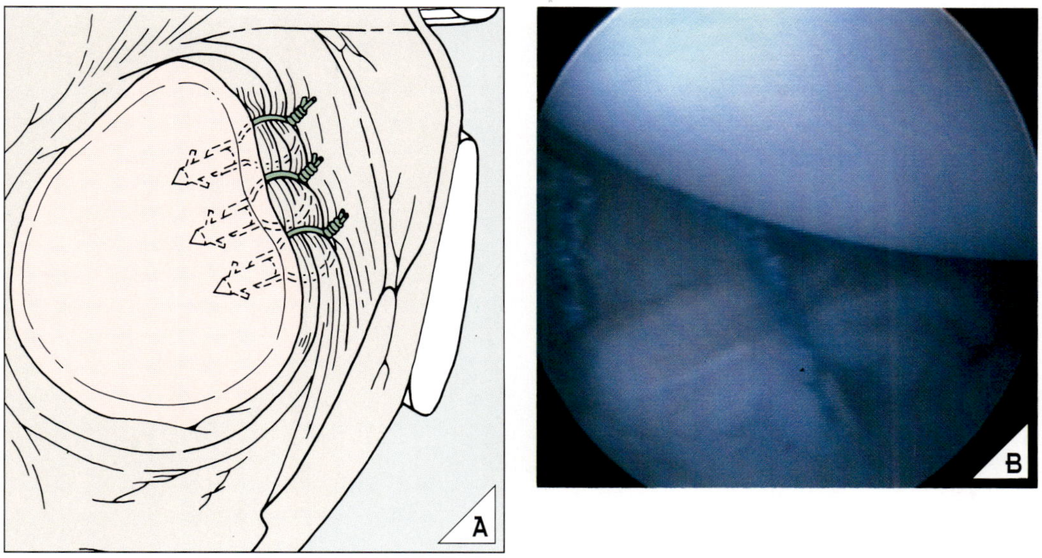

Figure 13.9
The completed procedure with three anchors and sutures in place (A). The buttress of the labrum has been reconstituted, and the inferior glenohumeral ligament–labrum complex retensioned. (B) Arthroscopic view.

REFERENCES

1. Bankart ASB. The pathology and treatment of recurrent dislocation of the shoulder joint. *Br J Surg.* 1939;26:23–29.
2. Symeonides PP. The significance of the subscapularis muscle in the pathogenesis of recurrent anterior dislocation of the shoulder. *J Bone Joint Surg.* 1972;54B:476–483.
3. Magnuson PB, Stack JK. Recurrent dislocation of the shoulder. *JAMA.* 1943;123:889–892.
4. DePalma AF, Cooke AJ, Prabhakar M. The role of the subscapularis in recurrent anterior dislocations of the shoulder. *Clin Orthop.* 1967;54:35–49.
5. Eden-Hybbinette R. Technique of Palmer and Widen. In: Crenshaw AH, ed. *Campbell's Operative Orthopaedics.* 1st ed. St. Louis, Mo: CV Mosby Co; 1;1971.
6. May VR. A modified Bristow operation for anterior recurrent dislocation of the shoulder. *J Bone Joint Surg.* 1970;52A: 1010–1016.

7. Moseley HF, Overgaard B. The anterior capsular mechanism in recurrent anterior dislocation of the shoulder: morphological and clinical studies with special reference to the glenoid labrum and the glenohumeral ligaments. *J Bone Joint Surg.* 1962;44B:913–927.
8. Turkel SJ, Panie MW, Marshall JL, Girgis RJ. Stabilizing mechanisms preventing anterior dislocation of the glenohumeral joint. *J Bone Joint Surg.* 1981;63A:1208–1217.
9. Galinat BJ, Howell SM. The containment mechanism: the primary stabilizer of the glenohumeral joint. Presented at the 54th AAOS meeting; San Francisco, Calif; January, 1987.
10. O'Brien SJ, Neves MC, Arnoczky SP, et al. The anatomy and histology of the inferior glenohumeral ligament complex of the shoulder. *Am J Sports Med.* 1990;18:449–456.
11. Torg JS, Balduini FC, Bonci C, et al. A modified Bristow-Helfet-May procedure for recurrent dislocations and subluxations of the shoulder: report of 212 cases. *J Bone Joint Surg* 1987;69A:904–913.
12. Hovelius L, Akermark C, Albrektsson B, et al. Bristow-Latarjet procedure for recurrent anterior dislocation of the shoulder. *Acta Orthop Scand.* 1983;54:284–290.
13. Hovelius L, Thorling J, Fredin H. Recurrent anterior dislocation of the shoulder: results after the Bankart and Putti-Platt operations. *J Bone Joint Surg.* 1979;61A:556–569.
14. Hawkins RJ, Angelo RL. Glenohumeral osteoarthrosis. *J Bone Joint Surg.* 1990;72A:1193–1197.
15. Rowe CR, Patel D, Southmayd WW. The Bankart procedure: a long term end-result study. *J Bone Joint Surg.* 1978;60A:1–16.
16. France EP. Technical report. Fixation strength evaluation of Mitek suture anchors: applications in the shoulder; October 1989.
17. Richmond JC, Fu FH. Presented at the AOSSM Meeting; Sun Valley, Id; July, 1990.
18. France EP. Fixation strength of double armed Mitek torpedo suture anchors: application in the shoulder. June, 1990.
19. Hawkins RB. Arthroscopic stapling repair for shoulder instability: a retrospective study of 50 cases. *Arthroscopy.* 1989;5:122–128.
20. Gross RM. Arthroscopic shoulder capsulorraphy: does it work? *Am J Sports Med.* 1989;17:495–500.
21. Zuckerman JD, Matsen FA. Complications about the glenohumeral joint related to the use of screws and staples. *J Bone Joint Surg.* 1984;66A:175–180.
22. Wolf EM. Arthroscopic anterior shoulder capsulorrhaphy. *Tech Orthop.* 1988;3:67–73.
23. Wiley AM. Arthroscopy for shoulder instability and a technique for arthroscopic repair. *Arthroscopy.* 1988;4:25–30.
24. Morgan CD, Bodenstab AB. Arthroscopic Bankart suture repair: technique and early results. *Arthroscopy.* 1987; 3:111–122.
25. Morgan CD. Presented at the Ninth Annual ANAA meeting; Orlando, Fla; April, 1990.
26. Wolf EM. Anterior portals in shoulder arthroscopy. *Arthroscopy.* 1989;5:201–208.

chapter Fourteen

Stapling: Arthroscopic Technique for Anterior Shoulder Instability

Stuart I. Springer

The basic premise of arthroscopic shoulder staple capsulorrhaphy is to reattach detached glenohumeral ligaments to the anterior glenoid with an arthroscopic staple. In order to perform this procedure successfully, an understanding of the anatomic and functional relationships between the glenoid labrum, the anterior capsule, and the inferior glenohumeral ligament is essential.[1–6] The inferior glenohumeral ligament is the primary anterior stabilizing structure of the glenohumeral joint, and the anterior labrum is the attachment area for the inferior glenohumeral ligament. So, a complete detachment of the anteroinferior labrum from the glenoid, also called a Bankart lesion, causes a loss of integrity of the inferior glenohumeral ligament –labrum complex and can result in instability. During the moment of dislocation, a compression-type injury to the articular cartilage of the posterior humeral head (Hill-Sachs lesion) may also occur.

The ligament and capsule repair system made by Instrument Makar has been available since 1982. The system was designed for acute repair and chronic reconstructions of a torn anterior cruciate ligament and for stabilization of anterior dislocation of the shoulder. As with any refinement of existing techniques, a learning curve is anticipated, and early complications can be expected. The stapling technique for anterior shoulder instability is technically demanding. However, attention to details and knowledge of anatomy enhances success of the procedure.

INSTRUMENTATION

The following instruments are used to perform arthroscopic shoulder stable capsulorrhaphy:

- Staple driver/extractor with staples of various sizes (Fig. 14.1)
- Wissinger rod and switching stick (Fig. 14.2)
- Motorized shaver and burr
- Hand instruments (grasping forceps, knives)

SURGICAL TECHNIQUE

Incision and Entry

The patient is placed in the lateral decubitus position. The shoulder is held in place by a pulley system with only 6 to 8 pounds of weight. The arm is monitored by somatosensory evoked potentials (Fig. 14.3).

To locate the incision area in the glenohumeral region, the posterior sulcus is palpated with the thumb. The area is located approximately one finger breadth inferior to the posterior margin of the acromion. By rotating the arm, the glenohumeral articulation can be located in most patients (Fig. 14.4). A deep incision is made with a #11 blade (Fig. 14.5).

The cannula and trocar of the arthroscope are passed into the glenohumeral joint anteriorly (Figs. 14.6, 14.7). The opposite long finger is kept on the coracoid process for appropriate direction. Once inserted, one may feel a slight "give" as both the cannula and trocar penetrate the capsule. The arthroscopic cannula should feel firmly surrounded by tissue, unlike when placing the cannula in the subacromial space. Entry into the shoulder joint can be confirmed by placing the arthroscope in the cannula (Figs. 14.8, 14.9).

The superior supraspinatus muscle approach is located between the acromion and clavicle. The bones meet in an inverted "V" and palpation of approximately one and a half finger breadths below its apex is the point of entry

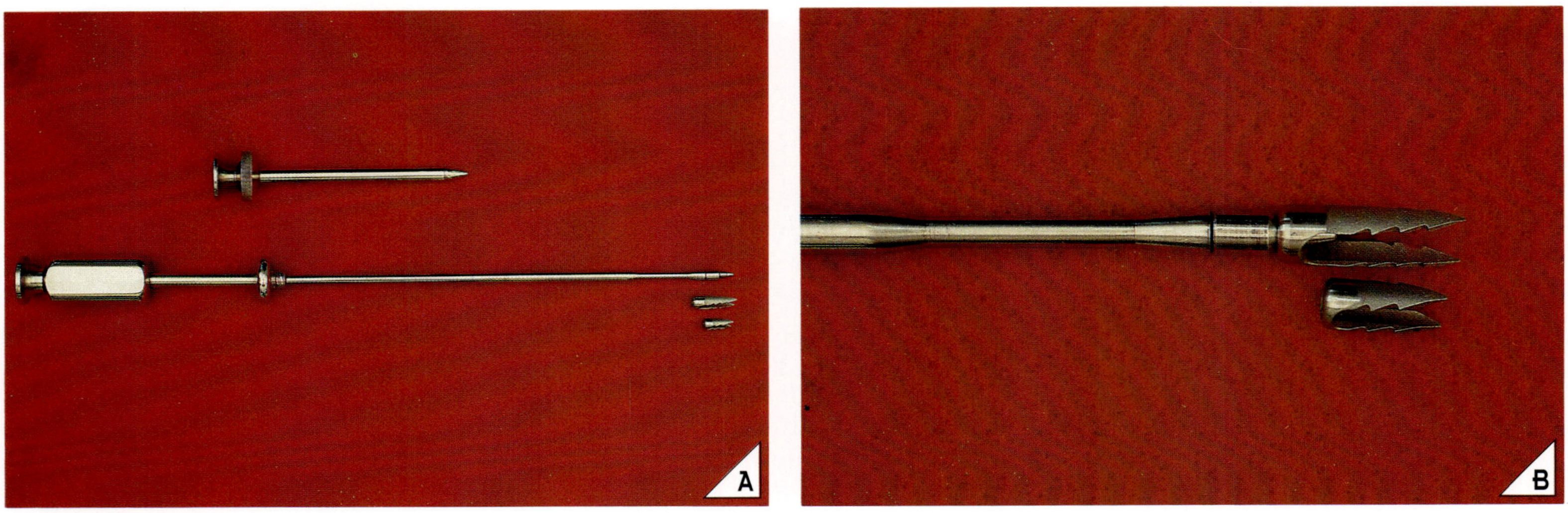

Figure 14.1
The Instrument Makar system. (A) From top to bottom: cannula and trocar, driver/extractor with staples. (B) Close-up of driver/extractor with staples.

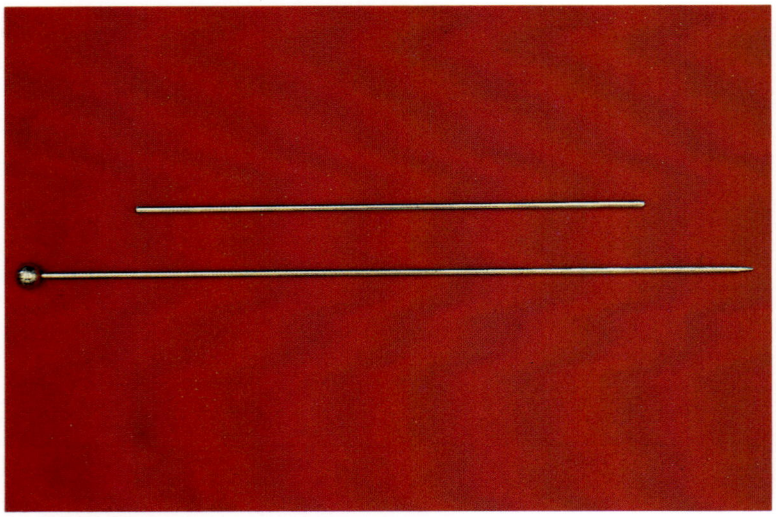

Figure 14.2
The Wissinger rod and switching stick.

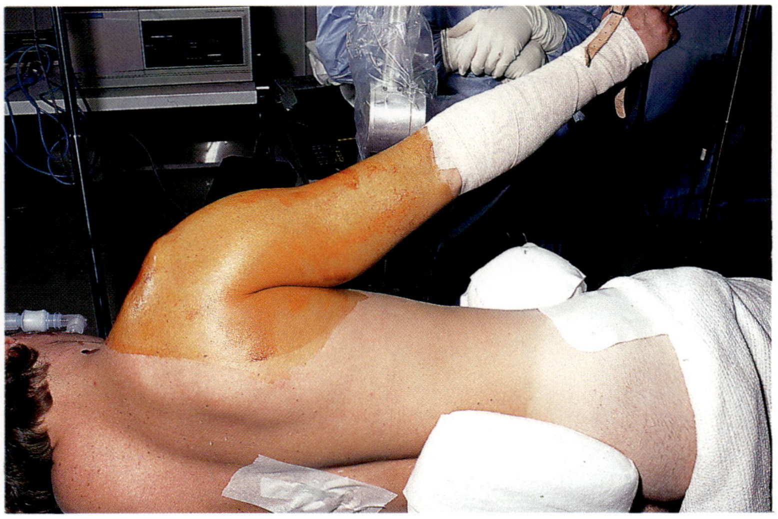

Figure 14.3
The patient is in the lateral decubitus position. A pulley system, using 6 to 8 pound weights, is used to hold the shoulder in place.

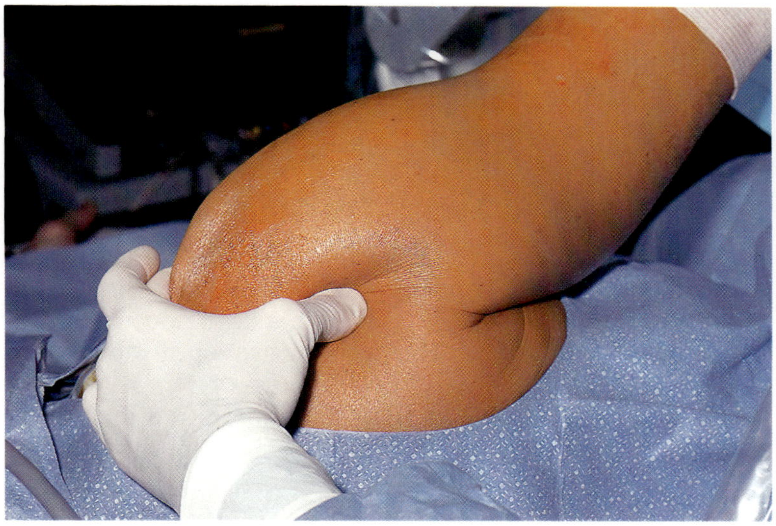

Figure 14.4

The posterior sulcus, which when palpated with the thumb, is located about one finger breadth inferior to the posterior margin of the acromion.

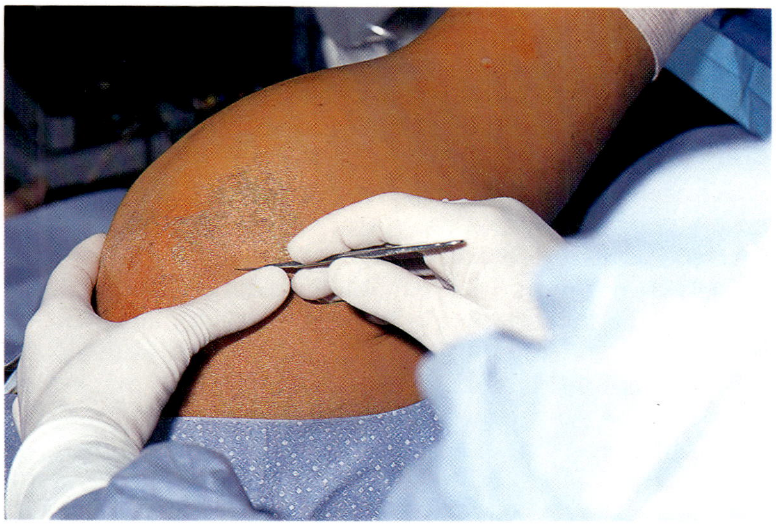

Figure 14.5

Once this area is located, a deep incision is made.

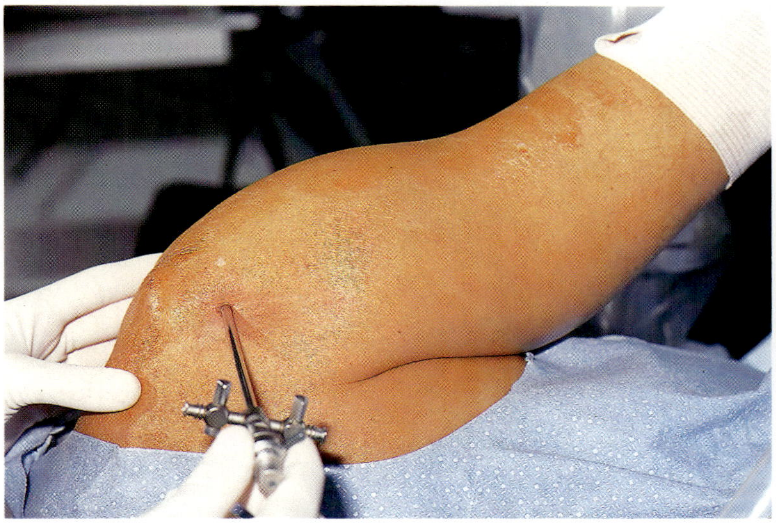

Figure 14.6

The arthroscopic trocar and cannula are prepared for insertion.

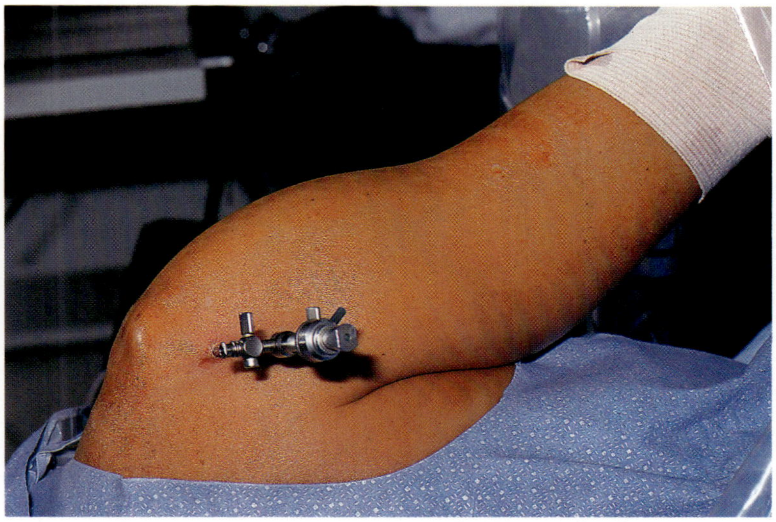

Figure 14.7

The arthroscopic trocar and cannula are passed into the glenohumeral joint anteriorly.

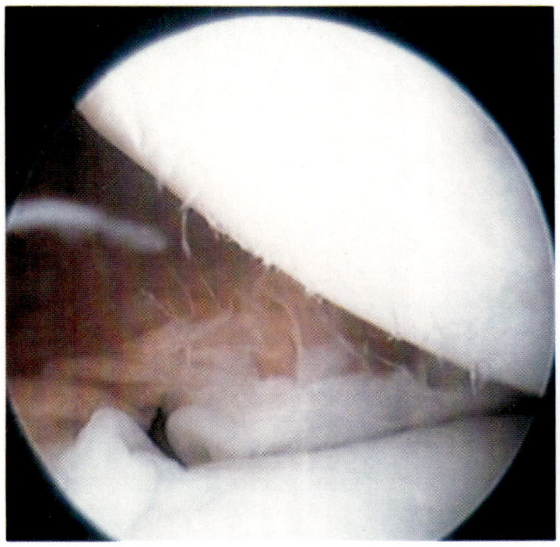

Figure 14.8

Arthroscopic view of a Bankart lesion.

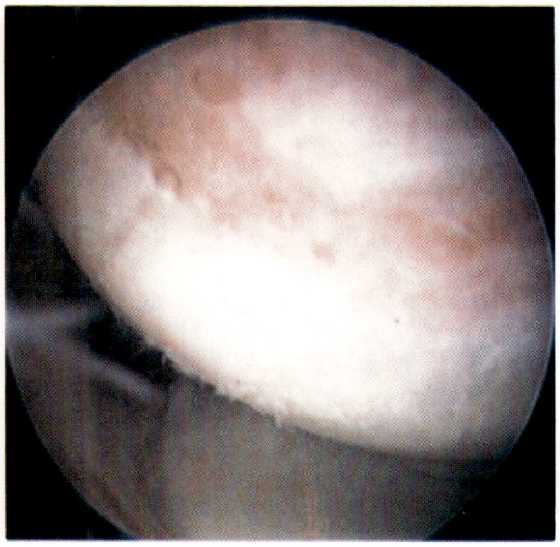

Figure 14.9

Arthroscopic view of a Hill-Sachs lesion.

(Figs. 14.10, 14.11). An 18-gauge needle is inserted at this point, and is pushed into the joint at a 45° angle anteriorly (Fig. 14.12). The 18-gauge needle is removed and replaced with the trocar and cannula (Figs. 14.13–14.15). The inflow is attached to the cannula (Fig. 14.16).

Although the anterior portal can be established with an 18-gauge needle, I prefer a Wissinger rod (Fig. 14.17). The rod is inserted into the arthroscopic cannula (Fig. 14.18) and pushed across the joint in the soft spot between the biceps tendon and the subscapularis tendon (Fig. 14.19), and then through the capsule and the subcutaneous tissue (Fig. 14.20). A skin incision is made over the tip of the Wissinger rod and the rod is pushed through the skin (Figs. 14.21, 14.22). A large-bore cannula is passed over the Wissinger rod, which will then go over the cannula of the arthroscope (Fig. 14.23). Finally, the Wissinger rod is withdrawn and the arthroscope is repositioned posteriorly.

Anterior Glenoid Neck Preparation

Preparation of the anterior glenoid neck with motorized equipment is essential in preparing the surface for the staple system (Figs. 14.24, 14.25). First, a high speed resector removes soft tissue from the anterior aspect of the glenoid neck (Fig. 14.26), followed by the burr system to remove cortical bone (Fig. 14.27). This facilitates fixation of the staple and healing of bone to tissue. A switching stick is

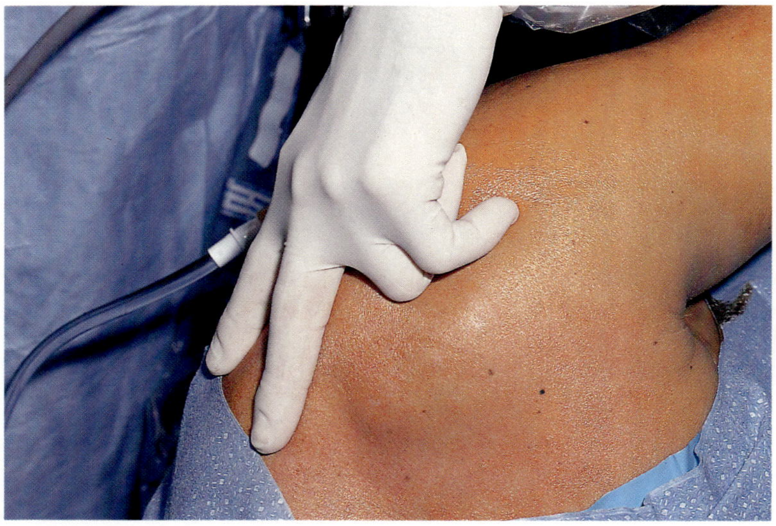

Figure 14.10
The supraspinatus approach.

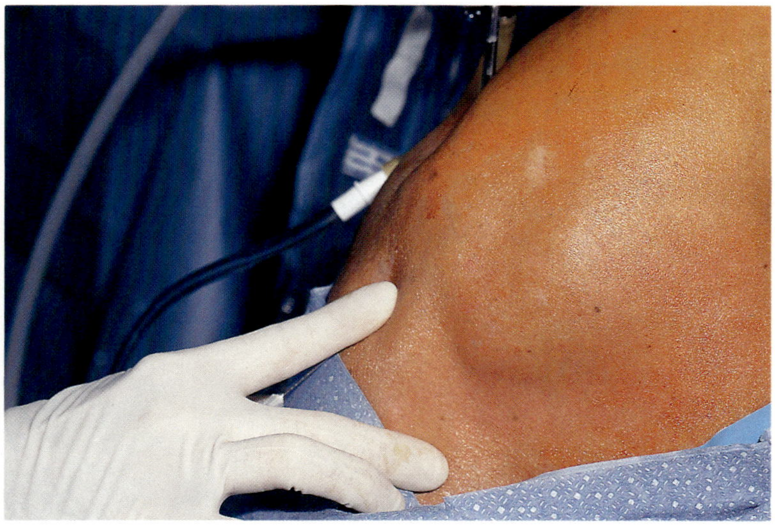

Figure 14.11
The point of entry can be located approximately one and a half finger breadths below the apex of the acromion and clavicle.

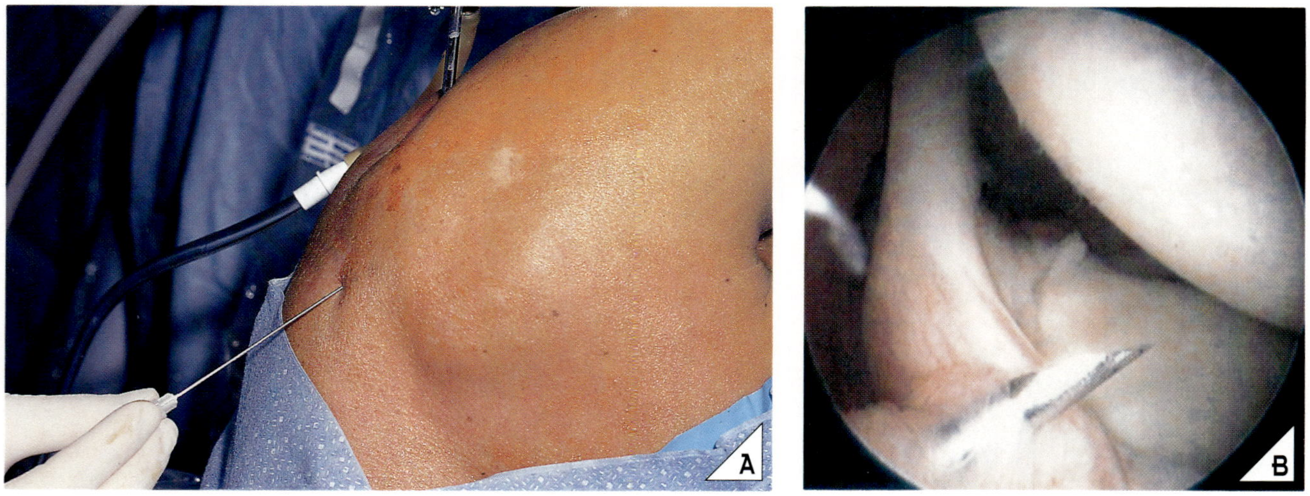

Figure 14.12
(A), An 18-gauge spinal needle is inserted at a 45° angle anteriorly. (B) The spinal needle's entry into the joint at the attachment of the biceps tendon will carry it to the humeral head posteriorly.

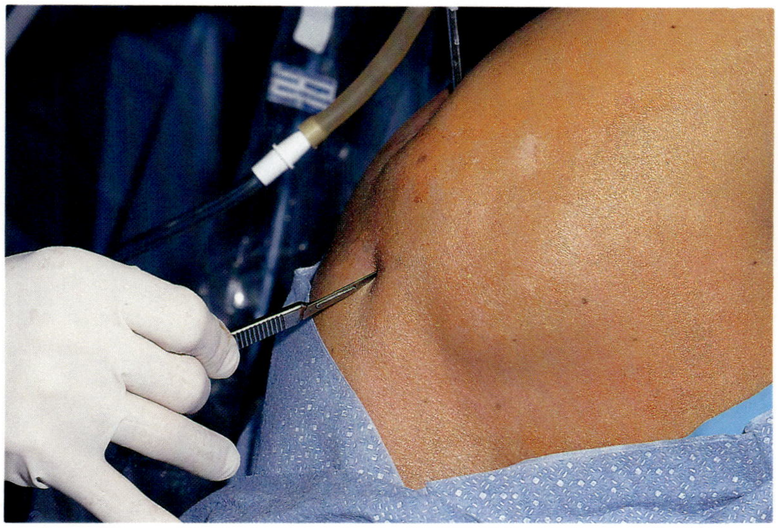

Figure 14.13
The skin is incised before introduction of the trocar and cannula.

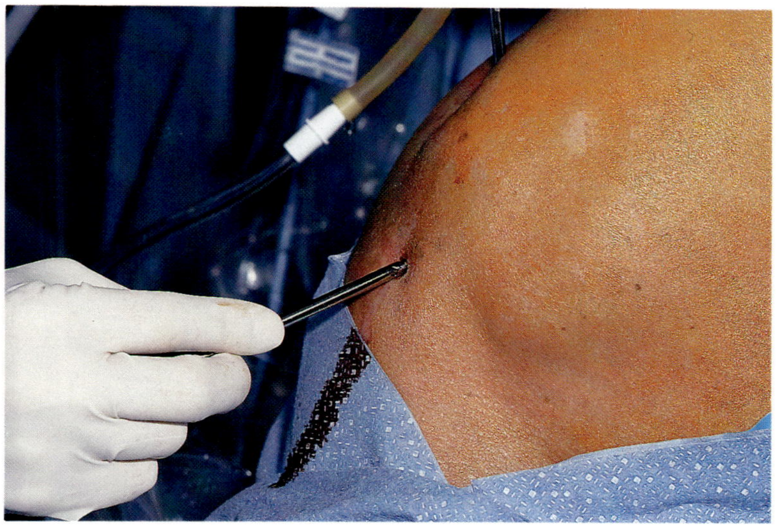

Figure 14.14
The trocar and cannula are substituted for the 18-gauge spinal needle after the skin is incised.

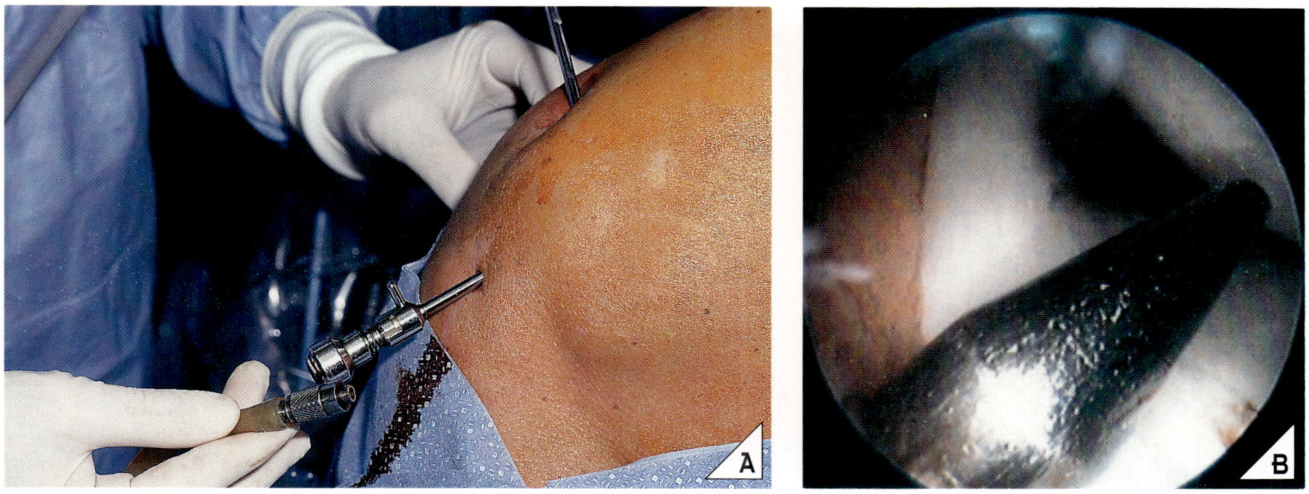

Figure 14.15
(A) The trocar and cannula are being introduced through the shoulder joint. (B) The cannula inside the joint.

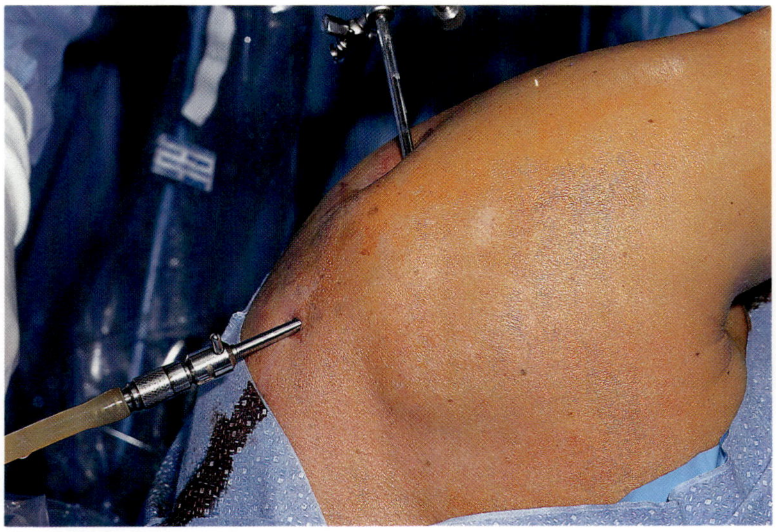

Figure 14.16
Irrigation fluid is attached to the inflow cannula.

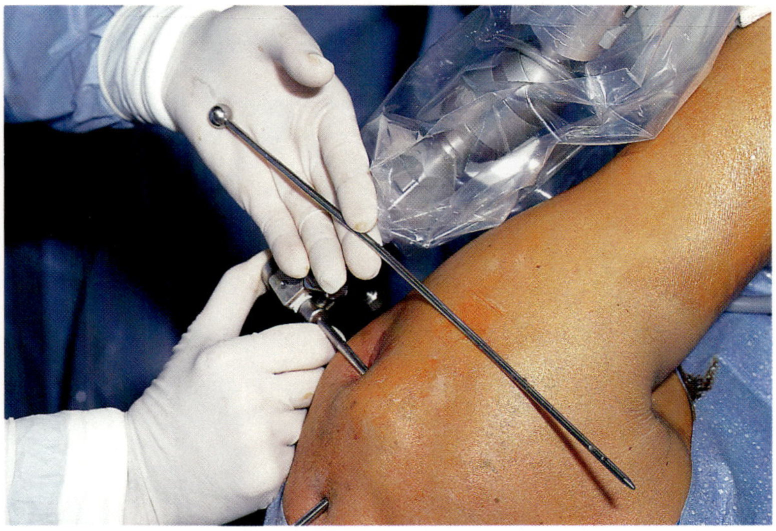

Figure 14.17
A Wissinger rod is used to establish the anterior portal. The surgeon is behind the right shoulder.

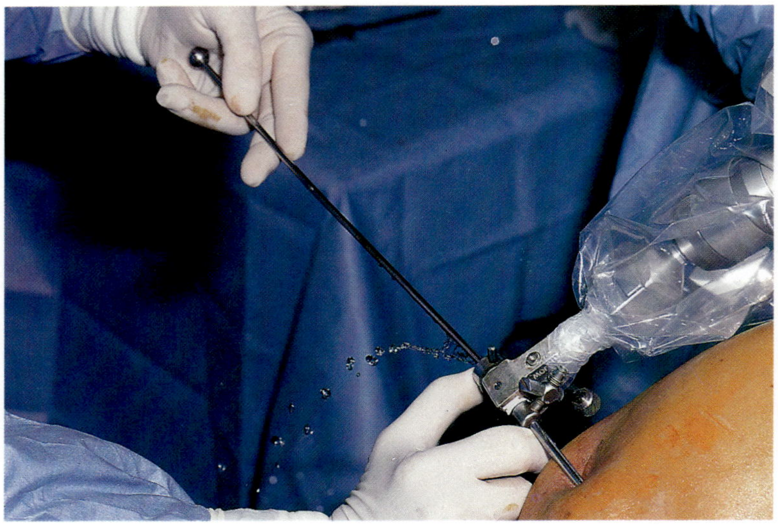

Figure 14.18

The Wissinger rod is inserted into the cannula.

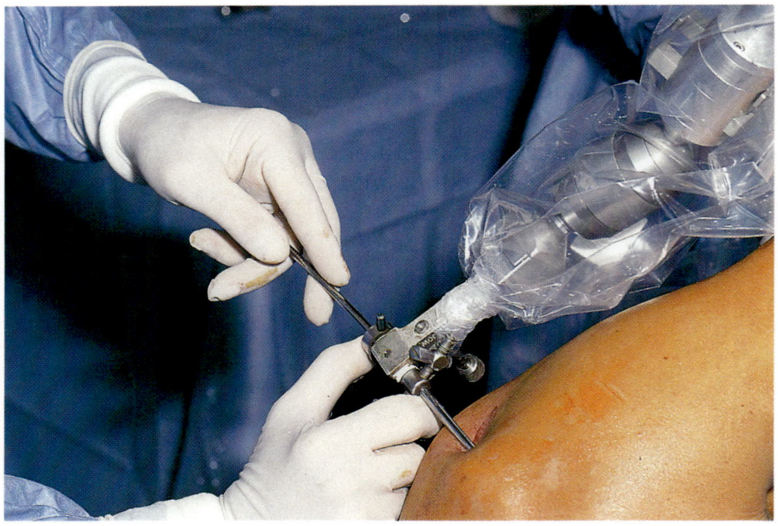

Figure 14.19

The rod is pushed across the joint in the soft spot between the biceps tendon and the subscapularis tendon.

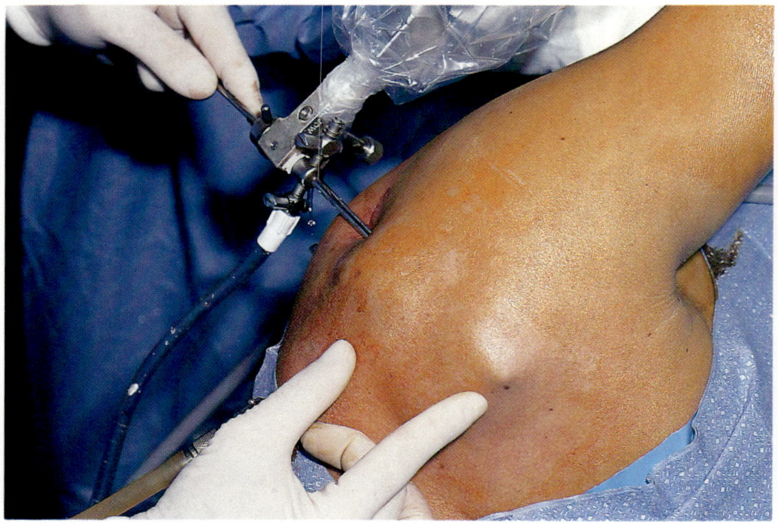

Figure 14.20

Anterior position of the tip of the rod through the capsule and subcutaneous tissue.

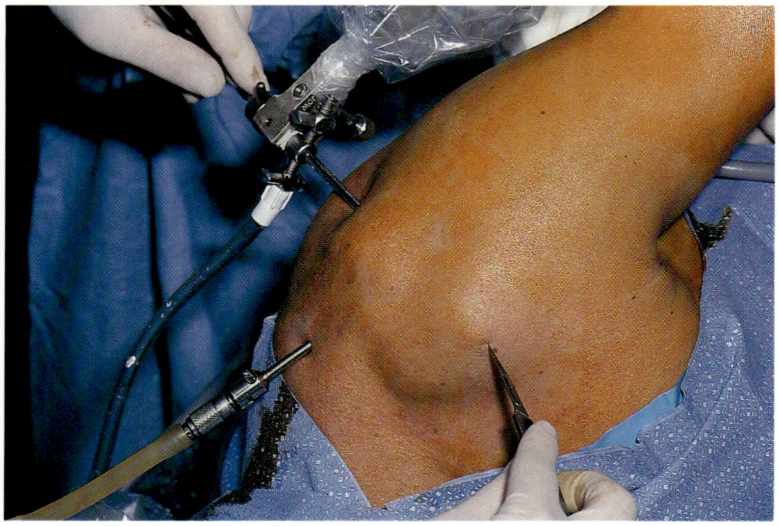

Figure 14.21

A skin incision is made over the tip of the Wissinger rod.

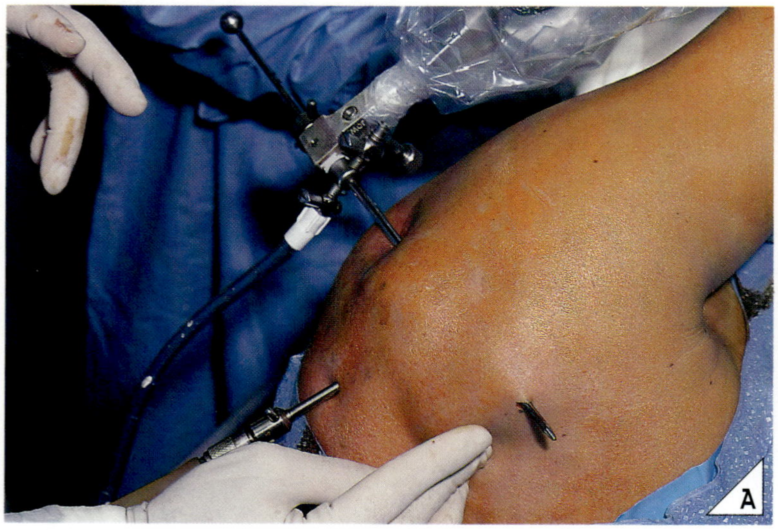

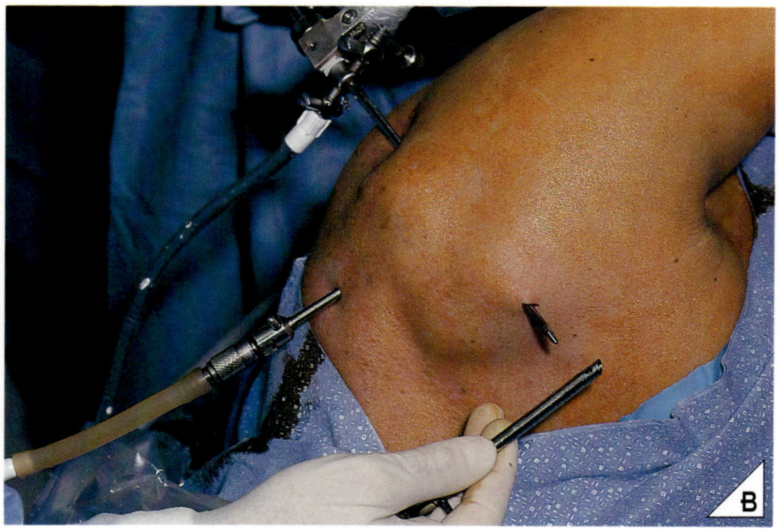

Figure 14.22

(A, B) The tip of the rod is pushed through the skin.

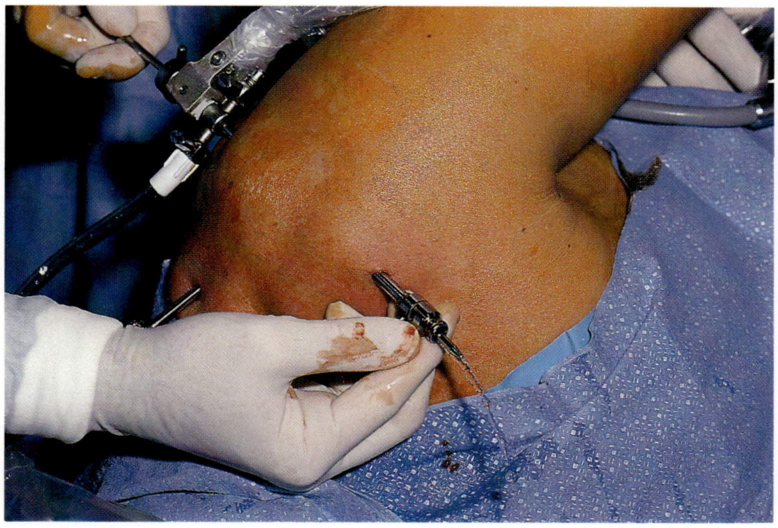

Figure 14.23
A large-bore cannula is passed over the Wissinger rod, which will also go over the arthroscopic cannula.

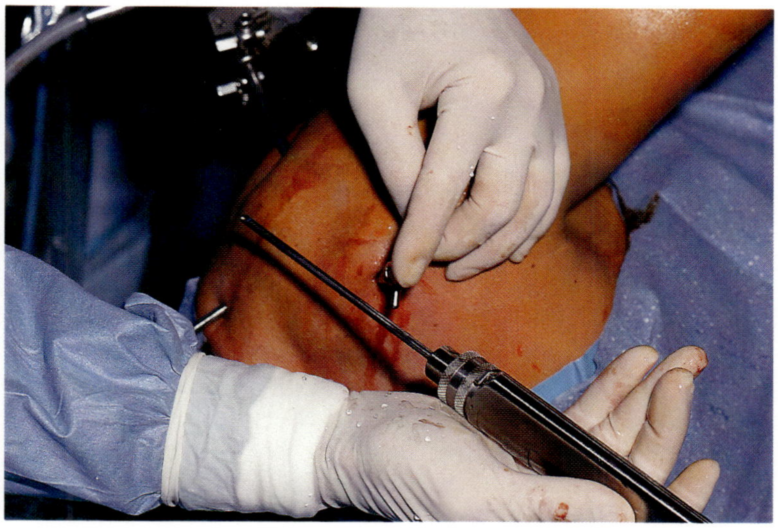

Figure 14.24
Motorized shaver before its placement through the large-bore cannula.

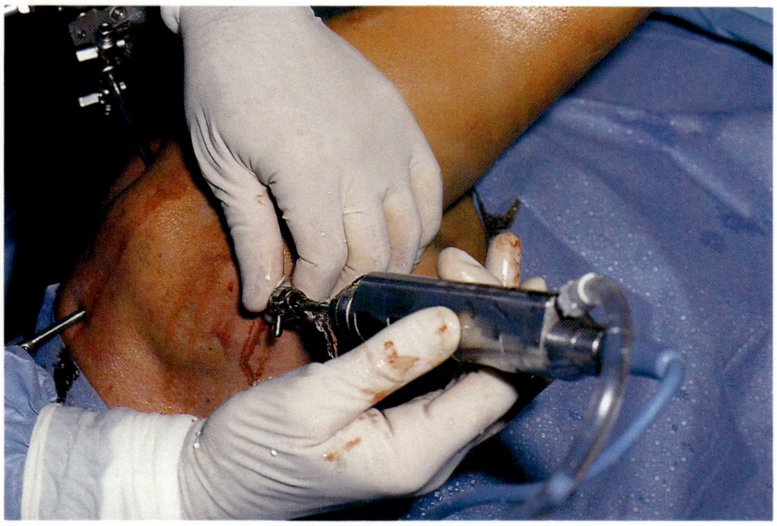

Figure 14.25
Motorized instrument being introduced through the joint anteriorly.

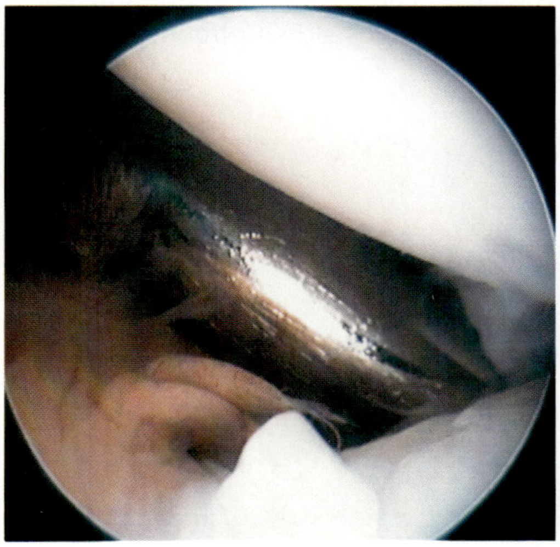

Figure 14.26
The high-speed resector removes soft tissue from the anterior aspect of the glenoid neck.

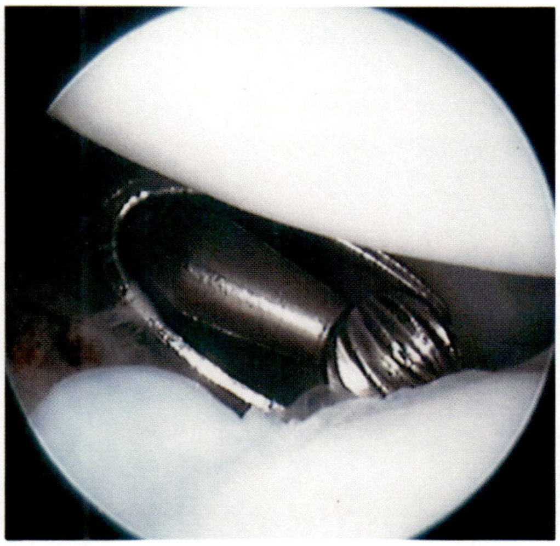

Figure 14.27
The burr is used to remove the outer cortex from the anterior glenoid.

used to change the standard arthroscopic cannula for the ligament and capsule repair system's cannula (Figs. 14.28–14.31).

Staple Insertion

After introduction of the ligament and capsule repair system into the joint, a staple is used to reattach the glenoid labrum (Fig. 14.32). The detached ligament is tensioned by rotating the staple 90° (Fig. 14.33).

To implant the staple, short firm strokes with a mallet are made into the glenoid neck below the surface (Fig. 14.34) until only the shiny part of the staple remains visible (Fig. 14.35). Before removing the driver/extractor, strong traction must be applied to insure that both legs of the staple are well fixed in the bone, or the staple might loosen. The driver/extractor may then be removed from the joint. A shift of the inferior capsule can be obtained by advancing superiorly the inferior glenohumeral ligament with the staple. To reduce the likelihood of staple irritation on the structures and damage to articular surfaces, the staple should be placed below the rim of the glenoid (Figs. 14.36, 14,37).

Postoperative Management

The patient is discharged on the day of surgery. A sterile dressing is applied and the shoulder is immobilized in a sling and swath for a minimum of 3 weeks. The sling is removed after 3 weeks. Isometric and progressive resistive exercises for adduction and internal rotation are started at this point. At 6 weeks, additional isometric and progressive resistive exercises, concentrating on extension, exter-

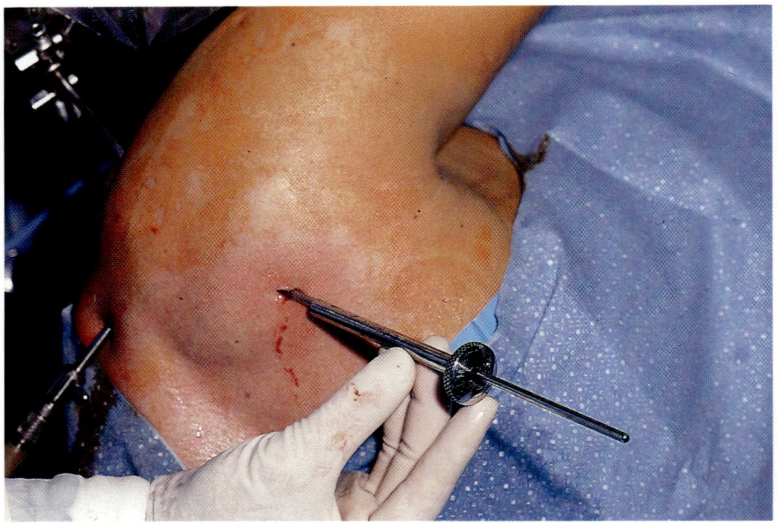

Figure 14.28
Switching sticks are used to change the standard arthroscopic cannula for the cannula of the ligament and capsule repair system.

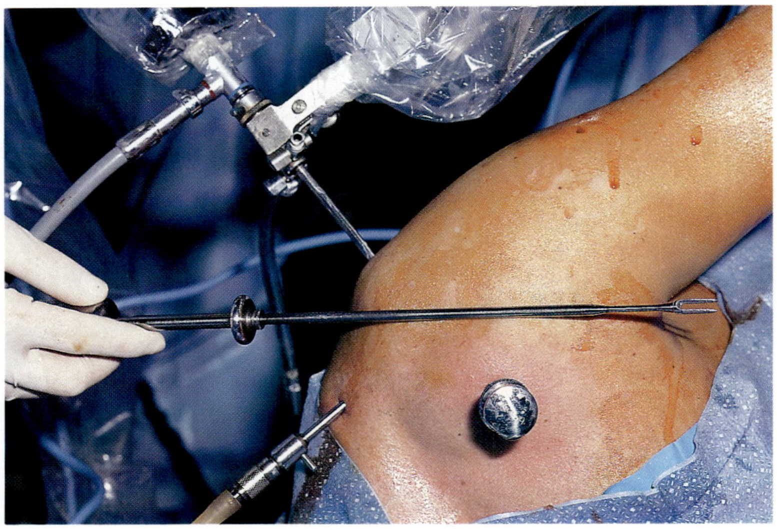

Figure 14.29
The Instrument Makar ligament and capsule repair driver/ extractor with its staple attached.

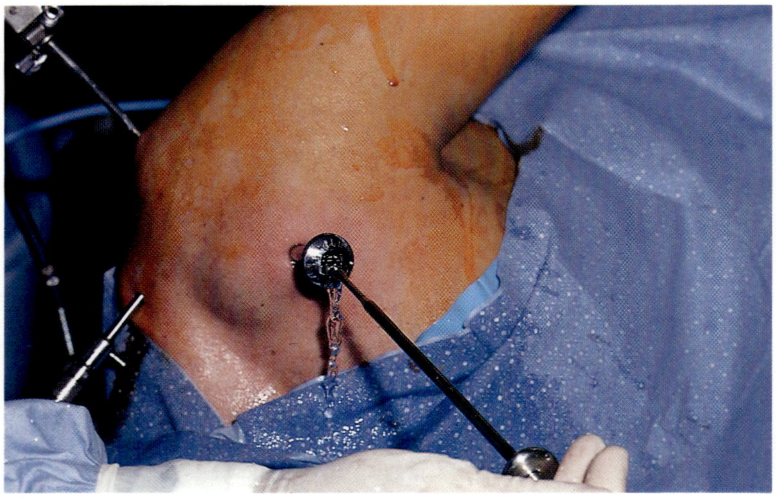

Figure 14.30
The ligament and capsule repair staple system passing down its cannula system into the shoulder joint.

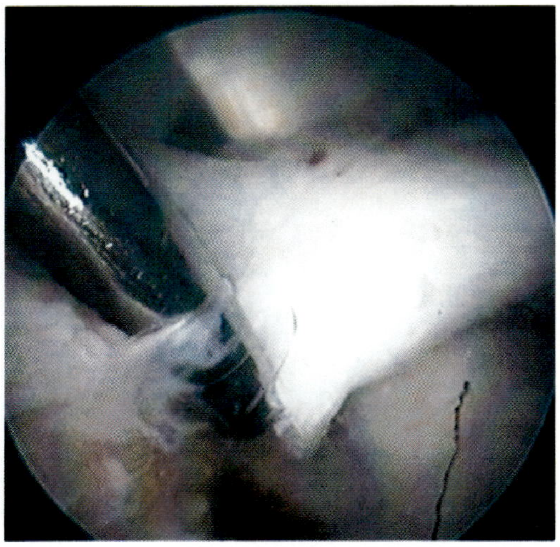

Figure 14.31
The cannula and trocar of the ligament and capsule repair staple system are brought into the shoulder joint.

nal rotation, and flexion, are performed. Competitive athletes will benefit from a physical therapy program. It is important to instruct patients to refrain from contact and overhead activities until full range of motion and strength have returned.

RESULTS

Among studies investigating the rate of redislocation in patients who have undergone shoulder staple capsulorrhaphy, Matthews et al.[3] noted that 12% of the patients (3 of the 25 shoulders studied) experienced postoperative recurrent anterior instability. Another investigation found a 16% rate of recurrent instability—8 shoulders out of the 50 studied during postoperative follow up.[2] It was felt that the lack of postoperative immobilization caused the majority of the shoulder instability in these patients. Detrisac and Johnson[1] recently reported a dislocation rate of 11% in a series of 148 patients with an average follow up of 4 years. Most of the failures occurred in patients who were immobilized for less than 3 weeks.

COMPLICATIONS AND PITFALLS

A major source of complications is the staple. Careful visualization and proper placement of the staple—perpendicular to the glenoid—during insertion is important to avoid malposition, loosening, bending, and even breaking. Erosion of the humeral head can occur if the staple is too close to the edge of the glenoid rim. Staple loosening can take place when the staple is not driven sufficiently into the glenoid. Recurrent dislocations are usually related to reducing postoperative immobilization time from 3 weeks to 2 weeks. Infections and/or neurovascular complications may occur, but these are fairly uncommon.

Complications of this technique can be minimized through a clear understanding of arthroscopic shoulder anatomy and continual education concerning advanced surgical techniques. Patients with traumatic anterior instability are good candidates for successful surgical outcomes. A postoperative immobilization regime of at least 3 weeks will enable the shoulder to heal properly without major complications.

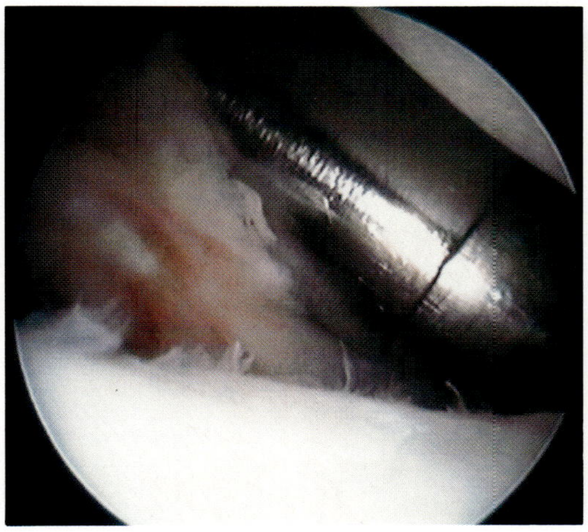

Figure 14.32
The ligament and capsule repair staple system is used to reattach the glenoid labrum.

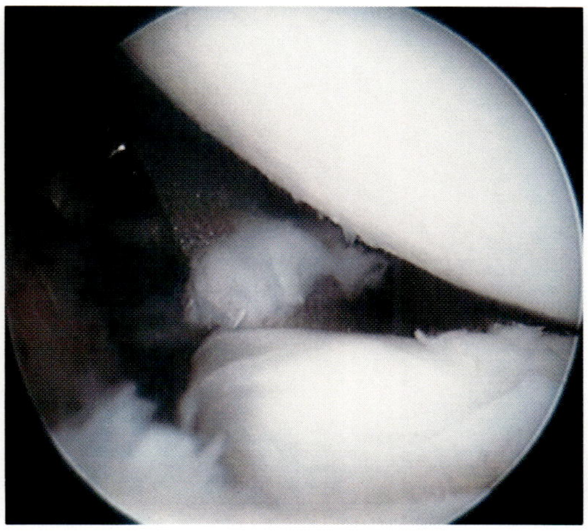

Figure 14.33
The ligamentous tissue is taut, with the staple rotated 90°.

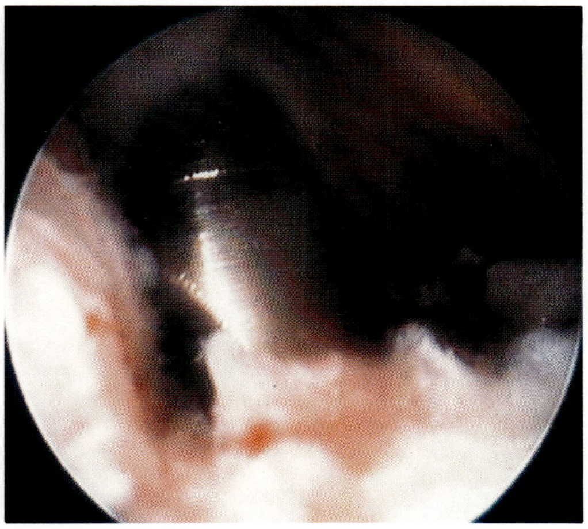

Figure 14.34
The staple is implanted with several short firm strokes of the mallet into the glenoid below the surface.

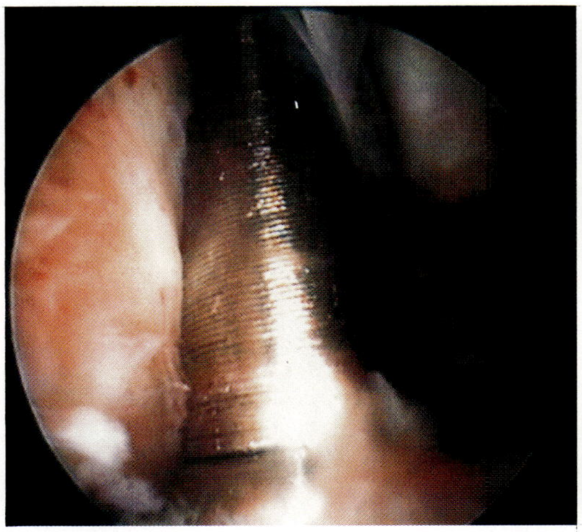

Figure 14.35
Impaction is continued until only the shiny part of the staple remains visible.

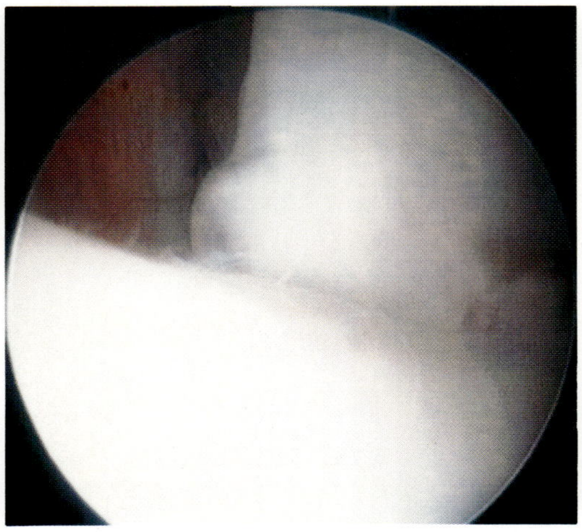

Figure 14.36
A view from the posterior portal after the repair is completed.

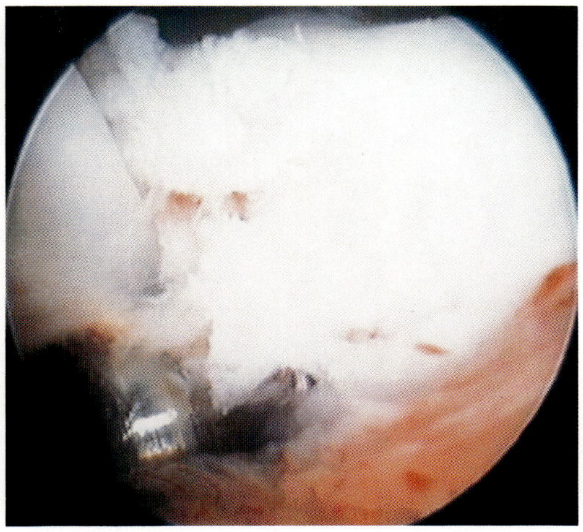

Figure 14.37
A view from the anterior portal reveals that the staple is below the rim of the glenoid.

REFERENCES

1. Detrisac DA. Arthroscopic shoulder capsulorrhaphy for traumatic anterior instability. In: McGinty JB, ed. *Operative Arthroscopy*. New York, NY: Raven Press; 1991:517.
2. Hawkins RB. Arthroscopic stapling repair for shoulder instability: a retrospective study of 50 cases. *Arthroscopy*. 1989; 2:122.
3. Matthews LS, Vetter WL, Oweida SJ, et al. Arthroscopic staple capsulorrhaphy for recurrent anterior shoulder instability. *Arthroscopy*. 1988;4:106.
4. Moseley HF, Overgaard B. The anterior capsular mechanism in recurrent anterior dislocation of the shoulder. *J Bone Joint Surg*. 1962;4B:913.
5. Turkel SJ, Ithaca MA, Panio MW, et al. Stabilizing mechanisms preventing anterior dislocation of the glenohumeral joint. *J Bone Joint Surg*. 1981;63A:1208.
6. Wiley AM. Arthroscopy for shoulder instability and a technique for arthroscopic repair. *Arthroscopy*. 1988;4:25.

chapter Fifteen

Techniques of Arthroscopic Acromioplasty

James C. Esch

Arthroscopic subacromial decompression is the arthroscopic equivalent of open surgical anterior acromioplasty. Rapid postoperative rehabilitation is one advantage of the arthroscopic procedure because the deltoid muscle is not detached. The ability to inspect and debride both surfaces of the cuff and the articular cartilage in the absence of a complete rotator cuff tear is another advantage (Fig. 15.1). After arthroscopic subacromial decompression, the rotator cuff can be repaired through a small deltoid-splitting incision.

Pathophysiology of Rotator Cuff Disease and Impingement

Ninety-five percent of rotator cuff disease is caused by compression of the cuff by the overlying acromion (Fig. 15.2), which leads to progressive fiber failure progressing from microscopic to gross partial tears and finally to complete tears of the rotator cuff. Impingement secondary to anterior or multidirectional instability accounts for the other cases of cuff disease, in which case surgical treatment should be directed toward the underlying instability.

Rotator cuff disease is divided into three phases[1]: Stage I is characterized by inflammation that responds to rest, medication, and exercise. It occurs in the 20- to 40-year-old age group. Stage II comprises rotator cuff fibrosis and tendinitis, including microscopic and partial tears. This sometimes responds to nonsurgical treatment. An advantage of diagnostic arthroscopy over open surgery is that an arthrotomy is not required to see articular side rotator cuff tears (Figs. 15.3, 15.4). Stage III is characterized by complete rotator cuff tears, which I prefer to divide into four categories: small (less than 1 cm), medium (1 to 3 cm) (Fig. 15.5), large (3 to 5 cm), and massive (Fig. 15.6).

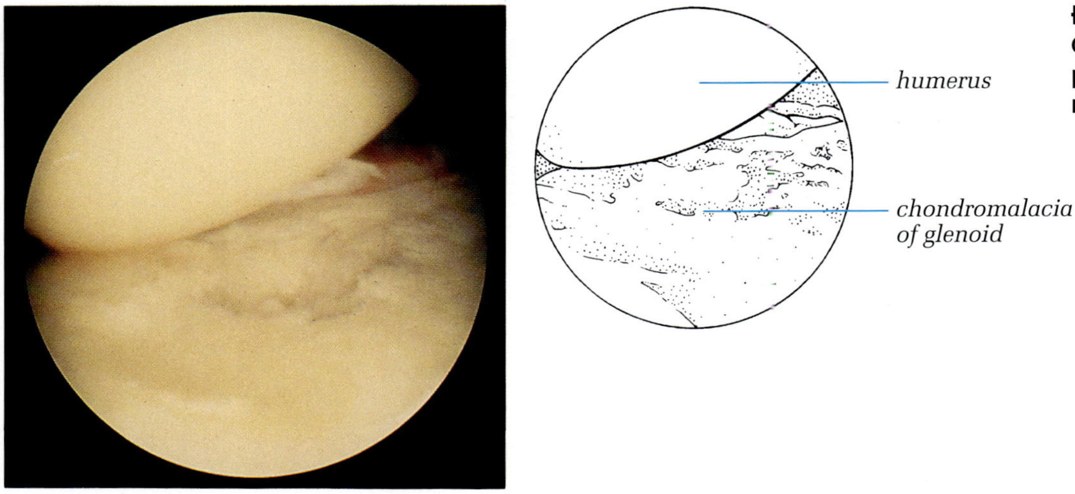

Figure 15.1
Glenoid labrum chondromalacia in a patient with impingement and an intact rotator cuff.

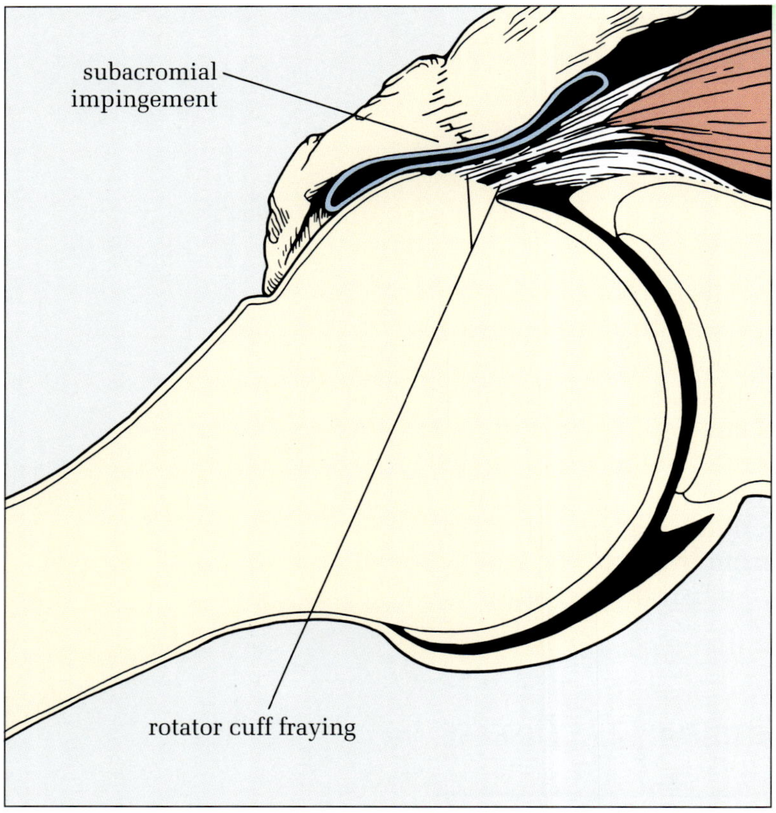

Figure 15.2
Impingement of rotator cuff against the acromion as the arm is abducted.

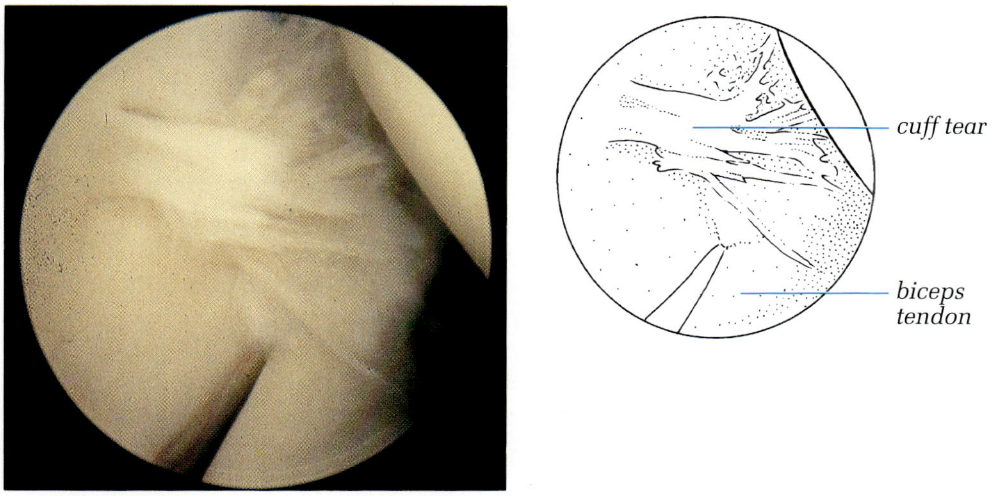

Figure 15.3
Small articular side partial rotator cuff tear.

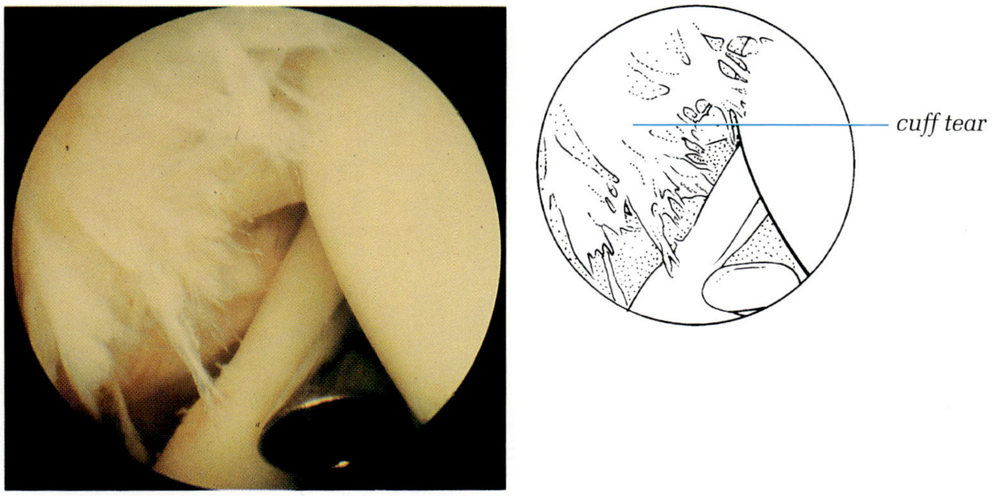

Figure 15.4
Large articular side partial rotator cuff tear.

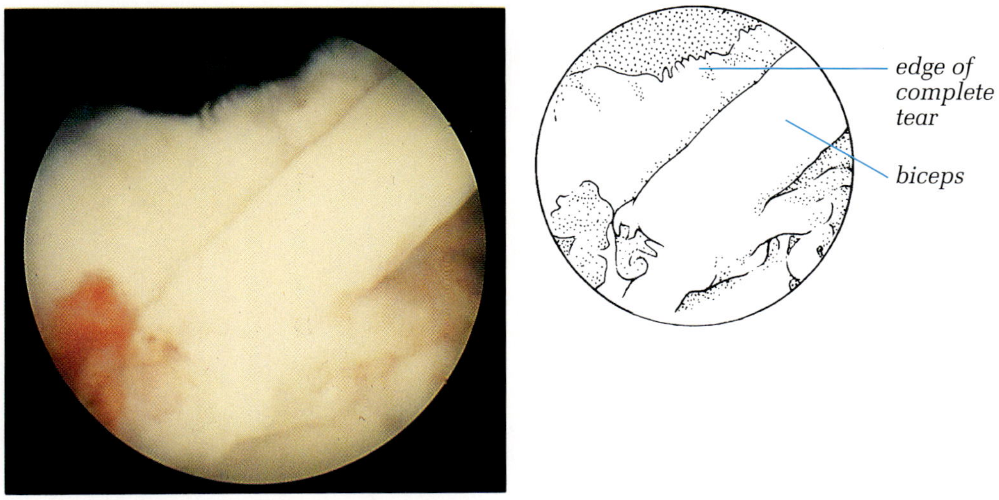

Figure 15.5
Medium-sized complete rotator cuff tear.

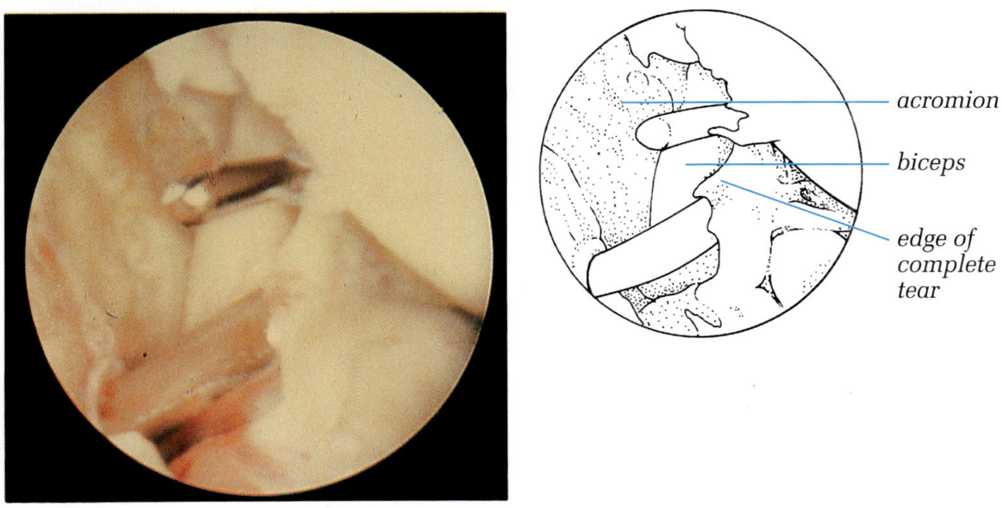

Figure 15.6
Massive complete rotator cuff tear.

The soft-tissue pathology (Fig. 15.7) includes: partial cuff tears with noticeable irregularity, scuffing, or flaps, on the articular and/or bursal surfaces; complete tears; fraying of the acromial attachment of the coracoacromial ligament; and thickening of the subacromial bursa.

The bone pathology (Fig. 15.8) usually consists of a type III acromion that has a 70% incidence of associated rotator cuff tears.[2,3] This acromion has a definite anterior hook. Next, there is a curved type II acromion that is associated with a 24% incidence of rotator cuff tear. Osteophytes on the inferior aspect of the acromioclavicular joint also contribute to this bone disease.

Glenohumeral arthroscopy and subacromial bursoscopy evaluate the articular surfaces, glenohumeral ligaments, both sides of the rotator cuff, the subacromial bursa, and the attachment of the coracoacromial ligament to the anterior acromion.

INDICATIONS

The primary indication for arthroscopic subacromial decompression is Neer stage II disease of the rotator cuff. Surgery is also indicated in selected patients with stage III disease.[4–8] These patients may have small to medium rotator cuff tears and no evidence of weakness or large tears that are deemed irreparable. Although many of these patients could be treated by open rotator cuff repair, they represent a group that is generally unwilling to participate in the necessary postoperative rehabilitation.

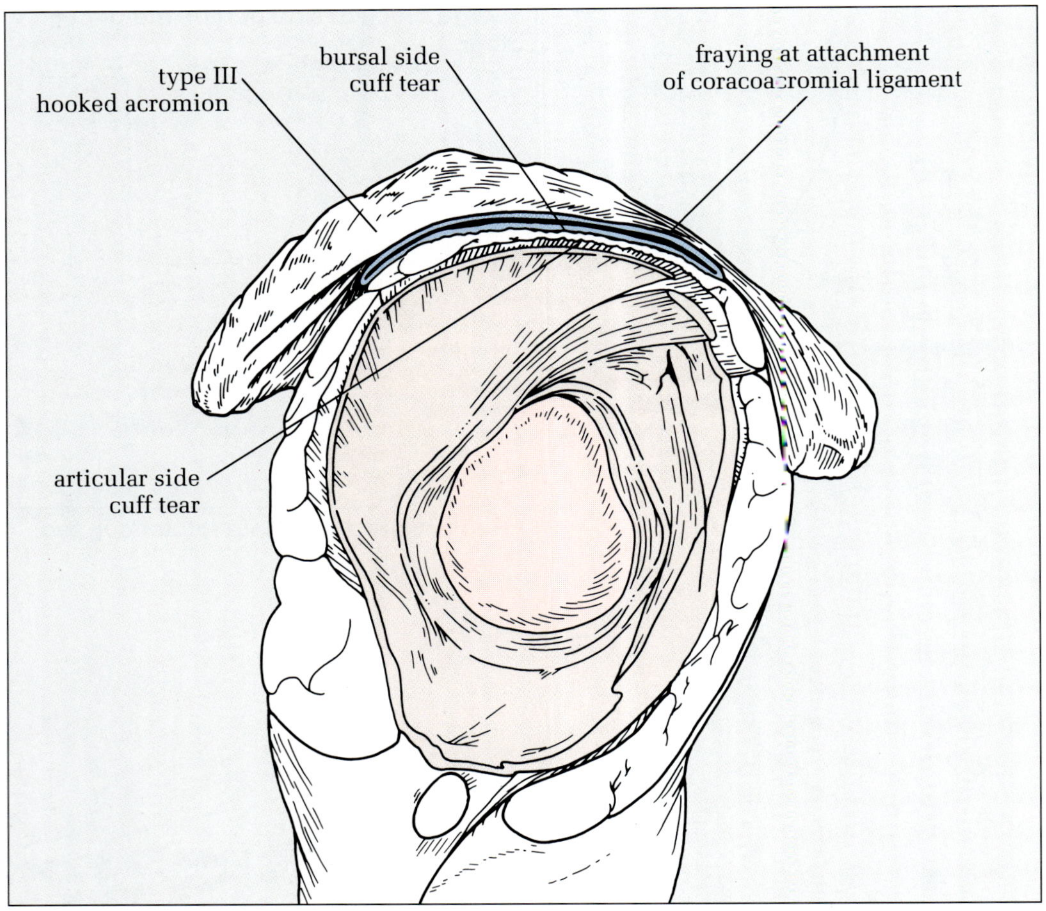

Figure 15.7
Soft-tissue and bone pathology. Rotator cuff tears on articular or bursal side, fraying at the attachment of the coracoacromial ligament. Type III acromion.

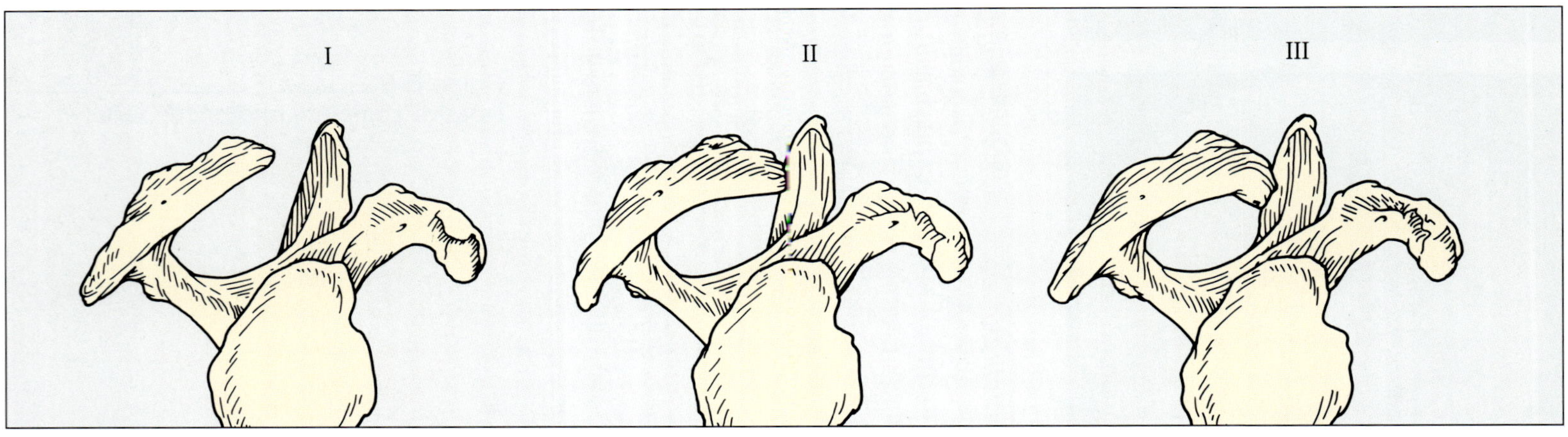

Figure 15.8
The three types of acromion. Type III has a 70% association with rotator cuff pathology.

Active patients of all ages who have complete tears, especially tears larger than 1 cm with associated weakness, can be treated with arthroscopic subacromial decompression followed by rotator cuff repair through a small deltoid-splitting incision.

The surgical goal is to decrease the volume of the unyielding subacromial space by removing the thickened subacromial bursa and loose fragments of the rotator cuff. The bone space is decompressed by excising the coracoacromial ligament and converting the hooked type III acromion to a type I acromion. This reduction of bone and soft tissue volume, similar to a carpal tunnel release, decreases compressive load and thereby provides a healing environment.

Surgical Technique

The surgery is performed in a free-standing, same-day surgery center.[9] An interscalene nerve block with bupivacaine HCl is given for postoperative pain control. The patient is then given a general anesthetic, placed in a lateral position, and tilted 30° posteriorly. The body is stabilized with a beanbag, and the involved arm is suspended by ten pounds in 30° of abduction and 15° forward flexion. A shoulder draping system is used. An electrocautery unit (Zimmer-Concept) is helpful for cutting the coracoacromial ligament as well as cauterizing small blood vessels. Open repair of the rotator cuff is easily performed through a deltoid-splitting incision while the arm remains suspended.

Some surgeons prefer the sitting "beach-chair" position, in which traction is provided by the assistant surgeon and the weight of the arm. However, I prefer the lateral suspension approach because the assistant does not need to manipulate the arm and transition to open cuff repair is easy.

I use an arthroscopic infusion pump with the pressure sensor and inflow attached to the side arm of the arthroscope. The pump pressure is maintained between 40 and 100 mm Hg. Reduction of blood pressure to less than 95 mm Hg is important to reduce bleeding.

Glenohumeral Diagnostic Arthroscopy

A posterior approach into the joint is followed by formation of an anterior portal using the Wissinger rod technique (Fig. 15.9). An accessory anterosuperior portal will provide additional inflow if a pump is not used. The intraarticular portion of the joint is systematically examined (Fig. 15.10). The status of the articular cartilage on the glenoid cavity and humeral head should be noted. Loose fragments and inflamed synovium are debrided. The biceps tendon is only minimally debrided because this tendon is an important depressor of the shoulder joint. A frayed or fragmented labrum should also be debrided. The underside of the rotator cuff is examined and any frayed areas are debrided. The patients with stage II disease may show either minor scuffing of the cuff or large cuff tears that extend extensively into the substance of the supraspinatus tendon. Loose cuff fragments are then trimmed.

A marking suture is placed in the exact location of the tear to identify it when the subacromial bursa is inspected. An 18-gauge needle is inserted from the lateral edge of the acromion through the tear. A monofilament suture is passed down the needle and grasped within the joint.

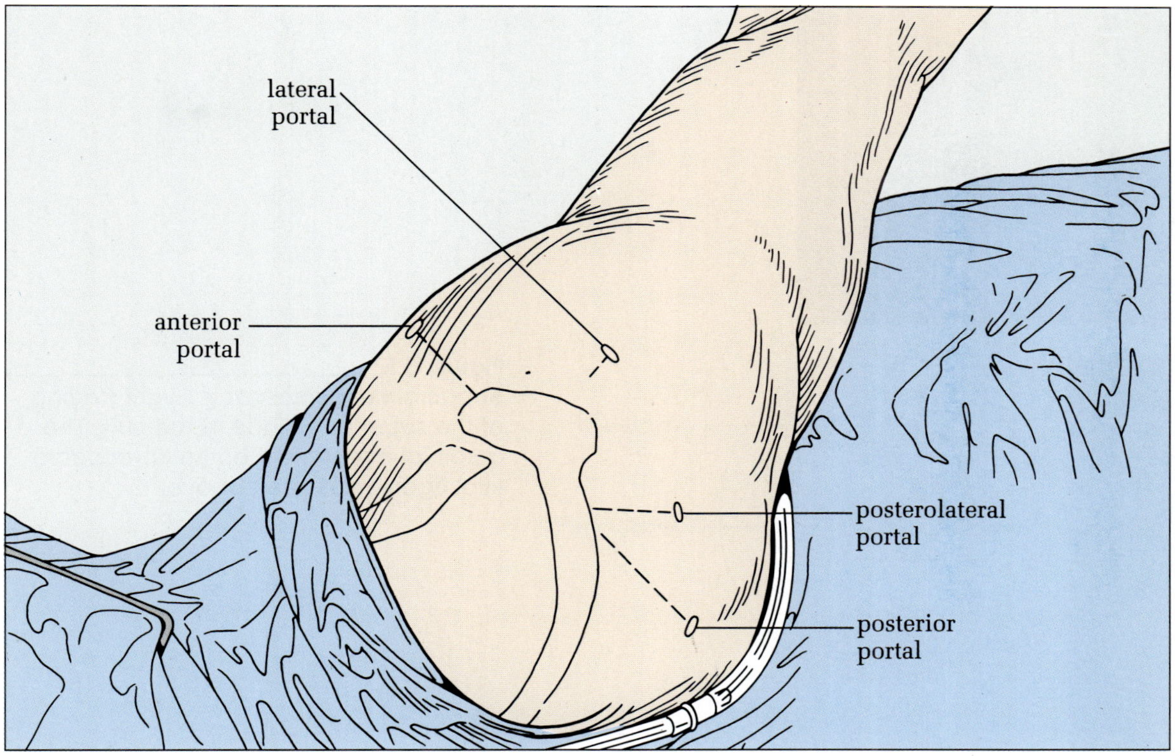

Figure 15.9 The primary posterior and anterior arthroscopic portals.

Subacromial Bursoscopy

The subacromial bursa is a well-defined structure bounded by the coracoacromial ligament anteriorly, the anterior half of the acromion superiorly, and the rotator cuff inferiorly (Fig. 15.11). The bursa has a definite posterior curtain and lateral margin.

The same posterolateral portal used for glenohumeral joint arthroscopy is used. The obturator is manipulated in order to puncture the subacromial bursa between the undersurface of the acromion and the subacromial space. A large 5.5-mm diameter arthroscopic sheath with a standard 4.0-mm, 30° arthroscope is used. I prefer an infusion pump (Zimmer-Concept) with a pressure sensor attached to the arthroscope.

As the bursa is entered, a definite change in tissue resistance will be felt. Common errors are entry too posteriorly or entry into the fatty tissue between the bursa and acromion. The bursa can usually be entered on a second try.

Create the lateral portal with a skin puncture 2 to 3 cm below and lateral to the anterolateral corner of the acromion (see Fig. 15.11). This portal is in line with the posterior aspect of the acromioclavicular joint. A small 4 mm

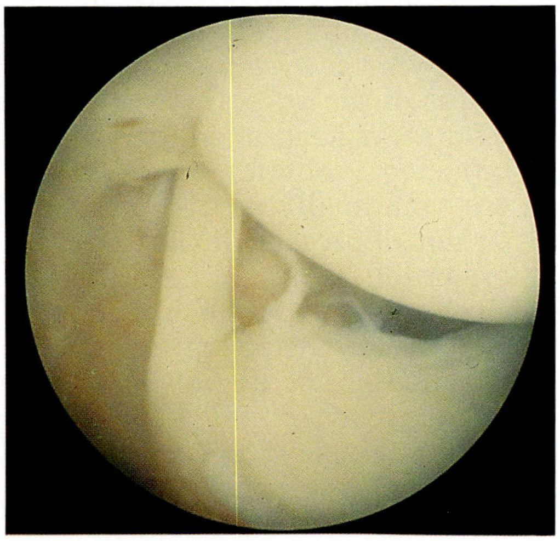

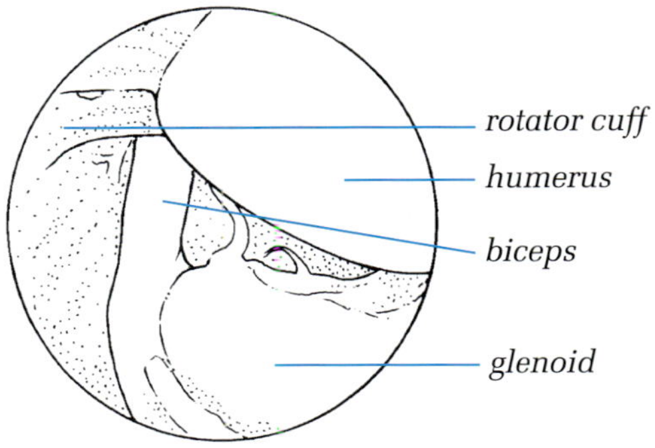

Figure 15.10
Normal glenohumeral arthroscopy. The articular surface of the rotator cuff is smooth. The biceps tendon wraps onto the posterosuperior labrum. The articular cartilage is smooth.

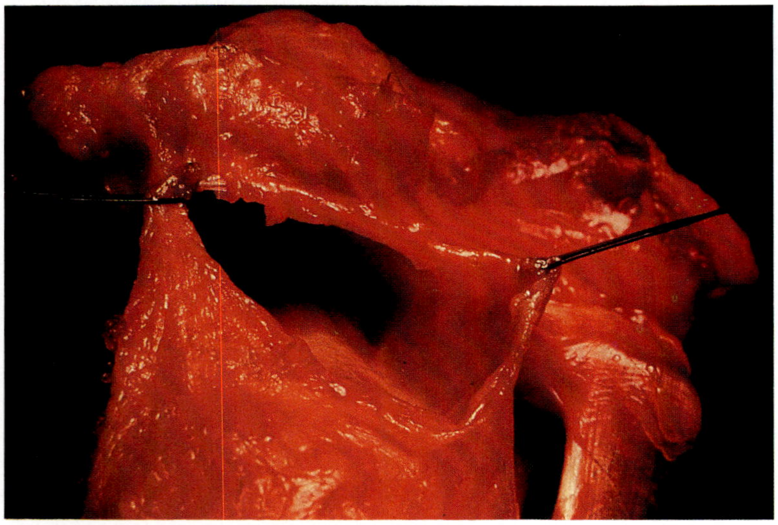

Figure 15.11
The subacromial bursa is an anterior structure. It is bounded superiorly by the anterior acromion and the coracoacromial ligament and inferiorly by the rotator cuff.

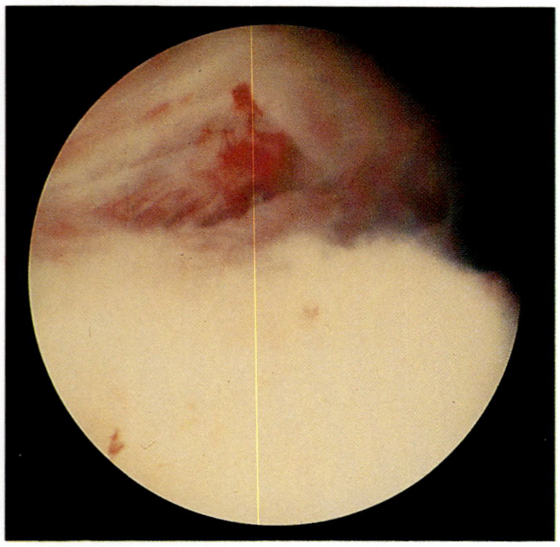

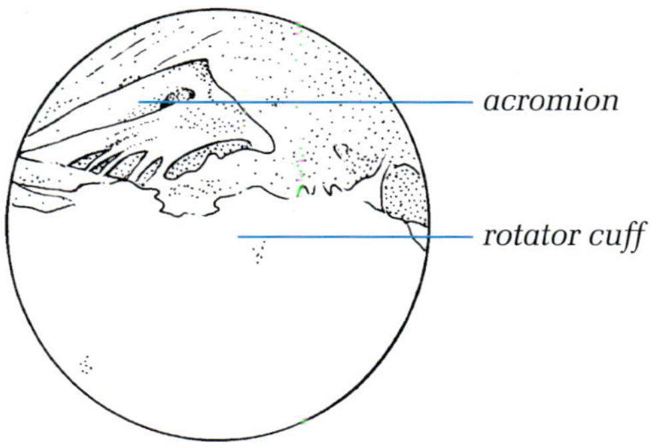

Figure 15.12
Subacromial bursoscopy. Slight fraying of the superior surface of the cuff. The acromial attachment of the coracoacromial ligament is seen above.

cannula should be moved into the subacromial space until fluid returns. Viewing may be improved by removing excessive bursal tissue with a small synovial resector.

Initial diagnostic bursoscopy is performed through the posterolateral portal while manipulating instruments through the lateral portal. The arthroscope is then switched to the lateral portal to view the posterior curtain of the subacromial space in order to obtain a different view of the underlying rotator cuff. The bone resection can be performed from either the lateral or the posterolateral portal.

The presence or absence of thickened bursal tissue, the articular surface of the rotator cuff, the anterior acromion, and the attachment of the coracoacromial ligament are all evaluated. Patients with stage II disease usually have significant fraying of the attachments of the coracoacromial ligament (Fig. 15.12). Patients with large rotator cuff tears also show this pathology of the anterior acromion. While viewing from the lateral portal, determine the shape of the acromion with a tool in the posterior portal.

A complete rotator cuff tear not only can be measured for size but can be grasped and guided to determine the ease with which open repair can be accomplished. Snyder has classified rotator cuff tears according to the surface, severity, and location (Fig. 15.13, Table 15.1).[10,11]

Cutting the Coracoacromial Ligament

At this time the surgeon must decide whether to cut the acromial attachment of the coracoacromial ligament or use a burr to peel its attachment off the undersurface of the acromion. The burr is an excellent way for the surgeon to define the bony margins of the acromion and the acromial attachment of the coracoacromial ligament.

I prefer to cut the coracoacromial ligament at its acromial attachment with an insulated electrocautery right

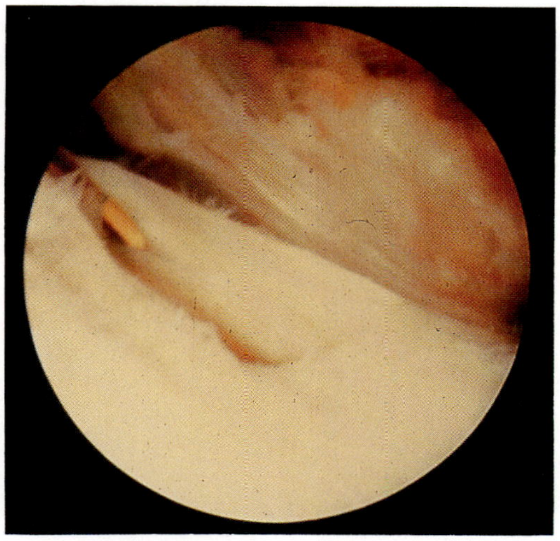

Figure 15.13
A probe is on the bursal surface of this rotator cuff tear.

TABLE 15.1
Rotator Cuff Classification System Based on the Surface, Severity, and Location of Tear

Surface of Tear	Severity of Tear	Location of Tear
A Articular surface of the rotator cuff	**0** Normal	**SS** Supraspinatus tendon
B Bursal surface of the rotator cuff (see Fig. 15.13)	**1** Superficial synovial or bursal irritation with mild fraying of the capsule without tendon fiber failure	**IS** Infraspinatus tenon
C Complete tear of the rotator cuff, which connects the articular surface and the bursal surface	**2** Minimal tearing of the tendon fibers with capsular fraying in area less than 2 cm	**RI** Rotator interval
	3 Moderate disruption of tendon fibers with fraying and fragmentation in 2 to 3 cm area	**SbS** Subscapularis tendon
	4 Severe fraying and fragmentation with splits and flap formation of cuff tendon in a large area, greater than 3 cm	

Examples of classification system:
A2 SS B1 C0 Minimal articular surface tear less than 2 cm in the supraspinatus region. Superficial bursal surface irritation. No evidence of complete tear.

Adapted from Snyder SJ, Pattee GA, 1991 and Snyder SJ, Pachelli AF, Del Pizzo WD, et al., 1991 angle knife (Figs. 15.14, 15.15). The knife is kept against the bone because the vessels are 5 to 8 mm from the bone. Any bleeding vessels are cauterized. After release of the ligament, a synovial resector or small burr is used to clean the inferior and anterior surfaces of the acromion and thus to define its margins accurately. Some surgeons prefer to define the anatomy by placing 18-gauge needles at the anterolateral aspect of the acromion and at the anterior aspect of the acromioclavicular joint.

Acromion Resection

The goal is to change the type III acromion to a type I acromion that can be verified by a postoperative office radiograph. The acromioplasty can be performed with a burr from either the lateral or posterior portal, although both portals are usually necessary.

Posterior Cutting

The arch of the acromion is delineated with the arthroscope in the lateral portal and the synovial resector in the posterior portal. The burr is placed along the posterior acromion and pushed anteriorly, using the posterior acromion as a planing jig to convert the curved or hooked acromion to a straight line.[12] This technique accurately defines the type I acromion as the endpoint.

Lateral Cutting

The anterior acromion can also be resected from the lateral approach. A full-thickness removal of the leading edge is begun at the anterior corner, which enables the surgeon to use the burr rapidly and efficiently to remove the anterior acromial osteophyte. The goal initially is to remove the anterior 5 to 10 mm of the acromion, which consists of the acromial osteophytes anterior to the leading edge of

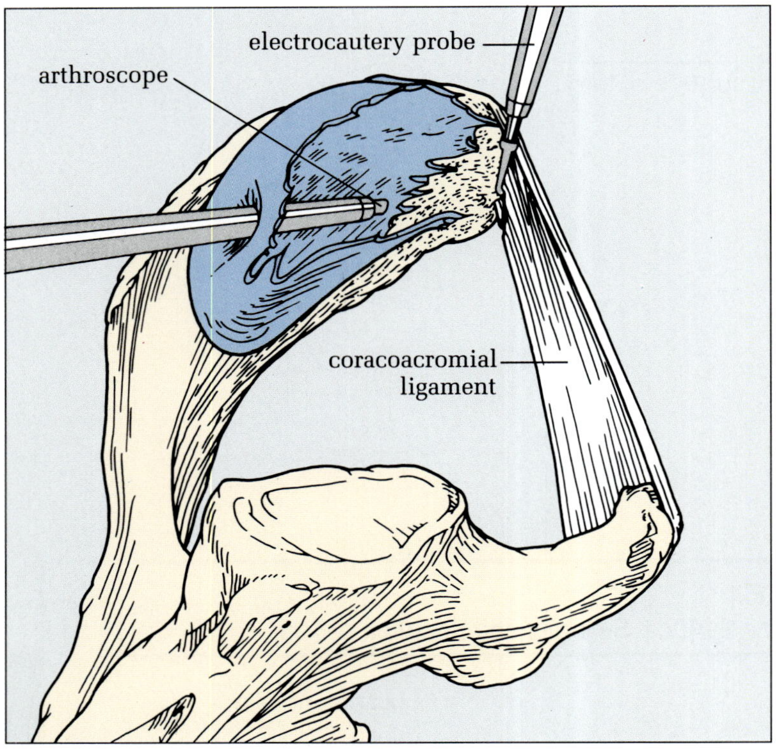

Figure 15.14
The coracoacromial ligament is cut at its bone attachment with electrocautery from the lateral portal while viewing from the posterior portal.

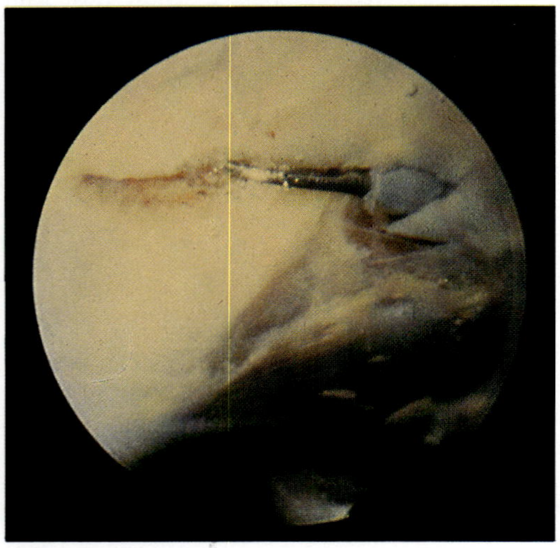

Figure 15.15
Cutting the coracoacromial ligament with the electrocautery insulated hook knife.

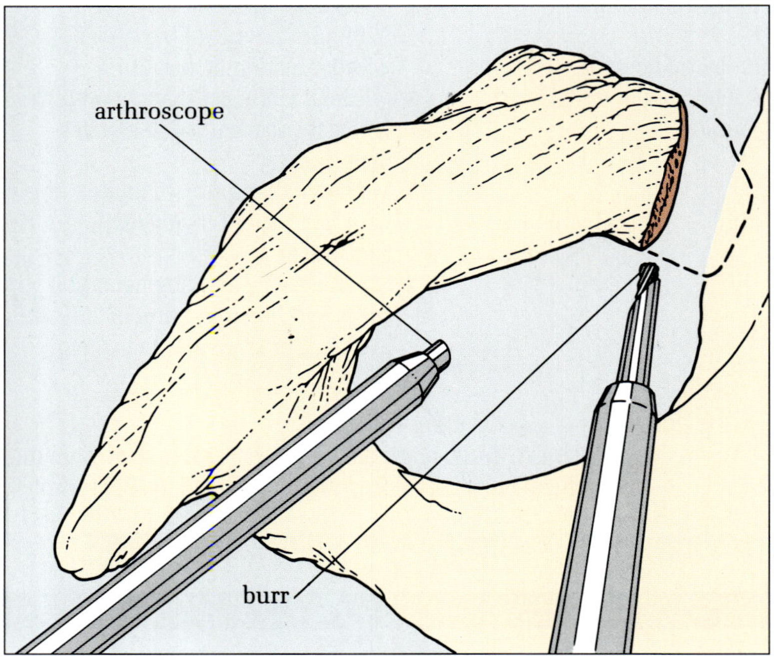

Figure 15.16
The anterior 5 to 8 mm of acromion are removed.

the clavicle. The bone is thinned for an additional 20 mm posteriorly to effect an acromioplasty. The depth of the resection is 2 to 4 mm. Final polishing is trimmed with an oval burr.

My Approach

At present, I prefer to resect the ligament and anterior osteophyte from the lateral portal, removing the anterior 5 to 8 mm of acromion (Fig. 15.16). The thickness and shape of the acromion are then determined by viewing from the lateral portal. The burr is laid along the posterior acromion and pushed anteriorly, using the posterior acromion as a planing jig to convert the curved or hooked acromion to a straight line (Fig. 15.17). The final planing of the anterior arch is accurately determined for size and thickness. This method is rapid and accurate, with a well-defined end point (Fig. 15.18). The postoperative arch radiograph provides a record of the surgeon's performance.

Acromioclavicular Joint

The undersurface of the acromioclavicular joint after the acromioplasty is then evaluated. This is the last step in the procedure, because troublesome bleeding frequently occurs from the synovial and bursal surfaces at the undersurface of this joint. Electrocautery is extremely helpful in this area. Many patients require resection of an inferior osteophyte to provide adequate clearance for the rotator cuff and to decompress the subacromial space.

A distal clavicle resection (Mumford procedure) can be done equally well by the arthroscopic or the open method. The resection burrs are manipulated from the anterior or superior aspect of the acromioclavicular joint. The best visualization is obtained with the arthroscope in the lateral portal and the resecting tool from the anterior portal in the plane of the acromioclavicular joint. The procedure is facilitated by downward pressure on the clavicle and a 70° arthroscope to look superiorly at the distal clavicle as the resection proceeds.

Rotator Cuff Evaluation

The rotator cuff is probed at the completion of the acromioplasty. The size, shape, and mobility of complete tears is examined. Significant partial tears may have widespread fragmentation of the cuff or may represent a 95% bursal side tear that appears normal from the articular side.

At this point the surgeon can choose whether or not to perform a deltoid-splitting incision to repair the cuff. The degree of cuff mobility will alert the surgeon to the potential difficulty of an open procedure.

Rotator Cuff Repair

A 3 inch deltoid-splitting incision, beginning at the anterolateral corner of the acromioplasty is used to repair the rotator cuff. Loose bursal tissue is removed with a rongeur to define the rotator cuff insertion. A firm #2 braided permanent mattress suture is inserted through the layers of the rotator cuff. The tendon is advanced and sutured into a bone trough at its normal insertion point. The rotator cuff suture repair kit (Zimmer-Concept) is extremely helpful in placing the sutures into bone. A roll pledget of 2 mm Gore-Tex, an expanded polytetrafluoroethylene soft-tissue patch (W.L. Gore), can be placed

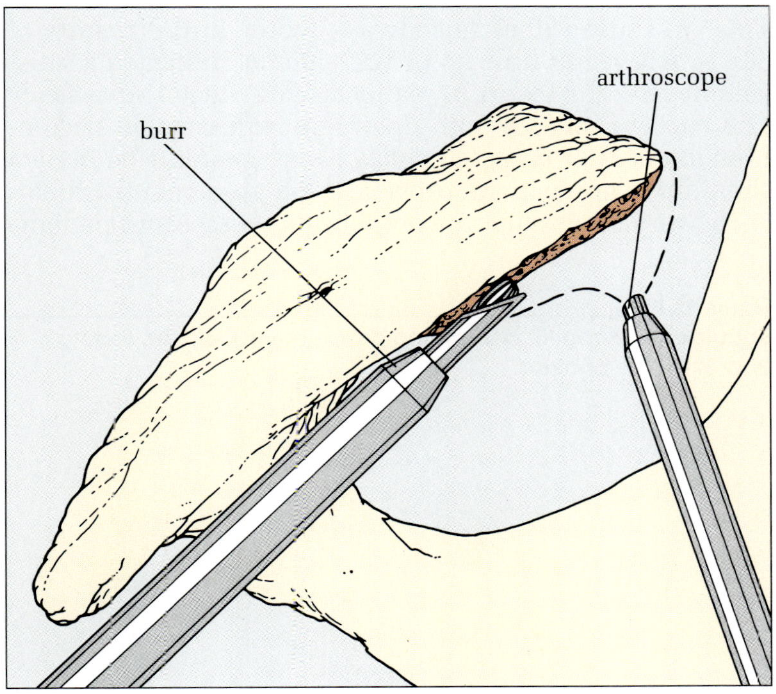

Figure 15.17
The acromion is trimmed and thinned from posterior to anterior while viewing from the lateral portal.

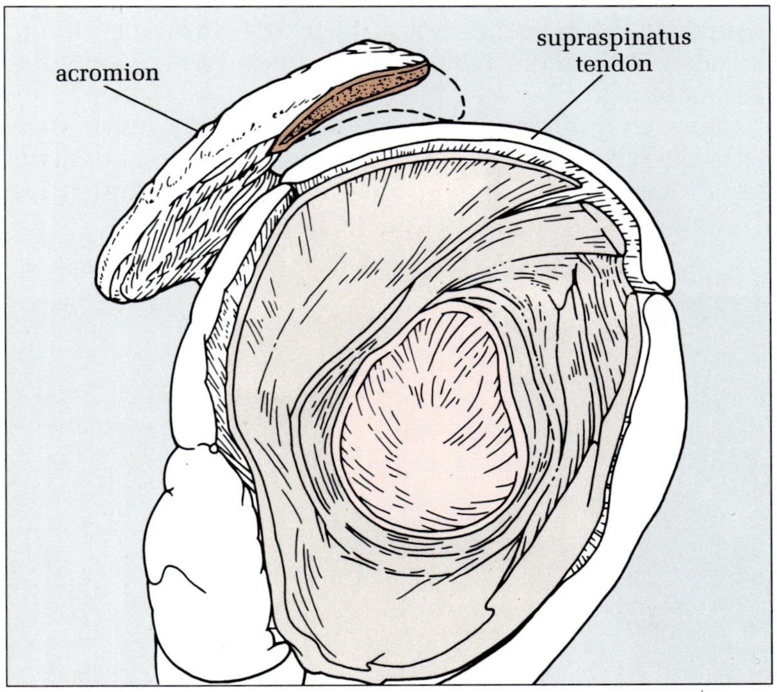

Figure 15.18
Lateral view of the final bone resection.

under the sutured knot to prevent the sutures from pulling out of osteoporotic bone.[13] A larger massive cuff tear can be exposed by an acromion osteotomy.[14]

Complications and Pitfalls

Inadequate surgical visualization due to hemorrhage or the surgeon's failure to enter the subacromial bursa is the main complication. Bleeding can be controlled by hydrostatic pressure applied through the infusion pump or by elevating the fluid bag. At the same time, the anesthesiologist should lower the patient's systolic blood pressure to less than 95 mm Hg. The initial debridement of the lateral bursa under posterior visualization prevents troublesome bleeding while medial tissue is being resected under the acromioclavicular joint.

Inadequate acromioplasty is another complication that accounts for poor results. The anterior acromion that lies anterior to the leading edge of the clavicle should be resected, followed by conversion of the hooked type III acromion to a smooth type I acromion. The use of the arthroscope laterally with the burr posteriorly allows the end point to be well defined.

Fractures of the acromion have been associated with excessive thinning of the acromion. I avoid this complication by inspecting the thickness of the anterior acromion after resecting the anterior acromion 5 to 8 mm. Excessive thinning is then avoided by resecting from posterior to the anterosuperior corner. A preoperative arch view x-ray can be used to determine the thickness of the acromion.

Instability of the acromioclavicular joint has been observed in several patients who began vigorous weight lifting within the first postoperative week. The symptoms subsided after several weeks of rest.

It is extremely important to recognize multidirectional instability. This occurs not only in the throwing athlete but also in workers who have an underlying congenital laxity of the joint.

Other complications include postoperative reflex sympathetic dystrophy and incorrect diagnosis. Some patients have unrealistic expectations because of preoperative stiffness, job stresses, and athletic stresses.

Postoperative Management

As noted above, postoperative care is simplified by having the anesthesiologist perform an interscalene block with bupivacaine HCl. Ice and analgesics are applied for relief of pain. Immediate passive forward flexion and external rotation exercises are demonstrated to the patient. Circumduction exercises are performed on the evening of surgery. I recommend the home use of a continuous passive motion machine for 6 to 8 hours daily during the first postoperative week. Active exercises are begun 1 to 6 weeks postoperatively. I also highly recommend immediate passive exercises with the use of an overhead bar-and-pulley exercise system. Isokinetic diagonal exercises with surgical tubing are begun as soon as painless motion is obtained.

Patients who have undergone repair of a complete cuff tear begin passive exercises immediately. Active assistive exercises are delayed until the sixth week.

The physician or physical therapist directs a home program consisting of overhead stretching exercises with a bar and overhead active and active assisted exercises with a door pulley. The final phase includes strengthening exercises in internal rotation, external rotation, and diagonals using elastic tubing. A shoulder therapy kit (STK Kit, Breg) enables the patient to perform exercises easily either at home or while traveling (Fig. 15.19).

Results

Partial Tears

This procedure does not always work! Initial results of our 1- to 3-year follow up of 102 patients indicated a satisfaction rate of 84% in 67 patients with stage II disease.[15] The success rate for both open and arthroscopic decompression is approximately 80%. Never guarantee a perfect shoulder to any patient, especially a high-demand athlete.

Be wary of workman's compensation cases and patients

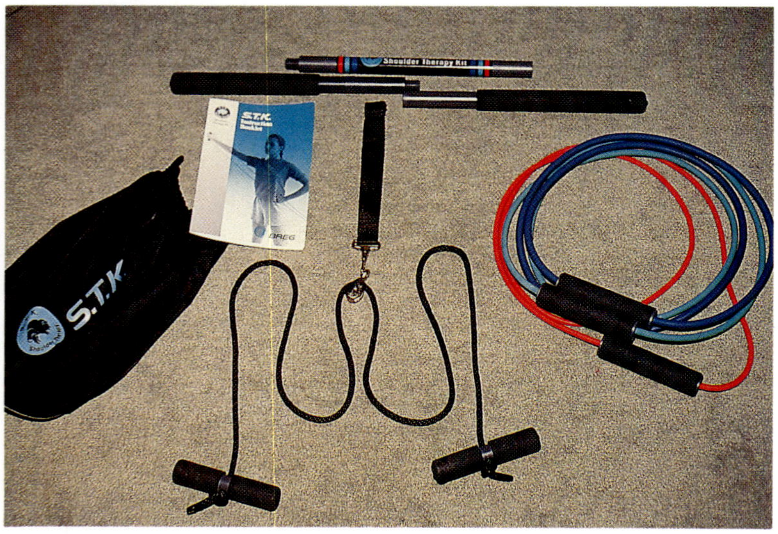

Figure 15.19
Shoulder therapy kit containing a bar, pulley, elastic tubing, and exercise booklet.

with preoperative stiffness, acromioclavicular joint pathology and, especially, multidirectional instability. I see this underlying instability not only in throwing athletes but in loose-jointed recreational athletes and workers.

The factors in surgical decisions include the patient's age, level of activity, pain, weakness, pathology, and response to nonsurgical treatment. Several options are available to treat partial tears of the rotator cuff, whether they are articular or bursal. This may include (Table 15.2):

- Debridement alone of articular side tears in young athletes.
- Debridement and arthroscopic subacromial decompression in most patients.
- Debridement and open subacromial decompression if you run into technical problems or are not comfortable with arthroscopy (there is nothing wrong with this approach).
- Excision and repair to bone of severe partial tears in high-demand individuals with greater than 75% thickness of their cuff involved.

Complete Tears

Arthroscopic subacromial decompression can be successful in some carefully selected patients with stage III complete rotator cuff tears. These are mainly elderly patients who have shoulder pain, especially at night, but no significant weakness. Open rotator cuff repair was performed in elderly patients with significant weakness.

Repair small tears, especially in the dominant arm, by arthroscopic subacromial decompression followed by open repair through a small deltoid-splitting incision. The exception is an elderly patient who has very low demands or will not participate in rehabilitation. At present, I repair medium and large tears of the rotator cuff, unless the individual is elderly with low demands whose chief complaint is pain without weakness.

Patients with massive tears may obtain some relief with arthroscopic decompression. Otherwise, they require open repair or prosthetic arthroplasty.

My treatment plan regarding complete tears of the rotator cuff depends on the size and mobility of the tear as well as the patient's age, demands, and expectations. Treatment options include (Table 15.3):

- Debridement and arthroscopic subacromial decompression alone, especially in the elderly or low-demand individual, when there is a small tear and the main complaint is pain.
- A mini-incision cuff repair after arthroscopic subacromial decompression. This is the most commonly performed procedure, especially in active individuals or patients with medium or large tears and significant weakness.
- A standard open repair for large tears that are difficult to mobilize.
- An open subacromial decompression without repair. I consider arthroscopic decompression without repair for massive tears in older patients whose main complaint is pain and who have active elevation and satisfactory external rotation.

CONCLUSION

Arthroscopic subacromial decompression is the arthroscopic equivalent of a standard open procedure. Although technically demanding, it facilitates early rehabilitation. The results with stage II disease are equal or better than those that can be achieved through open surgery.

The procedure is also useful in cases of stage III disease in which pain is the major complaint. Complete rotator cuff tears can be repaired into a bony trough through a small deltoid incision.

The arthroscope allows early detection and treatment of shoulder pathology in elderly patients and enables them to resume an active and healthy lifestyle.

TABLE 15.2
Decision Making for Partial Rotator Cuff Tears

Decision Making for Partial Rotator Cuff Tears
Debride
Arthroscopic subacromial decompression
Open subacromial decompression
Repair

TABLE 15.3
Decision Making for Complete Rotator Cuff Tears

Decision Making for Complete Rotator Cuff Tears
Arthroscopic subacromial decompression
Arthroscopic subacromial decompression with mini-incision cuff repair
Open repair
Open subacromial decompression

REFERENCES

1. Neer CS. Anterior acromioplasty for the chronic impingement syndrome in the shoulder: a preliminary report. *J Bone Joint Surg.* 1972;54:41–50.
2. Bigliani LU, Morrison DS, April EW. The morphology of the acromion and its relationship to rotator cuff tears. *Orthop Trans.* 1986;10:216–228.
3. Morrison DS, Bigliani LU. The clinical significance of variations in acromial morphology. Presented at the Third Open Meeting of the American Shoulder and Elbow Surgeons; San Francisco, Calif; January, 1987.
4. Ellman H. Arthroscopic subacromial decompression. *Arthroscopy.* 1987;3:173–181.
5. Ellman H. Diagnosis and treatment of incomplete rotator cuff tears. *Clin Orthop.* 1990;254:64–74.
6. Paulos LE, Franklin JL. Arthroscopic shoulder decompression development and application: a five-year experience. *Am J Sports Med.* 1990;18:235–244.
7. Esch JE, Ozerkis LR, Helgager JA, et al. Arthroscopic subacromial decompression: results according to the degree of rotator cuff tear. *Arthroscopy.* 1988;4:241–249.
8. Esch JC. Arthroscopic subacromial decompression: surgical technique. *Orthop Rev.* 1989;18:733–744.
9. Esch JC. Shoulder arthroscopy. basic setup. *Tech Orthop.* 1988;3:9–14.
10. Snyder SJ, Pattee GA. Shoulder arthroscopy in the evaluation and treatment of rotator cuff lesions. In: Paulos LE, Tibone JE, eds. *Operative Techniques in Shoulder Surgery.* Philadelphia, Pa: WB Saunders Co; 1991:45–55.
11. Snyder SJ, Pachelli AF, Del Pizzo WD, et al. Partial thickness rotator cuff tears: results of arthroscopic treatment. *Arthroscopy.* 1991;7:1–7.
12. Sampson TG. Precision arthroscopic acromioplasty: video supplement to *Arthroscopy.* 1990;2:2.
13. France EP, Paulos LE, Harner C, et al. Biomechanical evaluation of rotator cuff fixation methods. *Am J Sports Med.* 1989;17:176–181.
14. Kessel L. The transacromial approach for rotator cuff rupture. In: Bayley I, Kesell L, eds. *Shoulder Surgery.* Berlin, Heidelberg: Springer-Verlag, 1982:39–44.
15. Esch JC, Ozerkis LR, Helgager JA, et al. Arthroscopic subacromial decompression for partial and complete tears of the rotator cuff. Presented at the International Arthroscopy Association; Rome, Italy; 1989.

chapter Sixteen

Debridement of the Acromioclavicular Joint and Resection of the Distal Clavicle by Arthroscopy

Evan L. Flatow
Louis U. Bigliani

Resection of the distal clavicle has been reported to be a reliable treatment for acromioclavicular joint pain refractory to nonoperative management.[1–7] It is performed as an isolated procedure when the acromioclavicular joint is the only source of shoulder pain, as with osteolysis of the distal clavicle or post-traumatic acromioclavicular arthritis. More commonly, a painful acromioclavicular joint exists in combination with other conditions, such as subacromial impingement or inflammatory arthritis, so that resection of the distal clavicle is performed as part of a larger reconstructive procedure.

Since subacromial decompression is a common arthroscopic shoulder procedure, initial arthroscopic approaches to the acromioclavicular joint were often from below, via the subacromial bursa, especially when inferior protruding osteophytes on the acromioclavicular joint contributed to impingement.[8,9] However, in isolated acromioclavicular disease, there is no reason to violate the bursa. Johnson has described superior portals to the acromioclavicular joint through which the arthroscope and instruments are introduced directly into the acromioclavicular joint.[10] This superior approach allows resection of the distal clavicle under direct visualization, without the edema and bleeding of a bursal approach. Furthermore, this technique facilitates bone removal and contouring.

Clinical Indications

Simple excision of the distal clavicle is not appropriate for unstable acromioclavicular joints, such as those that are chronically dislocated. These cases are better treated with fixation of the coracoid and ligament reconstruction. Most chronic acromioclavicular disorders, for which resection of the distal clavicle might be considered, are due to osteolysis of the distal clavicle or to acromioclavicular arthritis.

Osteolysis of the distal clavicle may follow trauma to the acromioclavicular joint, especially type III intraarticular fractures of the distal clavicle and grade I or II acromioclavicular dislocations. It may also occur in association with repetitive stress (microtrauma) to the acromioclavicular joint, as in heavy weight lifting or gymnastics. Radiographs may show cysts and resorption of the distal clavicle, but the findings can be subtle (Fig. 16.1).

Acromioclavicular arthritis may cause pain directly or may contribute to impingement symptoms, if the undersurface of a hypertrophied joint diminishes the space under the coracoacromial arch.[11,12]

Acromioclavicular tenderness is the most reliable physical finding on clinical examination. Radiographs may underrepresent acromioclavicular disease.[13] Maneuvers that drive the scapula into the clavicle, especially horizontal adduction and internal rotation, compress the acromioclavicular joint and may also produce pain. Patients will often describe these positions as the ones that cause pain during functional activities (Fig. 16.2). They also have difficulty sleeping on the involved side.

Clinically, the ability of an acromioclavicular lidocaine injection to eliminate shoulder pain aids diagnosis, helps predict the possible value of surgical resection of the distal clavicle, and may be of therapeutic value if a steroid preparation is added. Multiple steroid injections should be avoided.

Most patients suffering from a tender, painful acromioclavicular joint will respond to nonoperative treatment, including heat, nonsteroidal antiinflammatory medication, activity modification, and cortisone injections. If not, resection of the distal clavicle should be considered.

Open Versus Arthroscopic Resection

Gurd[3] and Mumford[4] revived interest in open resection of the distal clavicle with their reports in 1941. Subsequent authors have consistently noted satisfactory results after this procedure for painful acromioclavicular disorders.[1,2,6,7,14,15]

Arthroscopic approaches to the acromioclavicular joint have been recently developed. Ellman[8] and Esch et al.[9] described approaching the acromioclavicular joint from the subacromial space in conjunction with arthroscopic anterior acromioplasty and resection of the coracoacromial ligament. Although this was performed primarily to remove inferior acromioclavicular osteophytes, full resection of the distal clavicle may also be performed. However, it is difficult to compare open and arthroscopic results with regard to the acromioclavicular joint when resection of the distal clavicle is performed together with acromioplasty, since it is only one portion of the reconstructive procedure.

To evaluate resection of the distal clavicle as an isolated procedure for a single diagnosis, we compared open and arthroscopic resections performed for osteolysis of the distal clavicle.[16] Bone removal was assessed by the difference between pre- and postoperative measurements

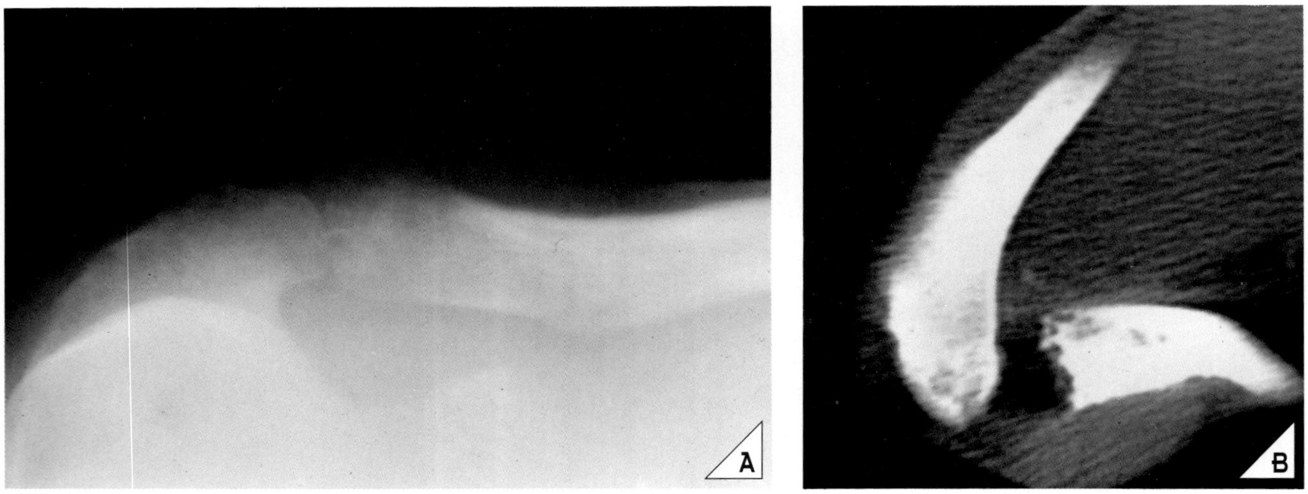

Figure 16.1
Although advanced cases of osteolysis of the distal clavicle are manifested in obvious radiographic resorption and cysts, in many cases the findings are more subtle. (A) This weight lifter with acromioclavicular pain has faint but unmistakeable cystic changes best appreciated on a cephalic tilt AP with reduced penetration (soft-tissue technique). (B) CT scans may demonstrate these findings in early cases where plain radiographs are more subtle.

of the acromioclavicular joint space on AP radiographs.[17] Bone removal averaged 18 mm in the open resections and 17 mm in the arthroscopic cases. The average hospital stay for the open procedures was 3 days. The arthroscopic procedures were performed on an outpatient basis. All patients in both groups had full return to all activities including athletics, full motion and strength, and no pain. However, full relief of pain and return to activities occurred on average 3.4 months sooner in the arthroscopic group. In the open group, two patients complained of skin numbness from transected cutaneous nerves and one patient complained of a keloid. All arthroscopic incisions healed without difficulty.

It is important to remember that these are preliminary results, and that long-term follow-up studies will be needed to fully define the arthroscopic indications. Nevertheless, it is clear that in bone removal arthroscopic procedures can achieve technical success comparable to traditional open techniques and with reduced morbidity. Pain relief and function appear comparable to that attained by open resection, with earlier return to activities and sport.

If there is significant disruption of the coracoclavicular ligaments after an acromioclavicular dislocation, an isolated resection of the distal clavicle, open or arthroscopic, should not be performed. In a chronic acromioclavicular dislocation with a damaged distal clavicular articular surface, we resect the distal clavicle in conjunction with internal fixation of the clavicle to the coracoid and reconstruction of the coracoclavicular ligaments, generally by transferring the acromial end of the coracoacromial ligament to the clavicle.[18]

SURGICAL TECHNIQUE

Arthroscopic approaches can be divided into indirect, bursal approaches[8,9,19,20] and direct approaches in which the arthroscope and instruments are inserted directly into the acromioclavicular joint.[10,16,21]

Bursal Approach

In bursal approaches, visualization and fluid flow are established in the subacromial bursa. Any soft tissue preventing visualization of the undersurface of the acromioclavicular joint is resected.[19] A 70° scope may improve the upward view of the distal clavicle.[20]

The burr is brought in anteriorly, and the distal clavicle resected. Visualization of the distal clavicle can be facilitated by manually pressing the distal clavicle down into the bursa (Fig. 16.3).[20] Alternatively, the instruments may be brought through a superior portal into the acromioclavicular joint while watching from below in the bursa.[22]

Gartsman, in a cadaveric study, demonstrated that arthroscopic distal clavicle excision from a bursal approach achieved bone removal comparable to that obtained by an open resection.[19]

Superior Approach

Superior acromioclavicular portals have been described by Johnson,[10] and allow direct visualization of the entire distal clavicular articular surface.

We began using this superior approach for arthroscopic

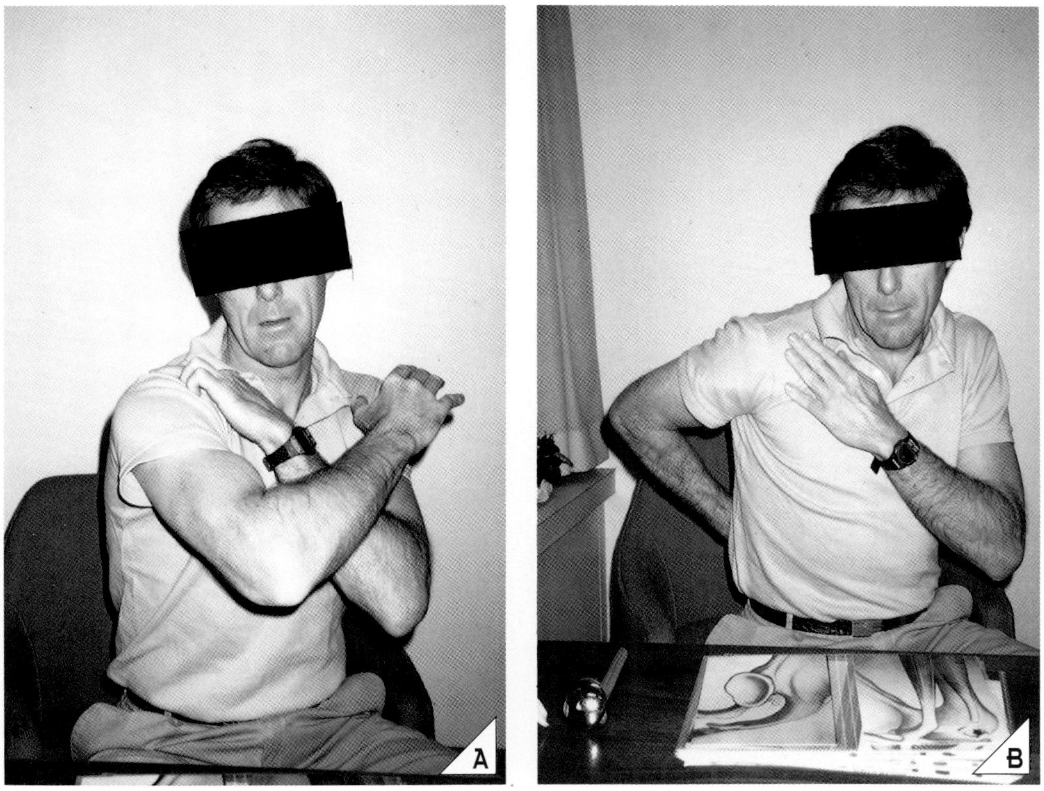

Figure 16.2
Horizontal adduction of the arm across the body drives the scapula toward the sternum, compressing the acromioclavicular joint. Patients with acromioclavicular disorders usually experience pain with this maneuver. (A) This patient is demonstrating a position he has found to be painful in his functional activities. (B) Internal rotation of the shoulder twists and compresses the acromioclavicular joint, which also produces pain, as the same patient has noticed. Although horizontal adduction and internal rotation are sensitive tests on physical examination for acromioclavicular disorders, they are not specific since other shoulder disorders, especially posterior capsular stiffness, may also produce pain with these maneuvers.

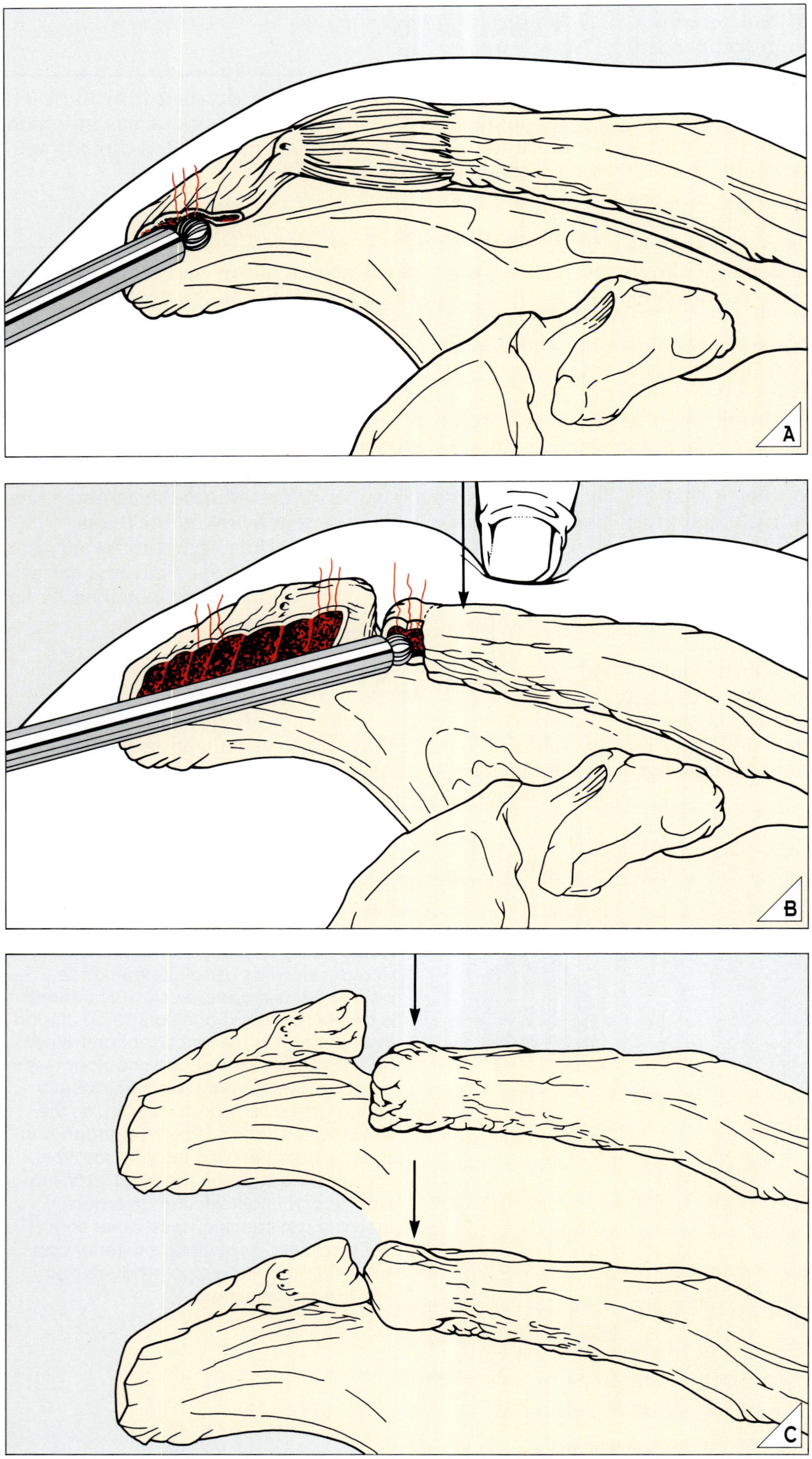

Figure 16.3
(A) A bursal approach for combined arthroscopic anterior acromioplasty and distal clavicle resection begins by thinning and flattening the acromion. If isolated resection of the distal clavicle is planned, a bursal approach may be more difficult because the intact acromion may obstruct access to the acromioclavicular joint. In addition, unnecessary bleeding and swelling will be introduced into the uninvolved bursa. (B) Visualization and resection of the distal clavicle are facilitated by manually pressing the distal clavicle down into the bursa. (C) If a tight or medially inclined distal clavicle cannot be depressed into the bursa, some authors recommend open resection.[27] An advantage of the superior approach for arthroscopic resection of the distal clavicle is that it does not depend on the specific inclination of the joint, since the inclination is determined with needles before the arthroscope and instruments are introduced in the plane of the joint. (Reproduced with permission from Meyers JF, 1991)

resection of the distal clavicle for isolated acromioclavicular disorders, such as osteolysis. It seemed logical to approach the pathology directly when other procedures in the glenohumeral joint and the subacromial space were not required. We have been pleased with the precise bone resection and contouring that direct visualization of the superior approach affords.

Regional anesthesia consisting of a scalene block is routinely employed.[23] Arthroscopy is performed in the sitting position.[24] Needles are used to determine the location and orientation of the joint (Fig. 16.4). This is critical as subtle variations in joint inclination can be difficult to appreciate.[25,26] Since the acromioclavicular joint is narrow, it is essential that the arthroscope and instruments be introduced in the plane of the joint surfaces.

The acromioclavicular joint is then insufflated with normal saline solution with 1:300,000 epinephrine added. Two portal sites are used, one anterior to the joint line and one posterior to the joint line (Fig. 16.5). One percent lidocaine with epinephrine is injected at the portal sites to reduce skin bleeding and provide comfort while the block is taking effect (see Fig. 16.5).

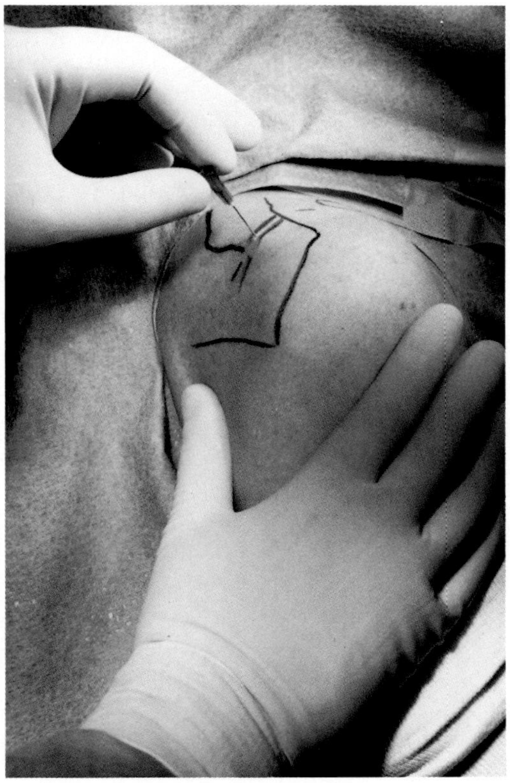

Figure 16.4
Needles (22-gauge 1.5 inch) are used to locate the acromioclavicular joint and determine its anteroposterior direction and its superior-inferior obliquity. This is a key step if proper introduction of instruments is to be accomplished.

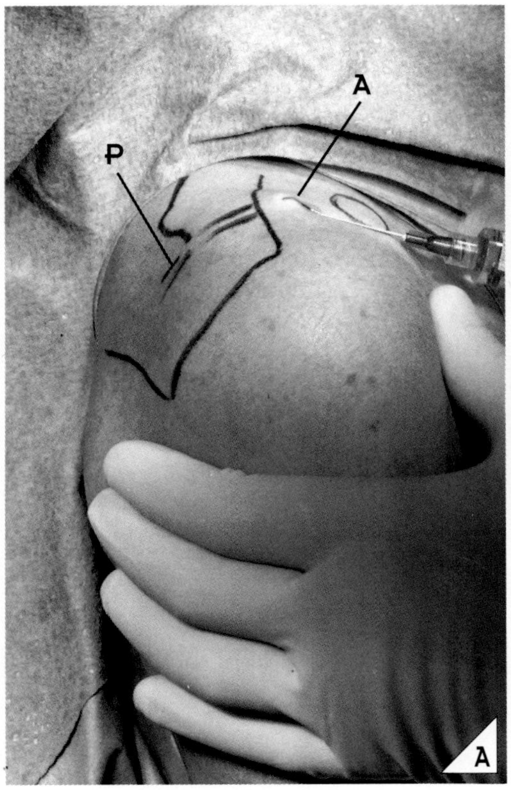

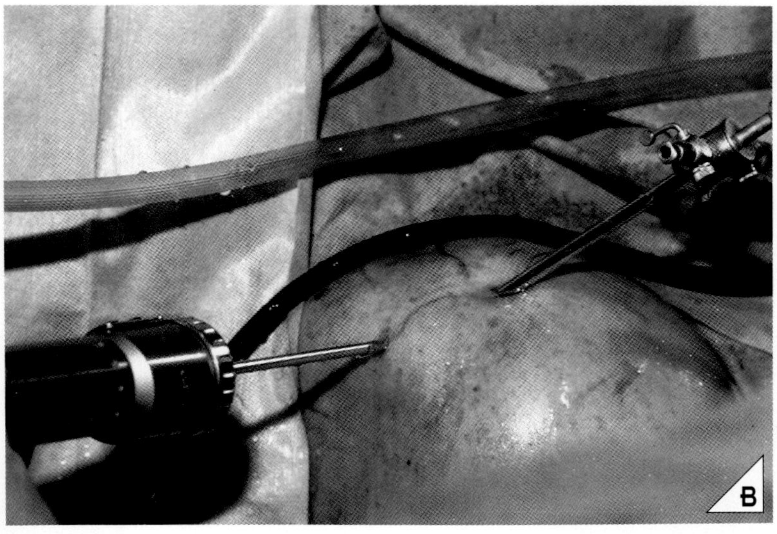

Figure 16.5
(A) Two portals are created, one just anterior (A) to the acromioclavicular joint and one just posterior (P). The portal sites are infiltrated with 1% lidocaine with epinephrine to reduce skin bleeding and provide comfort while the scalene block is taking full effect. (B) Since the arthroscope and motorized instruments are brought in at an angle, the anterior portal should be about 5 mm anterior to the anterosuperior edge of the acromioclavicular joint and the posterior portal about 5 mm posterior to the posterosuperior edge.

Initially a 2.7 mm wrist arthroscopy unit is used until adequate space is present for a standard 4.0 mm arthroscope. Normal saline with 1:300,000 epinephrine added is used for irrigation. Complete synovectomy is performed using a full radius resector (Fig. 16.6). A curette or rasp is then used to clean soft tissue and any remaining cartilage from the articular surface of the distal clavicle.

An electrocautery unit is used to shell out the distal clavicle, so the tube of soft tissue containing the acromioclavicular ligaments and the capsule are preserved (Fig. 16.7). It is also available to coagulate small bleeders if they occur. A small 2.0 mm burr is used to initiate bone resection, followed by larger 3.5 and 4.5 mm burrs (Fig. 16.8). The burr is switched from anterior to posterior portals to adequately remove bone under direct visualization. The final bevelling is performed with rasps. At the conclusion of the procedure, the joint is carefully examined with the arthroscope from both the anterior and posterior portals to insure that removal of bone is adequate and to check for loose fragments of bone or cartilage. It is essential to probe the edges to be sure that no overhanging ridges remain. This direct approach affords excellent visualization for such final "sculpting". After the instruments have been withdrawn, 0.25% Marcaine without epinephrine is injected into the joint to aid in postoperative comfort. The portal sites are closed with resorbable sutures in a subcuticular fashion.

Rehabilitation consists of immediate passive exercises, with active exercises beginning as soon as postoperative discomfort resolves, usually 3 to 5 days following the procedure. A sling is employed for comfort for only 1 to 2 days postoperatively.

Bursal Versus Superior Approach

The superior approach is ideal for arthroscopic resection of the distal clavicle in patients with isolated acromioclavicular disorders, such as osteolysis. These patients generally have complete though temporary relief of symptoms with a preoperative anaesthetic acromioclavicular injection, and it seems logical to confine the procedure to the clear source of symptoms. Because the pathology is approached directly, hemorrhage and swelling are not introduced into uninvolved subacromial bursa, reducing

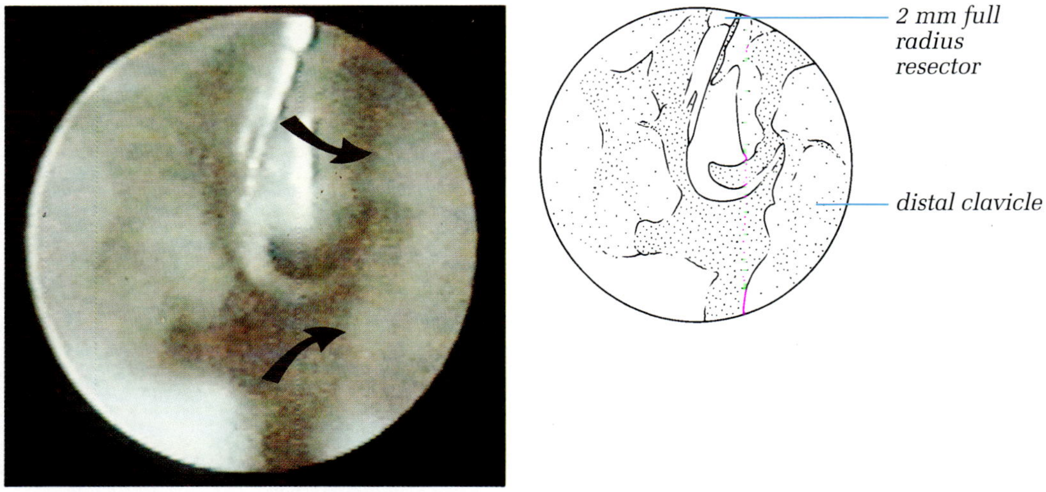

Figure 16.6 Initial view of a left acromioclavicular joint with a 2 mm arthroscope introduced through a posterosuperior portal. The distal clavicle is to the right (arrows). A 2 mm full radius resector has just been introduced from the anterosuperior portal.

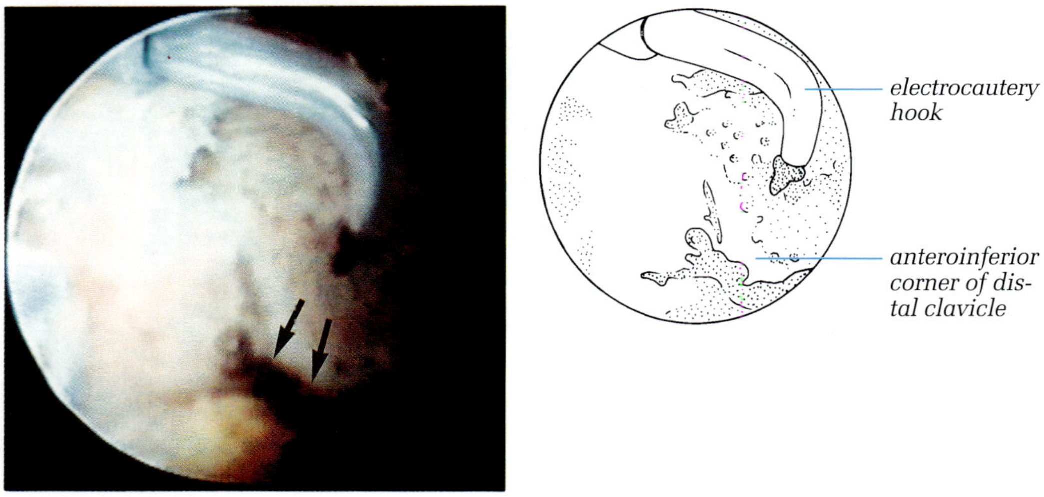

Figure 16.7 Initial bone resection widened this left acromioclavicular joint so a 4 mm arthroscope could be introduced from the posterosuperior portal. In order to avoid hollowing out the bone, which leaves shelves and ridges attached to the capsule and periosteum, the electrocautery has "shelled out" the bone (arrows: the anteroinferior rim of the distal clavicle), leaving a tube of intact soft tissues.

postoperative morbidity and allowing earlier return to sports and activities.

The majority of patients undergoing acromioplasty require at most an undersurface trimming of prominent inferior acromioclavicular osteophytes.[12] In cases with preoperative acromioclavicular pain and tenderness, complete resection of the distal clavicle at the time of acromioplasty is recommended. When resection of the distal clavicle is performed arthroscopically along with an arthroscopic acromioplasty, the superior approach may be preferable because time is not limited by additional swelling from a bursal approach to the distal clavicle. Also, precise contouring is more easily performed with the direct visualization afforded. The advantage of a combined bursal approach is that the two additional AC portals are not needed.

Acromioclavicular joints that are tight and inclined medially can not be easily depressed into the bursa and some surgeons, favoring a bursal approach, recommend open excision.[20] The superior approach, which does not require depression of the distal clavicle into the bursa, may be used in such cases.

Our first 15 cases of arthroscopic distal clavicle excision from a superior approach were followed for 12 to 30 months (average 18 months).[21] There results were: eight excellent, five good, one fair, and one poor. The poor result was due to inadequate bone resection early in our learning curve. Patients returned to full activity at an average of 8 weeks.

Degree of Bone Removal

Failure of open distal clavicle excision, because of abutment by the stump of the distal clavicle on the acromion with arm motion has been reported.[27] While it has been suggested that this may be due to inadequate bone removal, we have found that the relative motion between the distal clavicle and acromion may be a result of disruption of the ligaments by an open resection. The acromioclavicular ligaments are the prime restraints to anteroposterior motion, and the trapezoid ligament is the prime restraint against compression of the distal clavicle into the acromion.[28] Open resection of the distal clavicle may damage both of these ligament systems.

However, arthroscopic removal leaves both the coracoclavicular and acromioclavicular ligaments intact, preserving joint stability. We have noticed under arthroscopic visualization that only a "minimal" resection (4 to 5 mm) is needed to produce a space that will be maintained during range of motion of the arm, if the resection is even

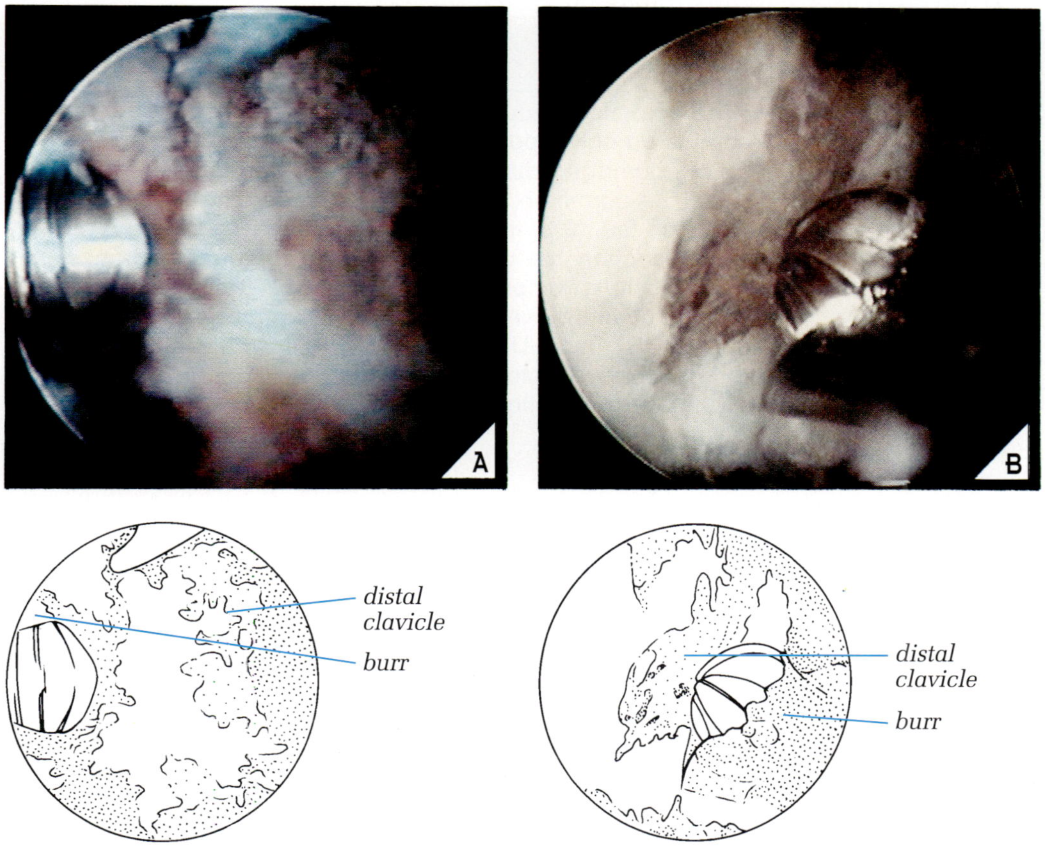

Figure 16.8
(A) A burr has been brought from the anterosuperior portal to further resect and sculpt the distal clavicle. The arthroscope has been moved to the anterosuperior portal. (B) The burr, now brought from the posterosuperior portal, is being used to resect the posteroinferior corner of the distal clavicle.

(Fig. 16.9), and we now routinely remove only this amount of bone (Fig. 16.10). Regrowth of bone has not been seen, but longer follow up will be needed to confirm this.

Complications and Pitfalls

It is important that burring be initiated with the burr in the acromioclavicular joint under direct visualization. If the burr is brought up from below toward the clavicle without clear visualization, a false channel may be cut in the clavicle, leaving a portion of the distal clavicle unresected. This may be avoided by starting the burr on the articular surface of the distal clavicle and progessing medially.

Retained ridges and corners may spoil the result. If attention is focused solely on the accessible central portion of the distal clavicle, burring may produce a central "valley", leaving behind a shell of the cortical bone on the periphery. Unlike the bleeding cancellous bone at the center, the white cortical margin may be confused with the attached soft tissues. Clear visualization of all four corners, combined with subperiosteal exposure of the entire rim with electrocautery, prevents such uneven resections.

Simple resections of the distal clavicle—either open or arthroscopic—require intact ligaments. Grade III acromioclavicular joint separation, when treated surgically, requires ligament reconstruction. However, even lesser degrees of instability may predispose to the failure of simple resection. In our current experience with 42 shoulders undergoing arthroscopic resection of the distal clavicle followed an average of 21 months, 31 of 34 (91%) patients with stable acromioclavicular joints had satisfactory results compared to only 3 of 8 (37%) patients with prior grade II acromioclavicular separations (unpublished data). So far, we have not seen clinical failure due to regrowth of bone or infection.

Future Directions

Operative treatment for painful acromioclavicular disorders has generally been complete excision of the distal clavicle. However, Taylor and Tooke[29] noted good results with meniscectomy and curettage of the cartilaginous end plates to raw, bleeding bone. Because of the poor correlation between radiographs and the extent of acromioclavicular disease and symptoms, it has been difficult to ascertain whether less than complete excision might be adequate in selected cases.

As information on soft tissue pathology is gained through direct arthroscopic visualization of the synovium, meniscus, and articular cartilage of painful acromioclavicular joints, a role for joint debridement without bone removal may be found.

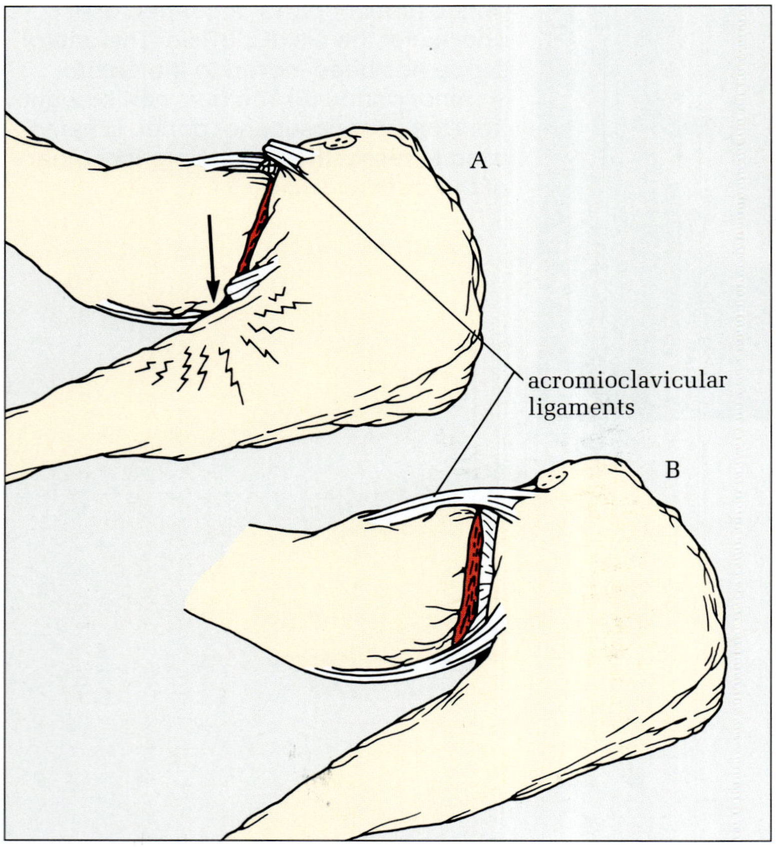

Figure 16.9

(A) The acromioclavicular ligaments and capsule are the prime restraints on anteroposterior motion of the distal clavicle. If they are damaged during open resection, the clavicle may hit against the acromion, even though a large amount of bone has been removed. (B) If the ligaments are preserved during arthroscopic resection, the clavicle will not touch the acromion, even though a smaller amount of bone has been removed, as long as the resection is even. (Reproduced with permission from Flatow EL, Bigliani LU. Arthroscopic acromioclavicular joint debridement and distal clavicle resection. Operative Techniques in Orthopaedics. Philadelphia, Pa: WB Saunders Co; 1992)

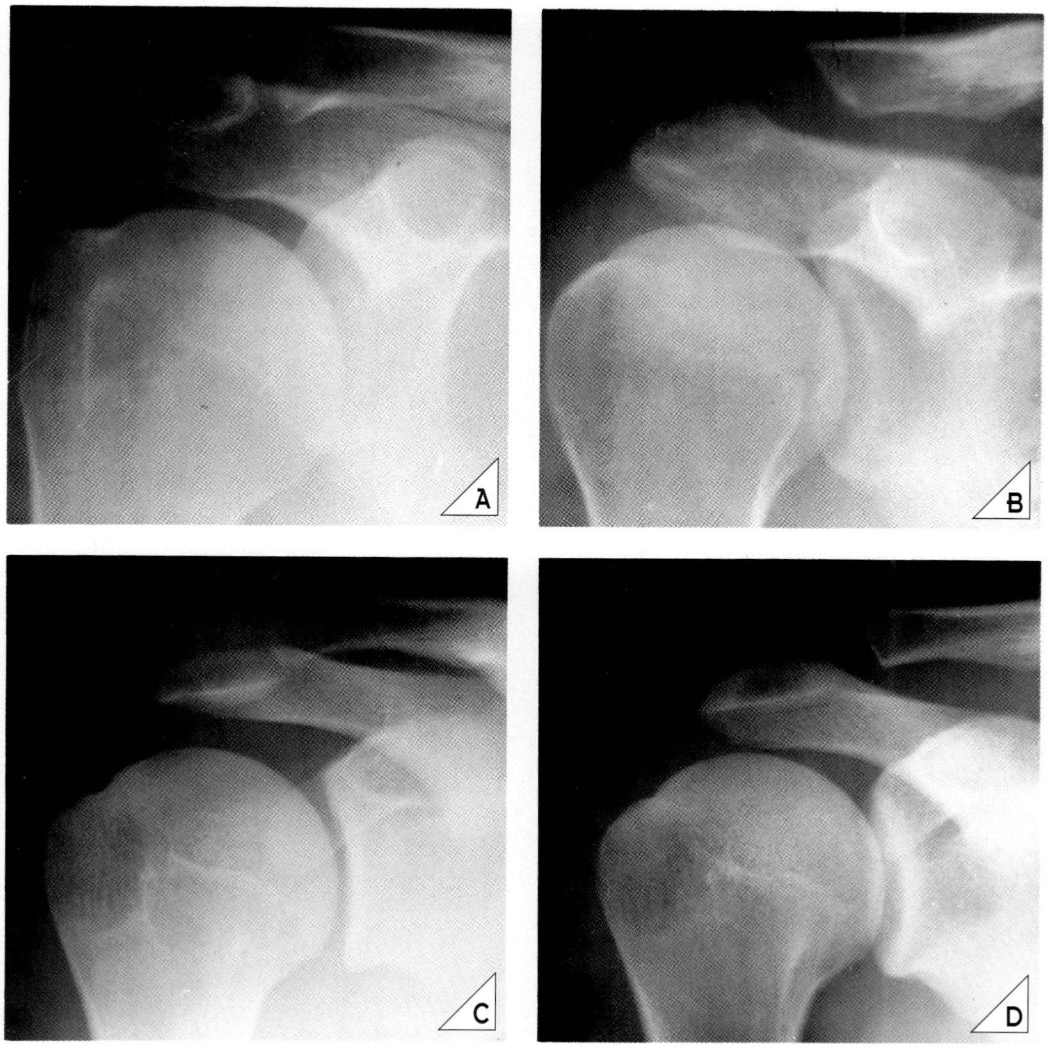

Figure 16.10

When we began performing arthroscopic distal clavicle excisions through a superior approach, we removed a generous amount of bone, as seen on these preoperative (A) and postoperative (B) radiographs of a patient early in our series. We now aim for a "minimal" but even resection of about 5 mm of bone, as shown on these preoperative (C) and postoperative (D) radiographs.

REFERENCES

1. Cook FF, Tibone JE. The Mumford procedure in athletes: an objective analysis of function. *Am J Sports Med.* 1988; 16:97–100.
2. Grimes DW, Garner RW. The degeneration of the acromioclavicular joint. treatment by resection of the distal clavicle. *Orthop Rev.* 1980;9:41–44.
3. Gurd FB. The treatment of complete dislocation of the outer end of the clavicle: a hitherto undescribed operation. *Ann Surg.* 1941;63:1094.
4. Mumford EB. Acromioclavicular dislocation: a new operative treatment. *J Bone Joint Surg.* 1941;23:799–801.
5. Petersson C. Resection of the lateral end of the clavicle: a 3 to 30-year follow-up. *Acta Orthop Scand.* 1983;54:904–907.
6. Wagner CJ. Partial claviculectomy. *Am J Surg.* 1953;85: 259–265.
7. Worcestor JN, Green DP. Osteoarthritis of the acromioclavicular joint. *Clin Orthop.* 1968;58:69–73.
8. Ellman H. Arthroscopic subacromial decompression: analysis of one- to three-year results. *Arthroscopy.* 1987;3: 173–181.
9. Esch JC, Ozerkis LR, Helgager JA, et al. Arthroscopic subacromial decompression: results according to the degree of rotator cuff tear. *Arthroscopy.* 1988;4:241–249.
10. Johnson LL. *Diagnostic and Surgical Arthroscopy.* St. Louis, Mo: CV Mosby; 1981.
11. Kessel L, Watson M. The painful arc syndrome: clinical classification as a guide to management. *J Bone Joint Surg.* 1977;59B:166–172.
12. Neer CS II. Impingement lesions. *Clin Orthop.* 1983;73:70–77.
13. Stenlund B, Marions O, Engstrom KF, et al. Correlation of macroscopic osteoarthrotic changes and radiographic findings in the acromioclavicular joint. *Acta Radiol.* 1988;29: 571–576.
14. Cahill BR. Osteolysis of the distal part of the clavicle in male athletes. *J Bone Joint Surg.* 1982;64A:1053–1058.
15. Murphy OB, Bellamy R, Wheeler W, et al. Post-traumatic osteolysis of the distal clavicle. *Clin Orthop.* 1975;109: 108–114.
16. Flatow EL, Cordasco FA, Bigliani LU. Arthroscopic resection of the outer end of the clavicle from a superior approach: a critical, quantitative, radiographic assessment of bone removal. *Arthroscopy.* 1992;8:55–64.
17. Petersson CJ, Redlund-Johnell I. Radiographic joint space in normal acromioclavicular joints. *Acta Orthop Scand.* 1983;54:431–433.
18. Weaver JK, Dunn HK. Treatment of acromioclavicular injuries, especially complete acromioclavicular separation. *J Bone Joint Surg.* 1972;54A:1187–1194.
19. Gartsman GM, Combs AH, Davis PF, Tullos HS. Arthroscopic acromioclavicular joint resection an anatomical study. *Am J Sports Med.* 1991;19:2–5.
20. Meyers JF. Arthroscopic debridement of the acromioclavicular joint and distal clavicle resection. In: McGinty JB, Caspari RB, Jackson RW, et al, eds. *Operative Arthroscopy.* New York, NY: Raven Press; 1991:557–560.

21. Flatow EL, Cordasco FA, Bigliani LU. Arthroscopic resection of the distal clavicle from a superior approach. Scientific Exhibit at the American Academy of Orthopaedic Surgeons, Fifty-Eighth Annual Meeting; March, 1991; Anaheim, Calif.
22. Snyder SJ. Arthroscopic acromioclavicular joint debridement and distal clavicle resection. *Tech Orthop.* 1988;3: 41–45.
23. Bigliani LU, Flatow EL, Weiss RA, et al. Interscalene block for shoulder arthroscopy: comparison with general anaesthesia. Presented at the Arthroscopy Association of North America; April, 1991; San Diego, Calif.
24. Skyhar MJ, Altchek DW, Warren RF, et al. Shoulder arthroscopy with the patient in the beach-chair position. *Arthroscopy.* 1988;4:256–259.
25. DePalma AF. *Surgery of the Shoulder.* Philadelphia, Pa: JB Lippincott; 1950.
26. Urist MR. Complete dislocations of the acromioclavicular joint. The nature of the traumatic lesion and effective methods of treatment with an analysis of forty-one cases. *J Bone Joint Surg.* 1946;28:813–837.
27. Rockwood CA Jr. Disorders of the acromioclavicular joint. In: Rockwood CA Jr, Matsen FA III, eds. *The Shoulder.* Philadelphia, Pa: WB Saunders Co; 1985: 449.
28. Fukuda K, Craig EV, An K-N, et al. Biomechanical study of the ligamentous system of the acromioclavicular joint. *J Bone Joint Surg.* 1986;68A:434–439.
29. Taylor GM, Tooke M. Degeneration of the acromioclavicular joint as a cause of shoulder pain. *J Bone Joint Surg.* 1977; 59B:507.

Section Three

The Ankle

chapter Seventeen

Techniques for Soft Tissue and Osteochondral Lesions

J. Serge Parisien

The arthroscope is a valuable tool in the management of many ankle disorders.[1–6] Arthroscopic surgery of the ankle is indicated for soft tissue disorders and osteochondral lesions. Less commonly, it is used to correct lateral instability and tibiotalar arthrodesis. Recent advances in miniature instrumentation facilitate the numerous arthroscopic surgical procedures, lessening the morbidity rate and enabling a more rapid, functional recovery for the patient than is possible with nonarthroscopic surgery.

INSTRUMENTATION

The following instruments are used for techniques related to soft tissue and osteochondral lesions:

- Video arthroscopes 25° to 30° oblique, 4 mm or 2.7 mm (Fig. 17.1)
- 70° arthroscope (see Fig. 17.1)
- Small motorized instruments (shavers and abraders) (Fig. 17.2)
- Hand instruments (various knives, basket forceps, scissors, rasps, curettes, grasping forceps, and pins) (Figs. 17.3–17.5)
- Gravity system or infusion pump for constant irrigation.

Distraction by mechanical means has been advocated by some surgeons not only to facilitate visualization but also to prevent scuffing of the articular cartilage (Fig. 17.6). However, some arthroscopists feel strongly that because of potential complications, mechanical distraction should only be reserved for selected cases, inasmuch as most lesions amenable to arthroscopic surgery are localized in areas readily accessible to arthroscopic instrumentation. Regardless of the controversy, there is no need for mechanical distraction in loose ankles, and its use is contraindicated in open epiphysis, reflex sympathetic dystrophy, and pyarthrosis.

PREOPERATIVE PREPARATION

General or regional anesthesia is used with a tourniquet applied on the thigh.

Choice of patient position is at the discretion of the surgeon. The patient can be placed in the supine position with a sandbag supporting the buttock on the operative side as suggested by Guhl.[3] A thigh holder to secure the knee in about 60° of flexion and an ankle holder to stabilize the ankle allow ready access to anterior and posterior portals (Fig. 17.7). The patient can also be placed in a

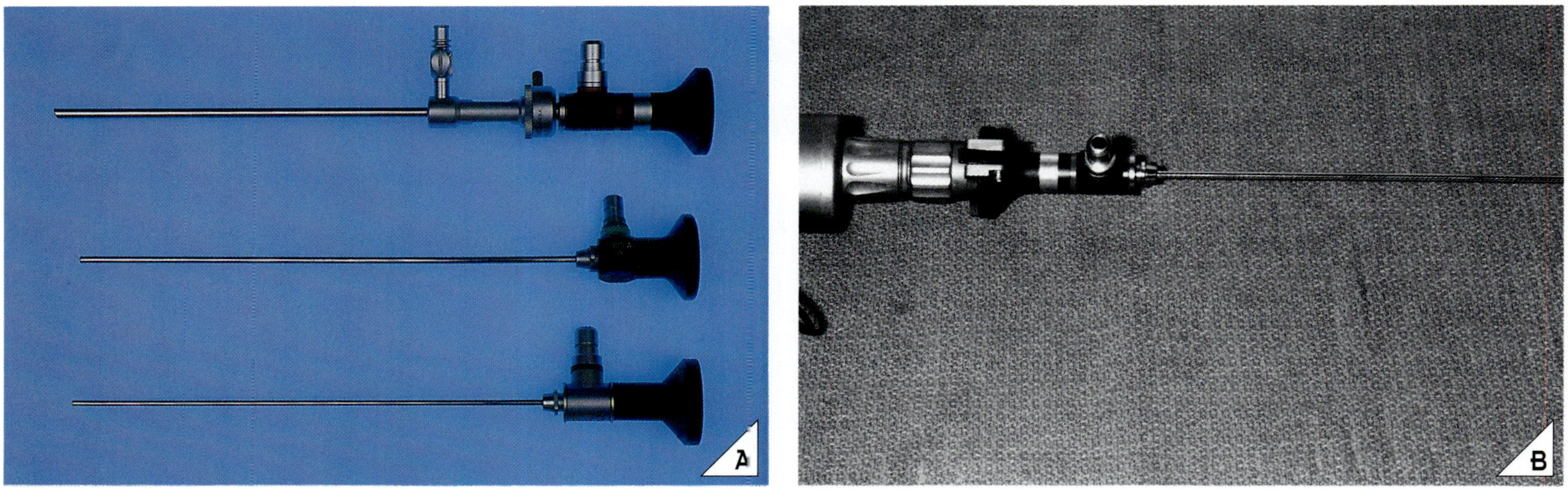

Figure 17.1

(A) Two 4 mm arthroscopes with 25° and 70° angulation and 2.7 mm arthroscope with 25° angulation. (B) Arthroscope with video camera.

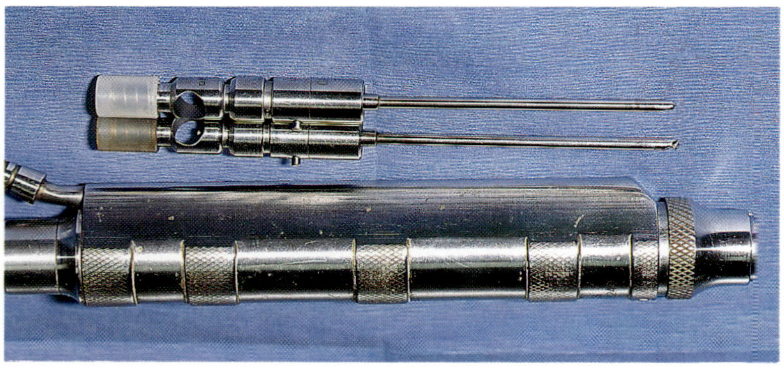

Figure 17.2

Motorized 2.8 mm resector and abrader.

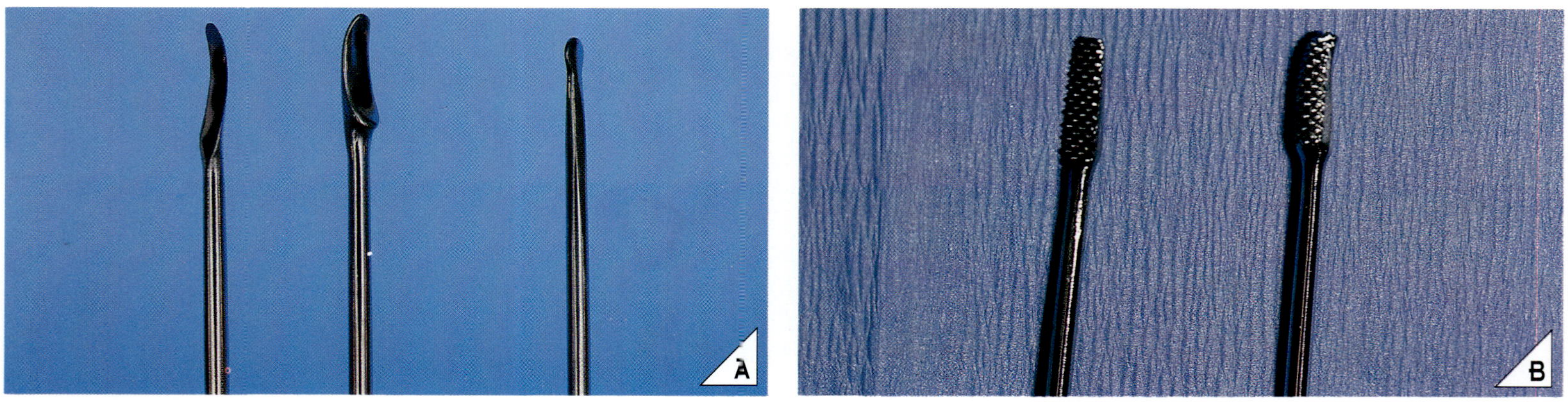

Figure 17.3

From left to right—knife, elevator, and probe (A) and small rasps (B) for ankle arthroscopic surgery.

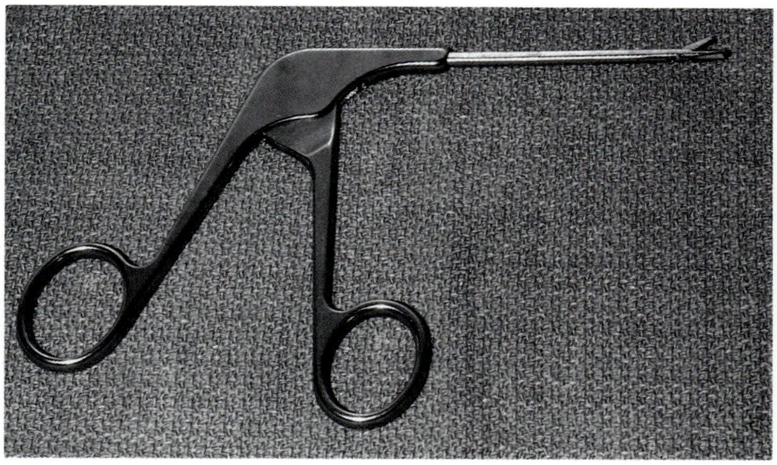

Figure 17.4
Basket forceps.

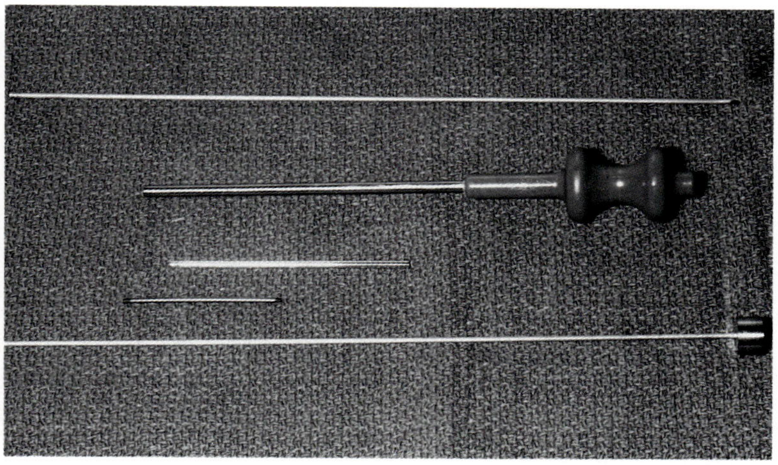

Figure 17.5
Biodegradable pin instrumentation.

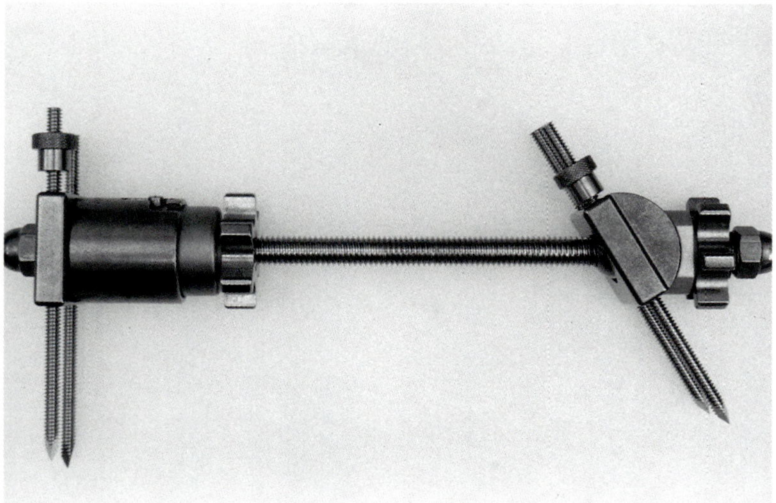

Figure 17.6
Mechanical distractor.

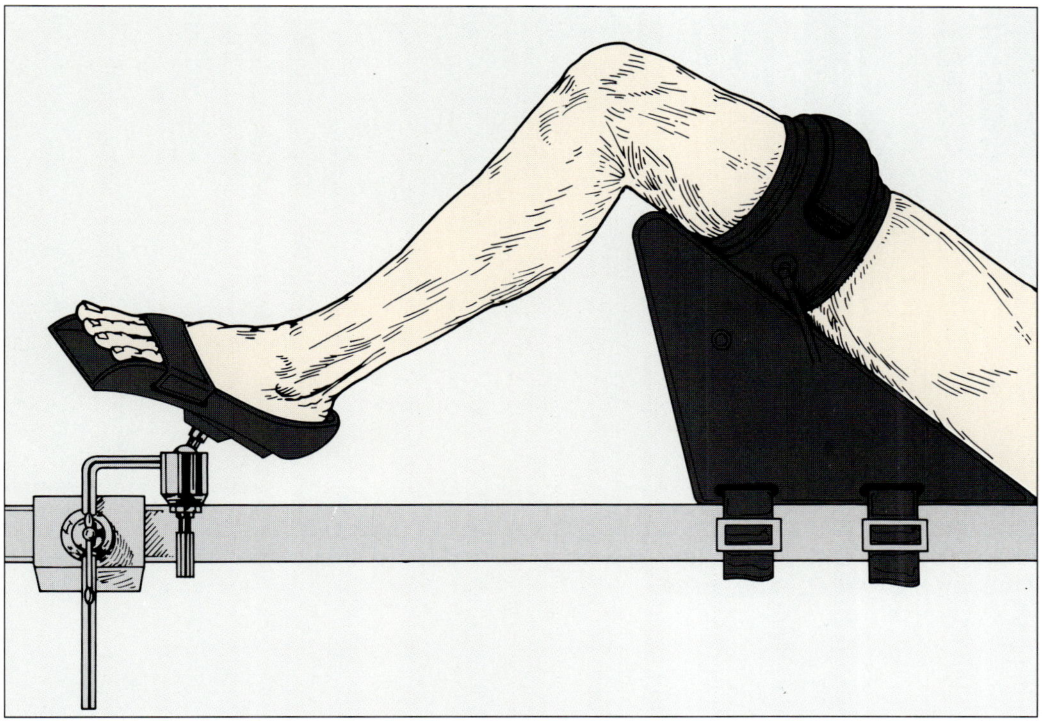

Figure 17.7
Surgical position of the patient. The knee and hip are flexed, and the foot is held in the plantigrade position in an ankle holder. (Modified from Guhl, 1988)

semisupine position with the leg elevated on a bolster and immobilized in a leg holder. Rotation of the lower extremity at the hip area allows easy access to the posterolateral aspect of the ankle (Fig. 17.8).

ANATOMY AND PORTALS

Knowledge of the extraarticular anatomy is important in order to prevent injury to the neurovascular and tendinous structures of the ankle. There are three anterior portals (Fig. 17.9A): anteromedial (medial to the anterior tibial tendon), anterolateral (lateral to the peroneus tertius tendon), and anterocentral. The anterocentral portal is not recommended because of its close proximity to the dorsalis pedis artery and the deep branch of the peroneal nerve.

Posteriorly, the posterolateral and the posteromedial portals, lateral and medial to the Achilles tendon respectively, are available (Fig. 17.9B). The posterolateral, which is approximately 1 inch proximal to the tip of the lateral malleolus, is used most often. The posteromedial portal, because of its proximity to the posterior tibial neurovascular bundle, is used with great caution.

SOFT TISSUE LESIONS OF THE ANKLE

The most common form of soft tissue pathology managed arthroscopically is soft tissue impingement. It can be present anterolaterally, anteromedially, or even posterolaterally. It is usually secondary to inversion injuries of the ankle and can be responsible for chronic ankle pain.

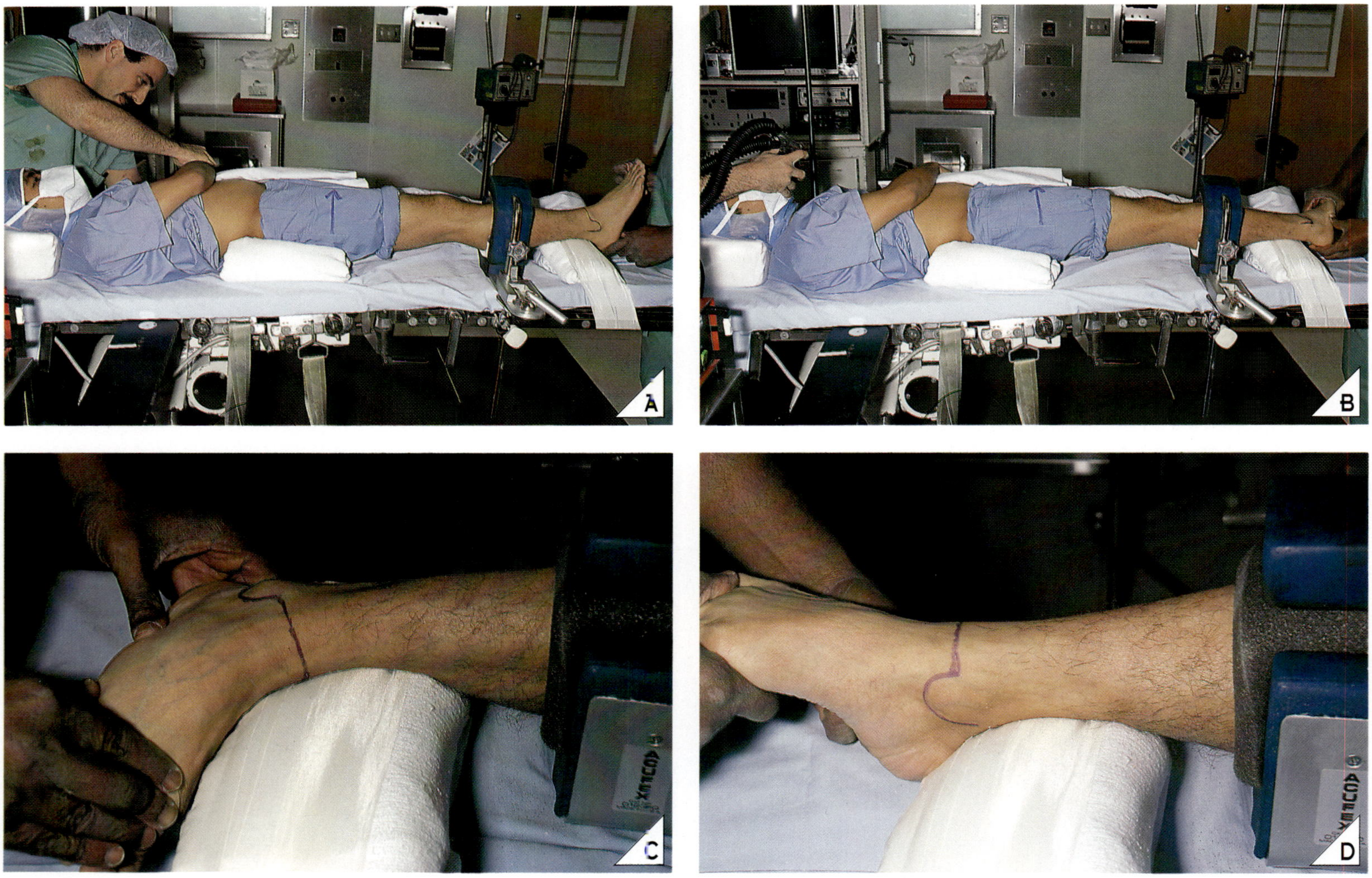

Figure 17.8
(A, B) Semisupine position. The leg is elevated on a bolster and immobilized in a leg holder. (C, D) Rotation of the lower extremity at the hip area gives access to the posterolateral aspect of the ankle.

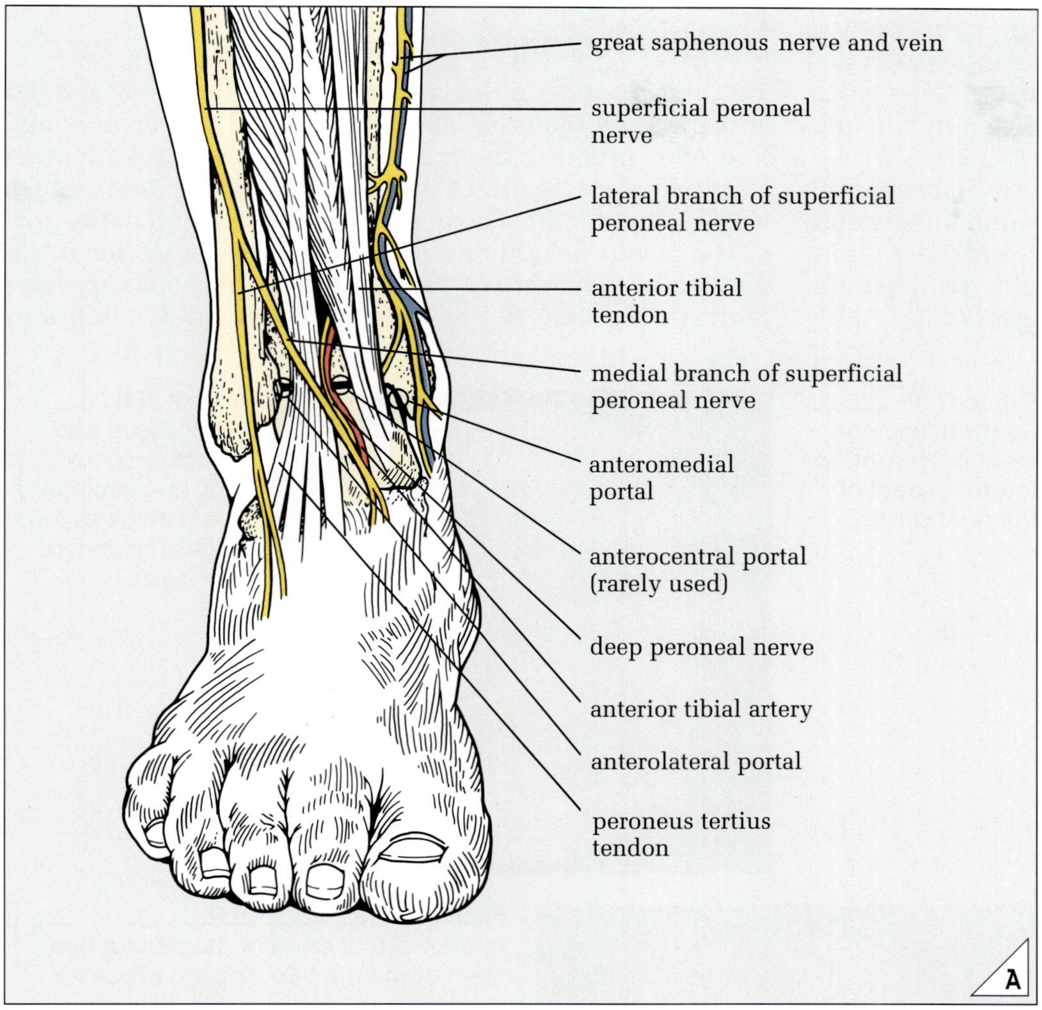

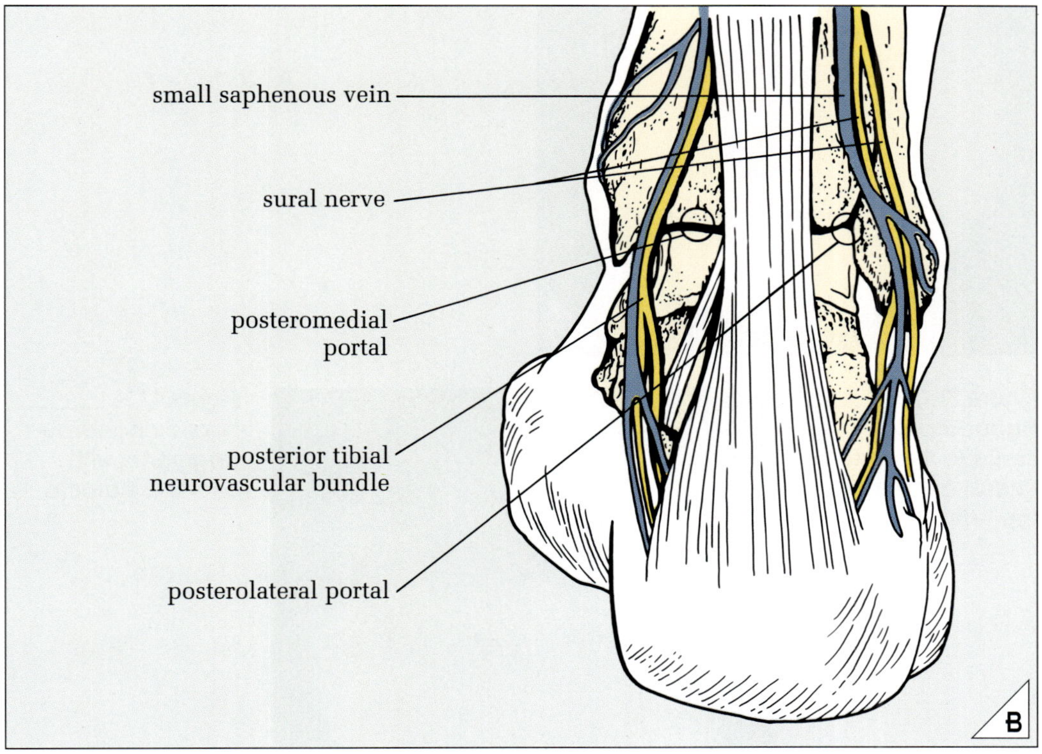

Figure 17.9
Recommended anterior (A) and posterior (B) portals.

Anterolateral soft tissue impingement is composed of entrapped, partially torn collateral ligaments associated with scar tissue and a reactive inflamed synovitis (Figs. 17.10, 17.11). Impingement can also be caused by the inferior slip of the tibiofibular ligament (Fig. 17.12).

Other soft tissue lesions amenable to arthroscopic surgery are adhesion formation, some rheumatologic conditions such as posttraumatic synovitis, synovial chondromatosis, pigmented villonodular synovitis, rheumatoid arthritis, and infectious synovitis (Figs. 17.13, 17.14).

Surgical Technique

Two portals are routinely established—the anteromedial and the anterolateral. The anteromedial portal is made first after inflating the anterior capsule of the joint with approximately 20 mL of normal saline using an 18-gauge needle (Fig. 17.15). The needle is removed, and at the area of the needle insertion a skin incision is made for introduction of the arthroscopic cannula with its smooth obturator, taking care not to injure the saphenous vein and

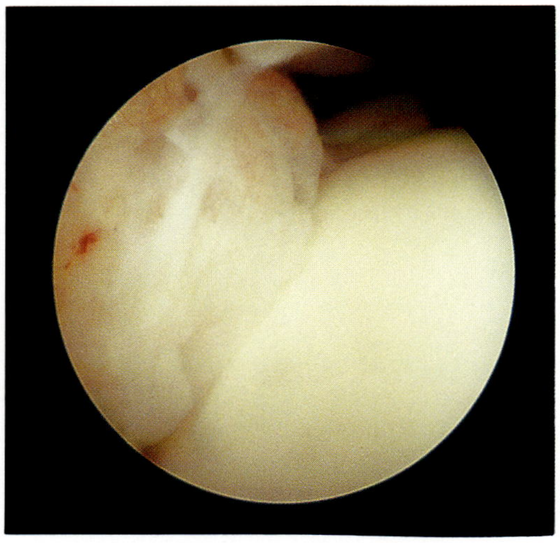

Figure 17.10 Synovial impingement of the anterolateral aspect of the right ankle.

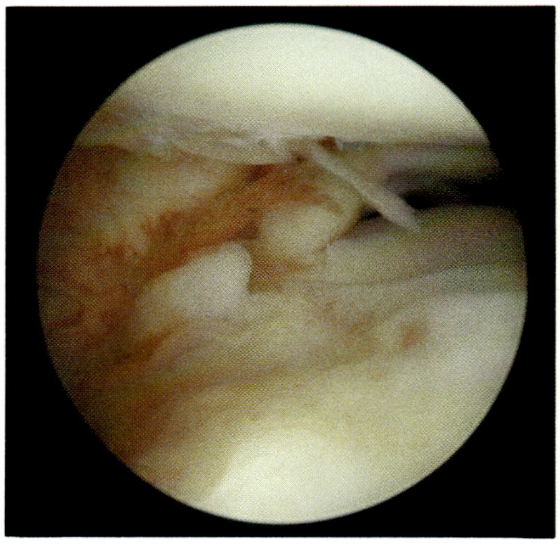

Figure 17.11 Scar tissue and reactive synovitis causing impingement in the anterolateral aspect of the ankle.

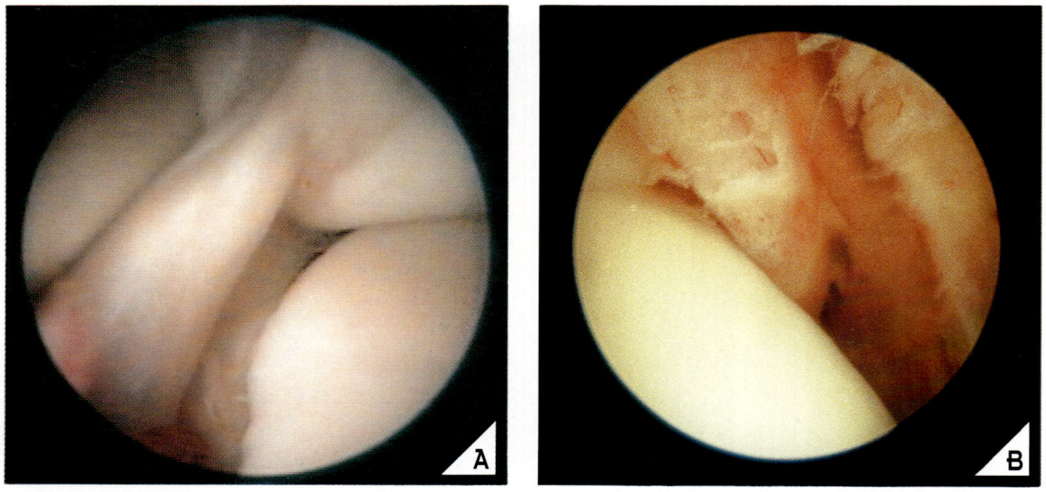

Figure 17.12 Inferior slip of anterior tibiofibular ligament of the right (A) and left (B) ankle.

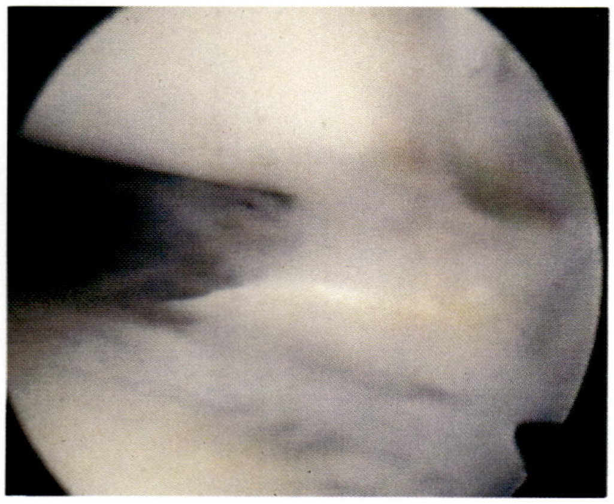

Figure 17.13 Hypertrophic scar tissue in the anterolateral aspect of the left ankle.

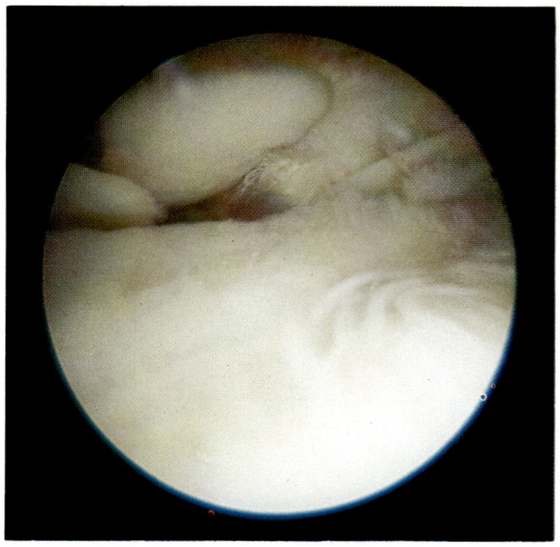

Figure 17.14 Loose chondral fragments with chondromalacia.

nerve (Fig. 17.16). The anterolateral portal is created through the anteromedial portal using a percutaneous spinal needle from the lateral aspect of the ankle under direct visualization or by tenting the skin of the lateral aspect of the ankle with the smooth obturator of the arthroscopic cannula. The branches of the superficial peroneal nerve should be identified before making the skin incision lateral to the peroneus tertius tendon (Fig. 17.17A). Constant irrigation with a gravity system is established. An infusion pump can also be used instead of a gravity system, making an accessory portal mandatory (Fig. 17.17B,C).

The ankle is methodically examined by visualizing the synovial pouch anteriorly over the talus, the small synovial recess above the anterior edge of the tibial plafond,

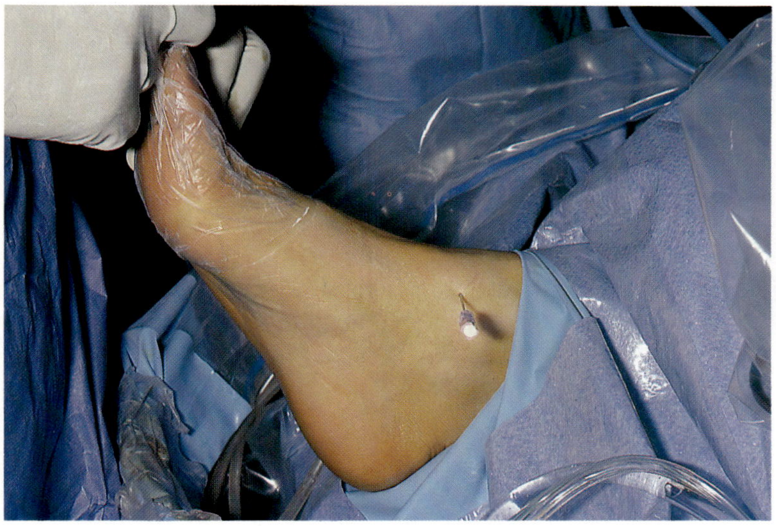

Figure 17.15

The spinal needle is placed medial to the tibialis anticus tendon of the right ankle to inflate the joint cavity with 30 mL of normal saline.

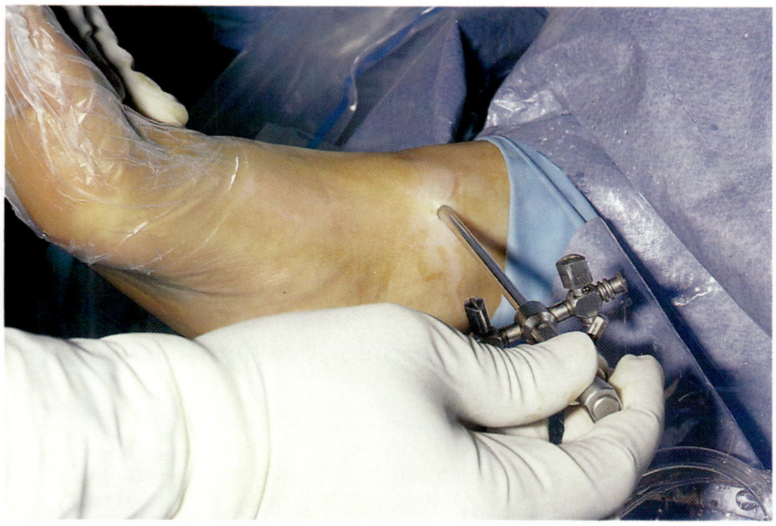

Figure 17.16

Placement of trocar for the 4 mm 25° arthroscope.

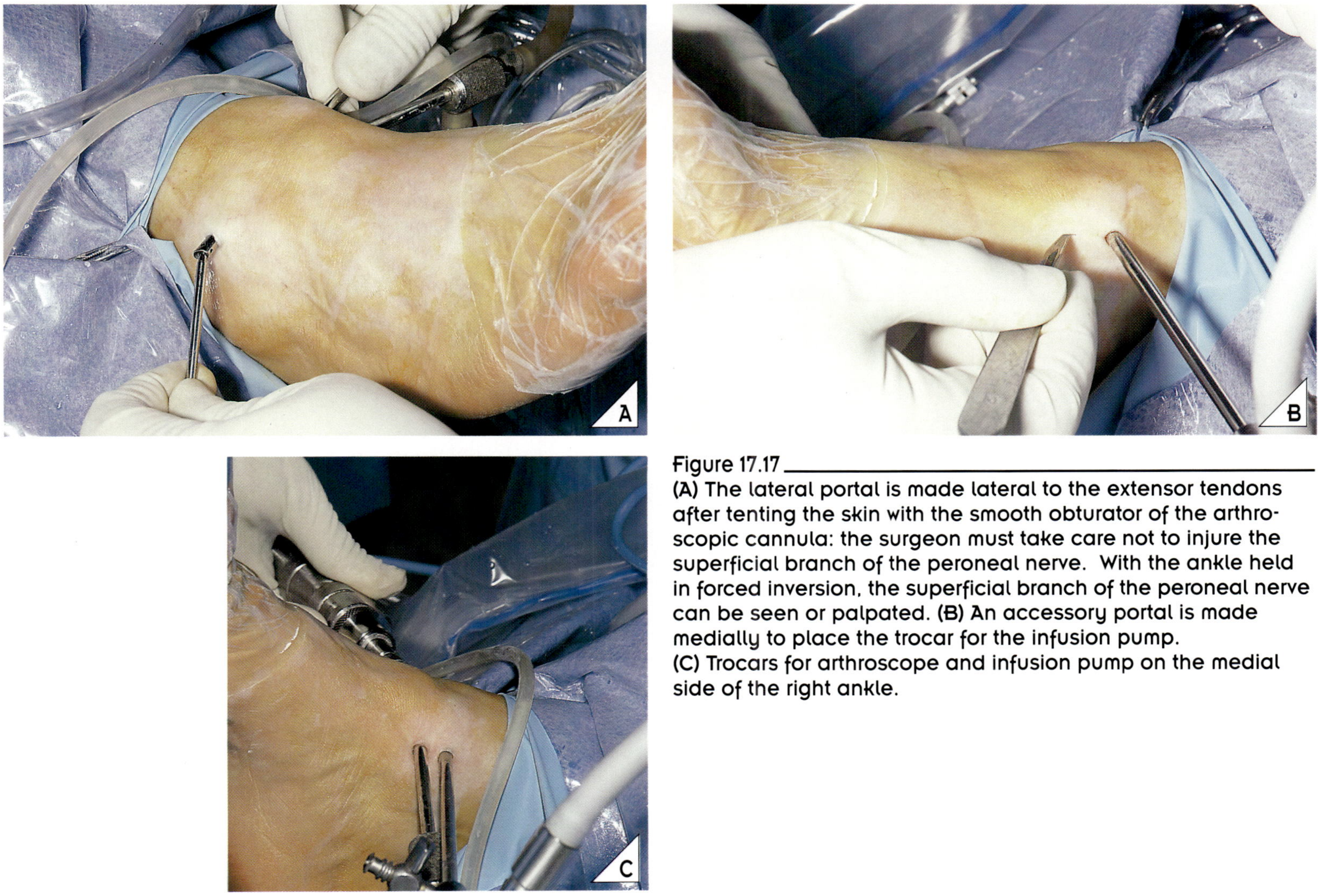

Figure 17.17

(A) The lateral portal is made lateral to the extensor tendons after tenting the skin with the smooth obturator of the arthroscopic cannula: the surgeon must take care not to injure the superficial branch of the peroneal nerve. With the ankle held in forced inversion, the superficial branch of the peroneal nerve can be seen or palpated. (B) An accessory portal is made medially to place the trocar for the infusion pump.
(C) Trocars for arthroscope and infusion pump on the medial side of the right ankle.

the articular cartilage of the talus and tibial plafond, the medial talomalleolar space, and the lateral talomalleolar space. Structures such as the anterior talofibular ligament should be visualized on the lateral aspect of the ankle (Fig. 17.18A). With the arthroscope placed through the anterolateral portal, the posterior talofibular ligament can be easily visualized. When the ankle is loose, manual distraction will facilitate visualization of the posterior aspect of the talocrural joint as well as the transverse tibiofibular ligament (Fig. 17.18B). If necessary, a posterolateral portal can also be used for visualization of the posterior aspect of the joint.

Power instruments in combination with basket forceps or scissors are the only instruments needed for arthroscopic surgery of soft tissue lesions of the ankle (Figs. 17.19, 17.20). A switch of portal is always necessary. As a rule, the surgical instruments are placed on the side of the lesion and the arthroscope is placed into the opposite portal. If the soft tissue lesion is associated with articular cartilage damage, chondroplasty can be performed at the same time.

Postoperative Management

The portals are closed with single sutures, and a compression dressing is applied. Patients are allowed to bear weight as soon as tolerated and encouraged to start range-of-motion exercises as soon as possible. Stitches are removed within 1 week and rehabilitation under supervision can be started when the presenting symptoms are loss of proprioception, laxity, and instability.

Osteochondral Lesions of the Ankle

Osteochondral lesions amenable to arthroscopic surgery of the ankle can be divided into the following categories: transchondral fractures or osteochondritis dissecans of the dome of the talus, loose bodies, impingement exostoses, chondral and osteochondral lesions of the tibial plafond and talomalleolar areas, and degenerative and posttraumatic arthritis of the ankle.

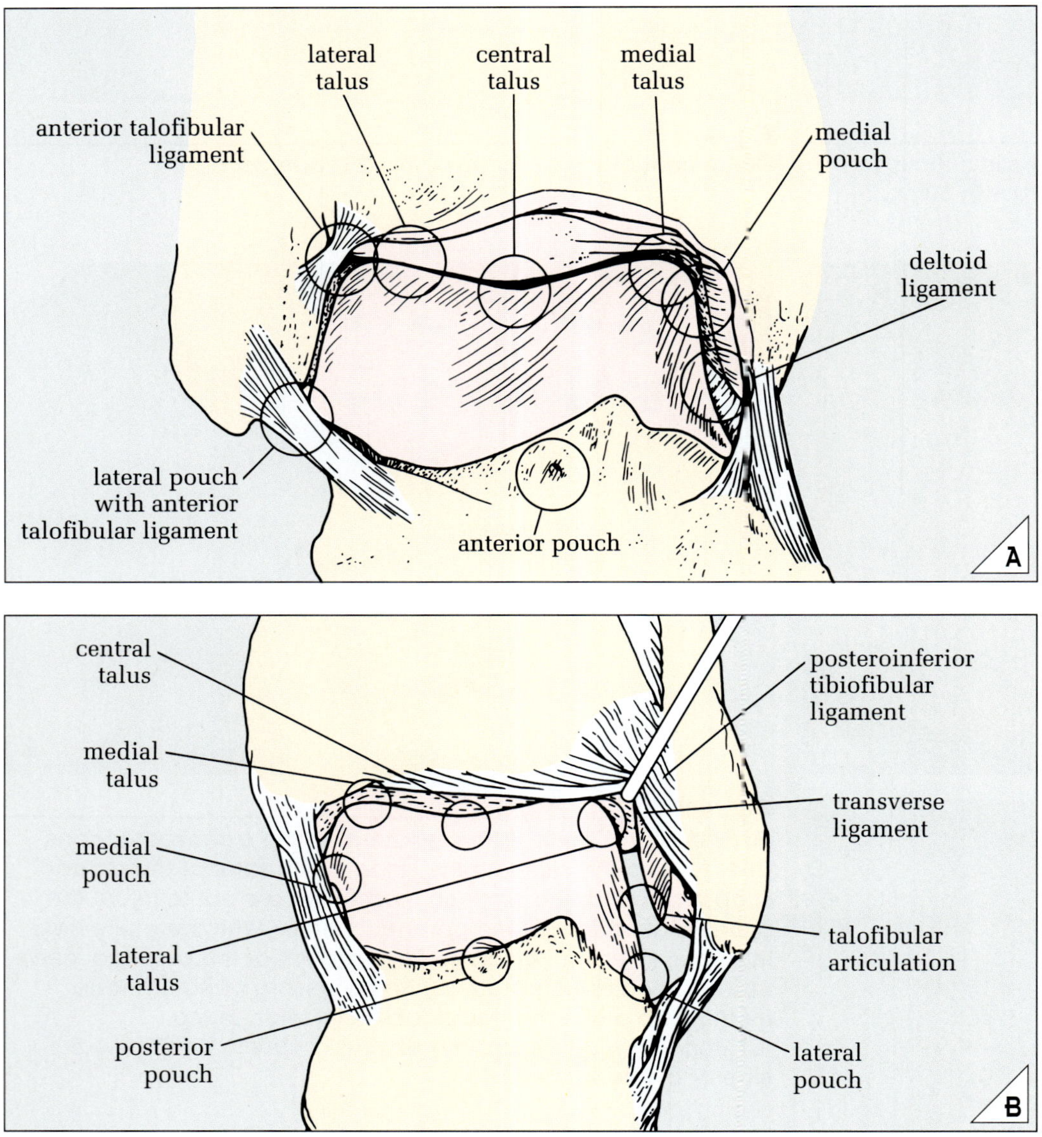

Figure 17.18 The anterior (A) and posterior (B) aspects of the ankle.

Transchondral Fracture of the Talus

Since there is a lack of correlation between the radiographic appearance of the transchondral lesions and the status of the articular cartilage lining, arthroscopic grading is of paramount importance (Fig. 17.21). After arthroscopic visualization and probing, the surgeon must choose among drilling, pinning, and excision. If the overlying articular cartilage is normal or shows minimal softening, the lesion can be drilled down to the subchondral bone. If the fragment is unstable but has a good articular surface, pinning is indicated. If advanced fraying and marked softening of the lesion exists, excision and curettage should be performed whether or not the lesion is stable.

Osteochondral Bodies

Loose osteochondral bodies in the ankle can be secondary to osteochondral fractures, part of a degenerative process of the joint, or secondary to synovial osteochondromatosis. When the loose fragments are located in the anterior pouch of the ankle, the excision requires use of the two

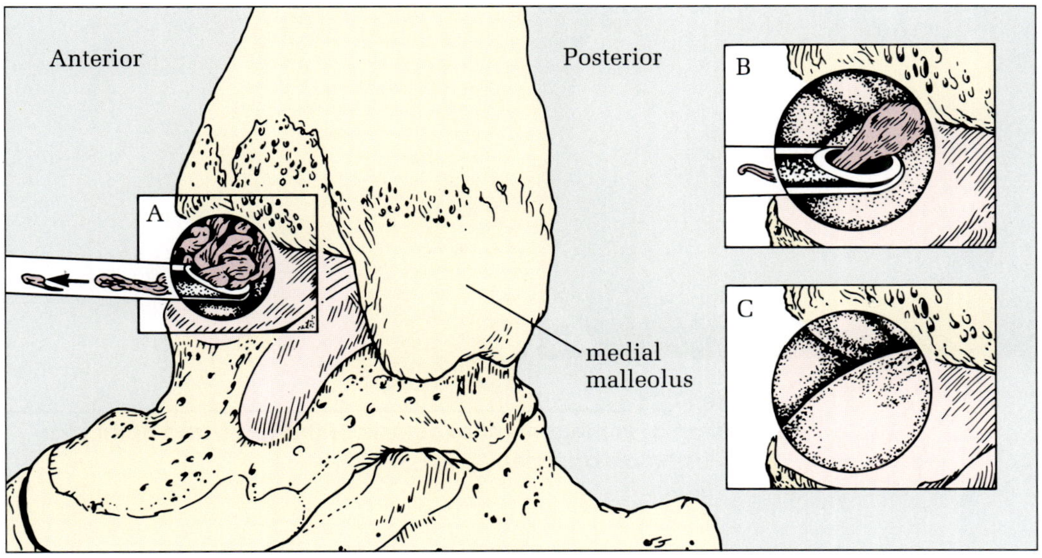

Figure 17.19
(A–C) Arthroscopic synovial resection in impingement.

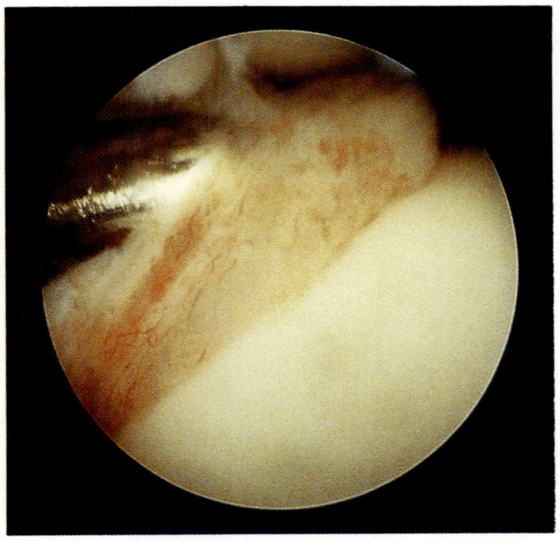

Figure 17.20
Excision of hypertrophic synovial tissue.

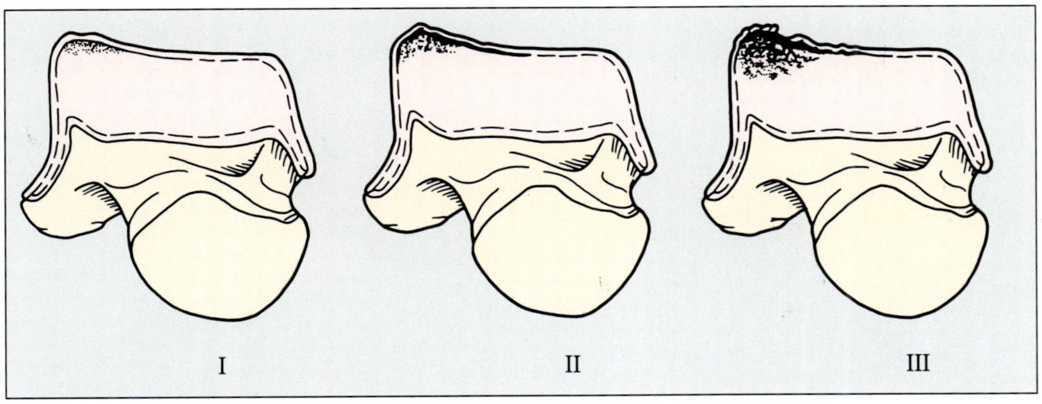

Figure 17.21
Arthroscopic grading of transchondral lesions of the talus.

anterior portals, anteromedial and anterolateral. When the loose fragments are mostly located posteriorly with a tight ankle, the patient can be placed in the prone position to enable use of posterior portals, or the patient can be placed in the supine position so a mechanical distractor can be used. It may be necessary to combine excision of the loose fragments with a partial synovectomy and chondroplasty of the damaged articular cartilage (Fig. 17.22).

Impingement Exostoses

Impingement exostoses can be found at the anterior lip of the tibial plafond and/or on the opposing surface of the

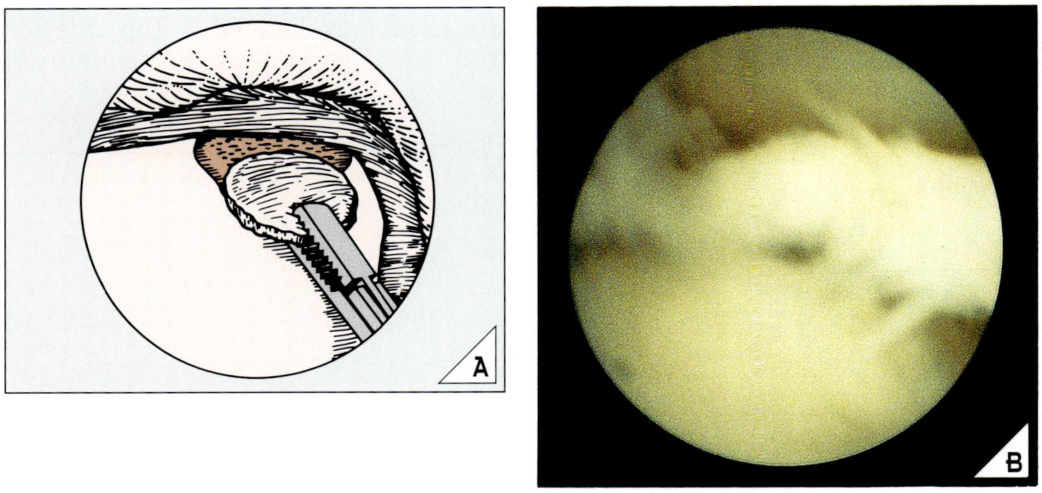

Figure 17.22
Schematic illustration (A) and arthroscopic view (B) of removal of a loose body.

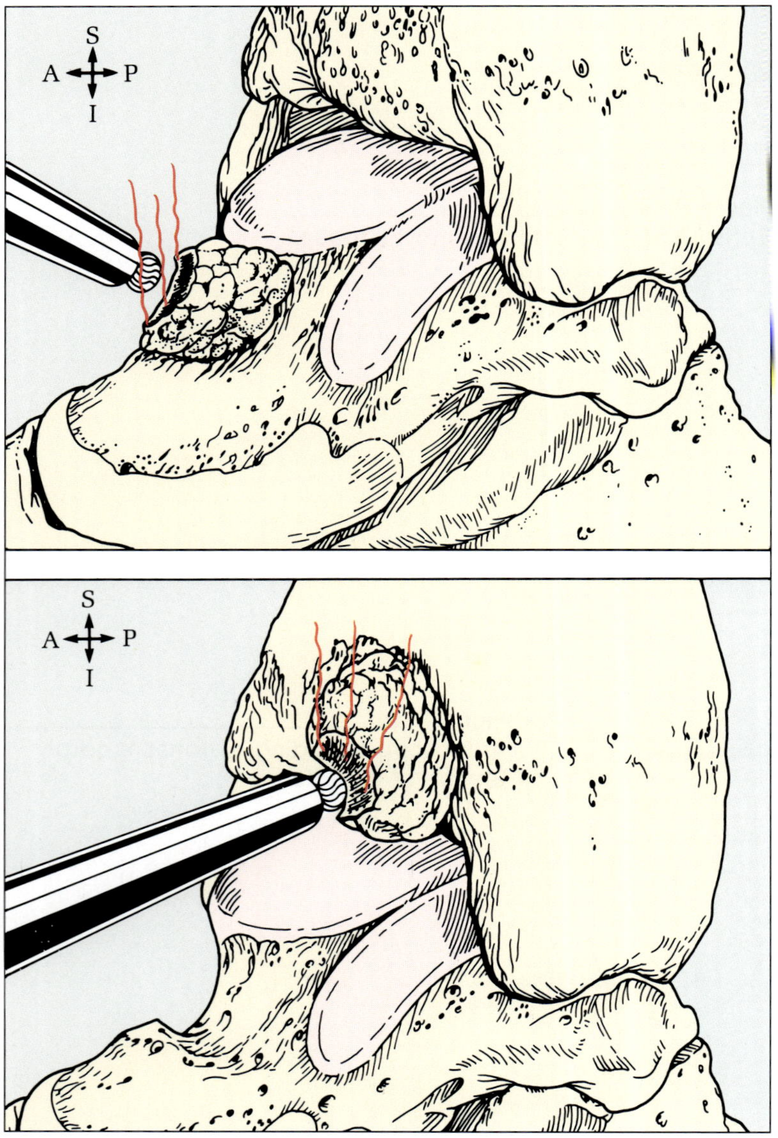

Figure 17.23
Excision of impingement exostosis of the talus and tibial plafond using an abrader.

talus. Exostoses can also be found in front of the malleoli. The excision can be performed through anterior portals. Usually partial synovectomy of the anterior aspect of the joint is necessary to improve visualization of the lesion. A combination of instruments—such as a small osteotome, a rasp, a curette, and a small abrader—are necessary for the procedure (Fig. 17.23).

Posterior impingement can be found in dancers. Excision of posterior impingement lesions requires a posterior portal with the patient in the prone position.

Chondral and Osteochondral Lesions of the Tibial Plafond

Depending on the location, chondral (Fig. 17.24) or osteochondral lesions of the tibial plafond may require anterior portals or a mechanical distractor. Anteriorly located lesions can be managed easily through two anterior portals. Posteriorly located lesions in a tight ankle usually require a distractor (Fig. 17.25). The distraction device affords better visualization while minimizing the risk of instrument breakage and articular cartilage scuffing.

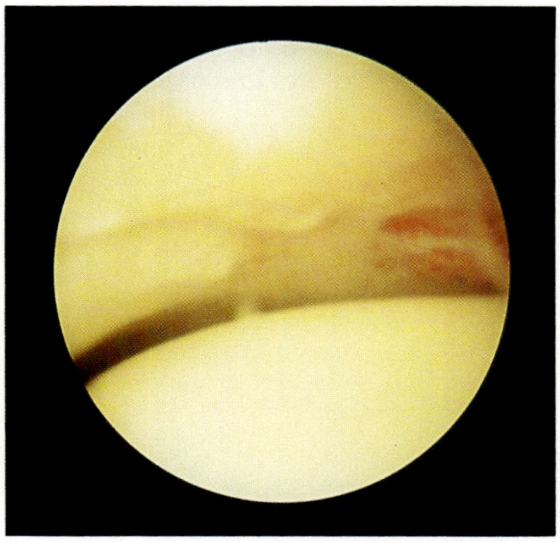

Figure 17.24
Chondromalacia of the tibial plafond.

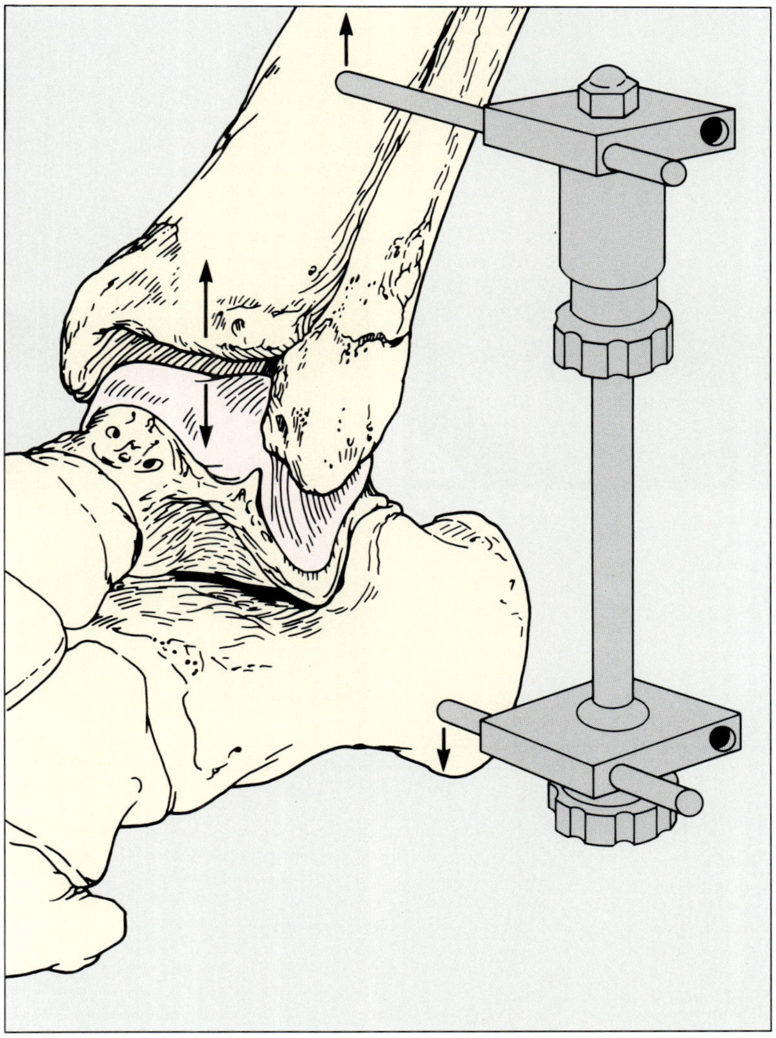

Figure 17.25
Application of a distractor. The proximal pin (3/16 inches in diameter) is placed above the ankle joint, laterally into the tibia behind the anterior tibial crest. The distal pin is inserted into the os calcis, 1/2 inch anterior to its posterior border and 1/2 inch proximal to its inferior border. A joint space opening of 8 mm can be obtained with distraction.

Osteochondral Lesions of the Medial Talomalleolar and Lateral Talomalleolar Spaces

Chondral and osteochondral lesions of the talomalleolar areas (Fig. 17.26) require using surgical instruments on the side of the lesion and a 70° arthroscope through the opposite arthroscopic portal. Chondromalacic areas, excstoses, loose bodies, and nonunited fragments of the tip of the malleoli can be handled successfully without a mechanical distractor.

Degenerative and Posttraumatic Conditions of the Ankle

In selected situations arthroscopic surgery benefits osteoarthritis of the ankle joint. Mechanical distraction is usually recommended to improve visualization and facilitate manipulation of the surgical instruments. A complete debridement of the joint requires a partial synovectomy, excision of the osteophyte, and chondroplasty with abrasion of the localized osteochondral defect. An infusion

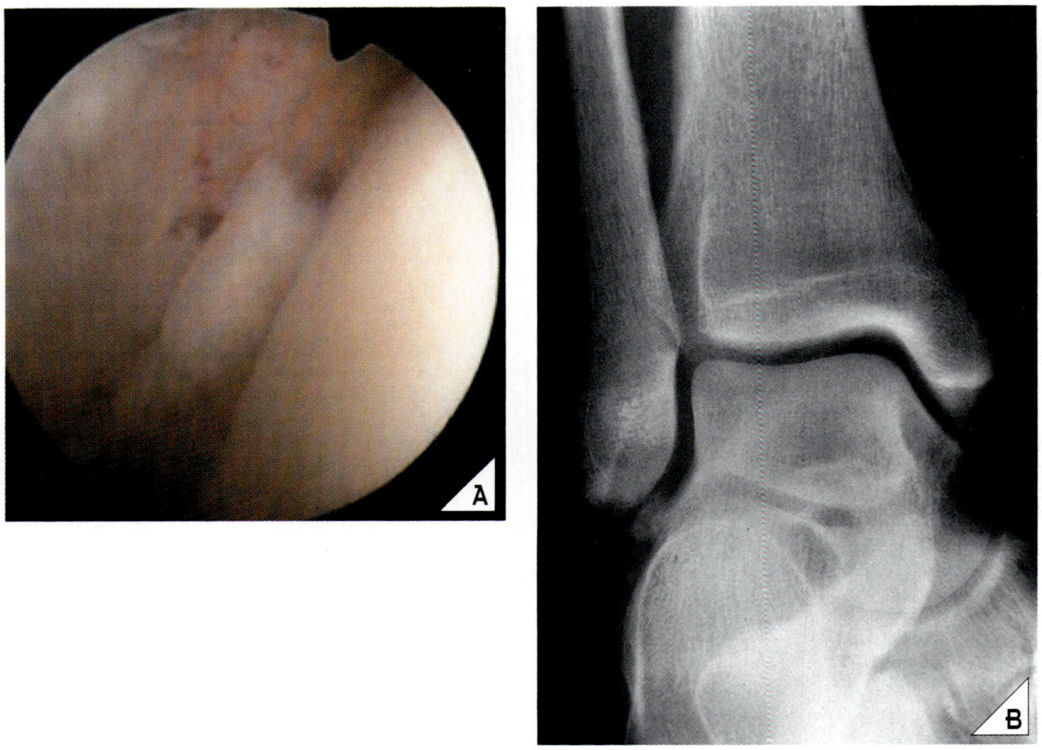

Figure 17.26
Arthroscopic (A) and radiographic (B) views of an osteochondral fragment in the lateral talomalleolar space.

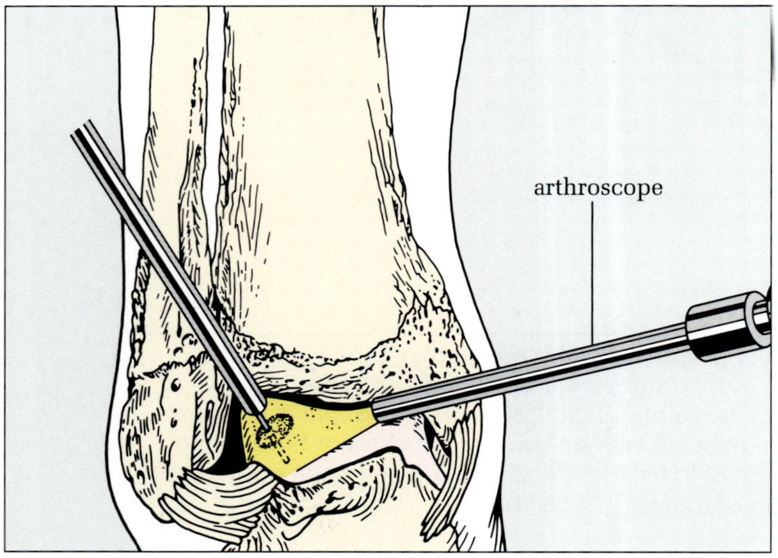

Figure 17.27
Drilling of an anterolateral lesion of the talus.

pump, if available, will allow better capsular distension and control of intraarticular bleeding.

Surgical Technique

Lesions located on the lateral aspect of the talus are usually anterior and, therefore, readily accessible for drilling. Two arthroscopic portals are necessary. The arthroscope is placed through the anteromedial portal and the operating instrument through the anterolateral portal. Kirschner wires, 0.062 mm in diameter, are used for drilling of the osteochondral lesion (Fig. 17.27).

Medial lesions are usually located on the posteromedial aspect of the ankle, and their location makes them very difficult to drill through an anterior portal. The transmalleolar portal may be used (Fig. 17.28). A guide facilitates placement of the Kirschner wire. With the wire in the desired position, multiple drill holes into the talus can be made by staying parallel to the initial wire and dorsiflexing or plantarflexing the ankle as needed.

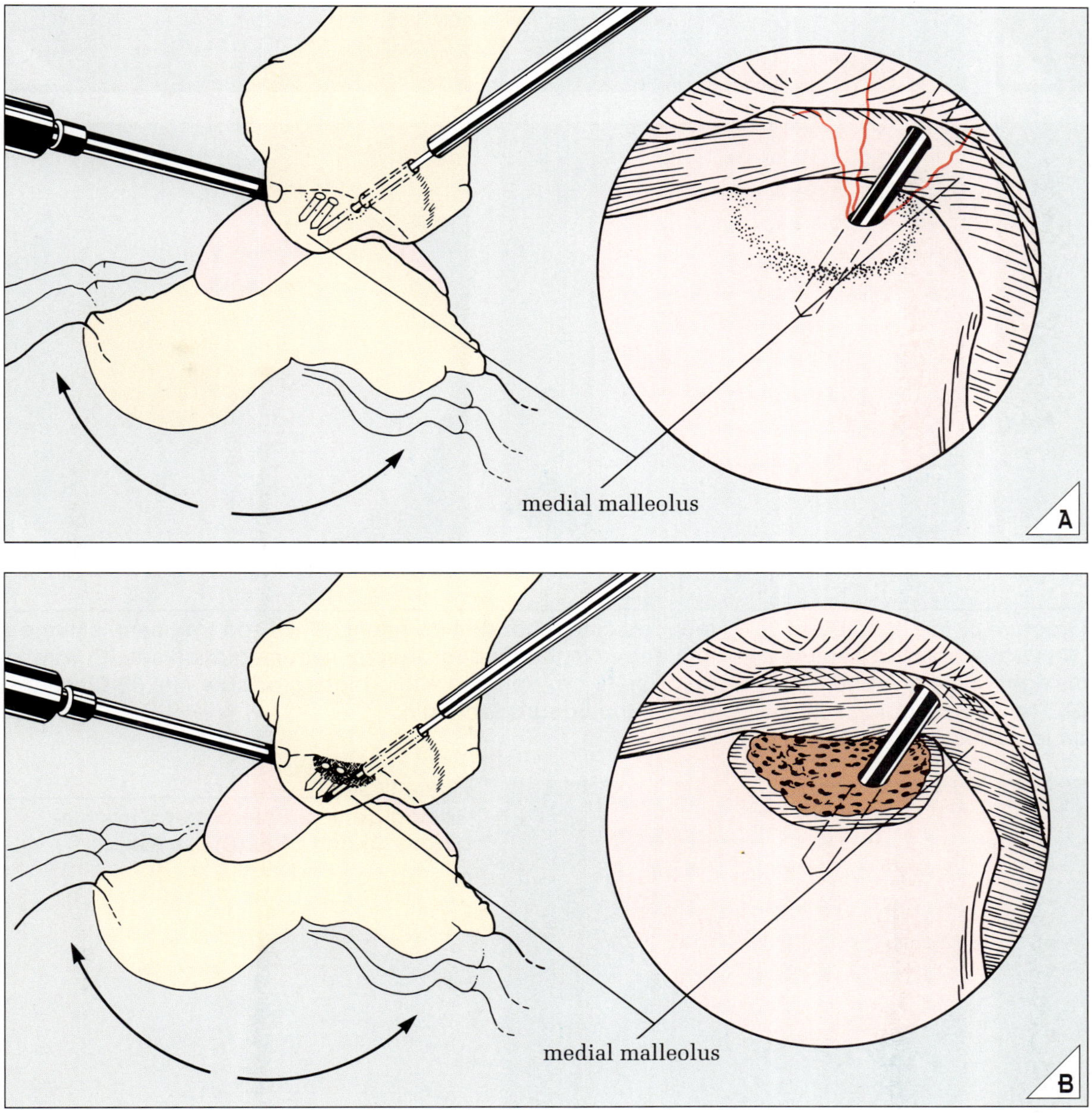

Figure 17.28 Transmalleolar drilling of a posteromedial lesion of a talus with an intact articular surface (A) and a posteromedial crater (B).

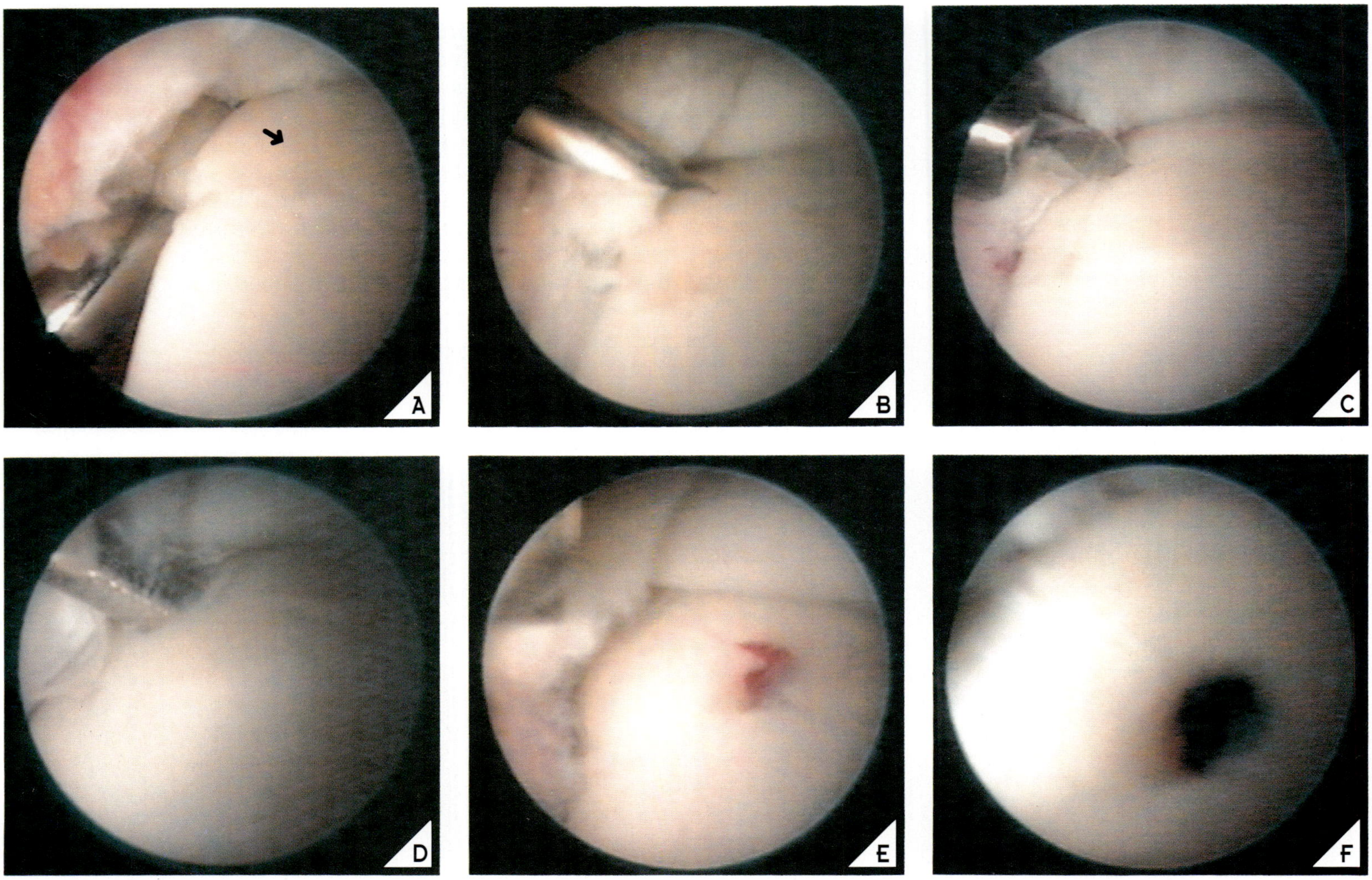

Figure 17.29

Pinning an unstable anterolateral fracture of the right talus (arrow) using biodegradable pins. (A) Osteochondral fracture of the anterolateral aspect of the talus right ankle is found to be viable and amenable to pinning. (B) The special guide of the biodegradable pins instrumentation is positioned over the reduced osteochondral fragment. (C, D) The fragment is pinned with wire from the biodegradable instrumentation set. (E) Wire is removed to be replaced with a biodegradable pin. (F) Close-up view of a biodegradable pin.

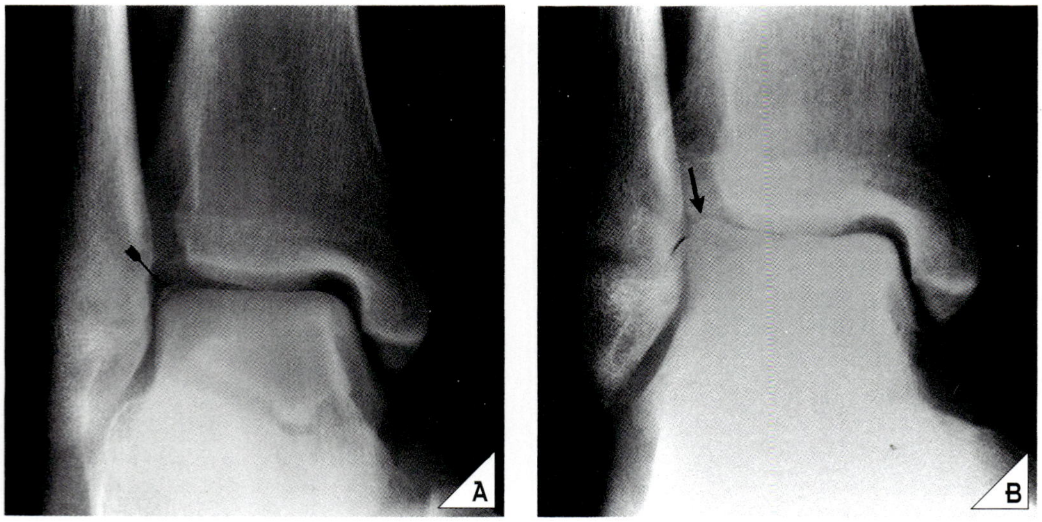

Figure 17.30

Radiographs of anterolateral fracture before (A) and after (B) fixation.

Pinning anterolateral lesions for drilling requires only two anterior portals (Figs. 17.29, 17.30). Pinning medial lesions can be performed through a tunnel made in the medial malleolus. Using a cannulated reamer, however, risks fracture of the medial malleolus. Biodegradable pins or small cannulated screws are used for fixation.

Excising an anterolateral lesion (Fig. 17.31) is quite easy. The arthroscope is placed medially and the surgical instruments laterally. Excision of the fragment is followed by curettage and drilling or abrasion of the osteochondral bed (Figs. 17.32, 17.33).

With proper instrumentation excision of a posteromedial lesion can be carried out without mechanical distraction (Figs. 17.34, 17.35). A small curved knife, a curved elevator, and a grasping forceps are necessary for the excision. Subsequently, curettage and abrasion can be performed.

Postoperative Management

Postoperative treatment consists of the application of a compression dressing, which is replaced by a light dressing the following day. Immediate active range-of-motion exercises with ice application are encouraged for the subsequent 4 to 5 days. Walking with full weight-bearing is recommended, if tolerated by the patient. When an osteochondral fragment has been pinned in situ, non-weight-bearing for a period of 6 to 8 weeks is advisable.

Conclusion

Since the portals in the ankle are in close proximity to tendons, nerves, and arteries, a good knowledge of the anatomy of the area is essential to avoid injury to these important neurovascular structures. Because of the restricted space, extreme care should be used to avoid both damage to the articular cartilage and instrument breakage within the joint. When mechanical distraction is selected, stress fracture of the tibia or calcaneus is a risk. A period of non-weight-bearing or a slow return to sport activities may be indicated in this situation.

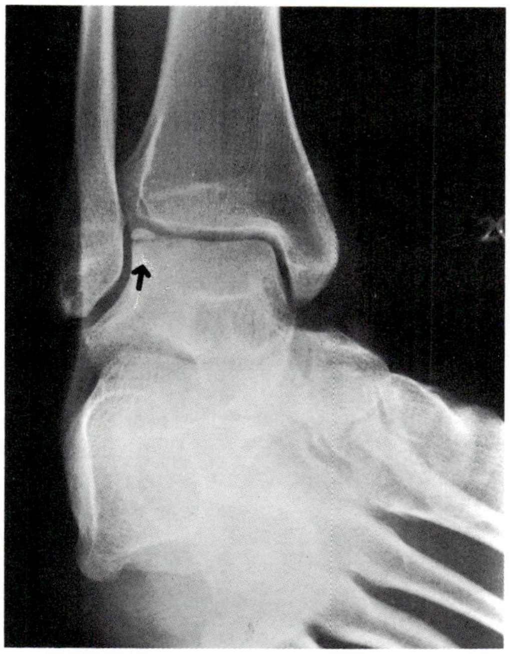

Figure 17.31
Radiograph of anterolateral transchondral fracture amenable to arthroscopic excision.

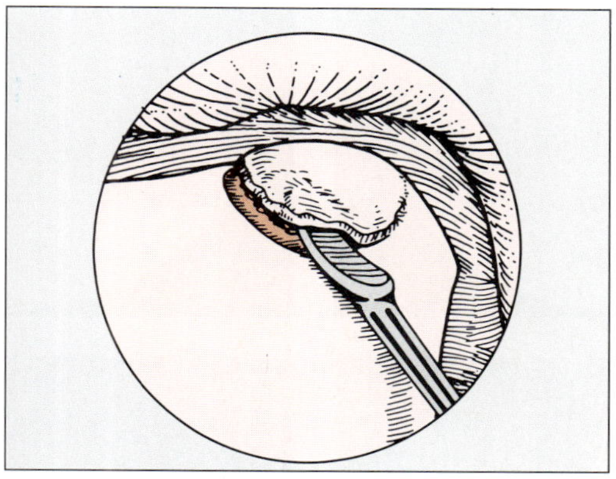

Figure 17.32
Excision of anterolateral fracture.

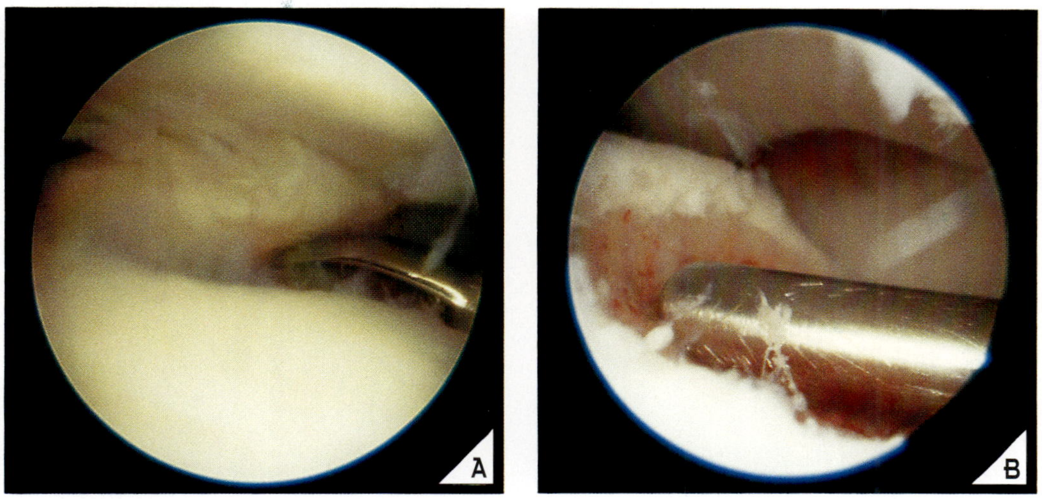

Figure 17.33
Mobilizing the fragment with a small elevator (A) and abrading the osteochondral bed with a small abrader after excision of the fragment (B) are the main steps in excision of an anterolateral fragment of the left ankle.

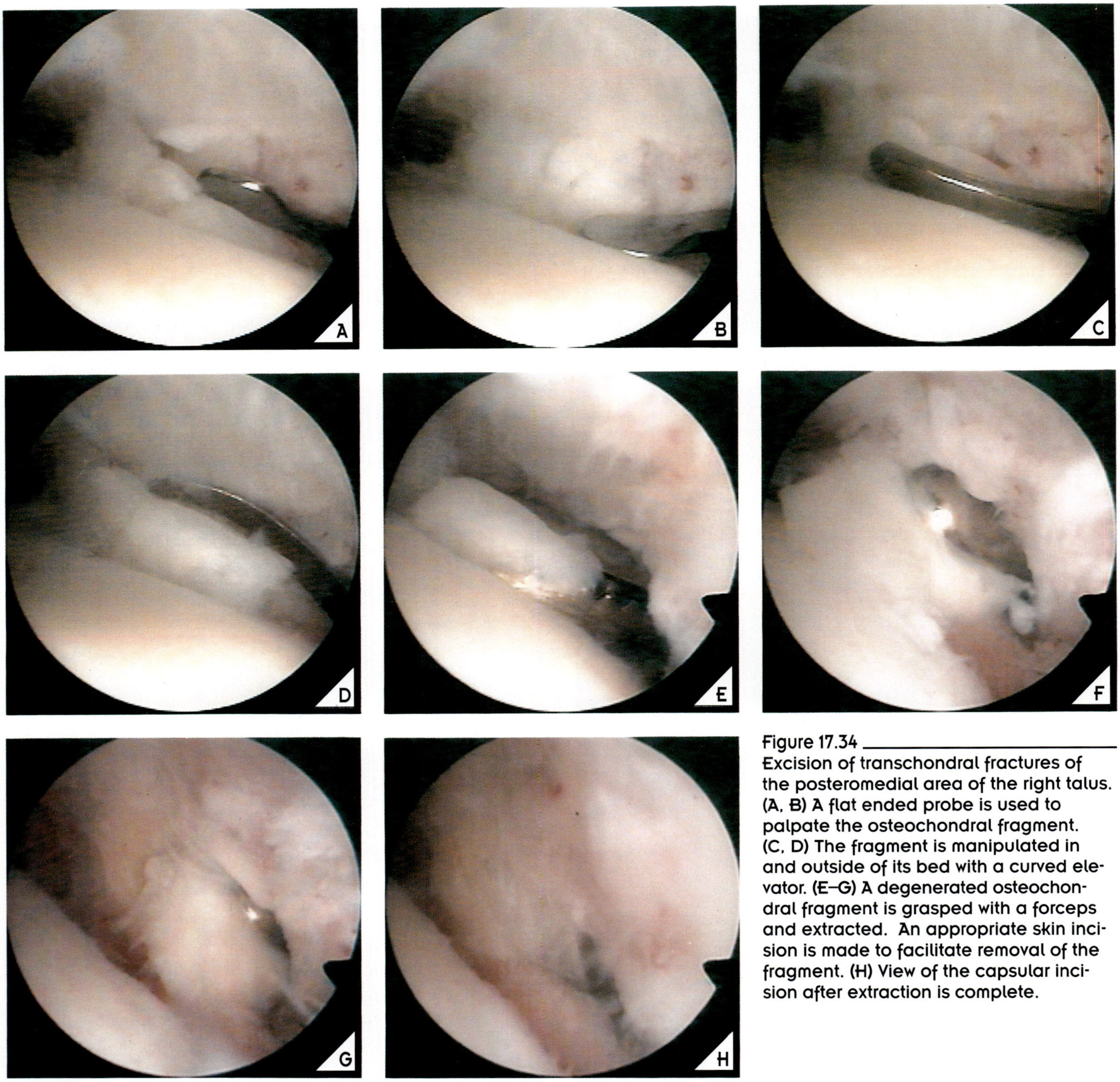

Figure 17.34

Excision of transchondral fractures of the posteromedial area of the right talus. (A, B) A flat ended probe is used to palpate the osteochondral fragment. (C, D) The fragment is manipulated in and outside of its bed with a curved elevator. (E–G) A degenerated osteochondral fragment is grasped with a forceps and extracted. An appropriate skin incision is made to facilitate removal of the fragment. (H) View of the capsular incision after extraction is complete.

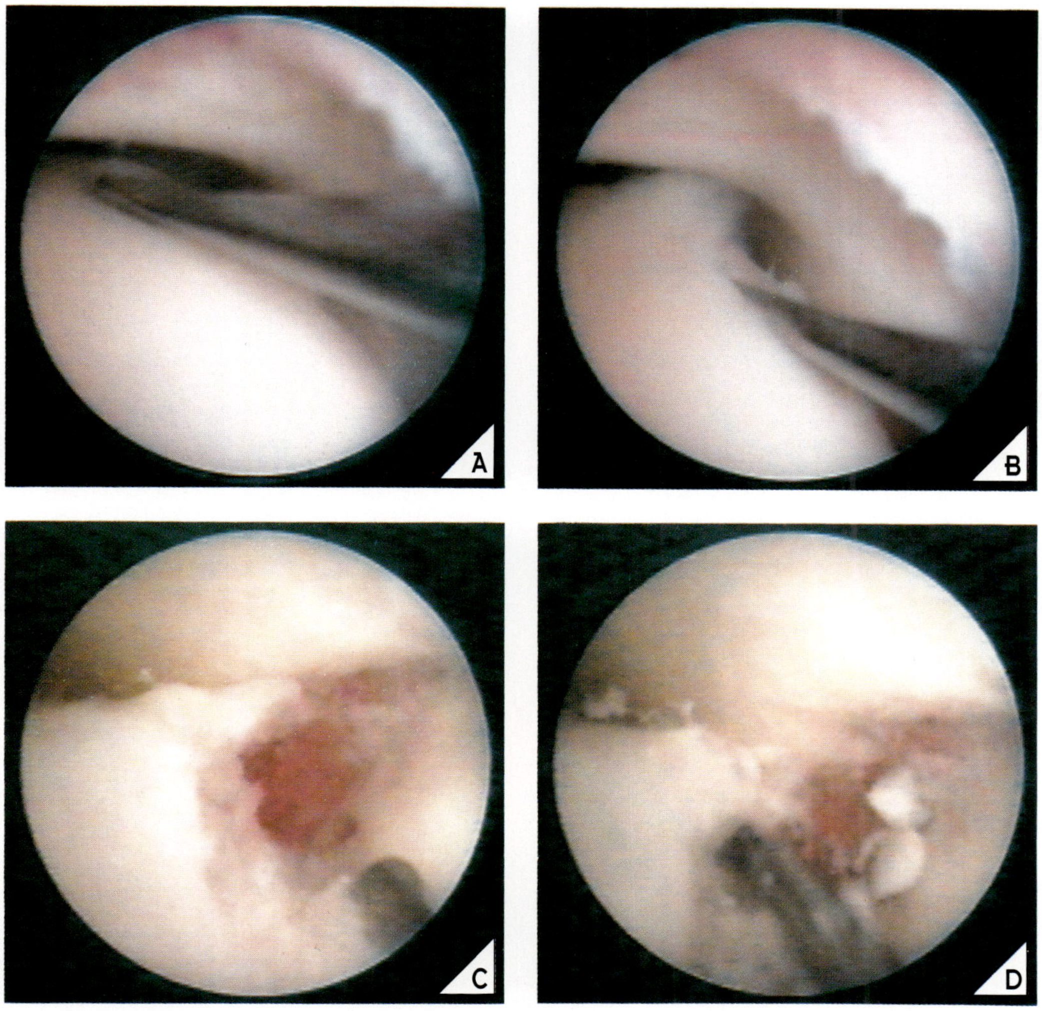

Figure 17.35

Excision of osteochondritis dissecans of the posteromedial area of the right talus. (A) Degenerated soft articular cartilage is probed with a flat ended probe. (B) An area of soft degenerated osteochondritis dissecans is shaved. (C, D) Curettage is performed on the osteochondral defect until bleeding bone is seen and articular debris is removed with suction.

REFERENCES

1. Baker CA, Andrews JR, Ryan JB. Arthroscopic treatment of transchondral talar dome fractures—arthroscopy. *J Arthro Rel Surg.* 1986;2:82–87.
2. Ferkel R, Karzel R, et al. Arthroscopic treatment of anterolateral impingement of the ankle. *Am J Sports Med.* 1991;19:440–446.
3. Guhl J. *Osteochondritis Dissecans in Ankle Arthroscopy: Pathology and Surgical Techniques.* Thorofare, NJ: Slack Inc; 1988:95.
4. Parisien JS, Vangsness T. Operative arthroscopy of the ankle: 3 years experience. *Clin Orthop.* 1985;199:46–52.
5. Parisien JS, Feldman R, Vangsness T. Diagnostic and surgical arthroscopy for the ankle: an experimental approach. *Clin Orthop.* 1987;224:228–236.
6. Parisien JS. Arthroscopic treatment of osteochondral lesions of the talus. *Am J Sports Med.* 1986;14:211.

chapter

Eighteen

Arthroscopic Surgery for Chronic Instability

J. Serge Parisien

Arthroscopic lateral ankle stabilization, in selected cases, is an alternative procedure to the well established open repairs and reconstructions (Bröstrom, Evans, Watson Jones, Christman-Snook) used for chronic instability of the ankle.[1–5] In this modification of the direct ligamentous repair proposed by Hawkins, the lateral aspect of the talus is abraded so the anterior talofibular ligament can be shortened via percutaneous stapling. Hawkins reported 24 cases with 2 to 5 years follow up. Of these, 23 patients were felt to be clinically stable.[6] From a review of these few reported cases and from our own experience, the Hawkins staple stabilization has been useful in patients with chronic lateral instability who have intermittent giving way, pain, and a positive anterior Drawer test and positive stress x-ray test.[6–8] This technique may be indicated for children so violation of the growth plate of the fibula can be avoided.

Surgical Technique

The instruments needed for this procedure are a 4 mm or 2.7 mm arthroscope with 25° angulation, a small motorized shaving system with a full radius blade and abrader, and small Instrument Makar staples with a driver-extractor. A 70° arthroscope is also very helpful to visualize the lateral aspect from the anteromedial portal (Fig. 18.1).

The ligament stabilization procedure can be done under general or spinal anesthesia with the patient in the semisupine position. A tourniquet is placed at the midthigh level and can be inflated if necessary. To stabilize the leg, a leg holder is used in the midcalf area. Three portals can be used to perform the procedure; the anteromedial portal, the anterolateral, and an accessory lateral portal (Fig. 18.2).

The lateral branch of the superficial peroneal nerve should be located under the skin (Fig. 18.3). After a complete exploration of the ankle joint to rule out any evidence of loose fragments and chondromalacia, partial synovectomy, removal of loose bodies and chondroplasty can be performed when appropriate. Subsequently, the lateral aspect of the joint is debrided with surgical instruments placed through an accessory lateral portal and the small arthroscope through the lateral portal. An area approximately 1 cm anterior to the tip of the fibula is then located on the vertical surface of the talus. With an abrader placed through the accessory portal, this area of the talus is denuded of approximately 8 mm of articular cartilage. If a 70° arthroscope is used medially, the need for an accessory portal can be avoided, and the anterolateral portal is used for the abrasion. To allow a right-angle entry of the staple into the prepared bed on the talus, a skin incision is made, with care being taken not to involve any sensory nerves in

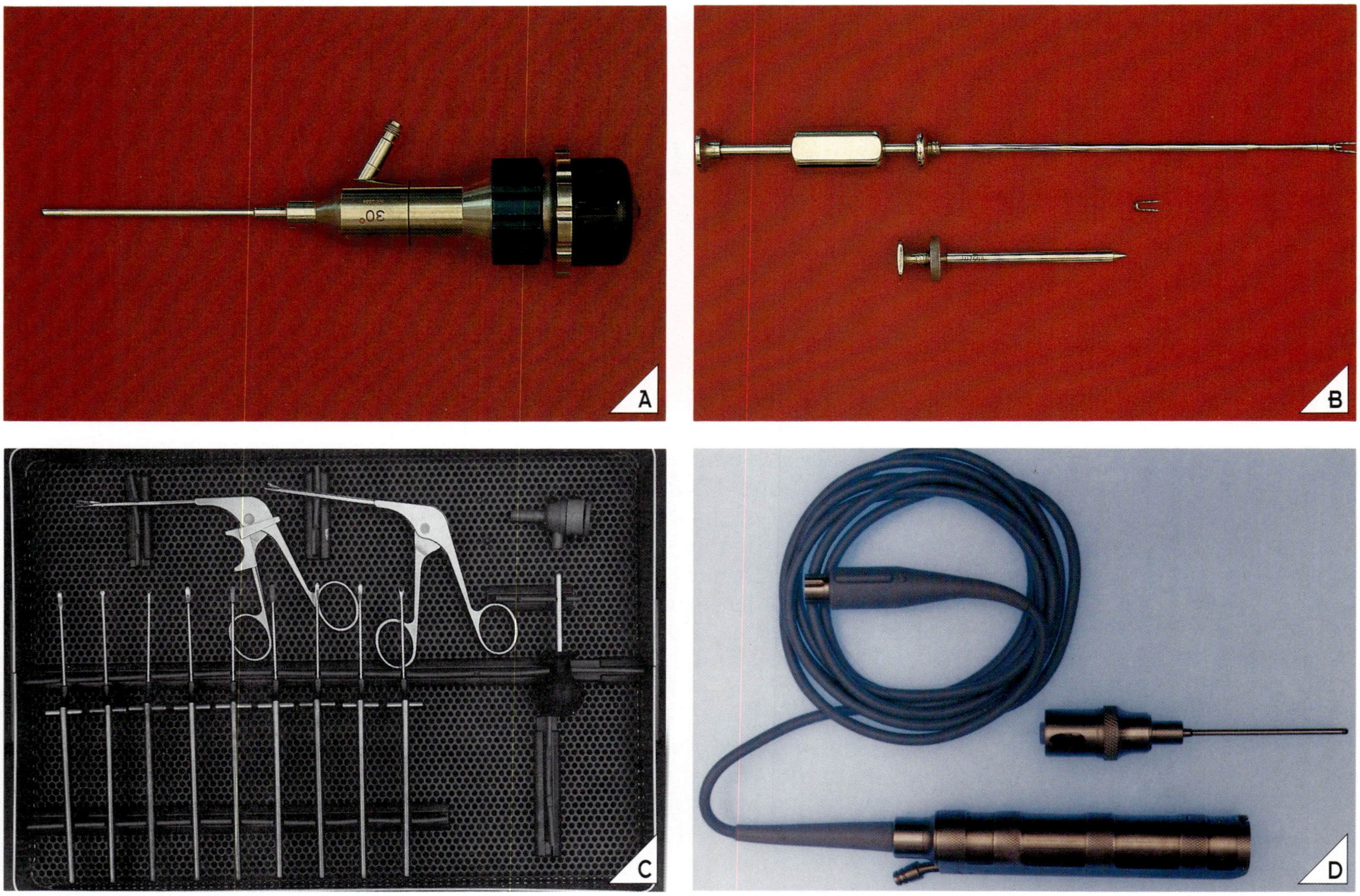

Figure 18.1
(A) Small camera with arthroscope that can be used for ankle arthroscopy (Dyonics). (B) Instrument Makar staples with driver-extractor. (C) Small instrument set with knives, basket forceps, curettes, and rasps. (D) Small motorized instrumentation.

this area. A spinal needle is used to guide the position of the staple inserter. A small hemostat is used to spread the skin down to the capsular tissue. The tines of the staple are pressed through the lateral capsule and the remaining fibers of the anterior talofibular ligament. With the ankle in neutral position, insertion of the staple is done with the inserter (Figs. 18.4, 18.5). The small 2.7-mm arthroscope can be used in the anterolateral portal to visualize the site of staple insertion at the end of the procedure.

Postoperative Treatment

After the portals are closed, a compression dressing is applied, and the leg is placed in a posterior splint in neutral position. After 1 week the sutures and the dressing are removed and the patient is placed in a short leg cast for approximately 6 weeks. Full weight-bearing is permitted as tolerated by the patient.

Complications and Pitfalls

Incorrect placement of a staple can cause impingement with dorsiflexion of the ankle. Intraoperative x-rays are necessary to confirm proper position of the staple. Numbness of foot and toes can be secondary to involvement of the sensory nerve fibers in the repair, particularly the lateral branch of the superficial peroneal nerve, hence the importance of locating the nerve before surgery. Staple protrusion into the joint may require staple removal at a later date.

The technique of arthroscopic lateral ligament stabilization of the ankle is not easy and should be attempted only by surgeons who have experience with arthroscopic surgery of the ankle. With future development of biodegradable materials, hardware may not be needed for intraarticular fixation of ligament to bone surfaces.

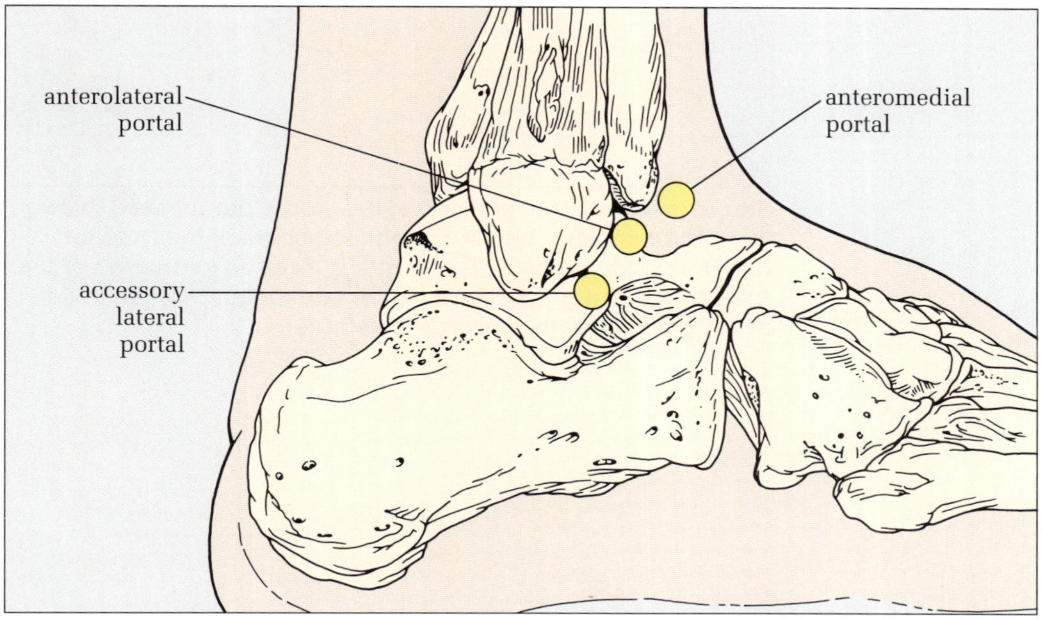

Figure 18.2
Arthroscopic portals.

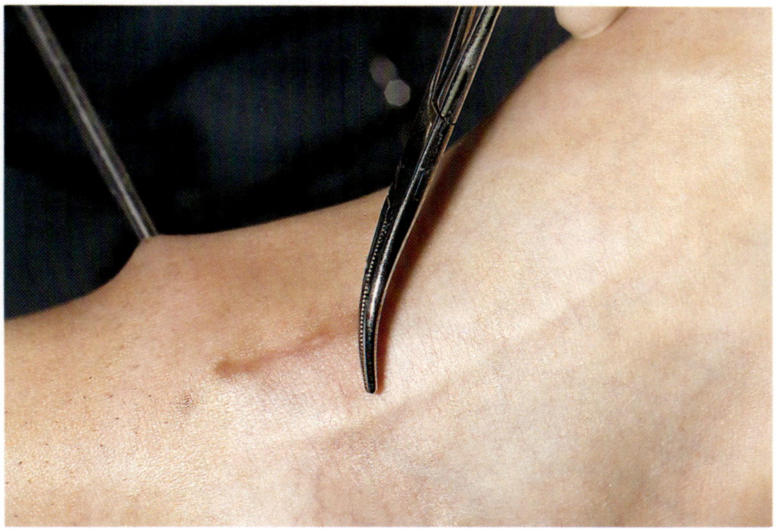

Figure 18.3
With inversion of the ankle, the lateral branch of the superficial peroneal nerve can be located under the skin.

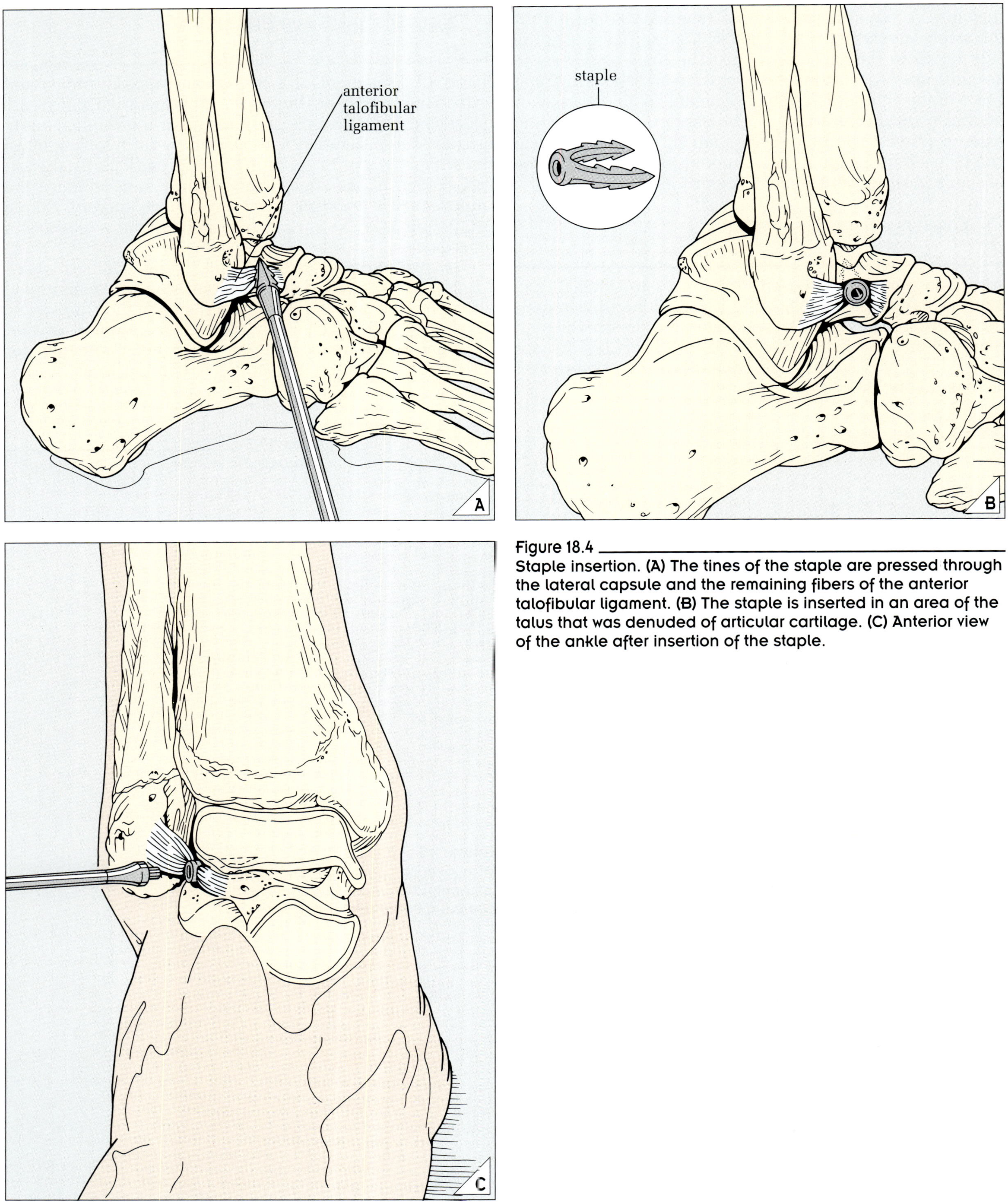

Figure 18.4

Staple insertion. (A) The tines of the staple are pressed through the lateral capsule and the remaining fibers of the anterior talofibular ligament. (B) The staple is inserted in an area of the talus that was denuded of articular cartilage. (C) Anterior view of the ankle after insertion of the staple.

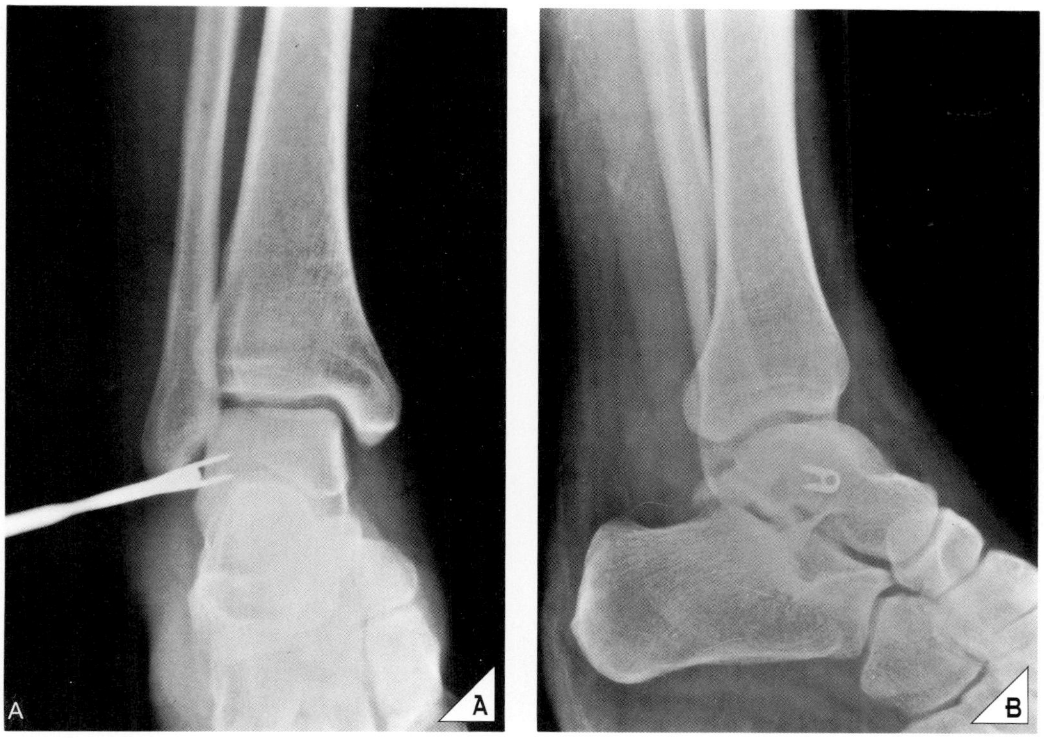

Figure 18.5
X-rays during (A) and after (B) staple stabilization of the ankle.

REFERENCES

1. Bröstrom L. Sprained ankles, IV: surgical treatment of "chronic" ligament ruptures. *Acta Chir Scand.* 1966;132: 551–565.
2. Chrisman OD, Snook GA. Reconstruction of lateral ligament tears of the ankle: an experimental study and clinical evaluation of seven patients treated by a new modification of the Elmslie procedure. *J Bone Joint Surg.* 1969;51A:904–912.
3. Evans DL. Recurrent instability of the ankle—a method of surgical treatment. *Proc R Soc Med.* 1953;46:343–344.
4. Peters JW, Trevino S, Renstrom PA. Chronic lateral instability. *Foot Ankle.* 1991;12:182–191.
5. Watson–Jones R. Recurrent forward dislocation of the ankle joint. *J Bone Joint Surg.* 1952;34B:519.
6. Hawkins RB. Arthroscopic reconstruction for chronic lateral instability of the ankle. In: McGuinty J, ed. *Arthroscopic Surgery Update.* Rockville, Md: Aspen Systems Corporation; 1985:175–181.
7. Hawkins RB. Arthroscopic stapling repair for chronic lateral instability. *Clin Podiatr Med Surg.* 1987;4:875–883.
8. Feldman R, Parisien JS. Clinical experience with arthroscopic ankle stabilization. Unpublished data.

chapter Nineteen

Arthroscopic Ankle Arthrodesis

James M. Glick
J. Serge Parisien

Severe degenerative arthritis of the ankle joint can be managed successfully by tibiotalar arthrodesis. Many surgical techniques have been described for obtaining a solid fusion. They include the use of a sliding graft involving the tibia or fibula, internal compression by plate or screws, and external compression pins.[1–5] All of these techniques have the potential for complications such as neurovascular injury, infection, or malunion. The incidence of pseudoarthrosis has been reported to be as high as 20%.[6] However, better results have been reported with limited open procedures involving internal compression screws and with the triangular external fixation method.[3,7,8] More recently, arthroscopic techniques have been used to perform ankle arthrodesis. A more rapid rate of union has been reported in the few available series.

The advantages of the technique seem to be decreased morbidity and a rapid rate of union, probably secondary to the preservation of the blood supply and to the small incisions.

INDICATIONS

Generally speaking, arthroscopic ankle arthrodesis is indicated to obtain relief of pain in disabling post-traumatic, degenerative, and inflammatory arthritis.

Other indications are hemophilic arthropathy, congenital deformities, rheumatoid arthritis, and a large area of osteochondritis dissecans with degenerative changes of the joint. This technique is without doubt appealing in patients with dermatologic and peripheral vascular problems, since the skin incisions are limited. The prerequisites for a successful arthroscopic ankle arthrodesis are the lack of significant sagittal and anteroposterior malalignment and the absence of significant bone loss, as is observed in avascular necrosis of the talus.[6,9–12]

SURGICAL TECHNIQUE

The following instruments are advisable: leg holder, distractor (either a pin or a strap fixator), full-radius resector and abrader, curettes, and cannulated 6.5 mm compression screws. An image intensifier is mandatory to verify the position of the fusion site and the placement of the percutaneous compression screws.

General or spinal anesthesia can be used. The patient is positioned supine on a standard operating table. The operative leg should be placed so that the ankle can be fluoroscoped with an image intensifier. If the leg holder is used, it should be placed over the thigh, as for knee arthroscopy. The foot and ankle should be positioned so the knee is over the end of the table (Fig. 19.1). The use of a tourniquet is optional.

The three traditional portals for ankle arthroscopy (anteromedial, anterolateral, and posterolateral) can be used (Fig. 19.2). An accessory anterolateral portal inferior to the usual anterolateral portal may be needed for debridement of the inferolateral aspect of the joint.

Distraction is accomplished with either skeletal or strap traction. When skeletal traction is used, an external half-frame fixation device with distraction capabilities is applied. For this procedure, medial pin distraction with pins placed in the talus and tibia is preferred because it allows dorsiflexion of the foot while maintaining parallel separation of the joint, and it does not obstruct the operative instrumentation placed from the anterior or posterolateral approach. In some cases with marked arthrofibrosis, initial joint distraction may be very difficult to obtain. In such a situation it is necessary to debride the joint anteriorly before applying distraction. With further debridement as more distraction is applied, more space will be available for visualization. If the ankle is contracted in an equinus position, a subcutaneous achilles tendon lengthening should be performed at the start of the procedure. Once this has been done, distraction during the procedure and reduction to a neutral position at the end can be easily accomplished.

All soft tissues (synovium, adhesive bands) are removed, followed by systematic excision of the degenerated articular cartilage from the talus, tibial plafond, and the medial and lateral malleolar spaces. A motorized resector and abrader are used for this task (Fig. 19.3).

During this debridement step, care is taken to maintain the normal bony contour of the talar dome and tibial plafond (i.e., talar convexity and tibial concavity) while cor-

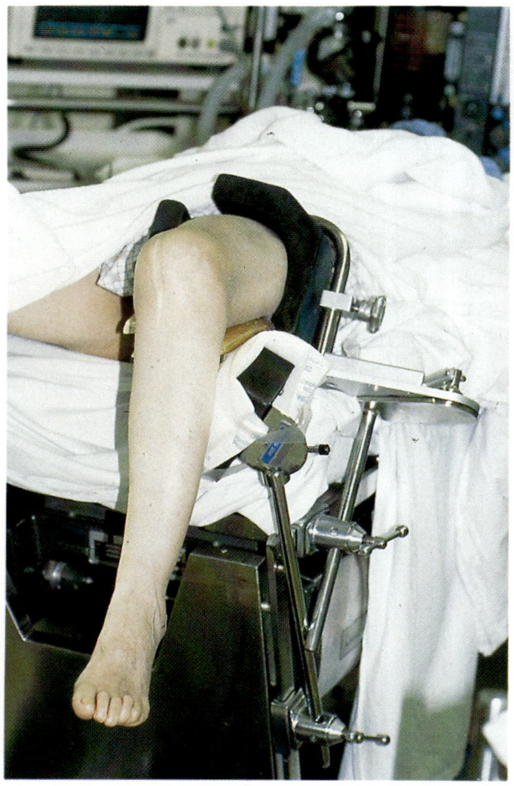

Figure 19.1
Position of the leg for ankle arthroscopy and arthroscopic arthrodesis. The thigh is fixed in a leg holder and the leg hangs over the end of the operating table.

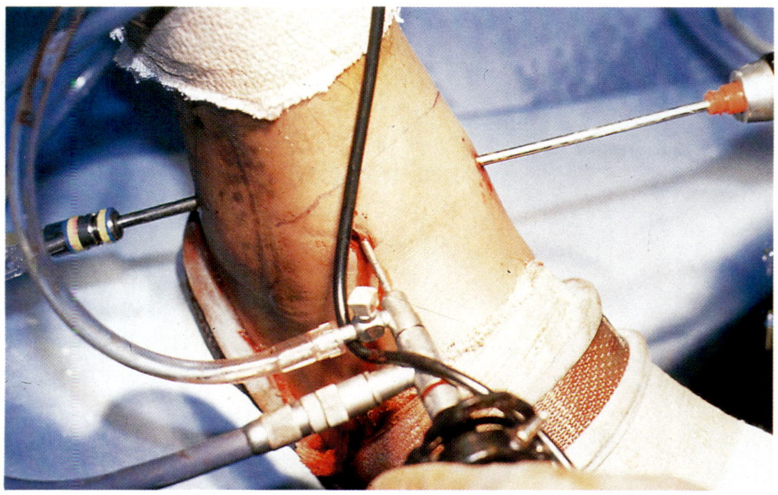

Figure 19.2
The three portals used for arthroscopic ankle arthrodesis (anteromedial, anterolateral, and posterolateral). Note the ankle strap used for distraction.

recting any mild varus/valgus deformity that may exist. Curettes are used to complete the debridement posteriorly if necessary.

Next, two screw guide pins, one through the lateral malleolus and the other through the medial malleolus, are placed from posterior to anterior at 45° to the long axis of the tibia and fibula. The tips of the screw guide pins directed towards the talus are visualized arthroscopically as they come through the tibia and fibula, respectively (Fig. 19.4). The pins are then placed flush with the tibial and fibular surfaces. The distraction mode is removed and the foot is placed in neutral dorsiflexion with 5° of hindfoot valgus (Fig. 19.5). The guide pins are drilled into the talus under fluoroscopic guidance to control the depth of penetration (Fig. 19.6). A small skin incision is then made around the guide pins to allow introduction of the correct size screws.

A compression dressing is applied on the ankle, followed by a splint. This arthroscopic technique can be modified, as suggested by Crosby, by adding bone marrow and demineralized bone matrix as a graft substitute.[6,12] In this situation, a 14-gauge Thomas needle with a heparin-coated glass syringe is used to aspirate bone marrow from the iliac crest. At least 50 mL of bone marrow are obtained and mixed with demineralized bone matrix. This mixture is then injected into the debrided tibiotalar and talomalleolar areas. Crosby, in a series of 16 patients followed for an average of 27 months, reported satisfactory results in all but two patients.[6]

Postoperative Management

At 3 to 5 days postoperatively, the splint is removed and a short leg walking cast is applied. Full weight bearing is allowed in 1 month. A walking fracture boot with the hinges locked can also be used. The cast is removed when fusion has occurred.

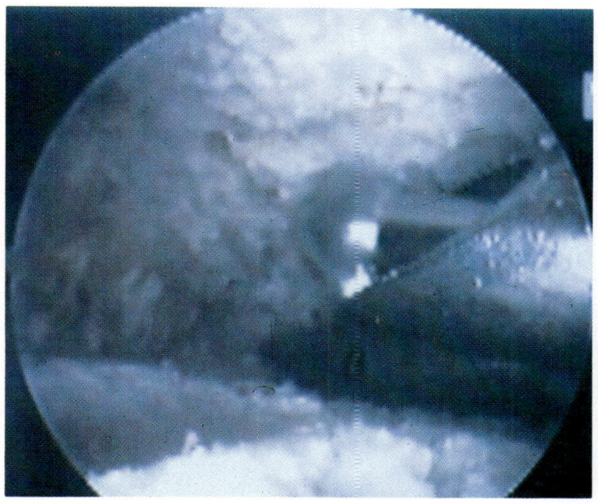

Figure 19.3
The motorized abrader debriding the tibial plafond.

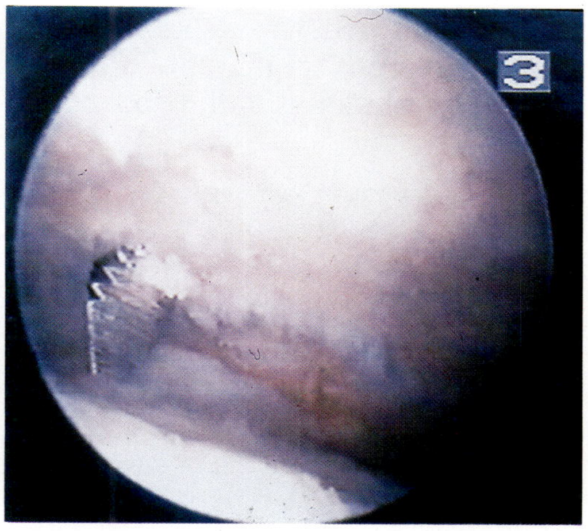

Figure 19.4
The tip of a screw guide pin penetrating the medial side of the tibial plafond and aiming toward the talar dome.

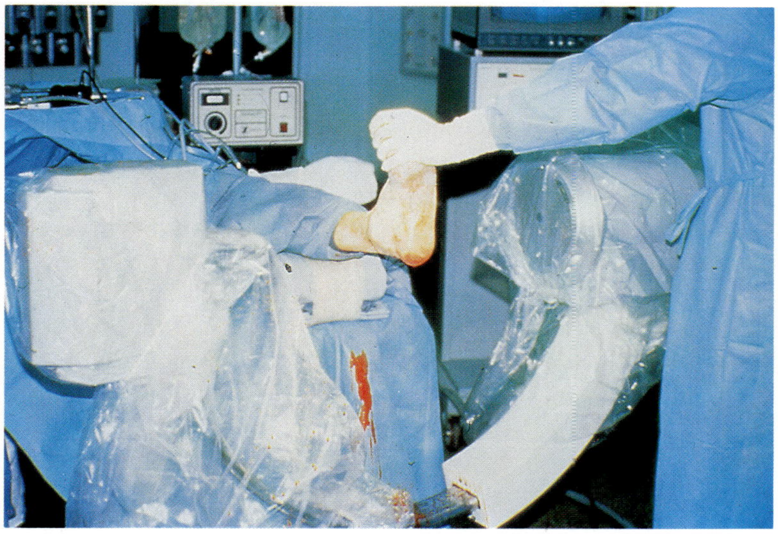

Figure 19.5
The arthroscopic portion of the procedure has been terminated. The ankle is being reduced using the image intensifier as a guide. (Reprinted with permission from Morgan CD. Arthroscopic tibiotalar arthrodesis. In: McGinty JB, ed. Operative Arthroscopy. New York, NY: Raven Press; 1991:696)

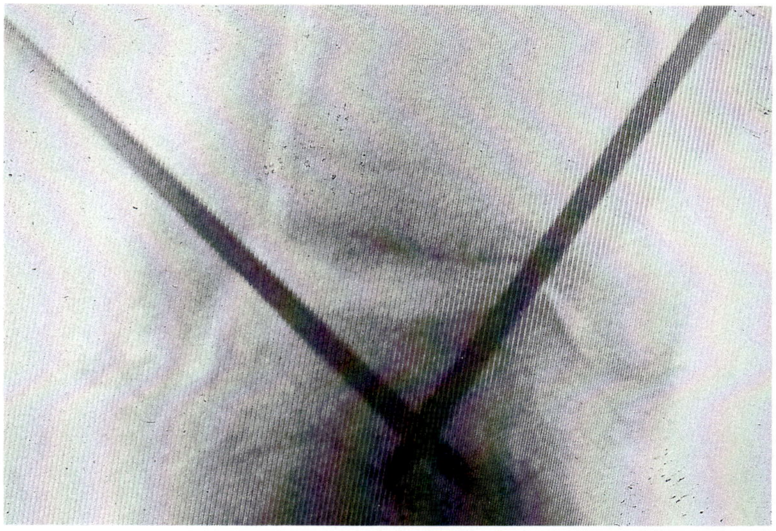

Figure 19.6
Position of the screw guide pins as seen on the image intensifier.

COMPLICATIONS AND PITFALLS

The major pitfall of arthroscopic ankle arthrodesis is the removal of too much bone, thus leaving large gaps in the ankle space. Such gaps do not appear to increase the chance of a nonunion but may prolong the time required for fusion. The complications are few and should be no different from those that might occur in any ankle arthroscopy procedure.

Sometimes pain persists long after the arthrodesis procedure. Fusion may appear to be progressing satisfactorily. A CT scan is helpful in determining the status of the fusion and also the appearance of the subtalar joint. Arthritis of the subtalar joint can explain persistent pain after a solid tibiotalar fusion has occurred.

CONCLUSION

Glick et al.[9] reported on 34 arthroscopic fusions performed between February 1984 and April 1989. In all but one ankle a secure fusion was obtained, radiographically documented by obliteration of the ankle's joint space and continuous bone trabeculae crossing from the tibia to the talus (Fig. 19.7). In the case of the nonunion, there were two errors made at surgery that we believe to have been the cause. First, smooth Steinmann pins (rather than threaded pins) were used for fixation. Second, an anterocentral portal was used. The patient developed a dorsalis pedis arterial pseudoaneurysm. When the cast was removed to fix the pseudoaneurysm, the two smooth pins pulled out of the ankle joint and the fixation was lost. The ankle later fused with an open sliding bone graft procedure. The complication occurred early in the series before screws were used. The average length of time until clinical and radiological union occurred was 9 weeks. In four cases, fusion was sufficient enough to discontinue immobilization in 6 weeks.

The fusion rate for arthroscopic ankle arthrodesis is high (97% according to Glick et al.[9]) and is comparable to the open arthrotomy series of Morgan et al.[3] Likewise, the complication rate is low as in any other arthroscopic procedure. The relatively rapid postoperative mobilization makes this approach particularly appealing in the debilitated or incapacitated patient.

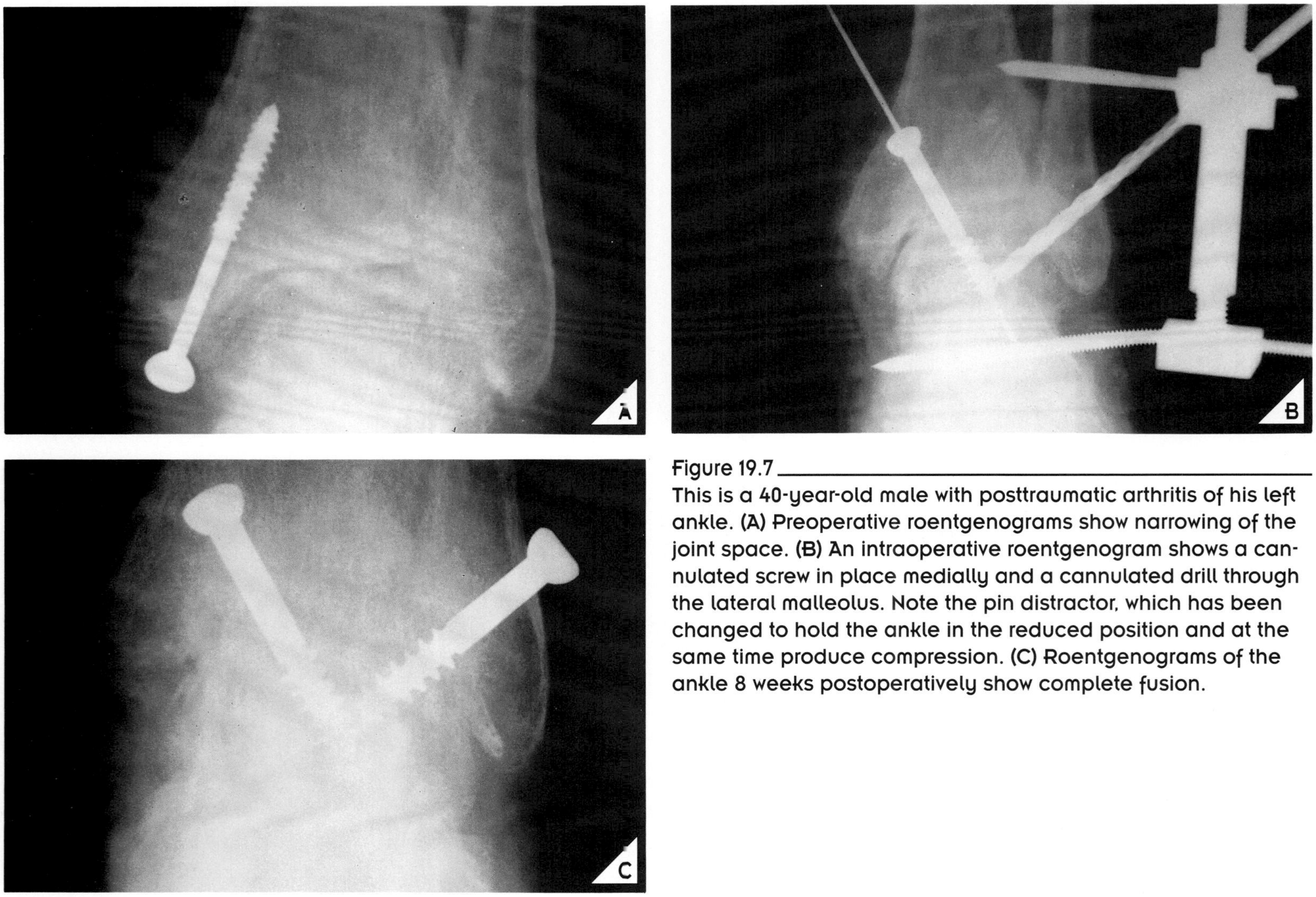

Figure 19.7

This is a 40-year-old male with posttraumatic arthritis of his left ankle. (A) Preoperative roentgenograms show narrowing of the joint space. (B) An intraoperative roentgenogram shows a cannulated screw in place medially and a cannulated drill through the lateral malleolus. Note the pin distractor, which has been changed to hold the ankle in the reduced position and at the same time produce compression. (C) Roentgenograms of the ankle 8 weeks postoperatively show complete fusion.

REFERENCES

1. Lance EM, Pavel A, Fries I, Larsen IN, Paterson RL. Arthrodesis of the ankle joint. *Clin Orthop Rel Res.* 1979;142:146–156.
2. Moeckel BH, Patterson BM, Inglis AE, Sculco TP. Ankle arthrodesis: a comparison of internal and external fixation. *Clin Orthop Rel Res.* 1991;268:78–83.
3. Morgan CD, Henke JA, Bailey RW, Kaufer H. Long term results of tibio-talar arthrodesis. *J Bone Joint Surg.* 1985;67A:546–550.
4. Myerson MS, Quill G. Ankle arthrodesis. A comparison of an arthroscopic and an open method of treatment. *Clin Orthop Rel Res.* 1991;268:84–95.
5. Scranton PE. An overview of ankle arthrodesis. *Clin Orthop Rel Res.* 1991;268:96–101.
6. Crosby LA, Fitzgibbons T, Formanek T. Arthroscopic ankle fusion utilizing demineralized bone matrix and bone marrow grafting. Scientific Exhibit at the annual meeting of the American Academy of Orthopaedic Surgeons; Washington, DC; February 20–25, 1992.
7. Malarkey RF, Binski JC. Ankle arthrodesis with the Calandruccio frame and bimalleolar inlay grafting. *Clin Orthop Rel Res.* 1991;268:44–48.
8. Maurer RC, Cimino WR, Cox CV, Satow GK. Transarticular cross-screw fixation: a technique of ankle arthrodesis. *Clin Orthop Relat Res.* 1991;268:56–64.
9. Glick JM, Myerson MS, Morgan CD, Sampson TG. Arthroscopic ankle arthrodesis. Presentation at the ninth annual meeting of the American Arthroscopy Association of North America; Orlando, Florida; April 1990.
10. Morgan CD. Arthroscopic tibio-talar arthrodesis. In: Guhl J, ed. *Ankle Arthroscopy, Pathology and Surgical Techniques.* Thorofare, NJ: Charles Slack; 1988: 119–123.
11. Myerson MS, Allon SM. Arthroscopic ankle arthrodesis. *Contemp Orthop.* 1989;19:21–27.
12. Tiedeman J, Connolly JF, Strates BS, Lippiello L. Treatment of nonunion by percutaneous injection of bone marrow and demineralized bone matrix: an experimental study in dogs. *Clin Orthop Rel Res.* 1991;268:294–301.

chapter Twenty

Arthroscopy of the Posterior Subtalar Joint and Great Toe

J. Serge Parisien

SUBTALAR JOINT

The talocalcaneal area is divided into two joint cavities: the talocalcaneonavicular joint or anterior subtalar joint and the posterior talocalcaneal joint or posterior subtalar joint. These two joints are separated by the tarsal canal and sinus tarsi. The *posterior subtalar joint* is formed by the posterior calcaneal facet of the talus superiorly and the posterior talar facet of the calcaneus inferiorly. This joint is directed upwards with a convex orientation, its long axis approximately 40° oblique to the midline of the foot. The joint capsule is reinforced by the lateral talocalcaneal ligament and the calcaneofibular ligament. In the posterior aspect of this joint, behind the lateral malleolus, the peroneal tendons, the sural nerve, and the small saphenous vein are located (Fig. 20.1).

Arthroscopy of the posterior subtalar joint may be helpful in chondromalacia, synovitis (rheumatoid or infectious), loose bodies, osteophytes, and arthrofibrosis. In chronic pain syndrome in the hindfoot, arthroscopic evaluation of the joint may be valuable to assess the status of the articular cartilage and to perform direct biopsy of the synovial lining as well.[1,2]

Diagnostic and arthroscopic surgery of the posterior subtalar joint can be performed as an outpatient procedure with minimal trauma to the joint. The technique is simple and is gaining wide acceptance in the management of some disorders of the hindfoot.

Surgical Technique

Small arthroscopes ranging from 1.9 to 2.7 mm in diameter with 25° to 30° of angulation are important to perform the procedure. Also needed are a small joint shaver set with 1.9 mm or 2.9 mm full-radius blade and abrader, an 18-gauge needle, and a 50 mL syringe (Fig. 20.2).

Local, spinal, or general anesthesia may be used. The patient is placed in the lateral decubitus position or in the semisupine position with a sandbag under the buttocks. A leg holder is optional, but when used should be placed far away from the fibular head. A tourniquet, applied over the thigh, can be inflated if necessary.

Two arthroscopic portals, anterior and posterior, are available for examination of the posterior subtalar joint.[1,2] The anterior portal is located approximately 2 cm anterior and 1 cm distal to the tip of the lateral malleolus. The posterior portal is located approximately at the level of the tip of the lateral malleolus between the lateral malleolus and the Achilles tendon (Figs. 20.3, 20.4). This portal should not be placed too close to the lateral malleolus, to avoid injury to the sural nerve and small saphenous vein. Anteriorly, an 18-gauge needle is used to inflate the joint with approximately 5 to 10 mL of normal saline. The needle is removed and a blunt obturator, followed by the arthroscope, is introduced through a stab incision made

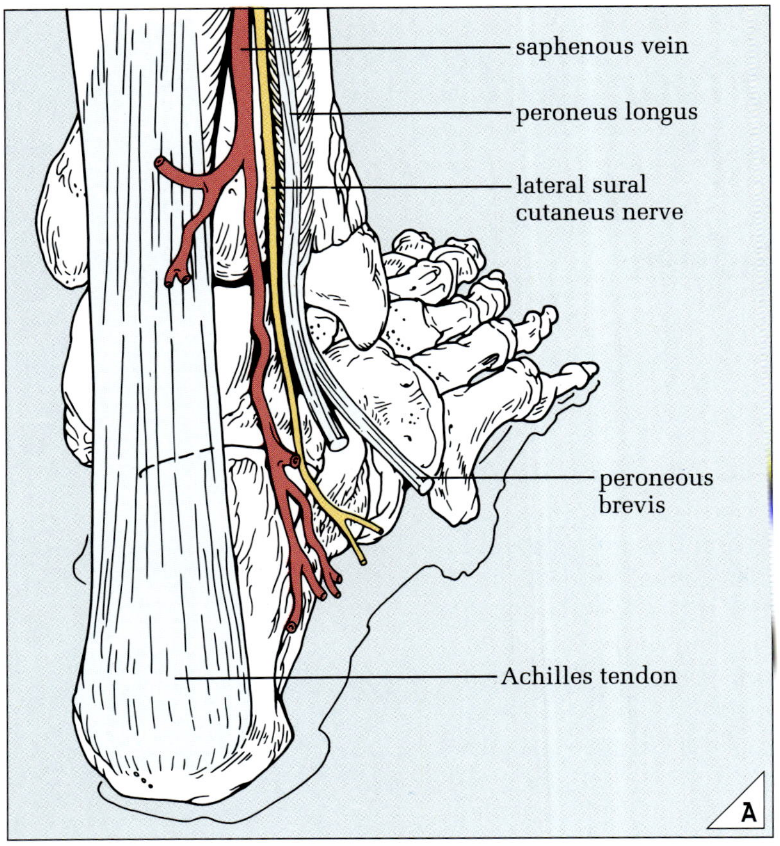

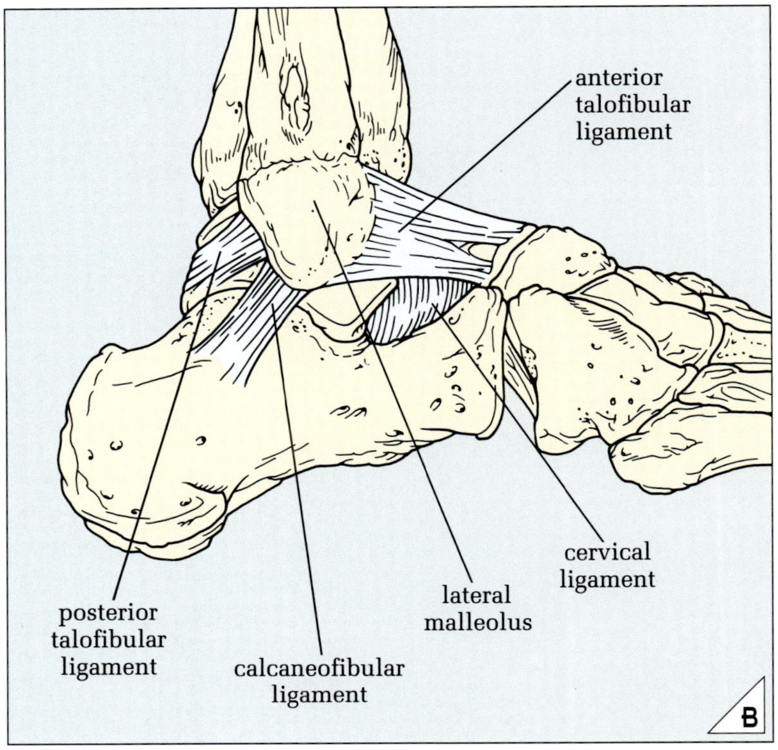

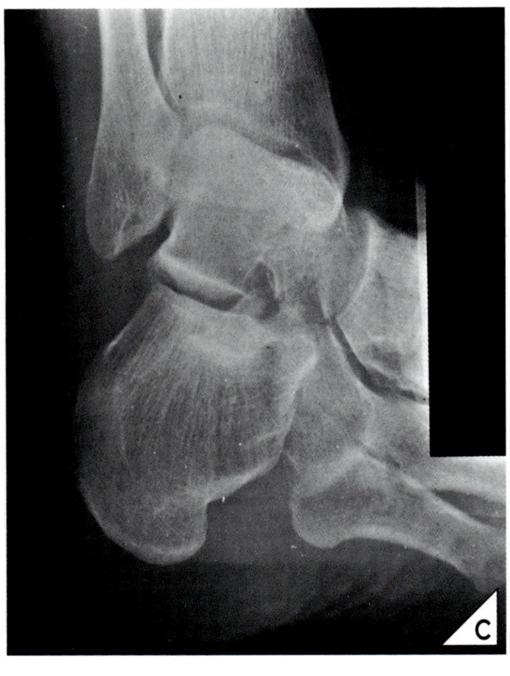

Figure 20.1
(A) Posterolateral aspect of the ankle and subtalar joint. (B) Posterior subtalar joint. (C) Radiograph of the posterior subtalar joint.

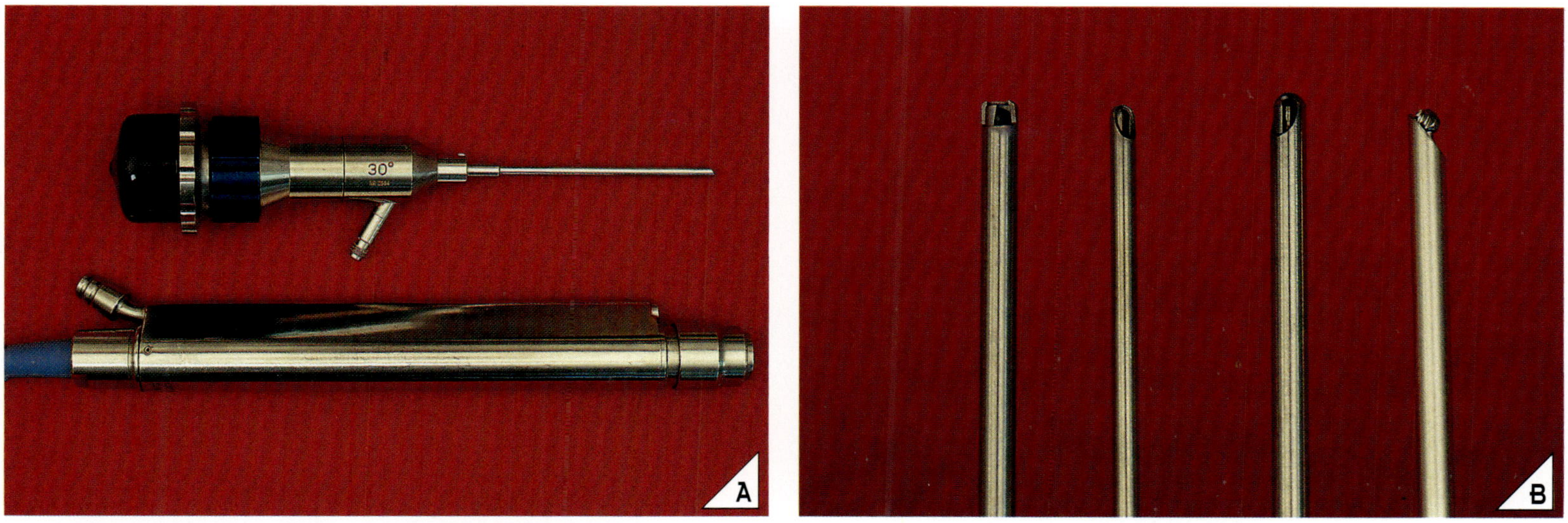

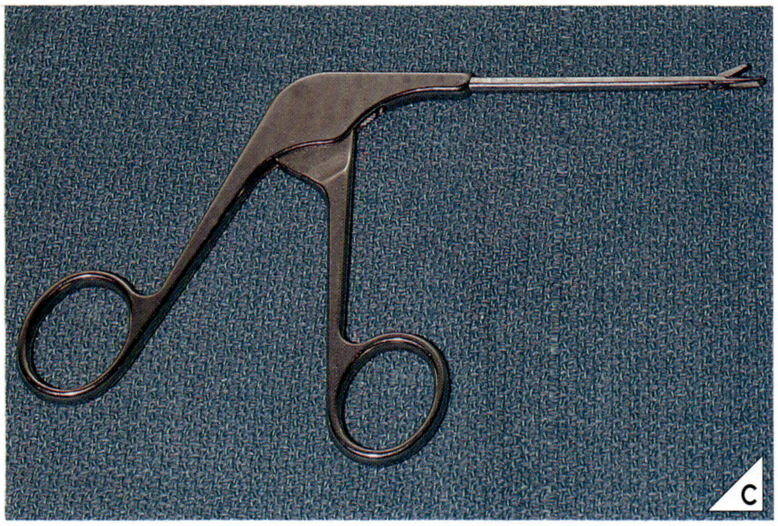

Figure 20.2

(A) Small arthroscope with camera used for arthroscopy of the subtalar joint. (B) Shaver and abrader blades for the small motorized instrumentation system. (C) Small basket forceps.

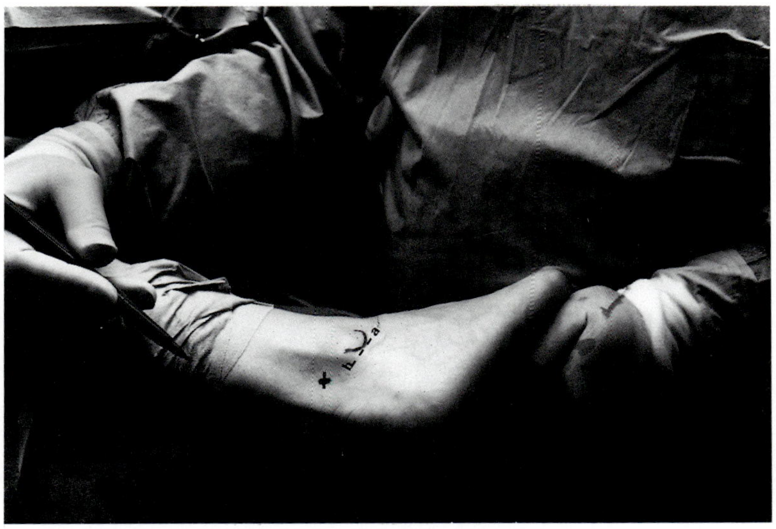

Figure 20.3

A and B show the anterior and posterior portals for subtalar joint arthroscopy. X indicates the location of the posterolateral portal for ankle joint arthroscopy.

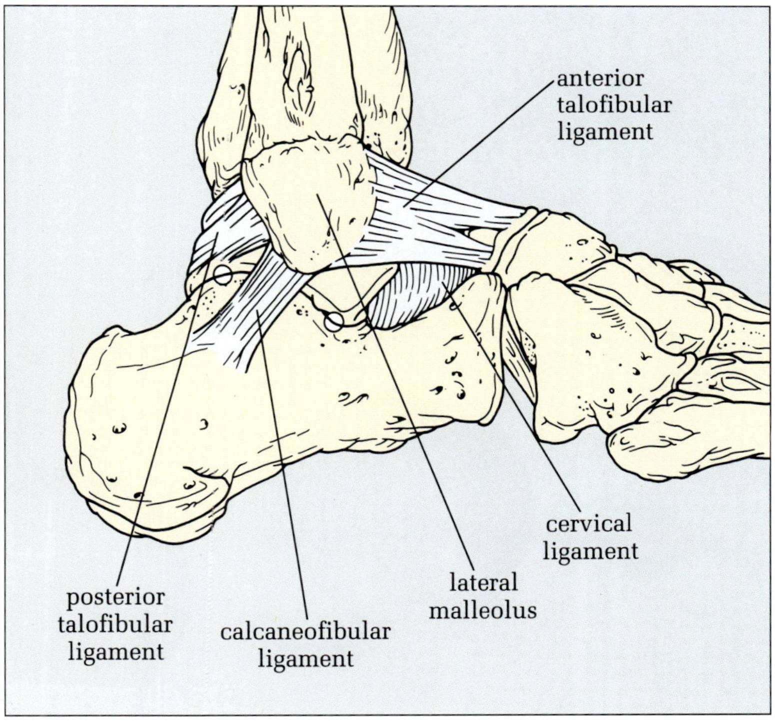

Figure 20.4

Schematic illustration of the posterior subtalar joint showing arthroscopic portals.

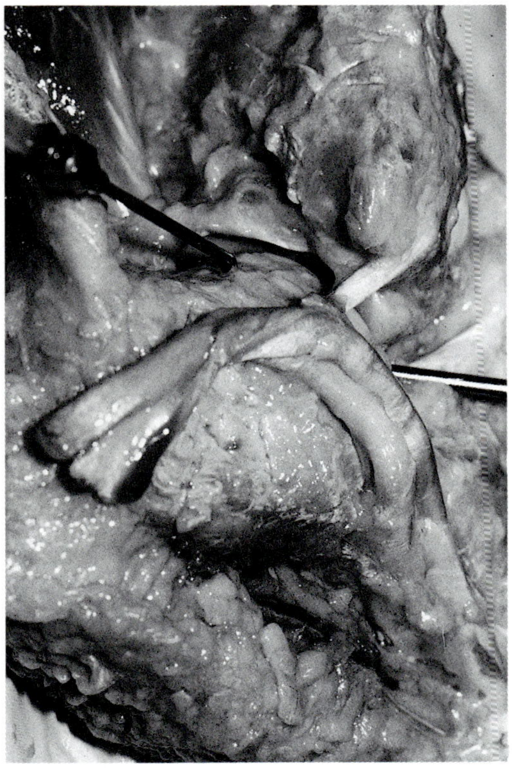

Figure 20.5

Cadaver specimen showing a scope at the anterior aspect of the posterior subtalar joint.

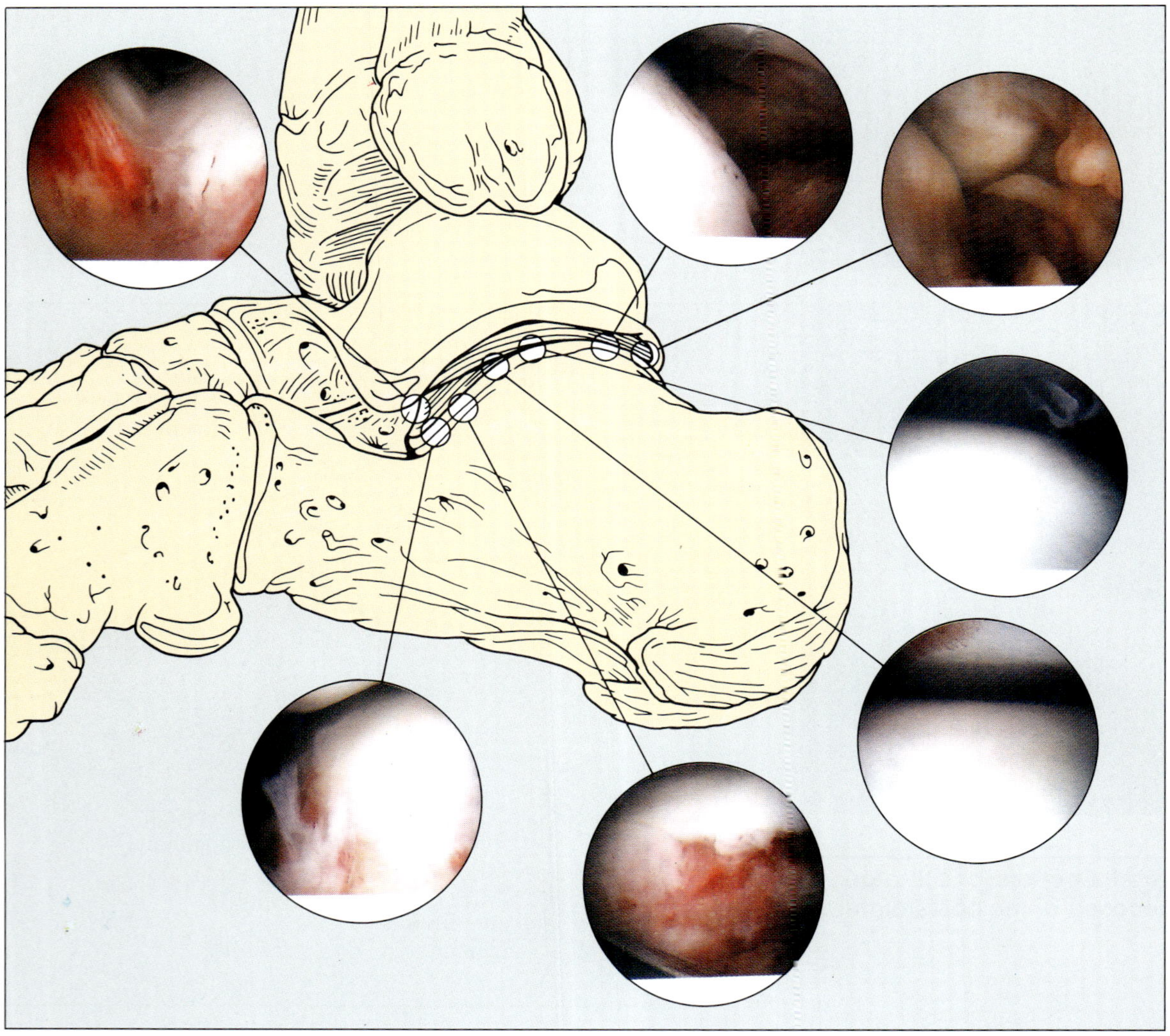

Figure 20.6

Diverse areas of the posterior subtalar joint left ankle in a patient with subtalar instability.

in the area of the needle insertion. With the joint inflated, another 18-gauge needle can be used to establish a posterior portal (Fig. 20.5). For diagnostic arthroscopy, constant irrigation can be provided with a 50 mL syringe filled with normal saline or Ringer's lactate solution, attached to the trochar sleeve by a plastic tube. Overhead irrigation is used when operative arthroscopy is contemplated.

From the anterior portal the following structures can be visualized: the synovial lining of the posterior aspect of the interosseous talocalcaneal ligament, the lateral capsule, the articular cartilage of the posterior facet of the talus, and the calcaneus. Maneuvering the arthroscope posteriorly will visualize the posterior pouch of the joint with its synovial lining (Figs. 20.6, 20.7). A more complete examination can be performed by switching portals, placing the arthroscope into the posterior portal and the inflow/outflow cannula anteriorly. Chondromalacic areas can be shaved, osteophytes and loose bodies removed,

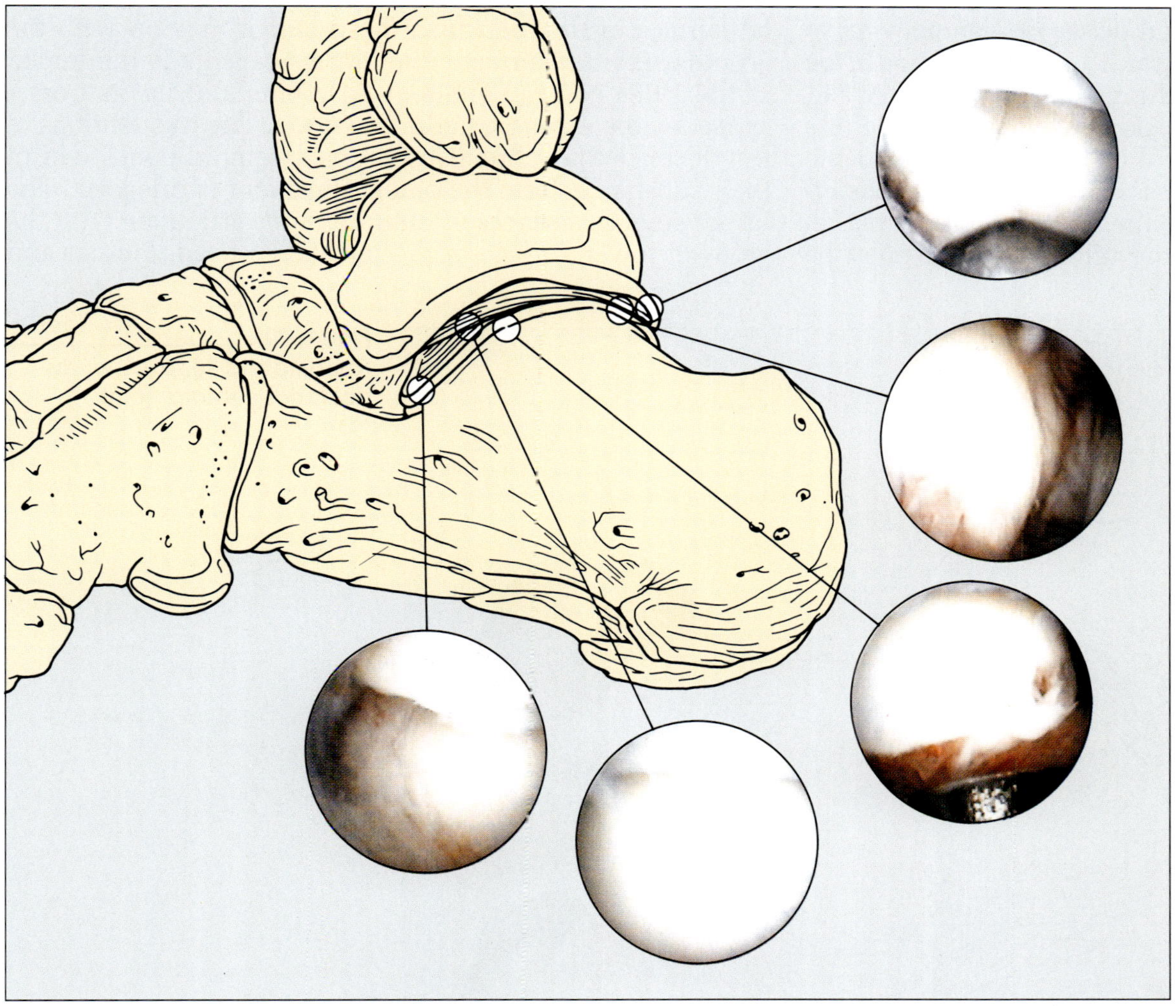

Figure 20.7 Several areas of the left posterior subtalar joint in a patient with ankle instability.

and partial synovectomy with excision of adhesions achieved using these two portals (Figs. 20.8–20.10). Postoperatively the portals are closed with nylon sutures or are left open for escape of the irrigating fluid. A compression dressing is applied and full weight-bearing is allowed as tolerated.

Complications and Pitfalls

A good knowledge of the hindfoot area anatomy will prevent damage to underlying neurovascular structures. The proximity of the sural nerve and lesser saphenous vein to the posterior aspect of the lateral malleolus should be kept in mind when making the posterior portal. A #11 blade can be used to make the skin incision. The use of a small hemostat to spread the skin incision down to the capsule will minimize neurovascular injury. If the posterior portal is placed proximal to the tip of the lateral malleolus, the posterior aspect of the talocrural joint may be entered instead of the posterior aspect of the subtalar joint. Infection can be avoided by the use of strict aseptic techniques.

GREAT TOE

The metatarsophalangeal joint of the great toe is a condyloid joint formed by the metatarsal head and the base of the proximal phalanx. The articular surface of the base of the phalanx articulates in extension with the articular distal surface of the metatarsal head and in flexion with the articular plantar surface. The fibrous capsule is reinforced at the sides by the collateral ligaments and on its dorsal aspect by the extensor hallucis tendon. The two tendons of the flexor hallucis brevis, with the sesamoid bones within their substance, form the plantar ligament of this joint. The upper smooth surfaces of the sesamoids articulate with the grooved lower surface of the metatarsal head. Plantar and

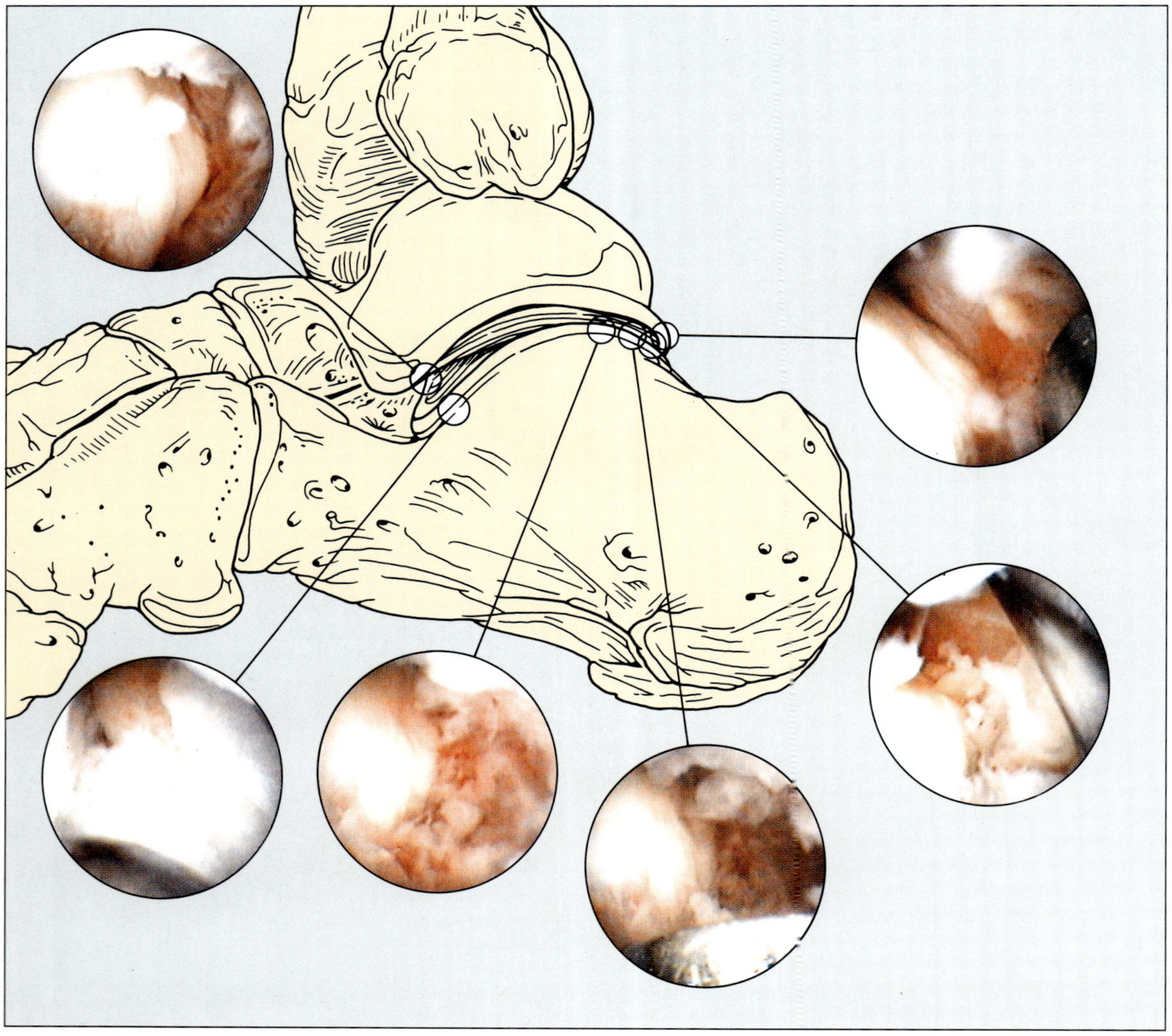

Figure 20.8
Rheumatoid synovitis of the posterior subtalar joint.

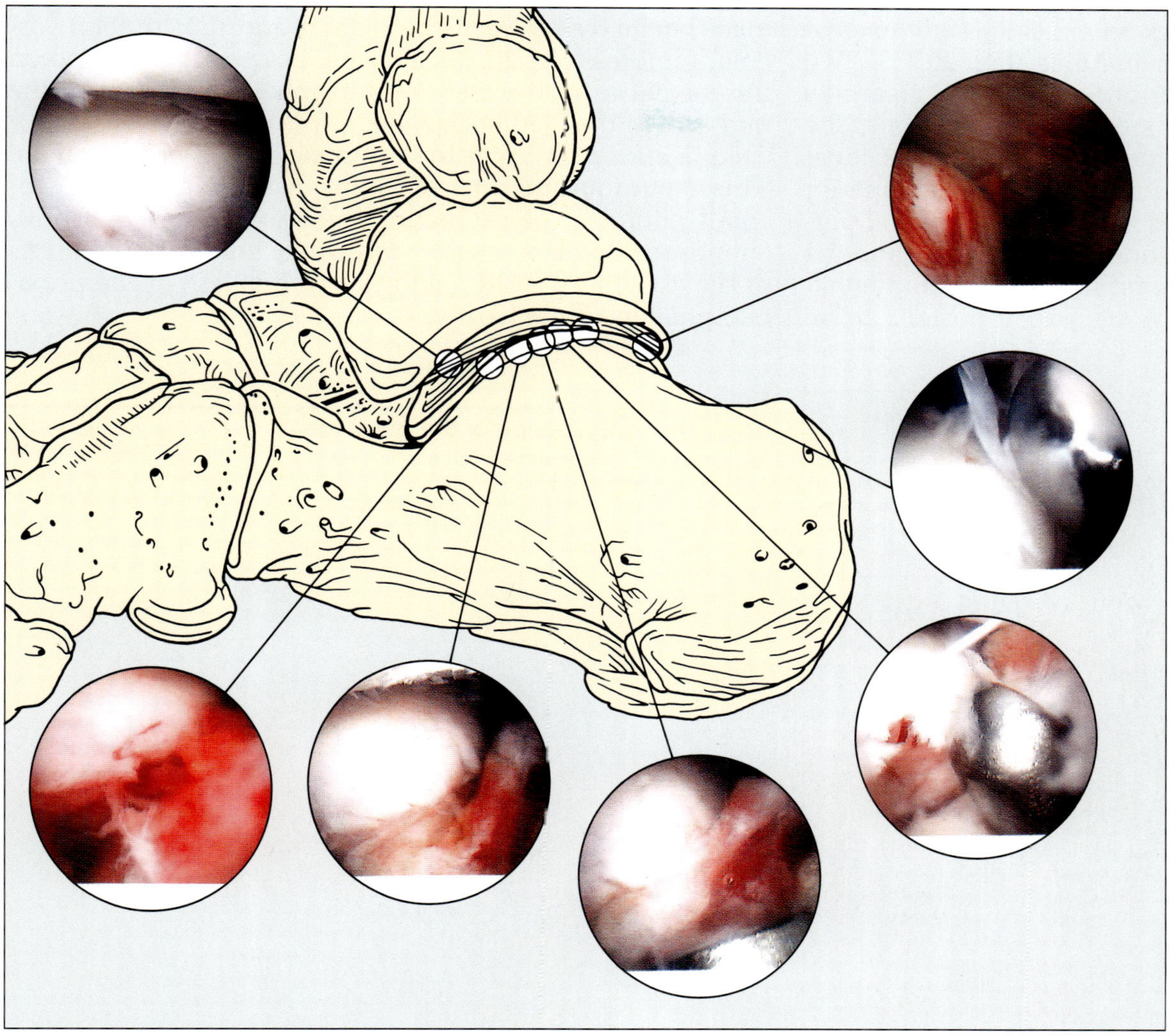

Figure 20.9

Adhesions and synovitis of the left posterior subtalar joint.

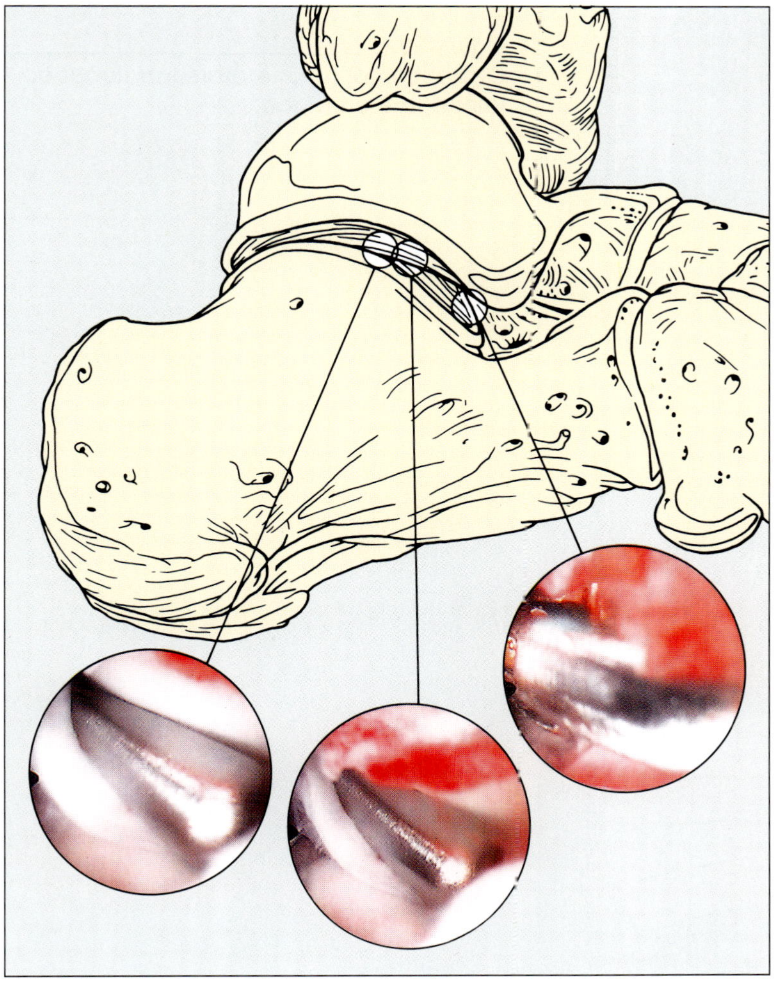

Figure 20.10

Synovitis and adhesions in the right posterior subtalar joint. A motorized shaver is seen performing debridement.

dorsal digital arteries and nerves on either side of the great toe make up the neurovascular bundles (Fig. 20.11). Two main portals are available for arthroscopy of the great toe: the superomedial portal and superolateral portal. The superomedial portal is localized at the joint line level medial to the extensor hallucis longus tendon and superior to the medial neurovascular bundle. The superolateral portal is lateral to the extensor hallucis longus tendon and the extensor hallucis brevis at the joint line away from the lateral neurovascular bundle. An accessory portal can be made medially between the plantar and dorsal neurovascular bundles (Fig. 20.12). This medial portal is located on the medial aspect of the metatarsophalangeal joint in the mid-area of the medial capsule.

Indications for great toe arthroscopy are not common. This technique may be of value in the management of small chondral or osteochondral fractures of the joint, chondromalacia, synovitis, and osteochondritis dissecans of the metatarsal head, and cysts of the base of the proximal phalanx of the hallux.

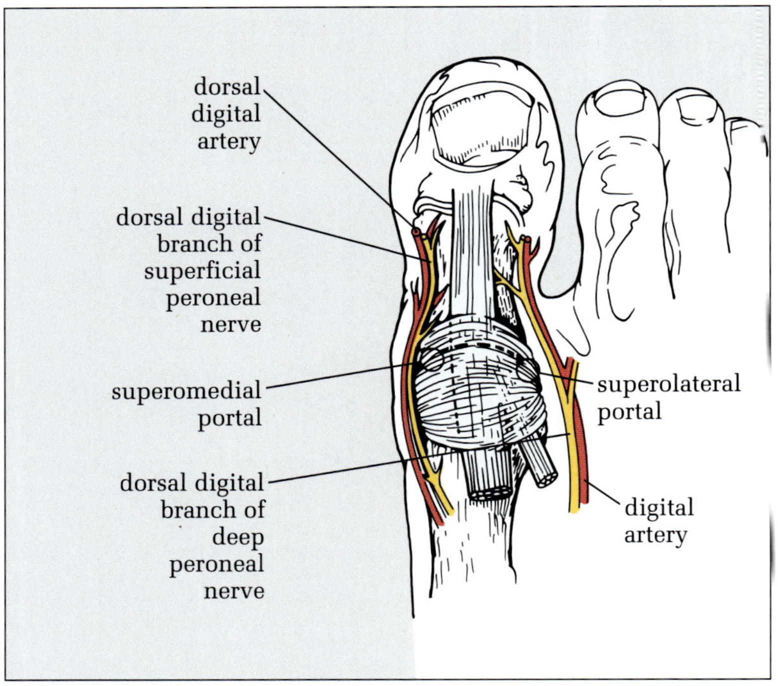

Figure 20.11
Portals for arthroscopy of the great toe.

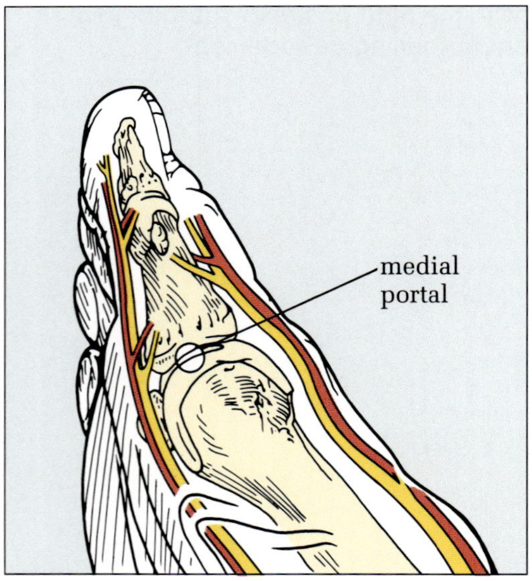

Figure 20.12
Medial portal for the great toe.

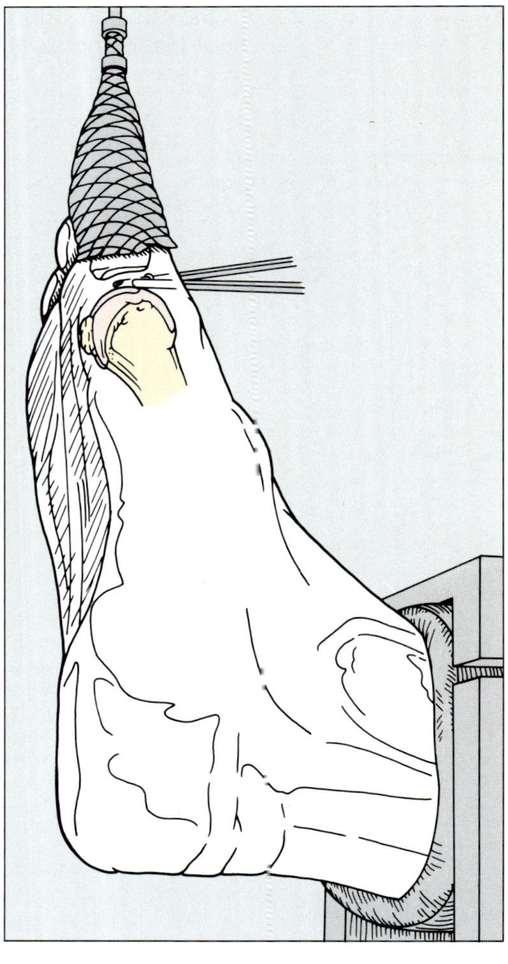

Figure 20.13
Distraction of the metatarsophalangeal joint of the great toe.

Surgical Technique

A 1.9 or 2.2 mm arthroscope with 30° angulation is necessary for the examination. A hand-held camera is used, as well as a small joint shaver system with a full-radius blade and abrader.

The procedure can be performed under general, spinal, or regional anesthesia. The patient is usually placed supine. No tourniquet is necessary around the thigh. The use of a leg holder to stabilize the lower extremity is optional. A Chinese finger trap applied to the distal phalanx of the great toe and suspended from an overhead pulley system can be used for distraction of the metatarsophalangeal joint (Fig. 20.13). An 18-gauge needle is used to inflate the joint cavity with approximately 3 to 5 mL of normal saline from either the superomedial or superolateral portal. From the opposite portal a #11 blade is used to make the skin incision and a small hemostat clamp is used to spread the incision down to the capsule to prevent injury to the adjacent neurovascular bundle. The arthroscope is placed through the superomedial portal with the outflow through the superolateral portal. An IV extension tubing attached to the arthroscope can give the necessary capsular distention. If surgery is indicated the motorized instrumentation can be placed through the portal opposite the scope with an overhead irrigation system connected to the arthroscope sheath. Any intraarticular pathology can be managed by use of these two portals. The accessory portal through the medial aspect of the joint can be established under direct vision if necessary, by means of a spinal needle. Complete exploration of the metatarsophalangeal joint can be performed, visualizing the dorsal recess of the joint, the articular cartilage of the phalangeal base and metatarsal head, and the inferior aspect with the medial and lateral sesamoids. Shaving of chondromalacic areas, removal of chip fractures, loose chondral or osteochondral fragments, excision of osteochondritis dissecans of the first metatarsal head, excision of a cyst of the proximal phalanx of the hallux, and debridement of some selected cases of degenerative arthritis of the great toe can be successfully performed (Figs. 20.14, 20.15).[3,4]

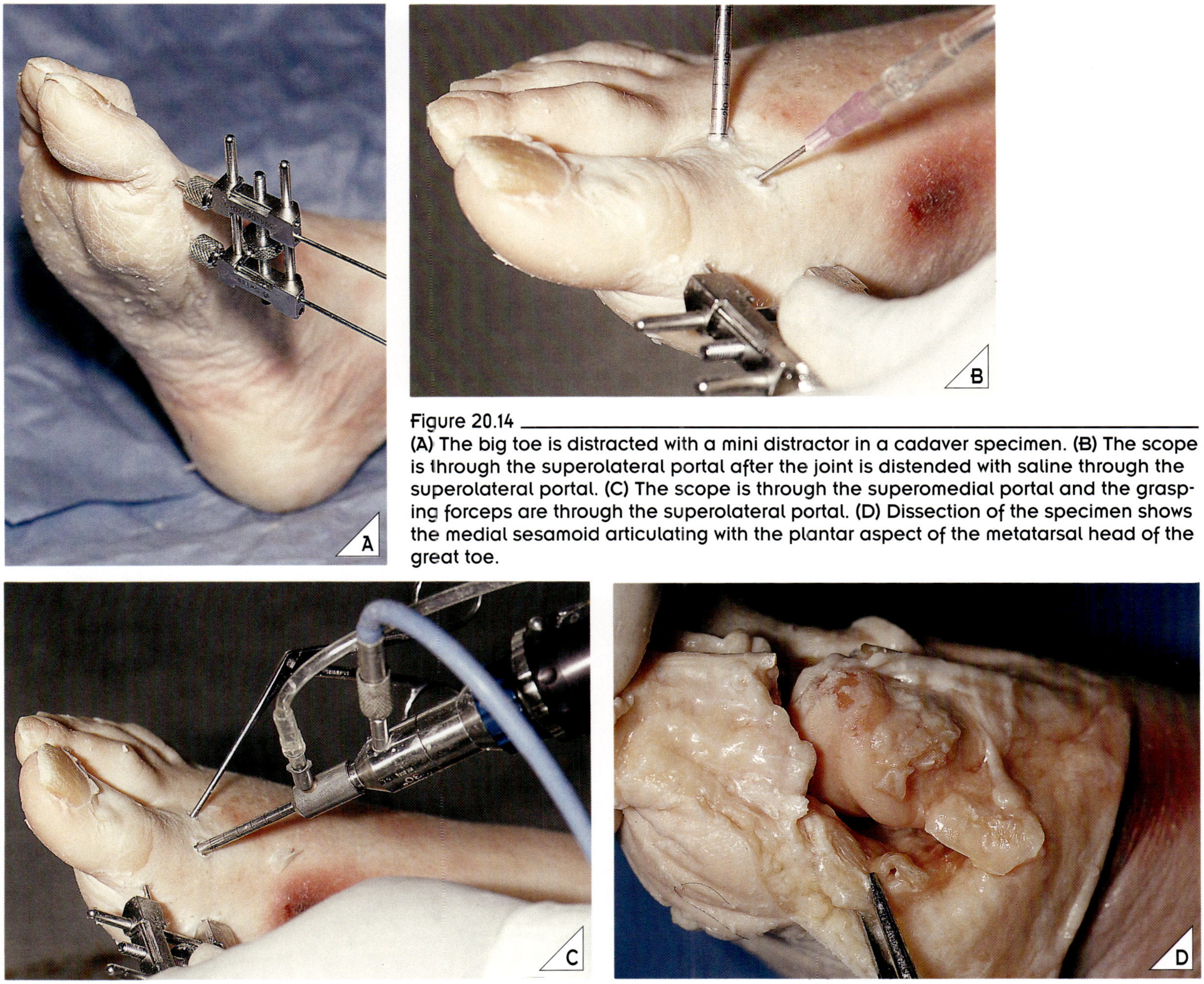

Figure 20.14
(A) The big toe is distracted with a mini distractor in a cadaver specimen. (B) The scope is through the superolateral portal after the joint is distended with saline through the superolateral portal. (C) The scope is through the superomedial portal and the grasping forceps are through the superolateral portal. (D) Dissection of the specimen shows the medial sesamoid articulating with the plantar aspect of the metatarsal head of the great toe.

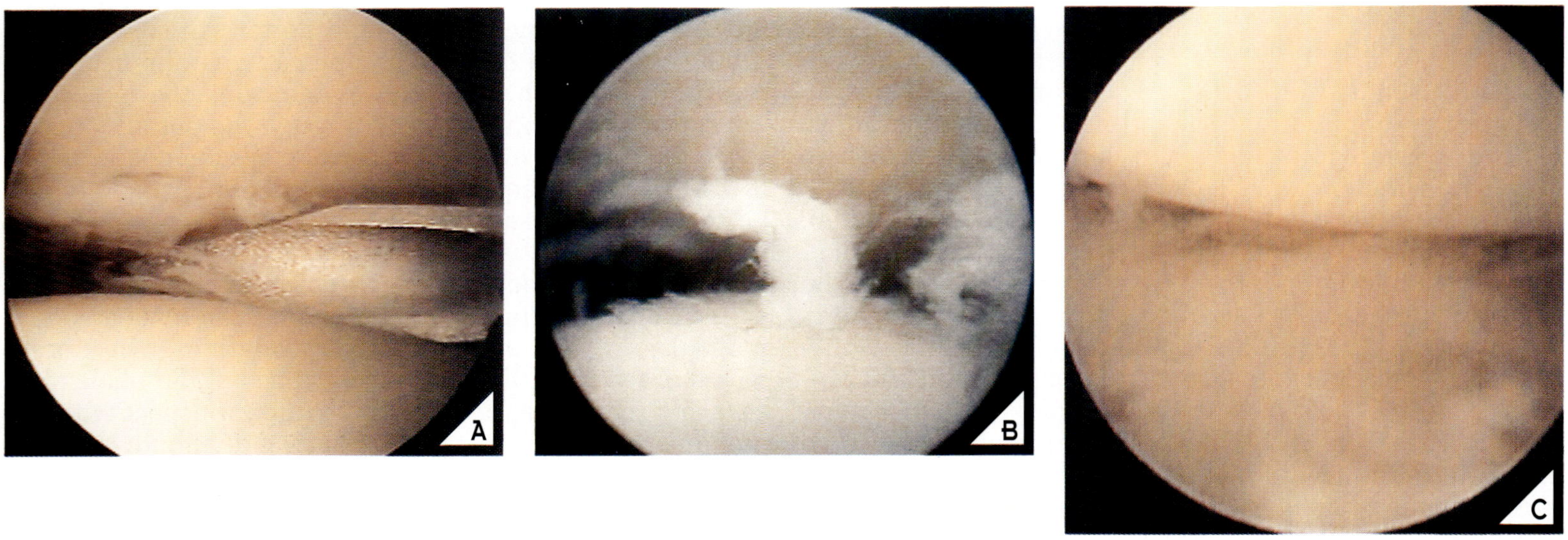

Figure 20.15

An arthroscopic view of the articulation of the great toe. (A) The needle is on the lateral side of the joint. The articular surface of the proximal phalanx is on top and the articular surface of the metatarsal head is at the bottom. (B) The metatarsal head is below and the proximal phalanx is on top. (C) The inferior aspect of the metatarsal head and capsule of the plantar aspect of the joint.

REFERENCES

1. Parisien JS, Vangness T. Arthroscopy of the subtalar joint: an experimental approach. *Arthroscopy.* 1985;1:53–57.
2. Parisien JS. Arthroscopy of the posterior subtalar joint: a preliminary report. *Foot Ankle.* 1986;6:219–224.
3. Ferkel RD, Van Buecken K. Great toe arthroscopy: indications, techniques and results. Abstracts of the 10th Annual Meeting of the AANA; San Diego, Calif; April 1991.
4. Barlett DH. Arthroscopic management of osteochondritis dissecans of the first metatarsal head. *Arthroscopy.* 1988;4:51–54.

Section Four

The Elbow

chapter Twenty One

Arthroscopic Surgery of the Elbow

J. Serge Parisien

Operative arthroscopy of the elbow is an effective and well-established procedure for treatment of various elbow disorders. The very narrow confines of the joint and the close proximity of the neurovascular structures to the arthroscopic portals (Figs. 21.1, 21.2), make meticulous technique mandatory to avoid serious potential complications.[1,2]

Based on my own experience and on a review of the available literature,[1–6] elbow arthroscopy can be useful in the following situations:

- Evaluation of chronic elbow pain when investigative procedures such as plain x-rays and MRI fail to give a proper diagnosis
- Removal of loose bodies
- Debridement of osteochondritic lesions of the capitellum
- Debridement and excision of osteophytes in posttraumatic disorders of the olecranon
- Synovitis
- Debridement in selected cases of osteoarthritis
- Management of posttraumatic or postsurgical arthrofibrosis.

Absolute contraindications for this procedure include bony or fibrous ankylosis that would make the introduction of the arthroscopic instruments into the elbow almost impossible. A relative contraindication is a previous anterior transposition of the ulnar nerve that would preclude use of the anteromedial portal.

INSTRUMENTATION

Video arthroscopes, 4 and 2.7 mm with 25° to 30° angulation, are used. Other equipment includes hand instruments (spinal needle, switching rod, basket forceps, grasping forceps, probe, rasp, curette) and small motorized instruments (synovial resector and abrader). The small 2.7-mm arthroscope is mostly helpful for visualization of the posterior aspect of the elbow.

POSITIONING OF THE PATIENT

General anesthesia, intrascalene block, or axillary block can be used at the discretion of the surgeon. A tourniquet placed high on the upper arm can be inflated as needed.

The patient is placed in a *supine* position with the elbow flexed at 90°. The hand and forearm are connected to an overhead suspension device (Fig. 21.3). The elbow can also be placed at the patient's side on an arm board. However, the first position, with the arm suspended, provides better access to both medial and lateral aspects of the elbow joint. The surgeon stands to the lateral side of the elbow, with the first assistant on the opposite side. Video equipment is placed opposite the surgeon (Fig. 21.4A).

Some surgeons have advocated a *prone* position for the patient to provide access to both the anterior and posterior aspects of the elbow.

I have described an *over the chest* position that can be used for examination of both the anterior and posterior compartments of the elbow or the posterior compartment alone. The patient is placed in supine position with the upper extremity draped free. The shoulder is at 90° with the forearm placed over the patient's chest. The hand is stabilized in a device attached to the opposite side of the operating table (Fig. 21.4B). This device can control flexion and extension of the elbow. The same arthroscopic portals can be used. If one prefers to perform the anterior compartment examination with the extremity connected to an overhead suspension, the arm can then be placed in the over the chest position to complete the posterior compartment examination (Fig. 21.4C). In that situation, the nonsterile part of the extremity should be wrapped in a sterile plastic sheet.

ANATOMY AND PORTALS

From an arthroscopic viewpoint, the elbow joint can be divided into two compartments: the anterior compartment, with a relatively large joint capsule that can accommodate a large 4-mm arthroscope, and the more shallow posterior compartment, which is better visualized with a smaller arthroscope. Two portals are described anteriorly, the anterolateral and the anteromedial. Three portals are available posteriorly, the straight lateral portal, the posterolateral portal, and the straight posterior portal. A proximomedial portal has been described recently.

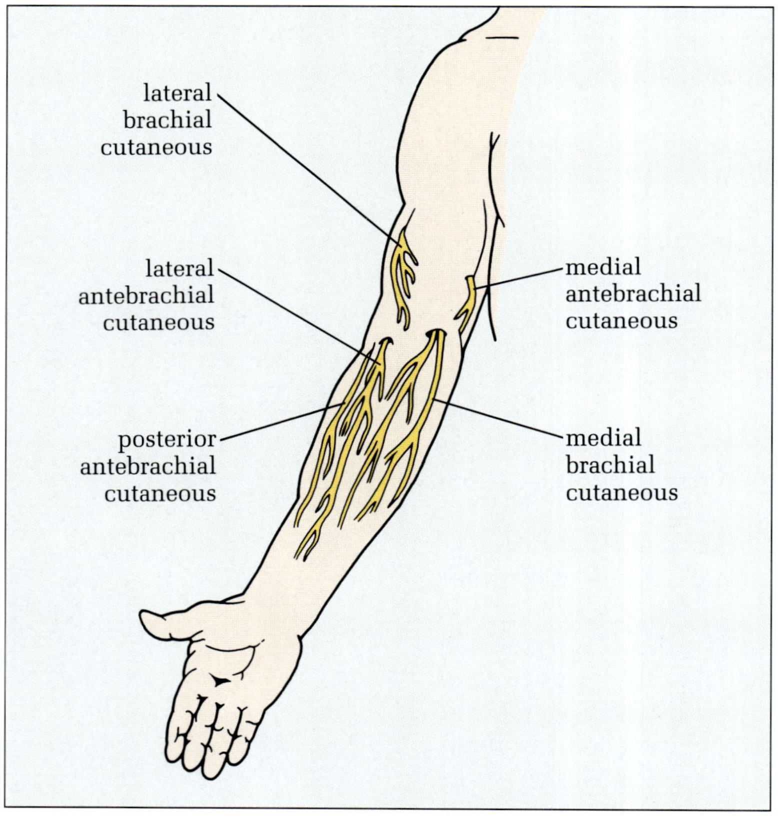

Figure 21.1
Cutaneous nerves of the anterior aspect of the elbow.

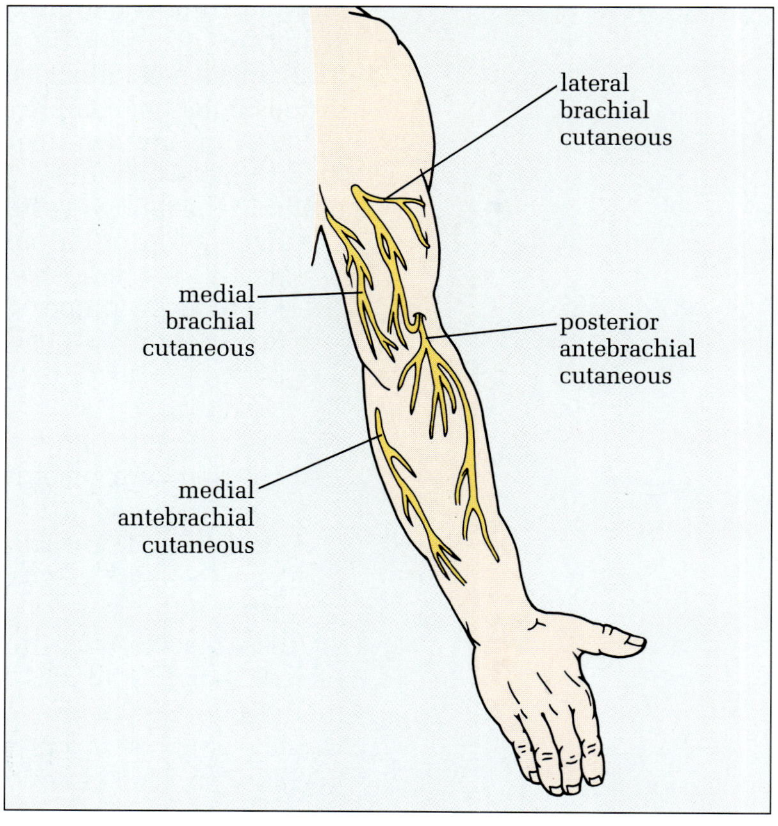

Fgure 21.2
Cutaneous nerves of the posterior aspect of the elbow.

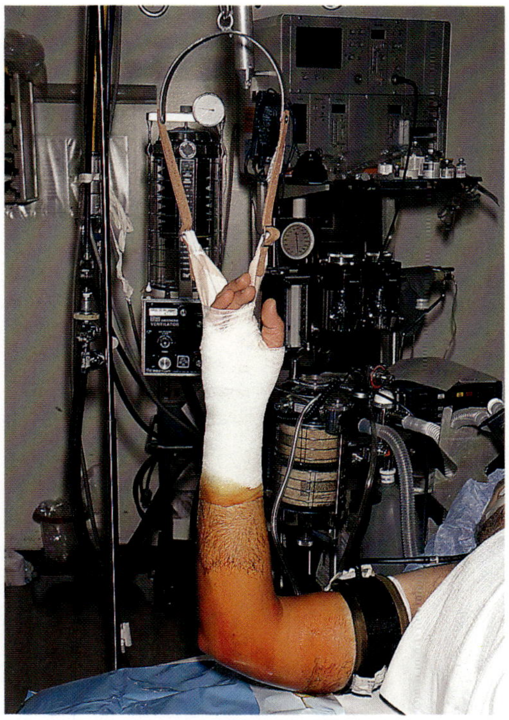

Figure 21.3
The patient is in the supine position with the elbow flexed at 90°. The hand and the forearm are connected to an overhead suspension device.

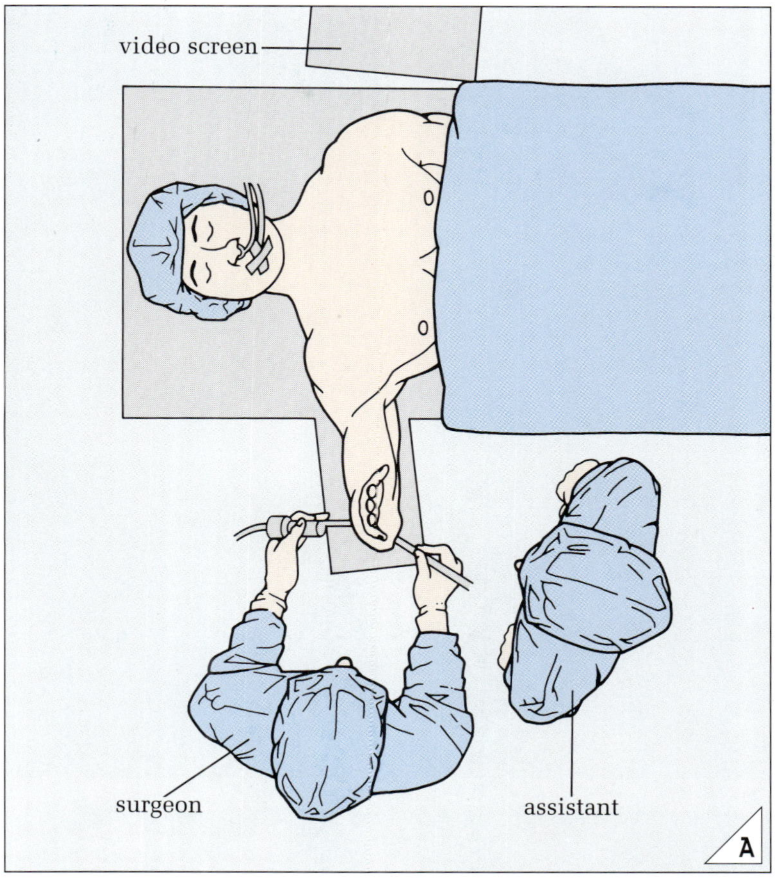

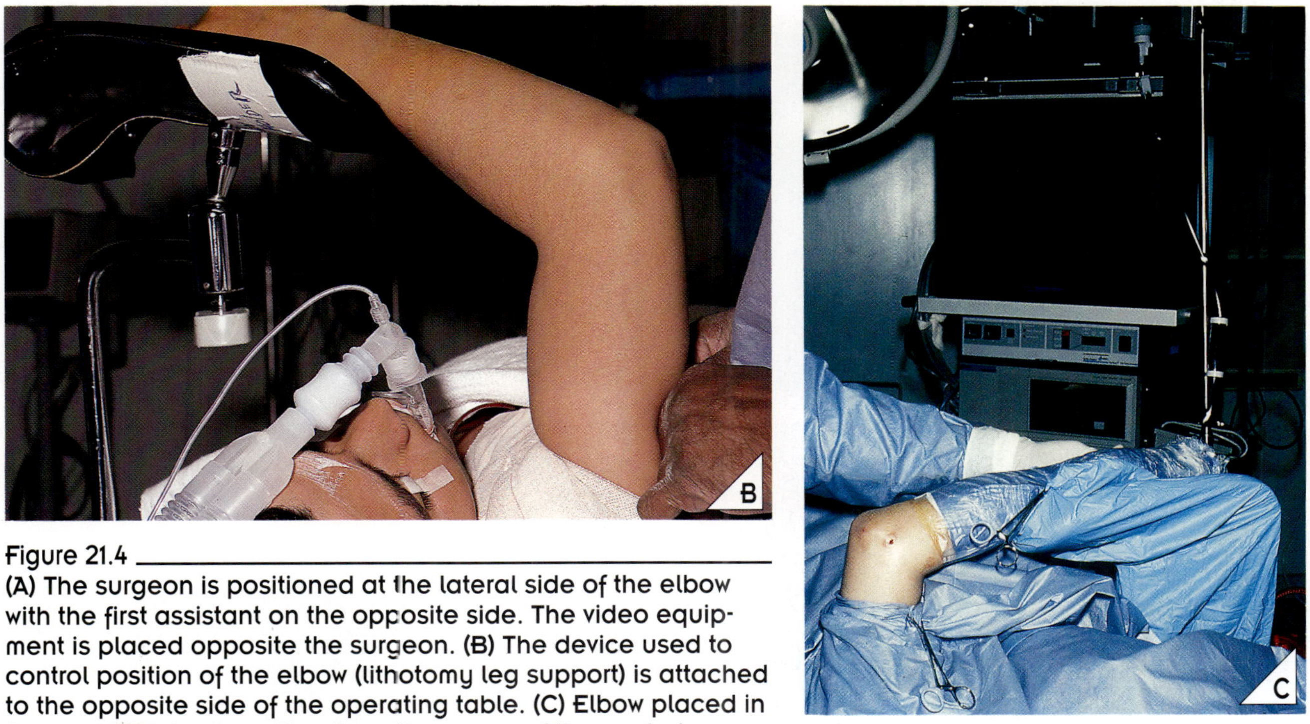

Figure 21.4
(A) The surgeon is positioned at the lateral side of the elbow with the first assistant on the opposite side. The video equipment is placed opposite the surgeon. (B) The device used to control position of the elbow (lithotomy leg support) is attached to the opposite side of the operating table. (C) Elbow placed in the over the chest position for arthroscopy of the posterior compartment. The device is covered with a sterile stockinet.

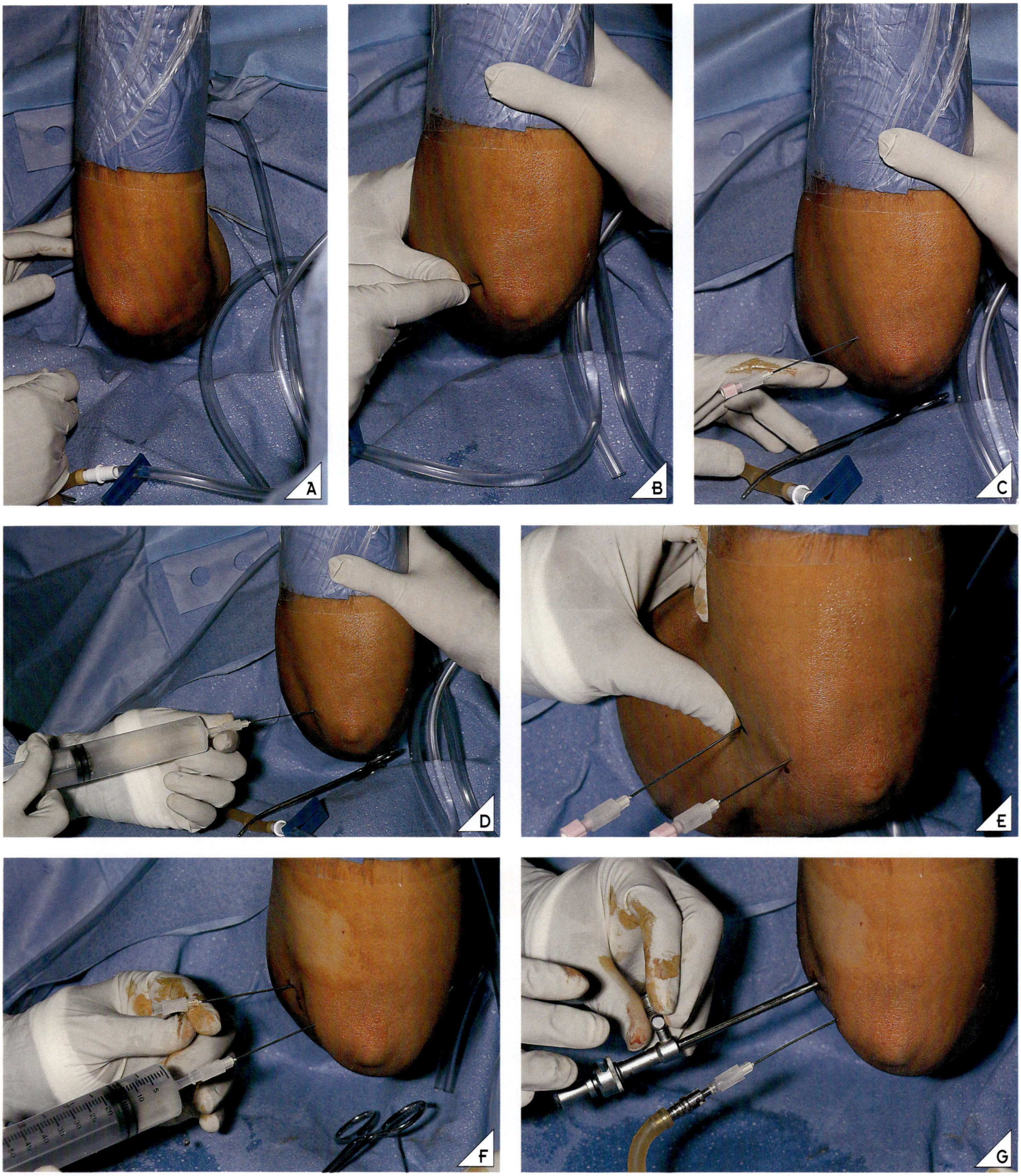

Figure 21.5

Steps used to develop the anterolateral portal. The patient is in the supine position with the elbow flexed 90°. (A) The portal is located above the radial head approximately 1 cm anterior to the lateral epicondyle. (B–D) An 18-gauge needle inserted in the area between the lateral epicondyle, radial head, and olecranon tip is used to inject saline into the posterior capsule. (E, F) A second 18-gauge needle is introduced 1 cm anterior to the lateral epicondyle. (G) A skin incision is made at the location of the second needle for introduction of a 4 mm trocar with its smooth obturator.

Anterolateral Portal

The anterolateral portal, usually the first arthroscopic portal established, is located above the radial head approximately 1 cm anterior to the lateral epicondyle (Fig. 21.5A). The anterolateral portal passes through the extensor carpi radialis brevis muscle, within a mean distance of approximately 4 mm from the radial nerve. However, as has been demonstrated by anatomic studies[1] with joint distention, the nerve moves an additional 7 mm anteriorly. Subcutaneous nerves at risk in developing this portal are the lateral and posterior antebrachial cutaneous nerves. The lateral antebrachial cutaneous nerve, which is the terminal branch of the musculocutaneous nerve, perforates the brachial fascia proximal to the joint and lateral to the biceps tendon. The posterior antebrachial cutaneous nerve, which is a branch of the radial nerve, perforates the brachial fascia in the distal two thirds of the arm.

To begin, an 18-gauge needle is inserted into the elbow joint in the triangular area located between the lateral epicondyle, the radial head, and the olecranon tip, and 30 mL of normal saline is injected into the posterior capsule of the joint (Fig. 21.5B–D). With maximal distention of the posterior capsule, distention of the anterior capsule is obtained (Fig. 21.6). Identification of the radial head is facilitated by pronation and supination of the forearm. A second 18-gauge needle is then introduced in front of the radial head approximately 1 cm anterior to the lateral epicondyle (Fig. 21.5E,F). This needle is directed towards the center of the joint and a reflux of fluid confirms proper penetration. After maximal distention of the anterior capsule is achieved, a #11 blade is used next to the anterior needle to make an incision for introduction of the arthroscope and cannular system. Continuous irrigation is obtained using the gravity system available for the knee joint. A hand-held camera is attached to the arthroscope for visualization. Arthroscopes ranging in size from 2.7 to 4 mm can be used (21.5G). The intraarticular structures best visualized through the portal are the trochlea, the distal humerus, and the coronoid process of the ulna (Fig. 21.7). However, by slowly retracting and rotating the scope, the medial aspect of the radiohumeral articulation can be seen.

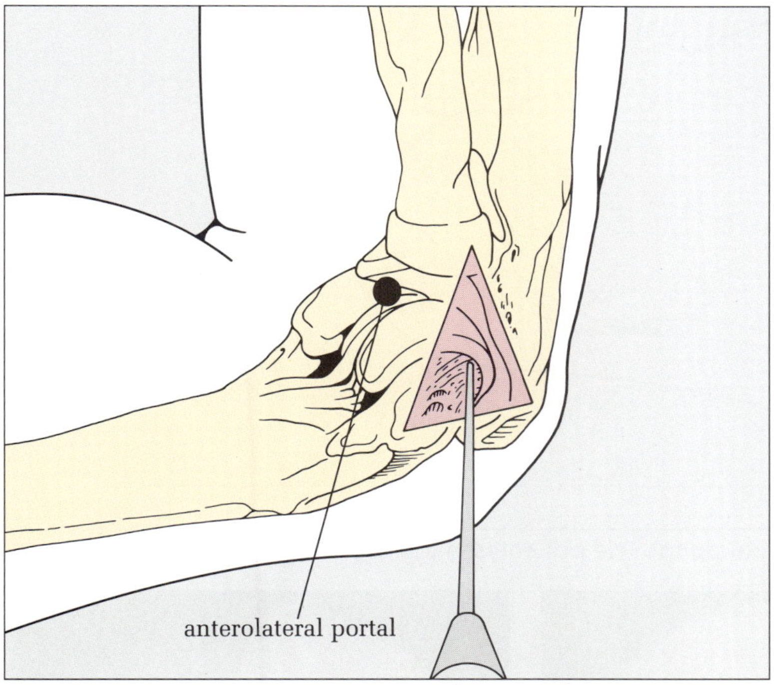

Figure 21.6
To begin the procedure, an 18-gauge needle is inserted into the elbow in the triangular area located between the lateral epicondyle, the radial head, and the olecranon tip. Normal saline (30 mL) is injected into the posterior capsule of the joint.

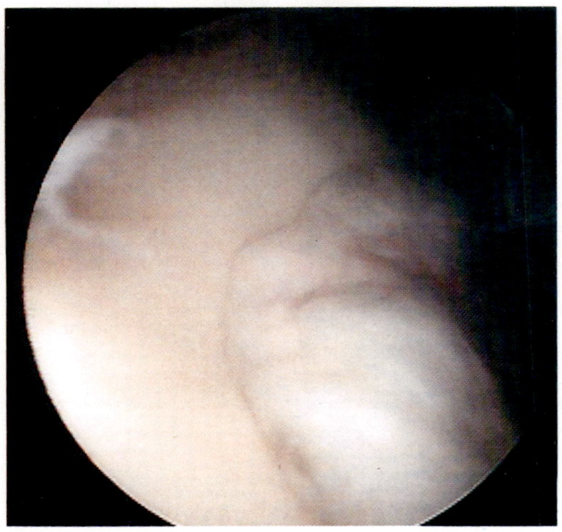

Figure 21.7
Visualization of the trochlea and the coronoid process of the ulna.

Anteromedial Portal

The anteromedial portal should avoid the medial antebrachial cutaneous nerve. This portal pierces the tendinous portion of the pronator teres and the radial aspect of the flexor digitorum superficialis within 6 mm of the median nerve and brachial artery. With distention of the elbow, it has been shown that the median nerve and brachial artery are displaced 10 and 8 mm anteriorly, respectively.[1]

The anteromedial portal is located approximately 2 cm anterior and distal to the medial epicondyle (Fig. 21.8). This portal can be established by using an 18-gauge spinal needle on the medial side. With the arthroscope placed anterolaterally, identification of the entry needle can be confirmed. An alternative way of achieving anteromedial entry is to insert a smooth rod through the sheath of the arthroscope and identify the tip of the rod through the tented skin medially. The anteromedial portal gives excellent visualization of the capitellum and radial head. This examination is maximized by pronating and supinating the forearm, as well as by flexing and extending the elbow. Before the incision is made on the medial side of the elbow, the ulnar nerve should be palpated in its groove at the posteromedial aspect of the elbow. It is important to remember that subluxation of this nerve anteriorly is not uncommon in the general population. Childress has shown, in a survey of 2000 supposedly normal elbows, a 16.2% incidence of recurrent dislocation of the ulnar nerve.[7]

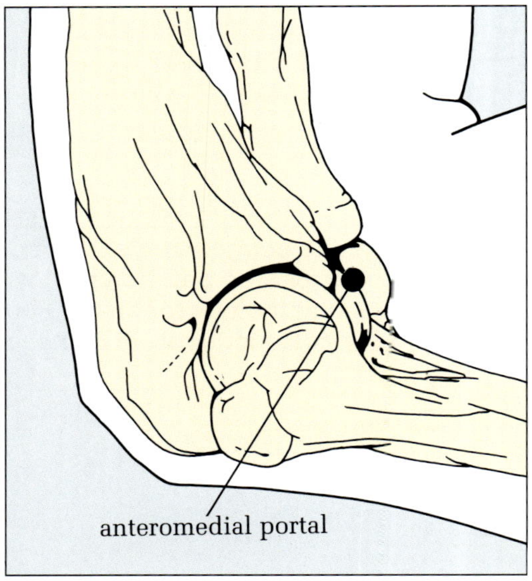

Figure 21.8
Anteromedial portal. The patient is in the supine position with the elbow flexed 90°.

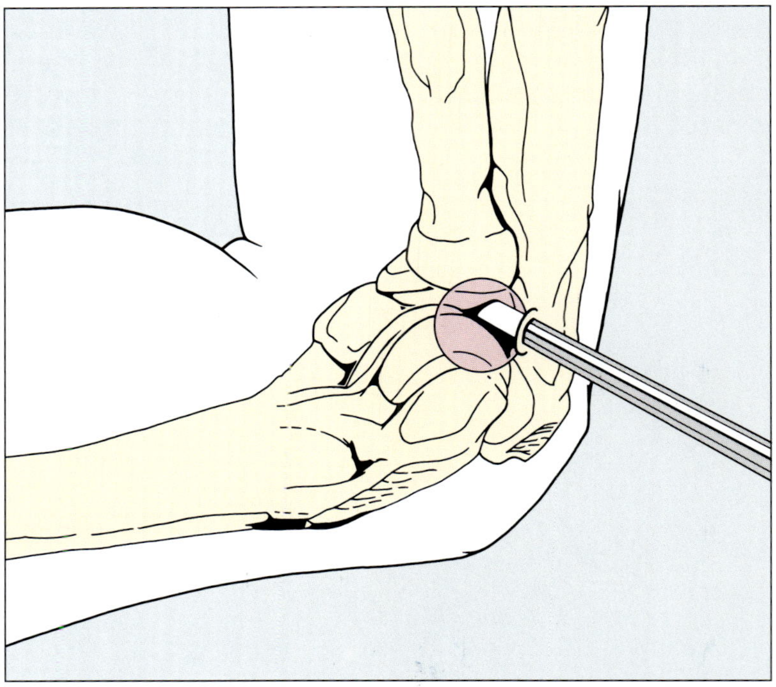

Figure 21.9
Straight lateral portal. The patient is in the supine position.

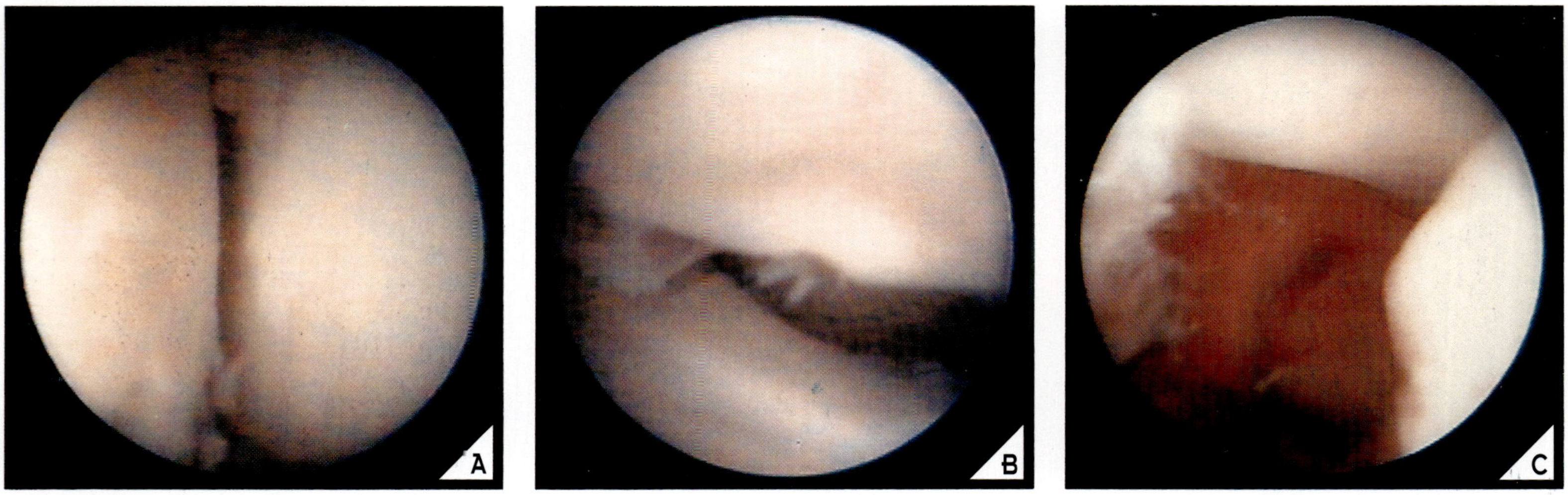

Figure 21.10
Arthroscopic images of the radiohumeral joint (the radial head is on the right) (A), the trochlear notch of the ulna (the ulna is at the bottom) (B), and the posterior compartment of the right elbow (the tip of the olecranon is on the right) (C).

Straight Lateral Portal

The straight lateral portal is located in the triangular area formed by the lateral humeral epicondyle, the radial head, and the olecranon (Fig. 21.9). This portal pierces the anconeous muscle. The posterior antebrachial cutaneous nerve is at risk with this portal. The straight lateral portal gives a good visualization of the radioulnar joint as well as the inferior surface of the radial head, the undersurface of the capitellum, and the trochlear notch of the ulna. If the scope is maneuvered posteriorly, visualization of the posterior compartment is possible (Fig. 21.10).

Posterolateral Portal

The posterolateral portal is located approximately 3 cm proximal to the olecranon tip and 2 cm lateral to the center of the triceps (Fig. 21.11). It provides excellent visualization of the olecranon fossa and the tip of the olecranon. To establish this portal, some extension of the elbow is necessary. The posterior antebrachial cutaneous nerve and the lateral brachial cutaneous nerve are at risk with this portal, which pierces the triceps muscle. When establishing this portal the surgeon should keep in mind that the ulnar nerve is located approximately 2.5 cm medial to the center of the joint.

Straight Posterior Portal

The straight posterior portal pierces the triceps tendon and is situated approximately 3 cm proximal to the olecranon tip but more towards the midline than the posterolateral portal (see Fig. 21.11). It provides good visualization of the posterior aspect of the elbow. When this portal is used the posteromedial position of the ulnar nerve should always be kept in mind.

Proximomedial Portal

The proximomedial portal is ordinarily used with the patient placed in the prone position (Fig. 21.12). This portal is located approximately 2 cm proximal to the medial humeral epicondyle and just anterior to the medial intermuscular septum. The arthroscopic cannula is directed towards the center of the elbow joint for safe insertion. Although the superomedial portal is

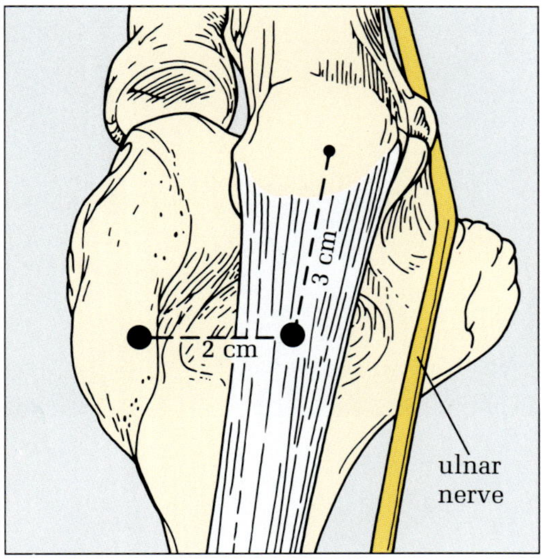

Figure 21.11
The posterolateral and straight posterior portals. The elbow is in the over the chest position.

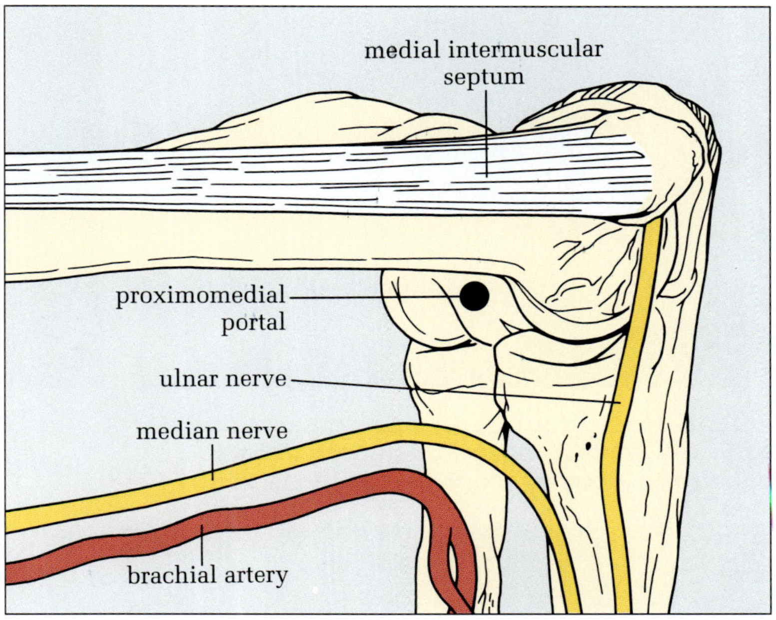

Figure 21.12
Proximomedial portal. The patient is in the prone position as described by Meyers.

very useful for simultaneous visualization of the medial and lateral aspects of the elbow, it is not as safe as the standard arthroscopic portals. It has been shown by Meyers[4] that the ulnar nerve is only 2 to 4 mm from the arthroscopic sheath, and with flexion of the elbow the ulnar nerve moves even closer to the medial intermuscular septum.

SURGICAL TECHNIQUE

Generally speaking, arthroscopic management of pathology in the anterior aspect of the elbow requires the use of the anterolateral and anteromedial portals. While the arthroscope is introduced through either the anterolateral or the anteromedial portal, the surgical instruments are placed through the opposite portal. Pathology on the lateral side of the elbow can also be approached through the straight lateral portal. Pathology of the posterior aspect of the elbow is best approached through a combination of a posterolateral portal and a straight posterior portal.

Removal of Loose Bodies

Loose bodies within the elbow probably represent the most common indications for operative arthroscopy of the elbow (Figs. 21.13, 21.14). Whether they are cartilaginous or osteocartilaginous, they can be secondary to an osteochondritic lesion of the capitellum, traumatic injuries with intraarticular fractures, or synovial osteochondromatosis (Figs. 21.15, 21.16). Loose bodies may be found in either the anterior or the posterior compartment of the joint (Fig. 21.17). The clinical diagnosis is usually based on a thorough history and physical examination and can be confirmed by plain x-rays, MRI, or CT arthrogram of the elbow. When the loose bodies are located anteriorly, removal can be achieved by using the two anterior portals (Fig. 21.18). At times it is necessary to perform a partial

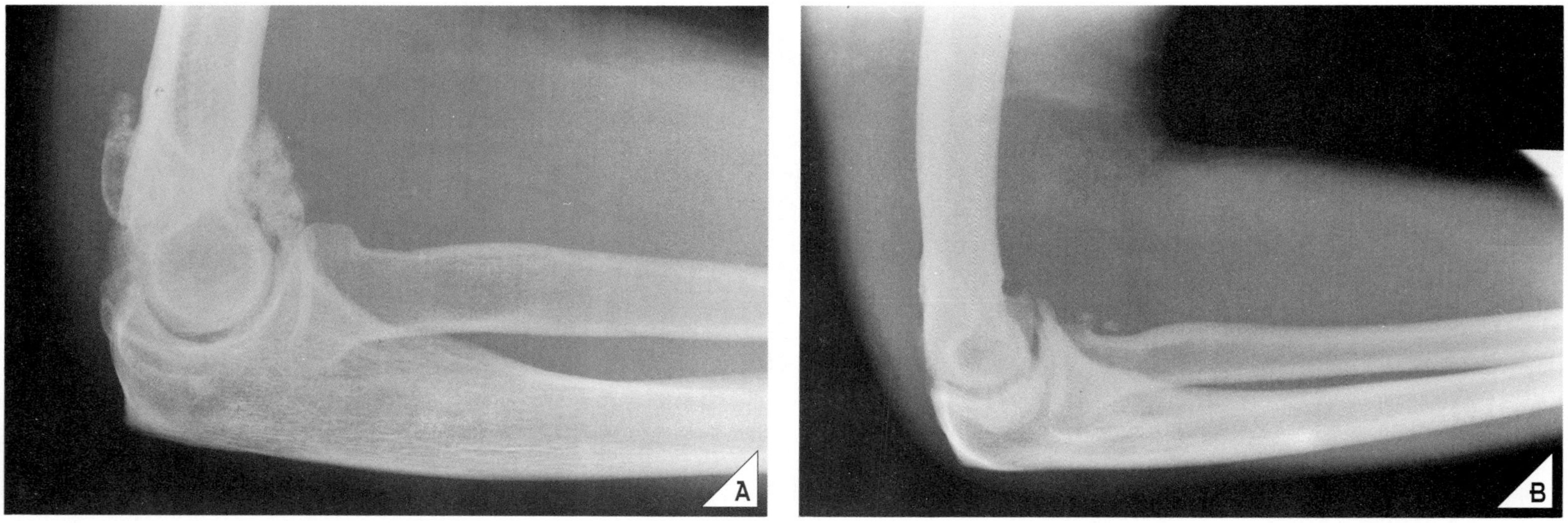

Figure 21.13
Radiograph of loose bodies in synovial osteochondromatosis (A) and the same elbow after arthroscopic excision (B).

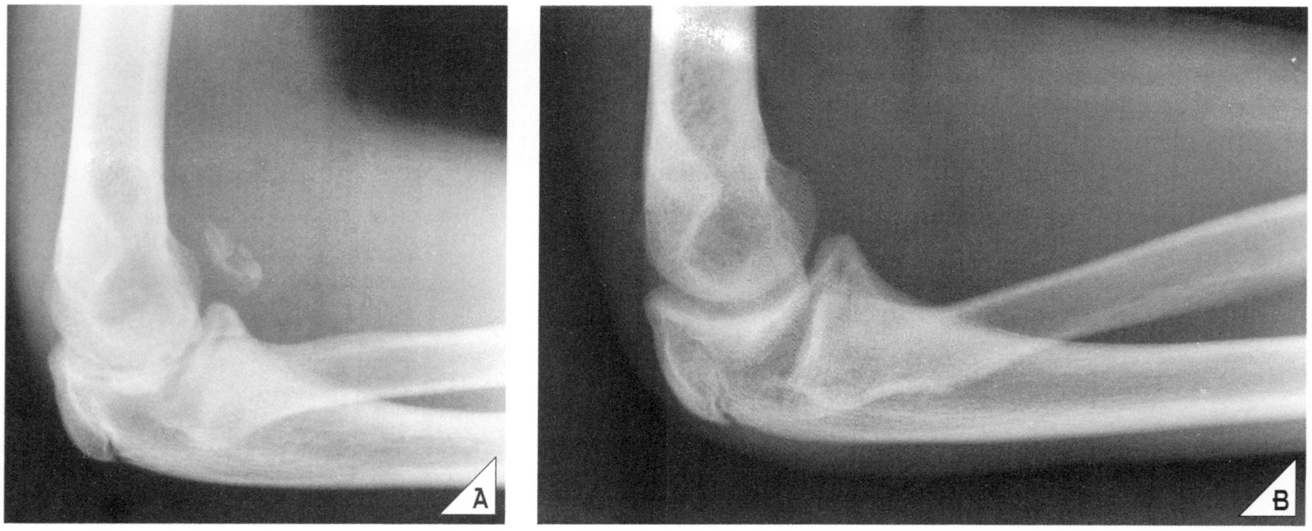

Figure 21.14
(A) A single loose body in the anterior compartment. (B) Results after arthroscopic excision.

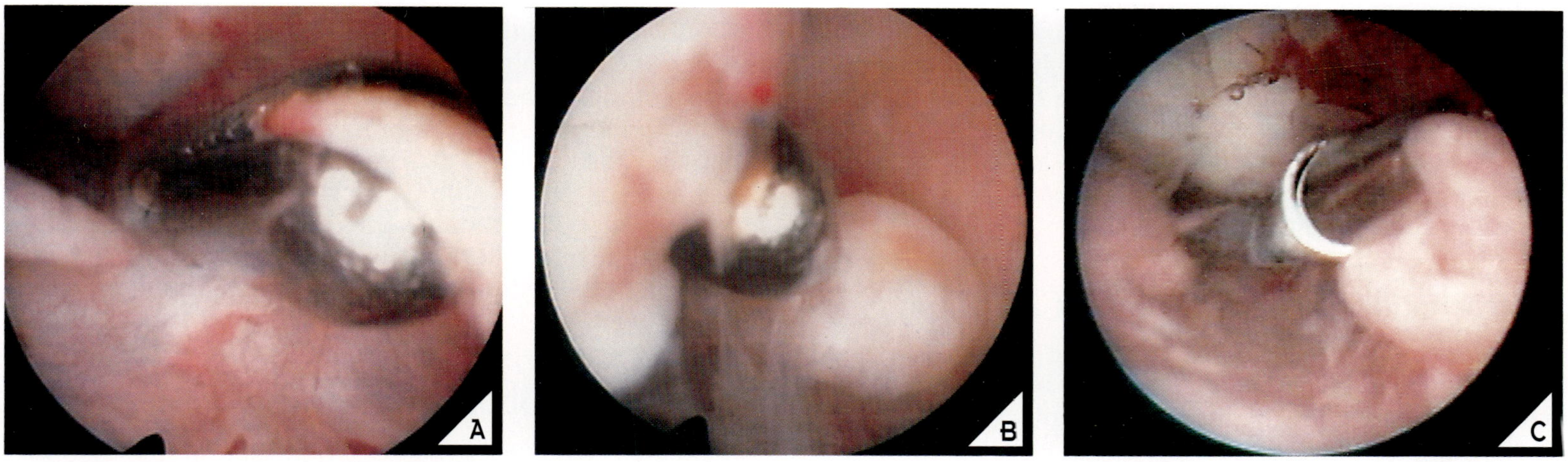

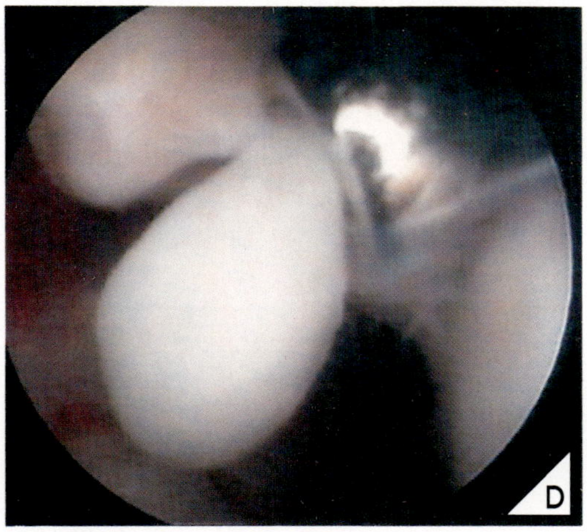

Figure 21.15
(A–D) Examples of loose bodies in synovial osteochondromatosis of the elbow.

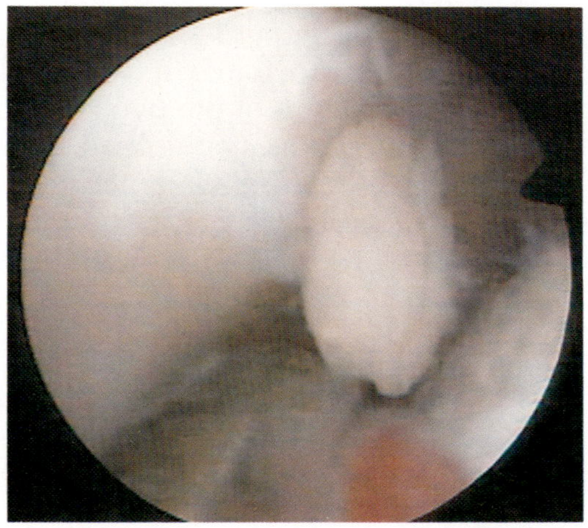

Figure 21.16
Loose body in the trochlear notch of the right ulna. The ulna is on the right.

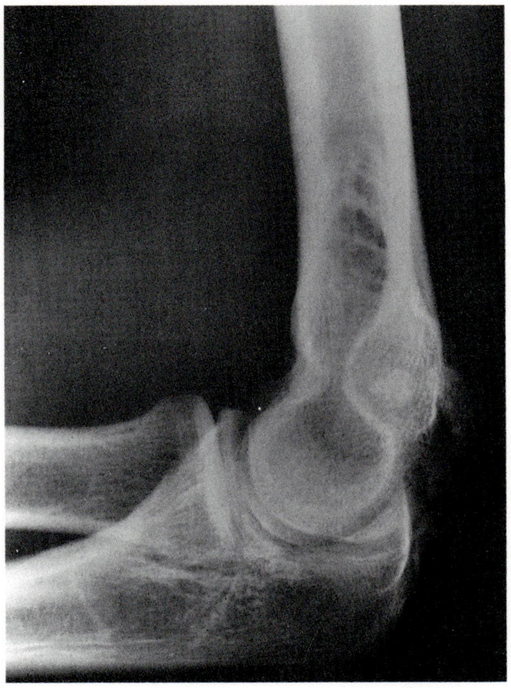

Figure 21.17
Loose bodies located in the posterior compartment.

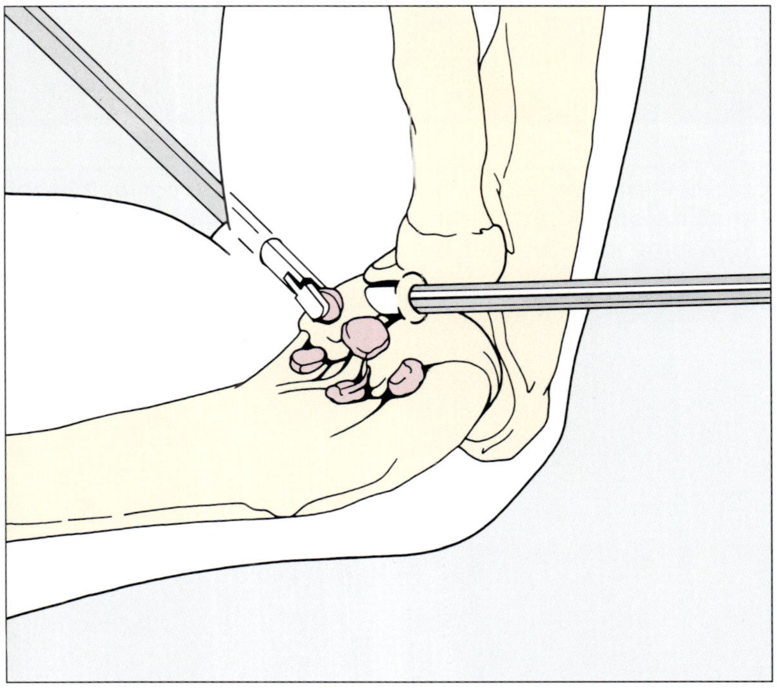

Figure 21.18
Removal of loose bodies via the medial and lateral portals, with the patient in the supine position.

synovectomy to evaluate the size and the number of fragments present in the joint (Fig. 21.19). Larger loose bodies are usually removed at the completion of the arthroscopic exploration to avoid extravasation of fluid into the soft tissue. Posteriorly located loose bodies are removed using the two posterior portals or a combination of the straight lateral and the posterolateral entrances.

Osteochondritis Dissecans of the Capitellum

After failure of conservative treatment for an osteochondritic lesion of the capitellum, arthroscopic surgery can be performed to remove a loose fragment, to drill a stable lesion with normal articular lining, or to debride a necrotic area with degenerative articular cartilage. A loose intraarticular fragment can be removed using the two anterior portals previously described. Drilling can be done using a combination of the two anterior portals or through a straight lateral portal combined with an accessory portal (Fig. 21.20). When the two anterior portals are used, visualization is preferably obtained with the arthroscope through the medial portal and the surgical instruments through the anterolateral portal. It is sometimes necessary to use a straight lateral portal combined with an accessory lateral portal to visualize and have access to the most distal area of the capitellum. Fixation of a viable osteochondral fragment can also be performed with small cannulated screws or biodegradable pins. With fragmentation and degeneration of the lesion, debridement and curettage of the base of the crater down to bleeding bone can be performed (Fig. 21.21).

Posttraumatic Disorders of the Olecranon

This group includes *posterior olecranon impingement* and the *valgus extension overload syndrome*. Patients with posterior olecranon impingement usually complain of pain on full elbow extension. Although x-rays are usually normal, at arthroscopy the pathology is commonly found to be posteriorly located and may represent a combination of synovial hypertrophy, articular cartilage degeneration, and presence of small bone spurs (Figs. 21.22, 21.23A,B).

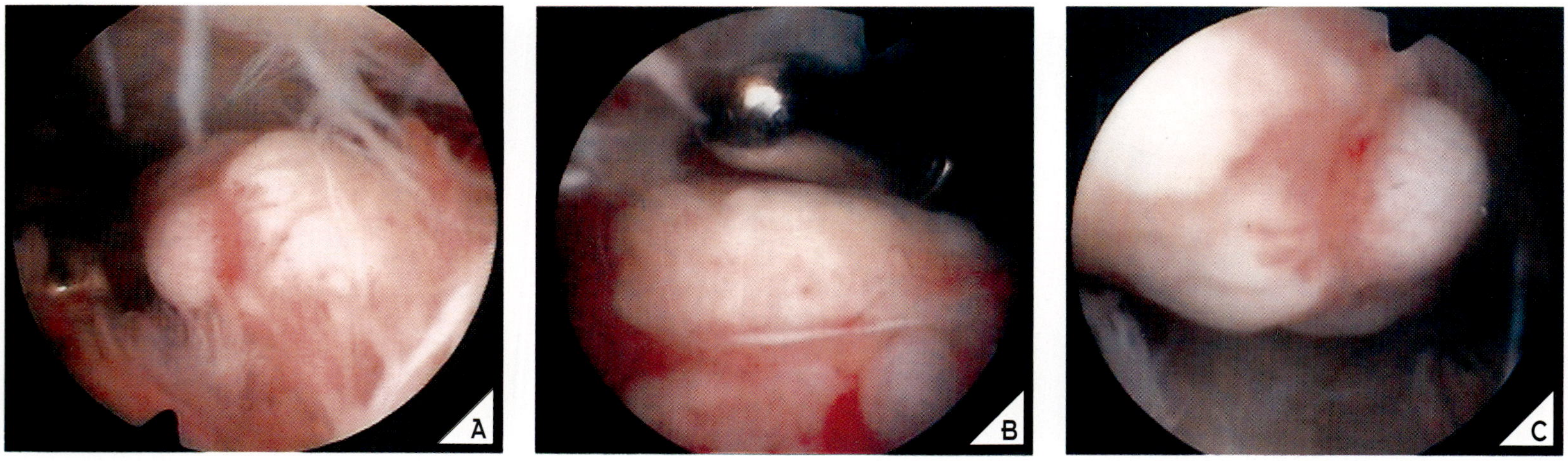

Figure 21.19
(A) Arthroscopic view of loose bodies located in the anterior compartment of the right elbow. (B) A small motorized instrument performs partial synovectomy to expose the loose body. (C) A large loose body in the anterior compartment of the right elbow.

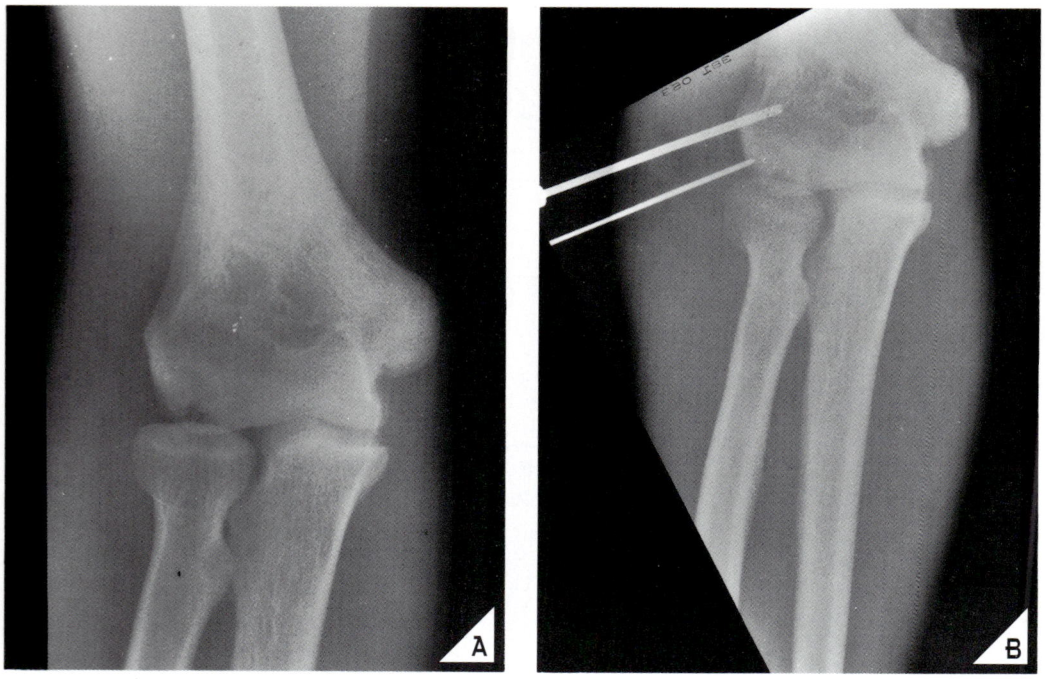

Figure 21.20
(A, B) Radiographs showing osteochondritis dissecans with drilling.

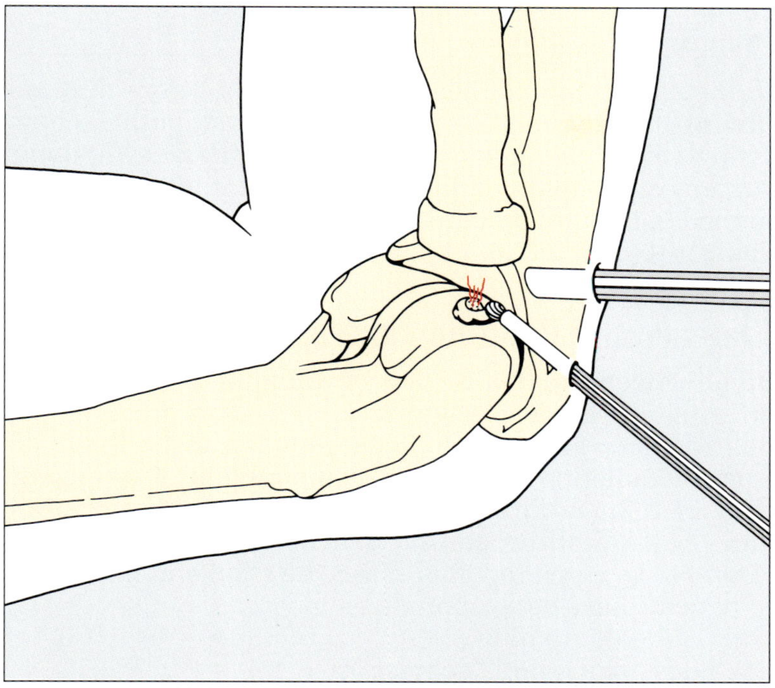

Figure 21.21
Arthroscopic portals (straight lateral and accessory lateral) used for the visualization and debridement of osteochondritis dissecans of the capitellum. The patient is in the supine position.

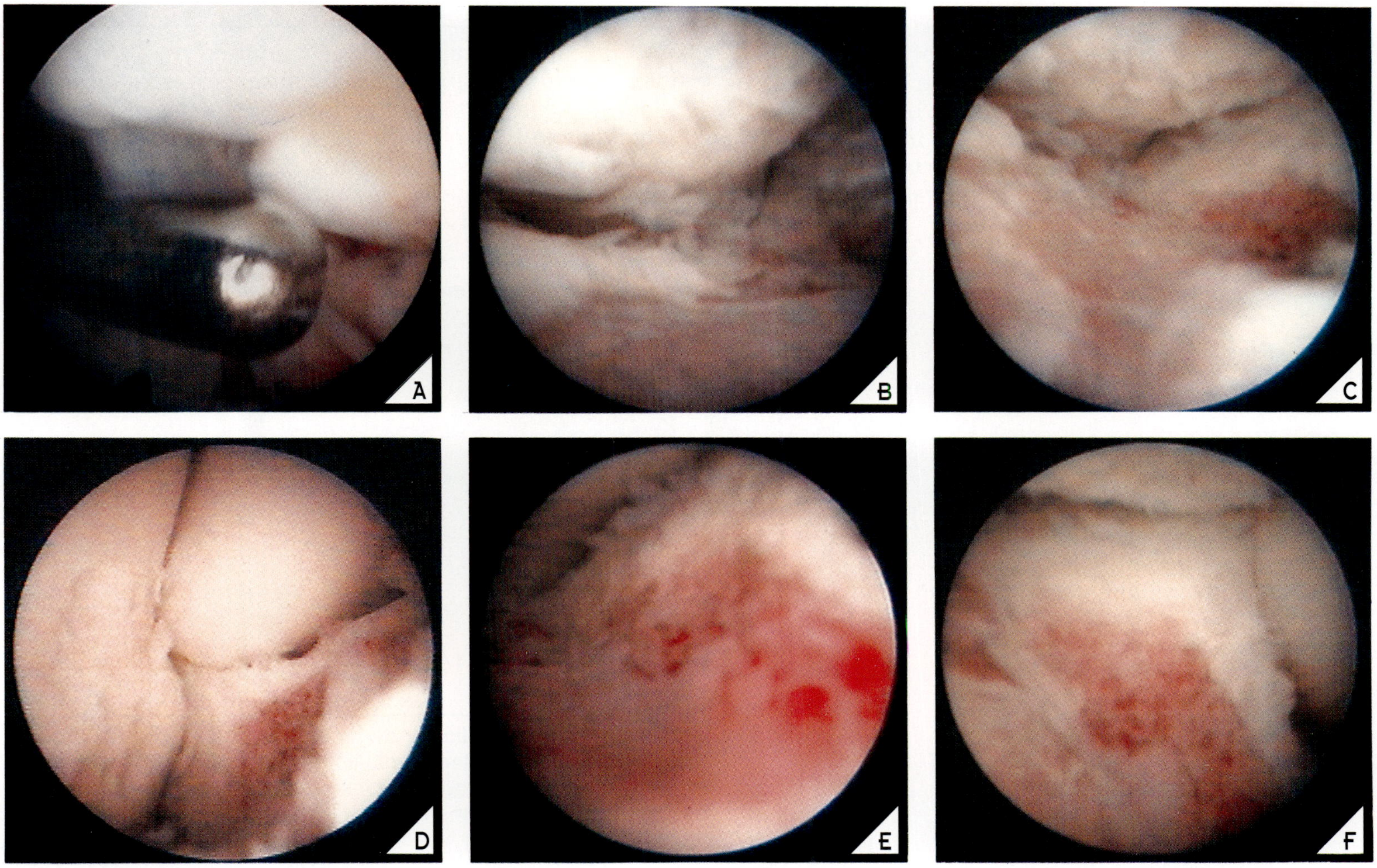

Figure 21.22
(A) Posterior compartment of the right elbow with exostosis of the tip of the olecranon. A surgical instrument is performing debridement. (B, C) Two views of articular cartilage degeneration of the ulnar notch of the right elbow. (C–F) Various views of an osteochondral defect of the lateral aspect of the ulna. The radial head is at the top in D.

Valgus extension overload syndrome is commonly seen in baseball pitchers. These patients have a limited range of motion of the elbow with pain secondary to the presence of posterior osteophytes in the olecranon area. Arthroscopically, chondromalacic changes of the olecranon fossa and posteromedial osteophytes are present. A combination of a posterolateral portal to evaluate the lesion and a straight posterior portal for the arthroscopic instrumentation is necessary (Fig. 21.23C). The small synovial resector and the small abrader are necessary to remove the osteophyte. Sometimes, the introduction of a small osteotome under direct vision can facilitate the excision. This procedure is technically demanding because of the location of the osteophyte close to the cubital tunnel.

Arthrofibrosis

Arthrofibrosis of the elbow can be secondary to either a traumatic injury or a postsurgical complication. Fibrous adhesions, usually located in the anterior compartment of the elbow, significantly limit the range of motion (Fig. 21.24). Removal of these adhesions can be performed through a combination of both anteromedial and anterolateral portals. After careful excision of the fibrous adhesions, manipulation of the elbow into extension is performed. Improvement in the range of motion can be obtained only when the procedure is followed by an aggressive program of rehabilitation, combined with use of a continuous passive motion apparatus, a Dynasplint, and anti-inflammatory medication.

Synovial Pathology

In the early stage of rheumatoid arthritis before destruction of the articular cartilage has occurred, arthroscopic synovectomy may achieve significant relief of symptoms. An almost complete synovectomy of the joint can be performed using the standard arthroscopic portals previously described (Figs. 21.25, 21.26).

Degenerative Posttraumatic Arthritis

Some selected cases of degenerative or posttraumatic arthritis can achieve temporary relief after arthroscopic debridement and lavage. Osteophytes can be removed from the anterior or posterior compartment of the elbow (Fig. 21.27). Old, malunited fractures of the radial head and the capitellum can be debrided arthroscopically. However, in a few reported series the results in this group of patients have been unpredictable.

Postoperative Treatment

A soft compression dressing is applied over the elbow after closure of the portals with sutures. To obtain immediate, reliable postoperative neurovascular assessment, it is advisable not to use local anesthesia for pain relief, since the anesthetic agent can leak into the soft tissue and cause temporary nerve block. Active range of motion of the elbow is begun as soon as possible.

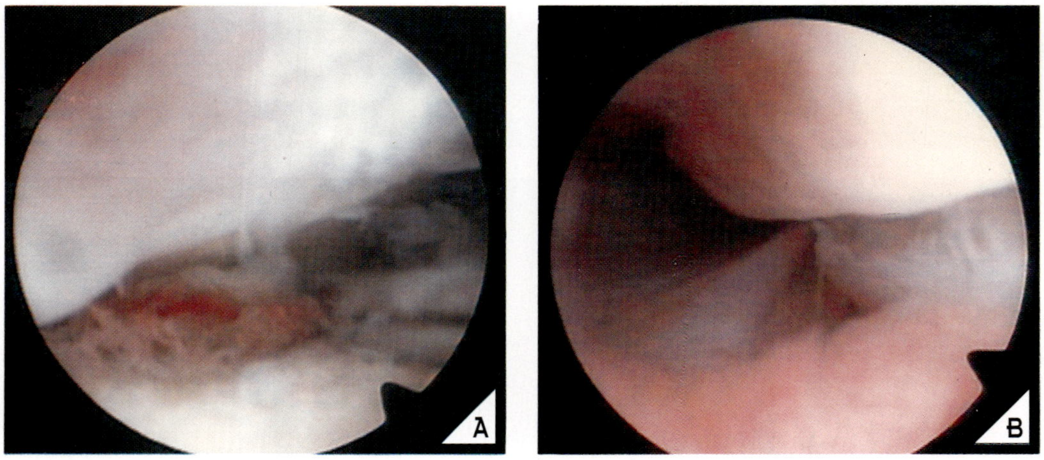

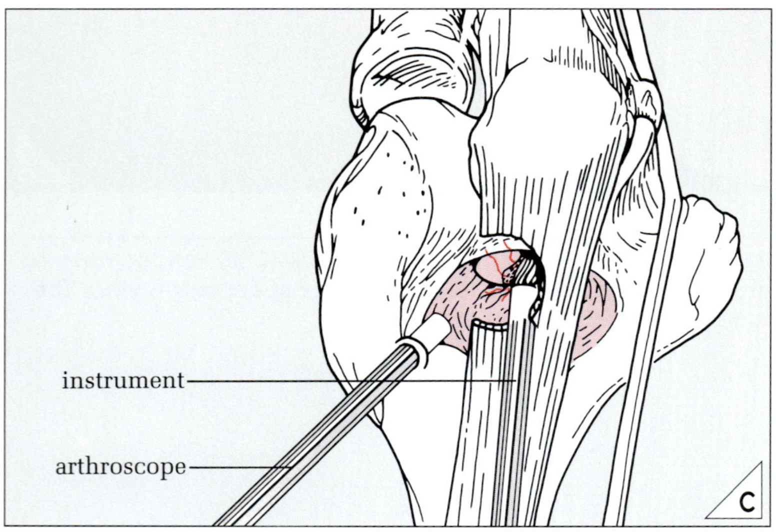

Figure 21.23
(A, B) Two views of articular degeneration and synovial hyper trophy in posterior olecranon impingement of the right elbow. (C) Arthroscopic portal used for surgery in the posterior compartment of the elbow with the elbow in the over the chest position.

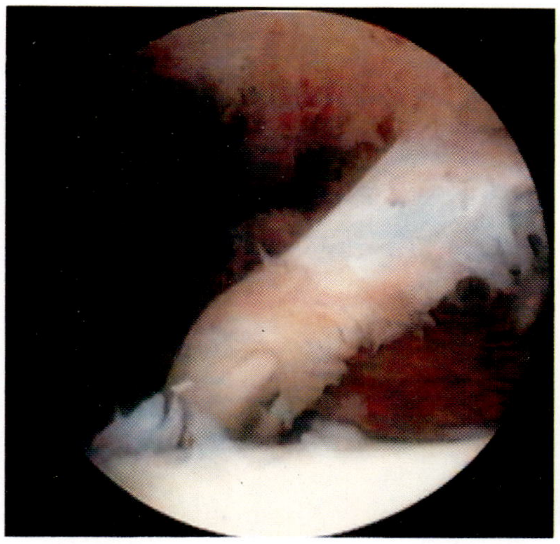

Figure 21.24

Fibrous adhesion in the anterior compartment of the elbow.

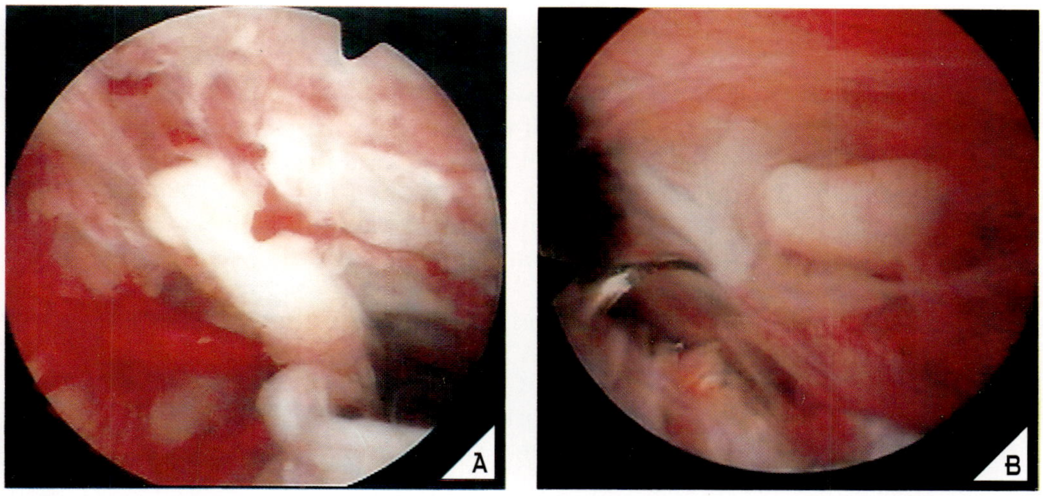

Figure 21.25

(A, B) Two views of synovitis of the elbow with a small resector performing synovectomy.

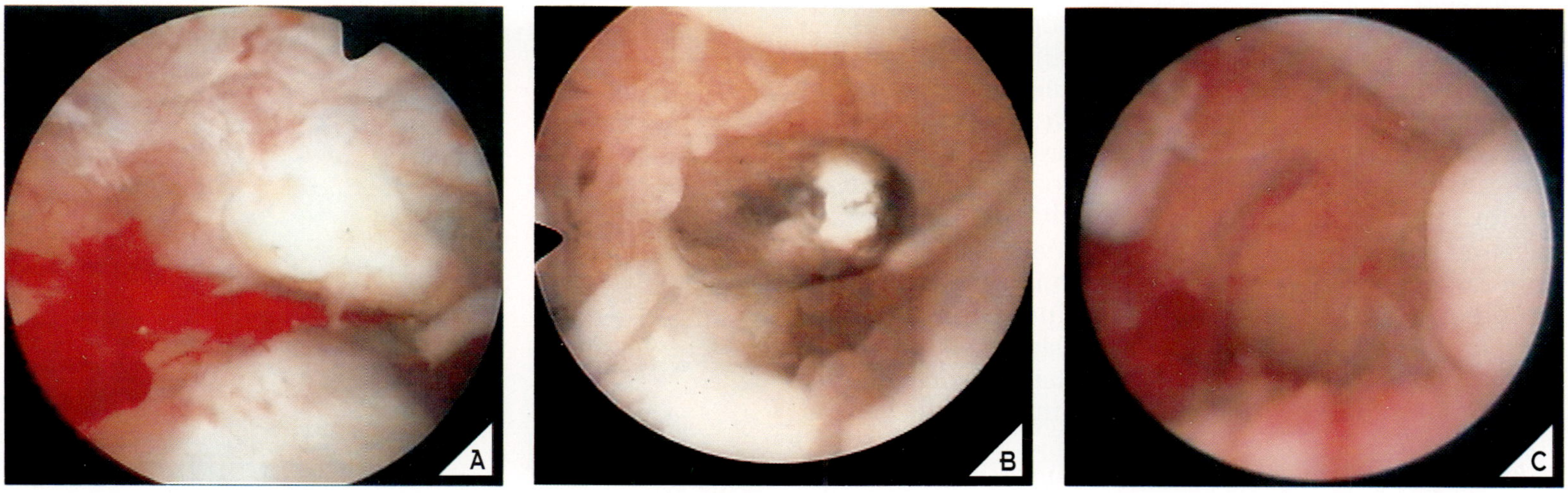

Figure 21.26

Views of synovitis of the anterior (A, B) and posterior (C) compartments.

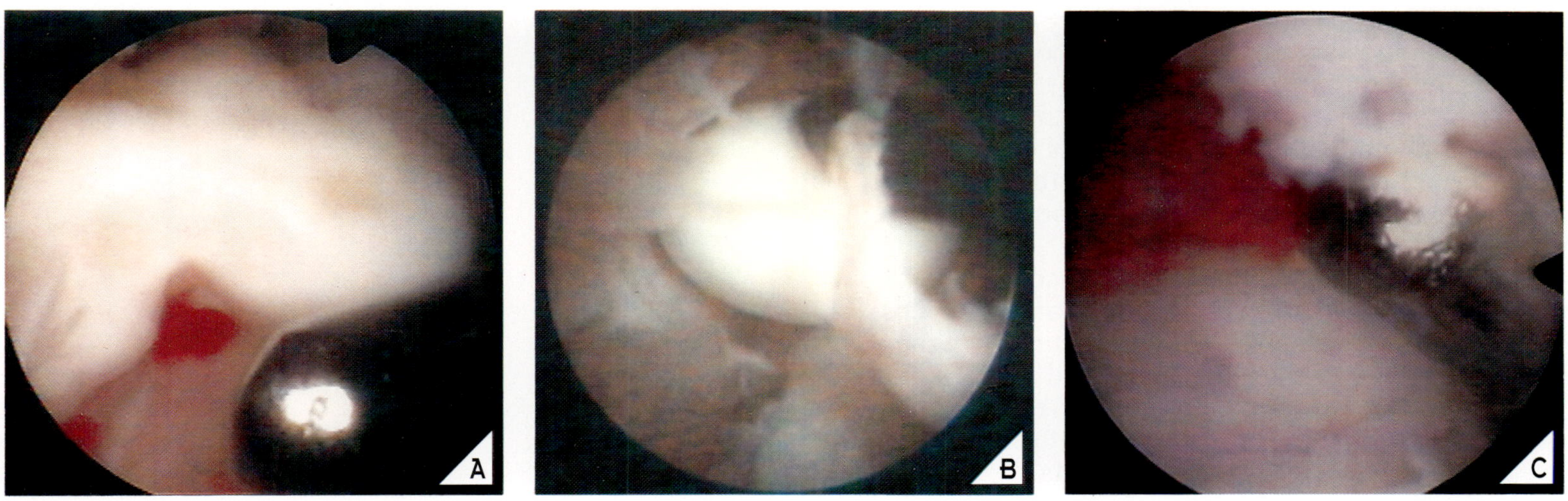

Figure 21.27

(A) Osteophyte in the anterior compartment in a patient with posttraumatic arthritis of the right elbow. (B) Loose osteochondral bodies in degenerative arthritis of the elbow. (C) Small motorized shaver performing debridement of degenerative arthritis of the elbow.

Complications and Pitfalls

Meticulous attention to the anatomy of the area and proper technique are essential to prevent serious potential complications of this procedure. Bone landmarks (radial head, lateral and medial epicondyle, tip of the olecranon), should be outlined with a marking pen before the procedure is begun.

Cutaneous neuroma can be avoided by spreading the subcutaneous tissue with a hemostat after incising the skin with a #11 blade during creation of the portals.

Radial nerve damage has been reported as a complication. However, extreme caution when performing the anterolateral entry should prevent this dreadful occurrence. The skin incision should be anterior to the radial head while the elbow is at 90° and the anterior capsule fully distended.

The *median* and *ulnar nerves* and the *brachial artery* can also be damaged during arthroscopic surgery of the elbow. Instruments should always be directed towards the center of the joint, while maximal distention of the joint will keep the neurovascular structures anteriorly displaced. When synovectomy of the anterior compartment is performed, extreme care should be taken to avoid penetration of the anterior capsule. Posteriorly, when motorized instruments are used an aggressive debridement of the posteromedial corner of the elbow can cause damage to the ulnar nerve. Localization and palpation of the ulnar nerve in the cubital tunnel before incising the skin for the medial portal are of the utmost importance, since anterior subluxation of the nerve is not uncommon in the general population.

Excessive extravasation of fluid into the soft tissue around the elbow can cause neurovascular compromise. To obtain overdistention of the posterior compartment of the elbow and to prevent extravasation of fluid through the anterior portals, it may be necessary to close these portals with sutures after completion of the anterior compartment examination.

Sterile technique coupled with intraoperative antibiotic therapy in some situations (history of previous surgery, complicated cases that may increase the operating time) will decrease the incidence of infection after elbow arthroscopy.

Although the indications for arthroscopic surgery of the elbow are limited, this procedure can be successfully applied in the treatment of various disorders of the elbow. The technique is very demanding, and successful results depend on a good knowledge of the regional anatomy, familiarity with the arthroscopic portals, and judicious use of the available surgical instruments.

References

1. Lynch GJ, Meyers JF, Whipple TL, Caspari RB. Neurovascular anatomy and elbow arthroscopy: inherent risks. *Arthroscopy.* 1986;2:191–197.
2. Thomas MA, Fast A, Shapiro D. Radial nerve nerve damage as a complication of elbow arthroscopy. *Clin Orthop.* 1987; 215:130–131.
3. Carson WG, Andrews JR. Arthroscopy of the elbow. In: Zarin B, ed. *Injuries to the Throwing Arm.* Philadelphia, Pa: WB Saunders Co; 1982:221–227.
4. Guhl JF. Arthroscopy and arthroscopic surgery of the elbow. *Orthopaedics.* 1985;8:1290–1296.
5. Meyers JF. Elbow arthroscopy: the supero-medial portal. In: Program and abstracts of the tenth annual meeting of the AANA; San Diego, Calif; 1991. Abstract.
6. Parisien JS. Arthroscopic surgery of the elbow. *Bull Hosp Jt Dis Orthop Inst.* 1988;48:149–158.
7. Childress HM. Recurrent ulnar nerve dislocation at the elbow. *J Bone Joint Surg.* 1956;38:978–984.

Section Five

The Hip

Chapter Twenty Two

Hip Arthroscopy: Lateral Approach

James M. Glick

Hip arthroscopy is performed infrequently because there are few indications for this procedure. As a result, perfecting a technique that requires frequent trials is difficult. With the help of my colleagues, I developed a direct lateral approach to the hip joint.[1–3] With the patient lying on the contralateral side and the use of traction to distract the hip, the arthroscope and arthroscopic instruments are directed through portals adjacent to the greater trochanter. This approach provides easy access to the hip. Complete visualization including the posterior compartment can be accomplished. My use of this method has been established by the performance of more than 125 hip arthroscopies. On the basis of my experience, I can share the indications, technique, and findings that will enable the surgeon to approach the task with confidence.

Indications and Contraindications

The primary indication for arthroscopy of the hip joint, as in other joints, is to obtain as much information as possible for planning treatment. In our experience, we have applied arthroscopy of the hip in the following situations:

1. Evaluation of unresolved pain after failure of conservative treatment.
2. Evaluation of the femoral head and acetabular involvement to help plan treatment for persistent arthritic hip pain. This is especially helpful for delaying arthroplasty in a young patient.

3. Exploration, debridement, and removal of loose bodies, including synovial chondromatosis and after fracture and/or dislocation of the hip. Epstein has reported on the importance of removing loose fragments and debris from fracture dislocations of the hip.[4,5]
4. Exploration and removal of foreign bodies.
5. Extraction of intraarticular cement in a total hip replacement.
6. Removal of a torn acetabular labrum.
7. Removal of an impinging ligamentum teres.
8. Evaluation and treatment of osteochondritis dissecans.
9. Synovectomy for synovitis. Pigmented villonodular synovitis also fits into this category.
10. Evaluation of the hip in conjunction with extracapsular procedures.

Other applications that have been described in the literature for hip arthroscopy include synovial biopsy and joint evaluation in chronic juvenile arthritis[6] and evaluation of the hip and other disorders in children, including congenital dislocated hips, Legg–Calvé–Perthes disease, neuropathic subluxation, residuals of prior sepsis, and a slipped capital femoral epiphysis.[7] Indications that have not been explored by this author are the treatment of pyarthrosis and an aid in reduction and fixation of selective fractures of the acetabulum.

The contraindications to hip arthroscopy are few. Advanced avascular necrosis of the femoral head, advanced osteoarthritis in the elderly, and congenital dislocation of the hip are relative contraindications. An absolute contraindication is ankylosis of the hip. Hogersson and co-authors evaluated a congenital dislocated hip in an infant with a small arthroscope.[6] Visualization in this case was limited. We were also unable to reach our objective by attempted arthroscopy in a patient with CDH, because an hourglass deformity of the capsule and the loss of landmarks made it impossible to enter the joint. In cases of avascular necrosis, arthroscopy merely added injury to insult. In this condition, the articular cartilage is completely stripped from the dead subchondral bone. On entrance into the hip joint with the arthroscope, we passed through the stripped articular cartilage and visualized the space remaining between the cartilage and the dead subchondral bone of the femoral head. Initially, the orientation could not be determined until this was appreciated. Complete debridement of the loose articular cartilage was difficult, and dead bone was left. The clinical results were poor.

SURGICAL TECHNIQUE

Specific equipment is necessary to help enter and reach all parts of the hip joint. The hip should be distracted at least 8 mm to safely and consistently assess the depths of the joint (Fig. 22.1). This is accomplished with either a fracture table (Fig. 22.2) or a newly developed apparatus

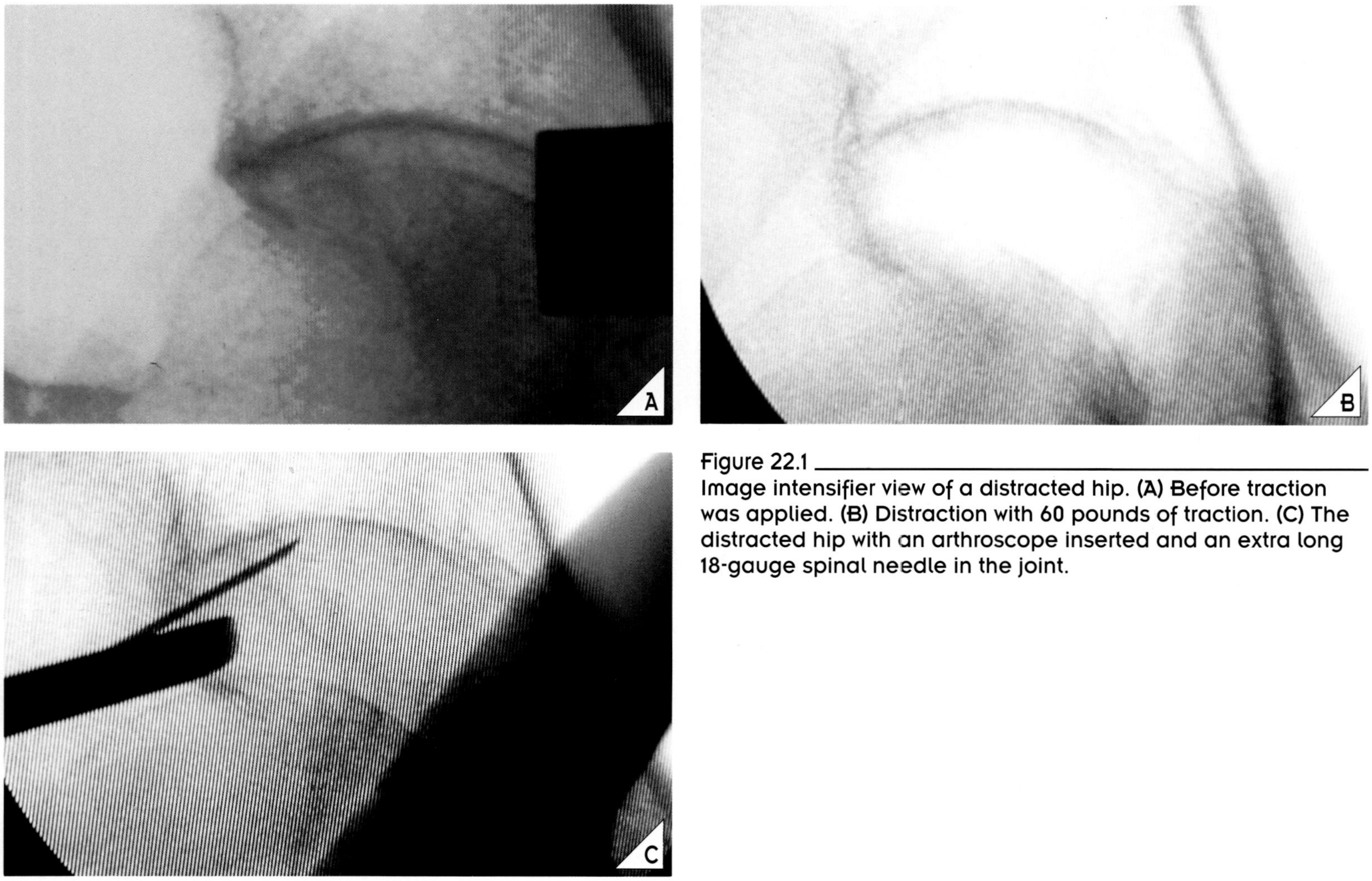

Figure 22.1
Image intensifier view of a distracted hip. (A) Before traction was applied. (B) Distraction with 60 pounds of traction. (C) The distracted hip with an arthroscope inserted and an extra long 18-gauge spinal needle in the joint.

known as a hip Distraktor (Arthronix) (Fig. 22.3).[1] The latter apparatus includes a well-padded perineal post for countertraction and a tensiometer to gauge the amount of traction applied. I have found this to be safer and more reliable then the fracture table. The hip Distraktor provides adequate distraction of the hip joint in all such operations. An image intensifier is used to verify the amount of distraction and to aid in directing the instruments into the joint.

In most hips, longer instruments are necessary to penetrate deep into the joint. These include 6 inch, 18-gauge spinal needles, extra long cannulas and sheaths (5 1/4 inch), a longer arthroscope, and longer motorized and hand instruments (Fig. 22.4). Telescoping cannulas (Fig.

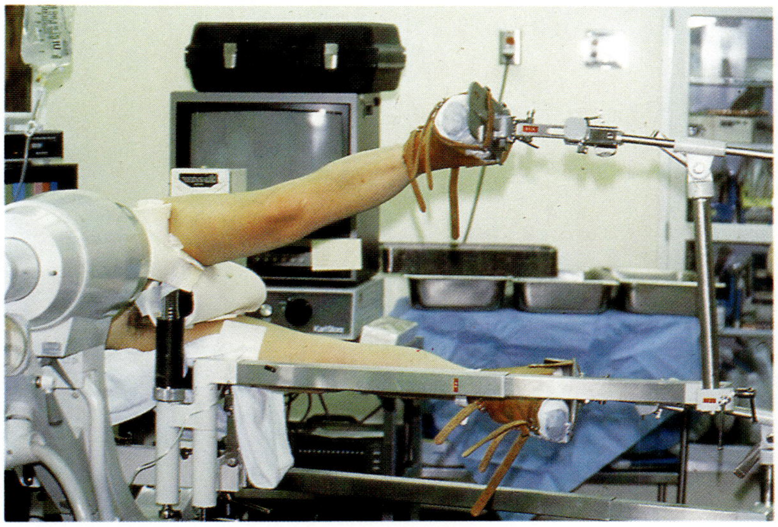

Figure 22.2
The patient in the lateral decubitus position on a fracture table. Note the well padded perineal post for countertraction.

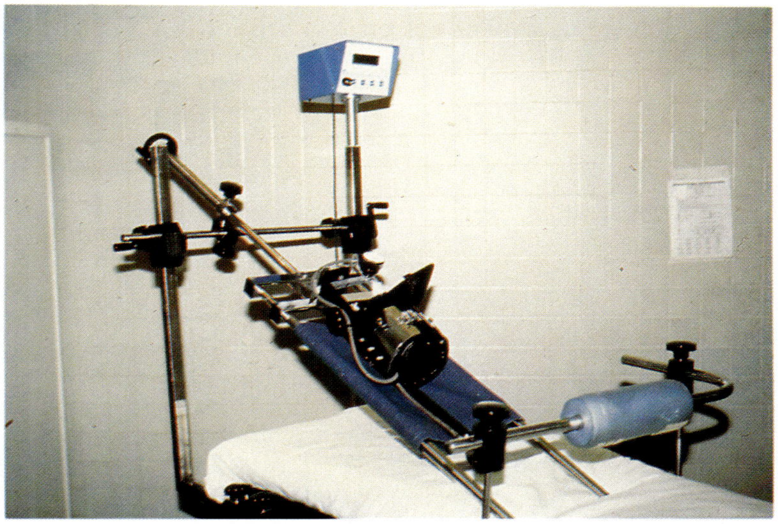

Figure 22.3
The hip Distraktor. The foot piece is attached to a stretcher for the attachment of the foot and leg. The crank to apply traction is at the end of the stretcher. The tensiometer is the box on top of the post on the right of the picture. Note the well padded perineal post. (Reprinted with permission from Glick JM, 1991)

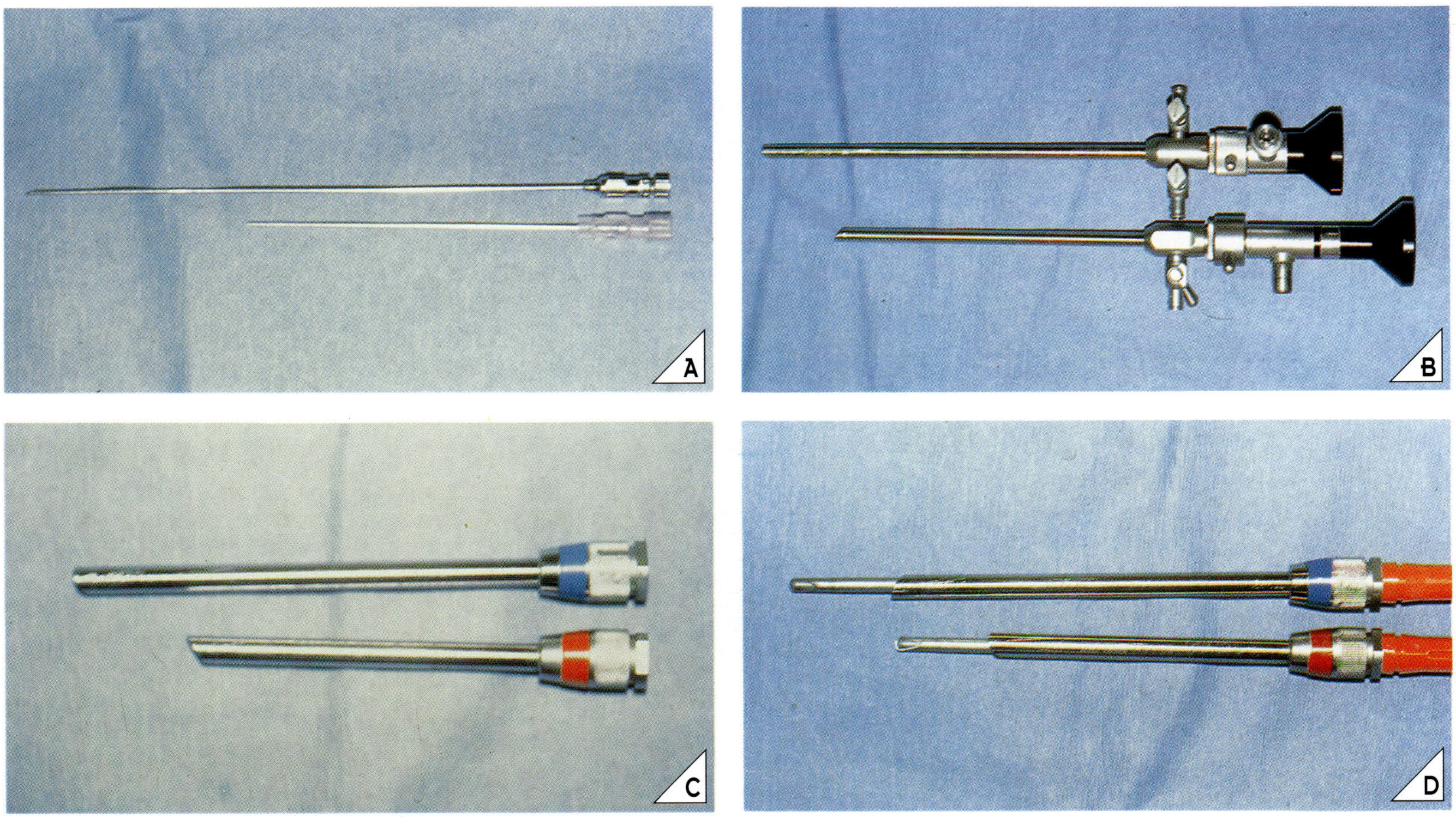

Figure 22.4
Extra long instruments: (A) 6 inch 18-gauge spinal needle next to a standard-size spinal needle. (B) A long arthroscope next to a standard-size arthroscope (1 1/4 inch difference in length). (C) A long cannula next to the standard cannula (1 1/4 inch difference in length). (D) A long full-radius resector next to a standard-sized resector (1 1/4 inch difference in length).

22.5) are used to maintain the portals when the instruments are initially inserted. The cannulas are hollow and consist of increasing diameter sizes that slide over one another. The smallest cannula is pointed on one end like a needle and is about the size of a large Kirschner wire.

The patient, under general anesthesia, is placed in a lateral decubitus position with the hip to be treated on top (Fig. 22.6). The leg is strapped into the hip Distraktor which places the leg in abduction. The amount of flexion and abduction is dependent on whether or not a contracture is present. If there is a hip flexion or adduction contracture, the hip must be left in that position so that it can be adequately distracted with a safe amount of traction. The perineal post placed between the legs is pushed upward against the medial portion of the thigh on the involved leg. This produces slight upward distraction and will keep the post away from the branch of the pudendal nerve that crosses over the pubic ramus (Fig. 22.7). Two portals are made over the greater trochanter and one directly anterior (Fig. 22.8). Additional portals can be

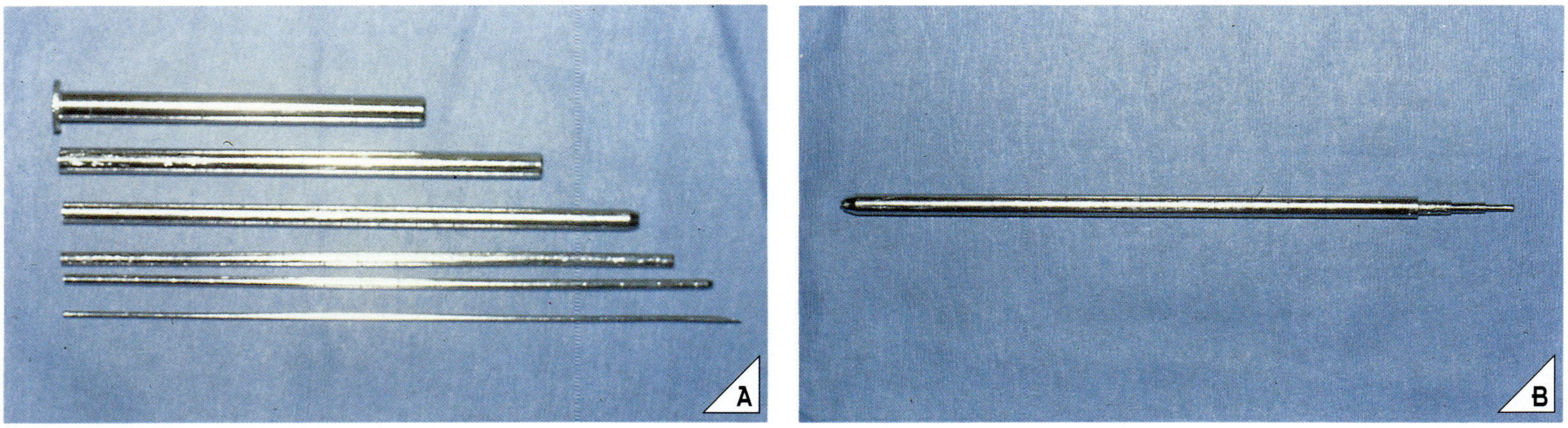

Figure 22.5
The telescoping cannulas. (A) The full set of six cannulas. Each larger cannula will fit over the next smaller size. The switching stick fits through the third largest cannula (third from the bottom). (B) Three cannulas nested together.

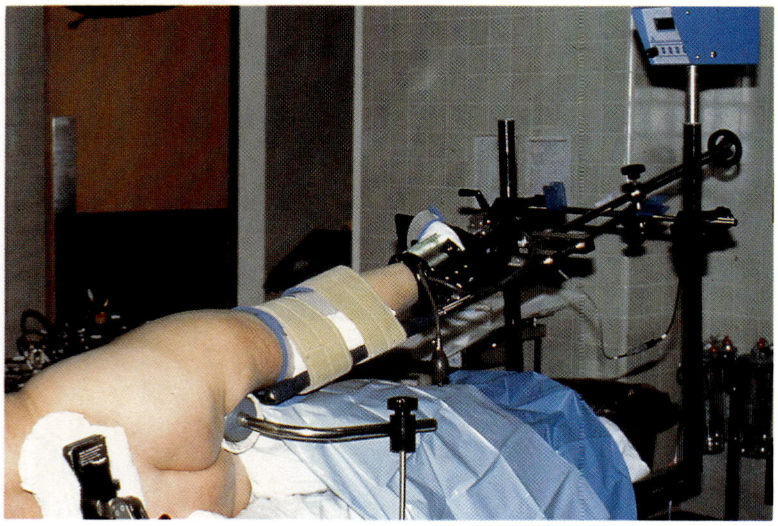

Figure 22.6
The patient is in the left lateral decubitus position with the right hip upward. The right leg and foot are strapped into the leg and foot piece of the hip Distraktor. Note the position of the perineal post.

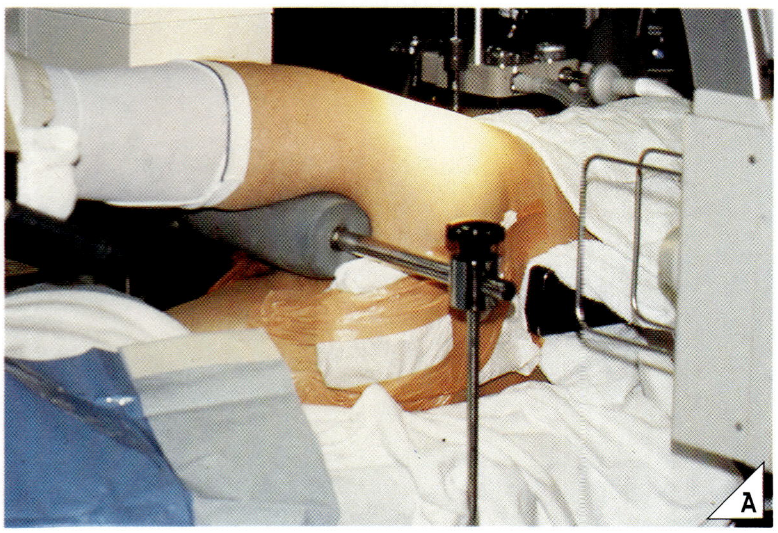

Figure 22.7
Position of the perineal post in the perineum. (A) The perineal post is pushed upward against the medial portion of the thigh to lever the head of the femur upward. (Reprinted with permission from Glick JM, 1991) (continued on next page)

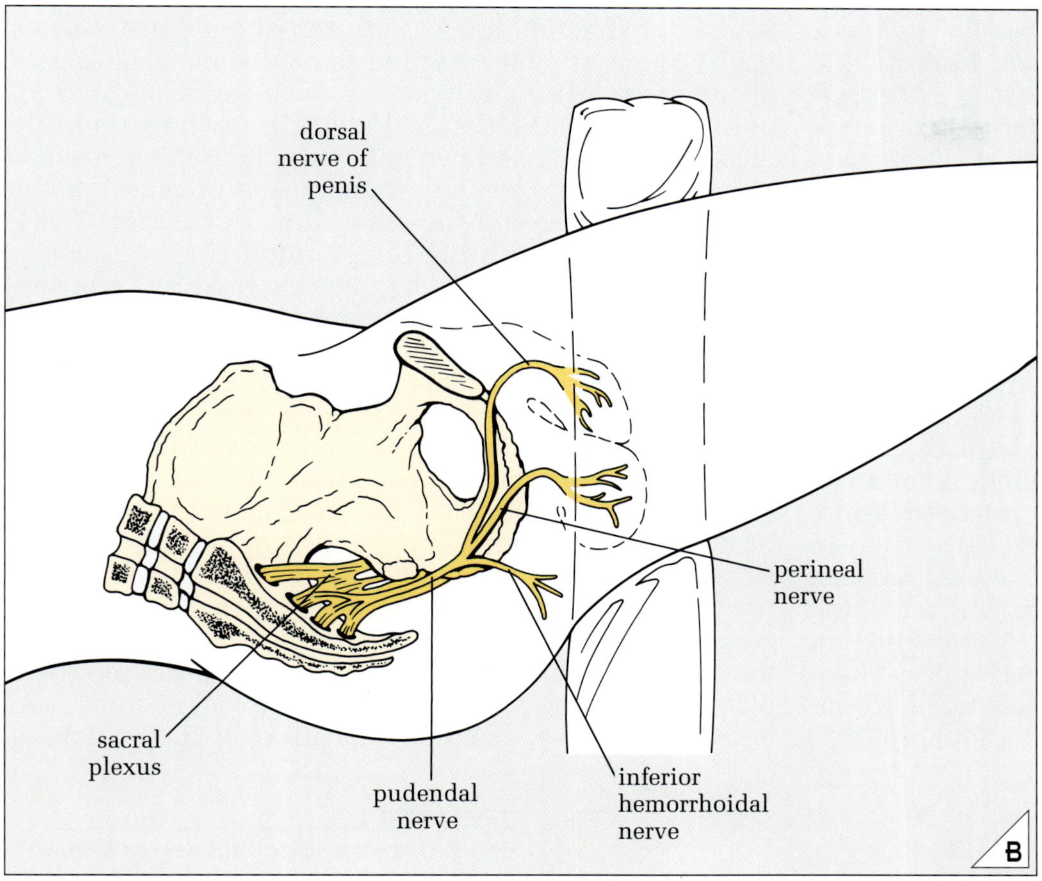

Figure 22.7 (continued)
(B) Diagram showing the position of the branches of the pudendal nerve between the patient's pubic ramus and the perineal post placed between the patient's legs.

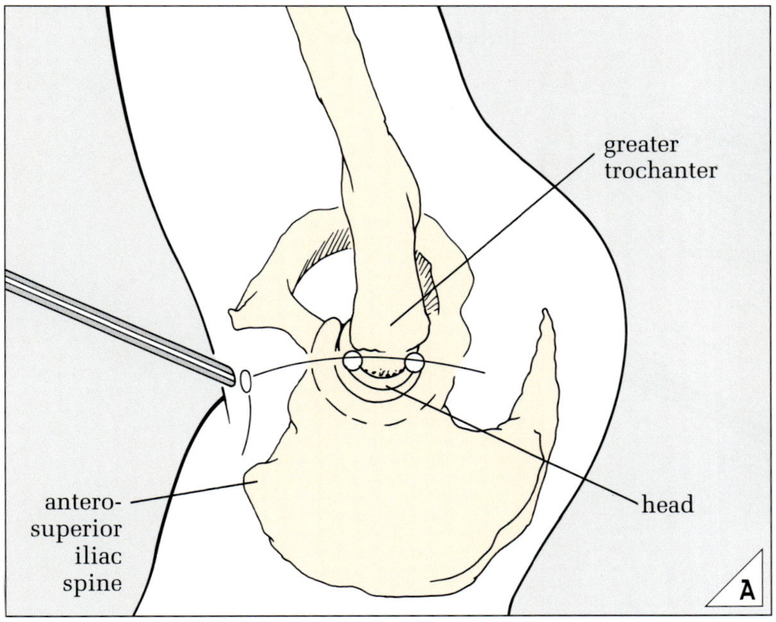

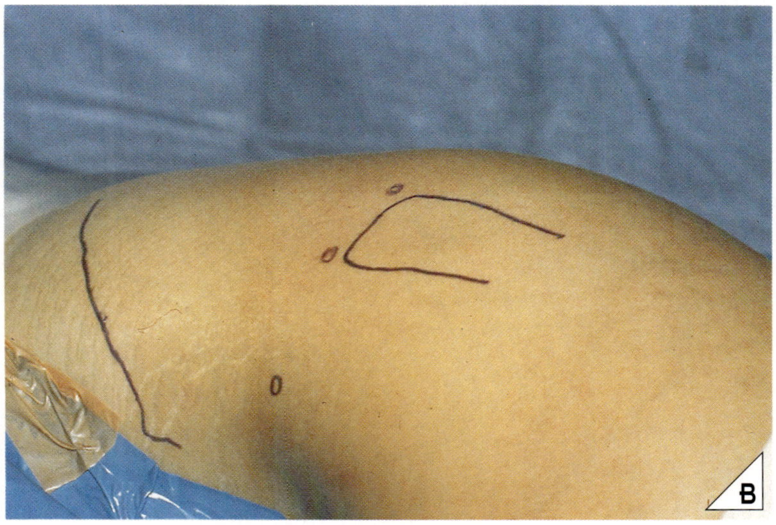

Figure 22.8
Portal placements in the direct lateral approach. (A) A diagram of a right hip. The greater trochanter and femoral head are marked. The circles are the portals of entry. B) Patient's right hip viewed from the front. The iliac crest and the greater trochanter are marked on the skin. The small circles mark the three portals most commonly used. The circles from anterior below to posterior above represent the direct anterior portal, the portal at the anterior edge of the greater trochanter, and the portal at the posterior edge of the greater trochanter, respectively.

made, but instrument crowding may become a problem. The extra long 18-gauge spinal needles are inserted into the skin at the planned portal sites to insure accurate placement of the incisions. Important arteries and nerves are safely away from the insertion sites (Fig. 22.9). Branches of the lateral femoral cutaneous nerve are near, but are not dangerously close to the direct anterior portal.

While the image intensifier is being sterilely draped, insert an extra long spinal needle over the anterior edge of the greater trochanter and advance it down the neck of the femur into the hip joint. A definite "give" is felt when the capsule is penetrated, and the needle is then stopped by the bony floor of the acetabulum. At this point, verify the position of the needle in the hip joint with the image intensifier. If the joint has not been entered, manipulate the needle into the joint under image intensification. Next, remove the stylet and with a syringe inject 10 to 15 mL of room air into the joint to break the suction seal. Once the suction seal is broken, the hip will relax and some distraction will occur. At this time, aspirate the hip to see if intraarticular fluid is present. Next, apply at least 50 pounds of traction and use the image intensifier to verify that sufficient distraction is present. Do not hesitate to apply more traction if necessary, but after all instruments have been inserted the traction should be reduced back to 50 pounds. After the traction is brought back to 50 pounds, the distraction will remain owing to muscle relaxation. Next, insert two more extra long spinal needles in a similar matter, one over the posterior aspect of the greater trochanter and the other directly anterior. Check the positioning with the image intensifier and verify entrance into the hip joint by injecting fluid into one needle and watching for it to emerge through the other.

Once the 18-gauge spinal needles are in place to mark the portal sites, the incisions are made. First, remove the needle over the anterior edge of the greater trochanter and make a skin incision at this point. Next, introduce the telescoping cannulas. The smallest cannula is inserted first and is directed into the hip joint under image intensification. The procedure is continued by placing the next larger size of cannula over the one in the joint and removing the first cannula. The procedure is repeated with progressively larger cannulas until adequate dilatation of the tissue around the incision is achieved (Fig. 22.10). Then, place a switching stick through the last telescoping cannula. Insert the arthroscope sheath over the switching

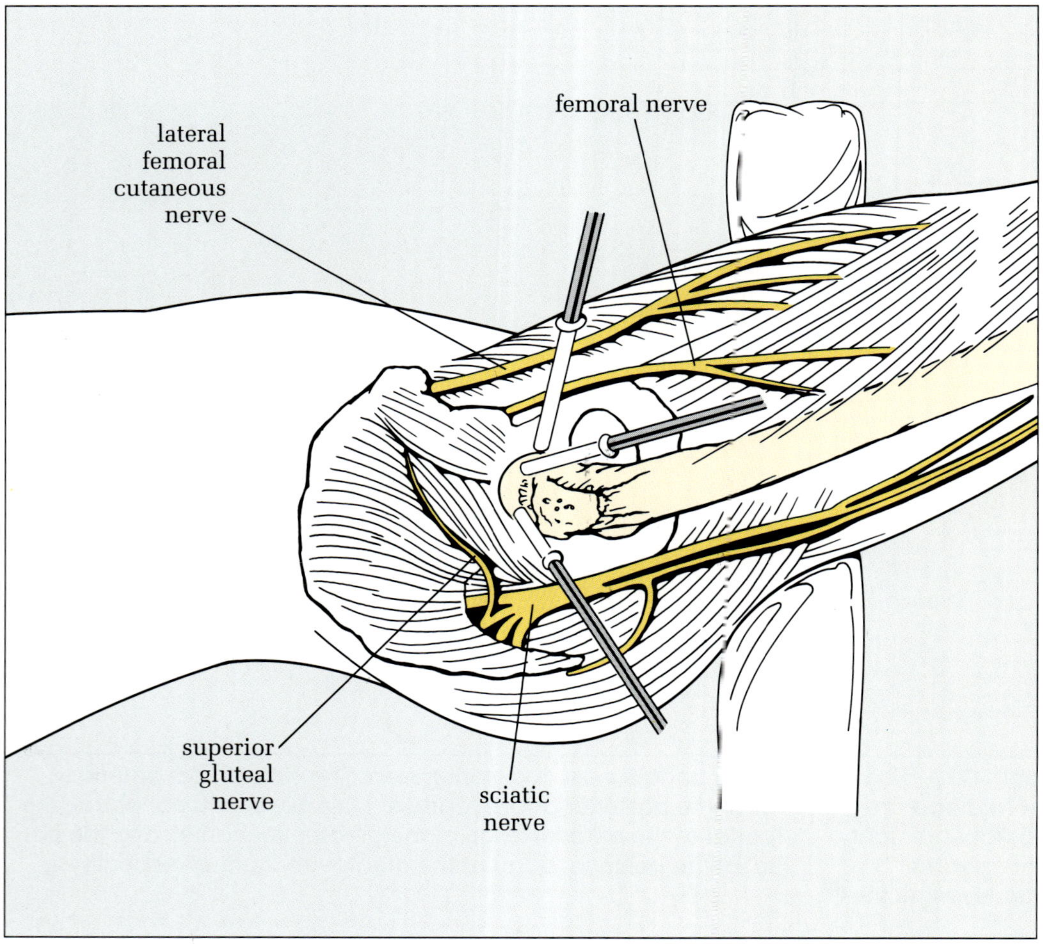

Figure 22.9
Diagram of the important nerves around the hip joint and their relationship to the portals used for hip arthroscopy by the lateral approach.

stick and into the hip joint and couple the arthroscope to it. The process is repeated for each portal. Place an inflow/outflow cannula into the direct anterior portal and a shaver sheath into the posterior portal. After the arthroscope is in the joint, telescoping cannulas are inserted under direct vision (see Fig. 22.10). When the portals have been completed and all instruments are in the joint, the image intensifier can be removed.

The last step is to widen the capsular portion of each portal to increase instrument mobility and to improve access to all portions of the hip joint. To do so, an arthroscopic knife is inserted under direct vision and the capsule is cut in all directions as far as possible (Fig. 22.11).

To visualize the periphery or capsular portion of the hip, pull the arthroscope back and reduce the traction until the head retracts into the acetabulum. Keep the contour of the femoral head in sight. Then, perform a capsulotomy with a motorized full-radius resector and a side-biting suction punch. Trim the capsule proximally and distally so that the junction of the head and the neck is

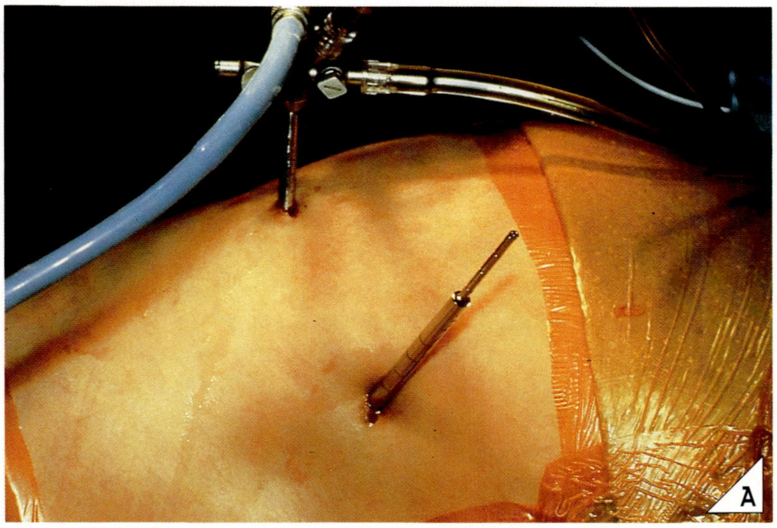

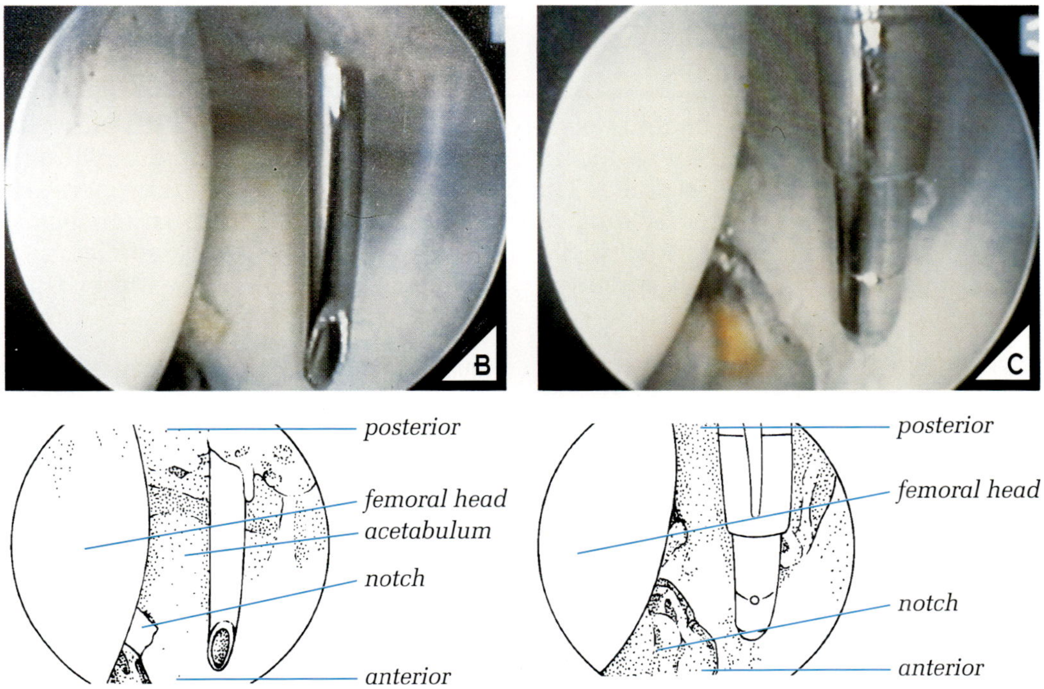

Figure 22.10
Telescoping cannulas inserted in the hip joint. (A) The telescoping cannulas as they appear in a portal adjacent to the arthroscope. (B) The first sharp cannula inside the hip joint. (C) The sharp cannula has been removed. The second can-nula is touching the acetabulum. The third cannula is telescoped over the second cannula.

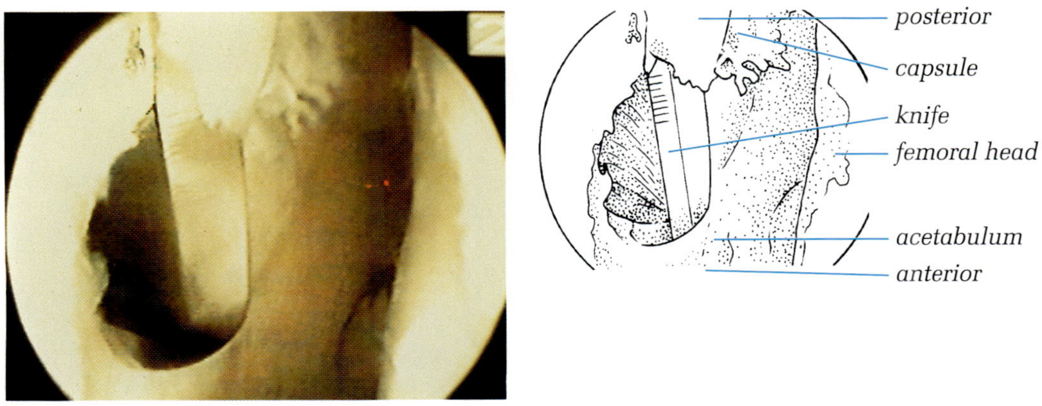

Figure 22.11
Cutting and elongating the left hip capsule with an arthroscopic knife. The knife is in the portal at the posterior edge of the greater trochanter and the arthroscope is viewing from the anterior portal. (Reprinted with permission from Glick JM, 1991)

easily visualized (Fig. 22.12). Debridement and synovectomy in this area are easily performed. Surgical instruments and the arthroscope can be interchanged among any of the portals. A complete view of the hip can be achieved by rotating, adducting, abducting, flexing, and extending the leg and transferring the arthroscope to each portal.

The lateral approach provides a safe route for the arthroscope. The vital structures are away from the actual insertion sites and are in jeopardy if the bony landmarks are not recognized (see Fig. 22.9). The palpable bony landmarks are the greater trochanter and the anterior superior iliac spine. The deep bony landmarks are the neck and head of the femur and the acetabulum. These are palpated with the spinal needle and the trocar as the joint is approached. The instruments pass through the gluteus medius and minimus muscles as they are directed into the hip joint. A definite "give" on either side is felt as the capsule is pierced, and the instrument is stopped by the bony floor of the acetabulum. If bone is not struck, the joint has not been entered. If bone is struck before the capsule appears to be penetrated, the instrument is placed too superior, striking the outer wall of the acetabulum, or too inferior, hitting the head of the femur. The vital adjacent structures include the sciatic nerve posteriorly and the lateral femoral cutaneous nerve anteriorly. The femoral artery and nerve anteriorly and the superior gluteal nerve are far removed from the portals of entry,[7] but their location should be kept in mind.

With the surgeon in the anterior position, the video camera is oriented to provide the same image that the surgeon sees through the arthroscope. On the video screen, the head of the femur appears on the side opposite to that operated on. (For example, in the right hip the femoral head is on the left, and in the left hip the femoral head is on the right; anterior is down and posterior is up in both the right and left hips.) The entire acetabulum can be seen by the direct lateral approach. Figure 22.13 is a diagram of the acetabulum in relation to the arthroscope. Figure 22.14 is an arthroscopic view of a normal hip joint. Note the orientation and the position of the ligamentum teres. This structure is best seen with the arthroscope directed to the medial aspect of the joint.

COMPLICATIONS AND PREVENTION

The complications attributable to this procedure are nerve traction palsy and scuffing of the joint surfaces.[8] The vital neurovascular structures, which include the sciatic nerve and the femoral nerve and artery, are a good distance from the portals. As long as the anatomic landmarks are observed, the vital structures can be avoided. A tensiometer on the hip Distraktor is a significant help in preventing neuropraxia. Safe continuous traction should be in the range of 50 pounds and, like a tourniquet, should be discontinued in 2 hours. Adequate distraction of the hip is important not only to visualize the confines between the femoral head and acetabulum but also to prevent scuffing. The arthroscope and the arthroscopic instruments can be easily brushed against the chondral surfaces, resulting in scuff marks if the hip is not distracted sufficiently. Adequate distraction should be at least 8 mm for ease of entrance. In our experience, instrument breakage occurred once, and the piece was removed arthroscopically. Infections and pressure necrosis of the foot and scrotum were not noted.

CONCLUSION

The benefits of hip arthroscopy are well established. The need for dislocating the hip to reach intraarticular pathology is avoided. The procedure produces little postoperative morbidity and can be performed on an outpatient basis. Prompt recovery from the operation is also beneficial, particularly for elderly patients. Distraction of the hip by trac-

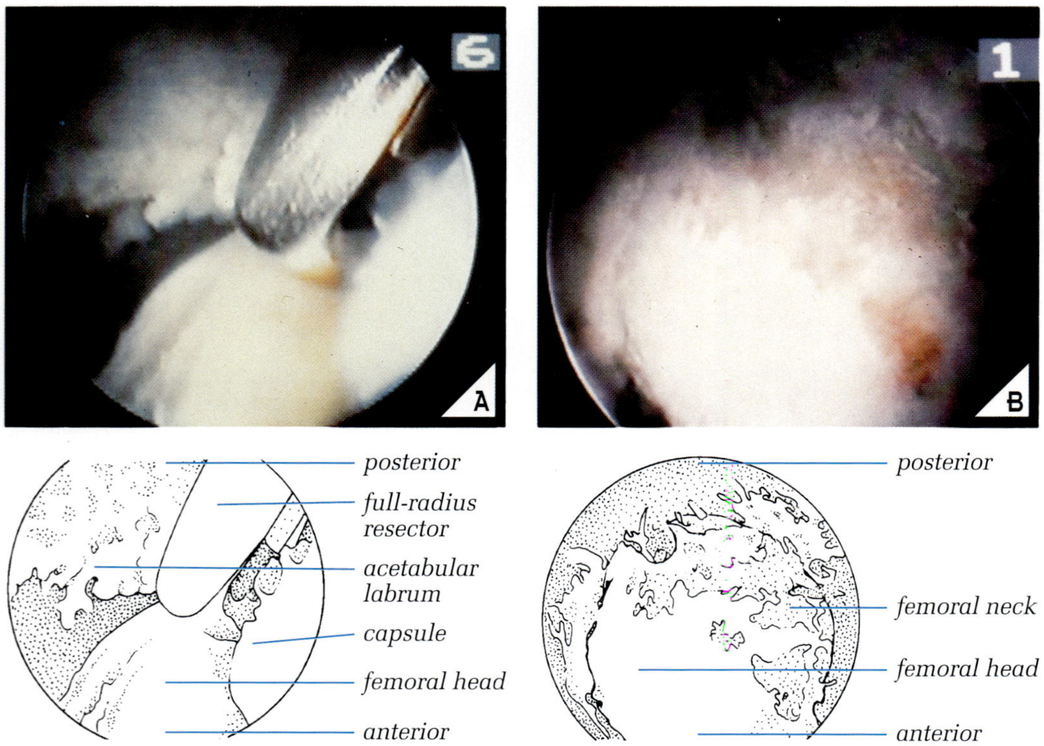

Figure 22.12
Views of the periphery of the hip joint. (A) Trimming the capsule around the periphery of the left hip with a motorized full-radius resector at the anterior edge of the greater trochanter. The arthroscope is viewing from the posterior portal. The traction has been reduced. (B) View of the head-neck junction after the capsule was resected.

tion is necessary. To accomplish this safely, special precautions are necessary. A tensiometer is required to determine the amount of traction to be applied. The foot piece and perineal post should be well padded and adjustable. Safe continuous traction should be about 50 pounds. The traction time should be limited to 2 hours. Enough traction should be applied to sufficiently distract the femur out of the acetabulum at least 8 mm. Suggested indications for this procedure include synovectomy and synovial biopsy, removal of loose bodies and foreign bodies, removal of debris after a closed reduction of a fracture dislocation, evaluation and treatment of osteochondritis dissecans, removal of entrapped cement in total hip arthroplasties, evaluation for arthroplasty, debridement for osteoarthritis, removal of a torn labrum or an impinging ligamentum teres, treatment of infection, and unresolved hip pain. Arthroscopy of the hip joint by the lateral approach is a valuable addition to the evaluation and treatment of hip disorders.

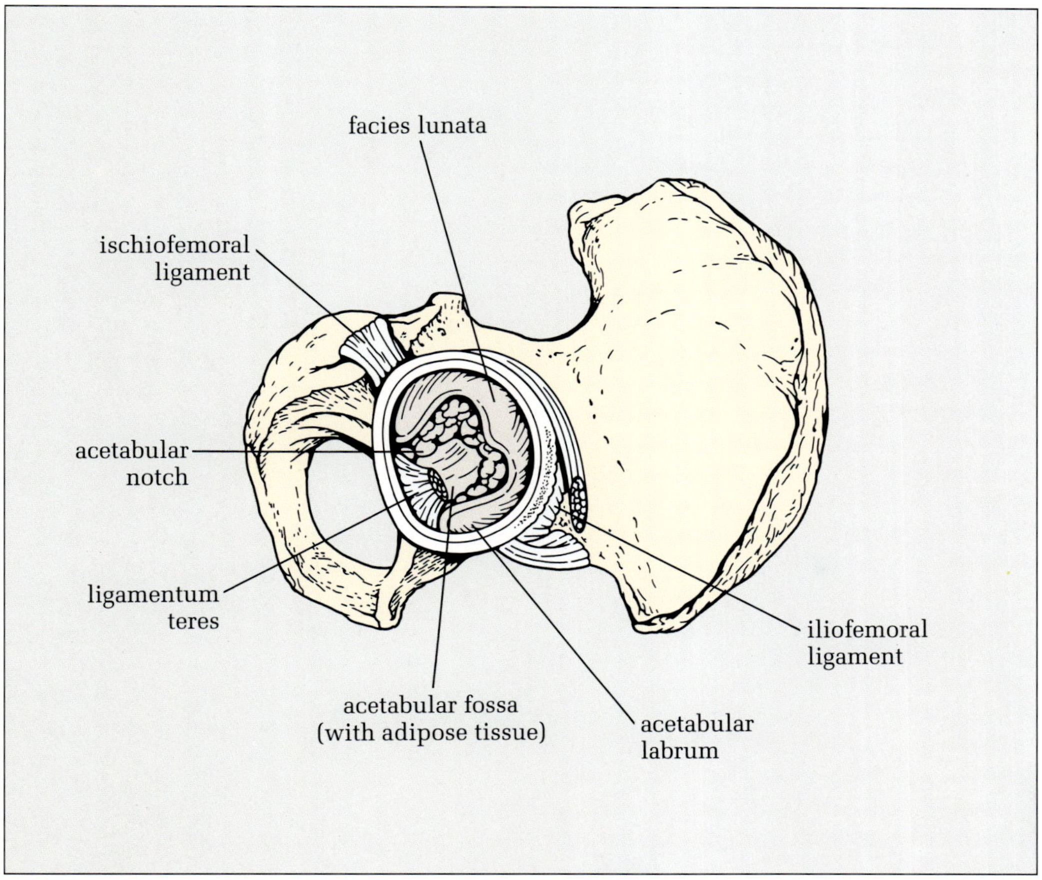

Figure 22.13 Diagram of the right acetabulum with the surgeon standing in front of the patient.

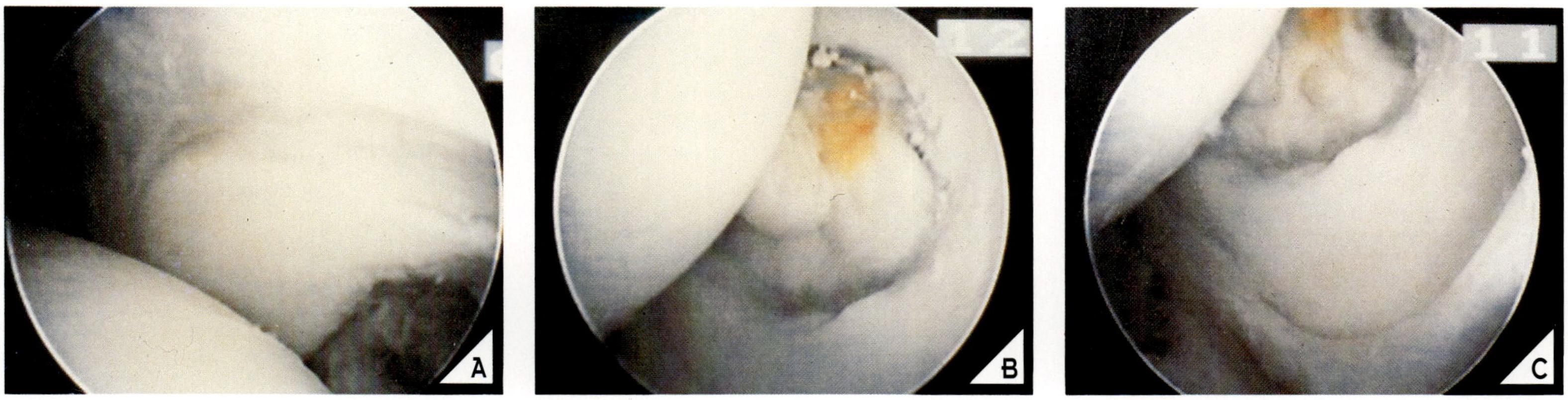

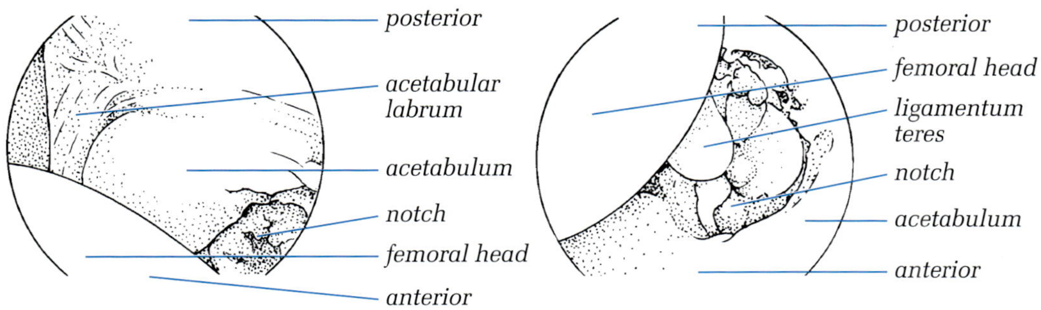

Figure 22.14 The right hip joint. (A) The posterior aspect of the hip joint. (B) Acetabular notch. The ligamentum teres is noted deep in the notch. (C) The anterior aspect of the hip joint.

REFERENCES

1. Glick JM, Sampson TG, Gordon RB, Behr JT, Schmidt E. Hip arthroscopy by the lateral approach. *Arthroscopy.* 1987;3:4–12.
2. Glick JM. Hip arthroscopy using the lateral approach. American Academy of Orthopedic Surgery: Instructional Course Lectures. 1988;19:223–231.
3. Glick JM. Hip arthroscopy. In: McGinty JB, ed. *Operative Arthroscopy,* 1st ed. New York: Raven Press; 1991:663–675.
4. Epstein HC. Posterior fracture-dislocations of the hip: comparison of open and closed methods of treatment in certain types. *J Bone Joint Surg.* 1961;43A:1079–1098.
5. Epstein HC. Posterior fracture-dislocation of the hip. *J Bone Joint Surg.* 1974;56A:1103–1127.
6. Hogersson S, Brattstrom H, Mogensen B, Lidgren L. Arthroscopy of the hip in juvenile chronic arthritis. *J Pediatr Orthop.* 1984;1:273–278.
7. Foster DE, Hunter JR. The direct lateral approach to the hip for arthroplasty. *Orthopaedics.* 1987;10:274–280.
8. Glick JM. Complications of hip arthroscopy by the lateral approach. In: Sherman OH, Mikoff J, eds. *Arthroscopic Surgery.* 1st ed. Baltimore, Md: Williams & Wilkins; 1990:193–201.

chapter Twenty Three

Hip Arthroscopy: Supine Position

J. Serge Parisien

Techniques of hip arthroscopy with the patient supine, with or without traction, have been refined and allow adequate visualization of the joint in most clinical situations.

ANATOMY

The hip joint is a ball-and-socket synovial joint formed by the femoral head and the acetabulum (Fig. 23.1). The femoral head, except for the fovea, which provides an attachment to the ligament of the head, is covered with hyaline articular cartilage. The fibrocartilaginous labrum is attached to the rim of the acetabulum, which it deepens. At the inferior aspect of the acetabular notch the labrum is completed by the transverse acetabular ligament. Through the foramen, located between the transverse ligament and the acetabular notch, vessels supply the fat pad and the ligament of the head (ligamentum teres). The articular capsule is attached superiorly to the rim of the acetabulum beyond the labrum and inferiorly it reaches the anterior intertrochanteric line. Posteriorly the attachment is less distal, leaving the posterior third of the femoral neck without capsular coverage. Some thick longitudinal fibers reinforce the capsule and are named, according to their pelvic origins, the iliofemoral, ischiofemoral, and pubofemoral ligaments.

The iliofemoral ligament or ligament of Bigelow, also called the Y ligament because of its shape, is the strongest of all the ligaments. It covers almost all of the anterior aspect of the joint and becomes very tight when the hip joint is hyperextended. Zona orbicularis is located around the neck of the femur and is formed by a circular ring of fibers.

INDICATIONS

From a review of the literature and on the basis of my own experience, hip arthroscopy is useful in the following situations[1–22]: removal of loose chondral or osteochondral bodies; debridement of osteochondritis dissecans of the femoral head; debridement of torn labrum; evaluation of the articular cartilage with synovial biopsy or partial synovectomy in cases of juvenile chronic synovitis or pigmented villonodular synovitis; assessment of the joint cavity with removal of loose fractured fragments in cases of traumatic injuries of the hip joint (fracture dislocation of the hip); and visualization of an artificial hip joint for removal of cement fragments or loose metallic fragments and biopsy for purpose of histologic examination of tissue material to rule out infection before reimplantation.

HIP ARTHROSCOPY WITH AND WITHOUT DISTRACTION

Dorfmann et al.[3] describe an anterolateral arthroscopic portal that does not require the use of a fracture table or x-ray control. From an arthroscopic point of view, he divides the examination into two zones, superficial (synovium, neck, labrum, and two thirds of the circumference of the femoral head) and deep (acetabulum and remainder of the femoral head). The point of entrance is midway on the line joining the anterosuperior iliac spine and greater trochanter. The arthroscope is directed towards the center of the femoral head. Dorfmann et al.[3] feel that this technique allows only examination of the superficial zone, in which most conditions of the hip are located.

Klapper and Silver[15] also feel that traction is not necessary during hip arthroscopy, since most surgical procedures that can be performed with the arthroscope do not require complete visualization of the acetabulum. These authors use an anterolateral portal located at a point two fingerbreadths above the anterior margin of the greater trochanter and two fingerbreadths lateral to the anterosuperior iliac spine. The second portal used for instrumentation is lateral to the femoral pulse. The authors claim that placing the "draped-free" lower extremity through a range of motion will improve visualization of the femoral head.

When visualization of the confines of the acetabulum is desired, distraction of the hip joint is mandatory. The hip joint can be distracted by applying traction to the leg. Fifty pounds of traction force is necessary to open the joint approximately 8 to 10 mm.[7]

PORTALS

Three portals are available: *lateral, anterolateral,* and *anterior* (Figs. 23.2, 23.3).

The landmark for the *lateral* portal is the greater trochanter. This portal is placed above the greater trochanter laterally. It is far away from the sciatic nerve posteriorly

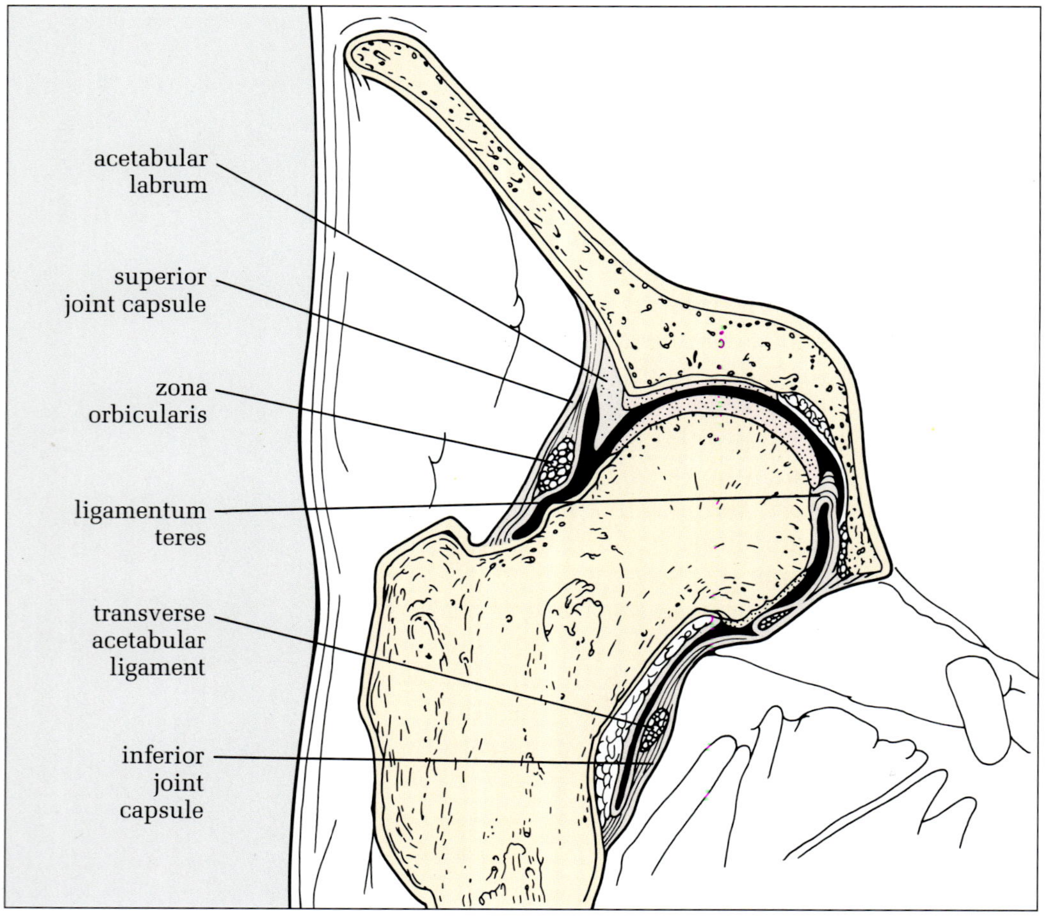

Fig. 23.1
Hip anatomy and capsular attachment.

and from the femoral nerve and artery anteriorly. The lateral femoral cutaneous nerve is located anterior to this portal and passes over the sartorius muscle approximately 2.5 cm below the anterosuperior iliac spine.

The landmarks for the *anterolateral* portal are the anterosuperior iliac spine and the anterior border of the greater trochanter. This portal is midway on the line joining the anterosuperior iliac spine and the greater trochanter. To develop this portal, a spinal needle is directed medially and posteriorly at approximately a 45° angle towards the femoral head. The lateral femoral cutaneous nerve is at risk because of its proximity to this portal.

The *anterior* portal can be made by carefully palpating the femoral artery. It is located approximately 4 cm lateral to the artery and 1 cm distal to the inguinal ligament. When a spinal needle is inserted through this portal, a return of fluid confirms its proper insertion into the joint.

INSTRUMENTATION

The necessary instruments include a 25° arthroscope (2.7 or 4 mm) with sharp and smooth obturators, an extra long spinal needle with a 50 mL syringe, plastic tubing for irri-

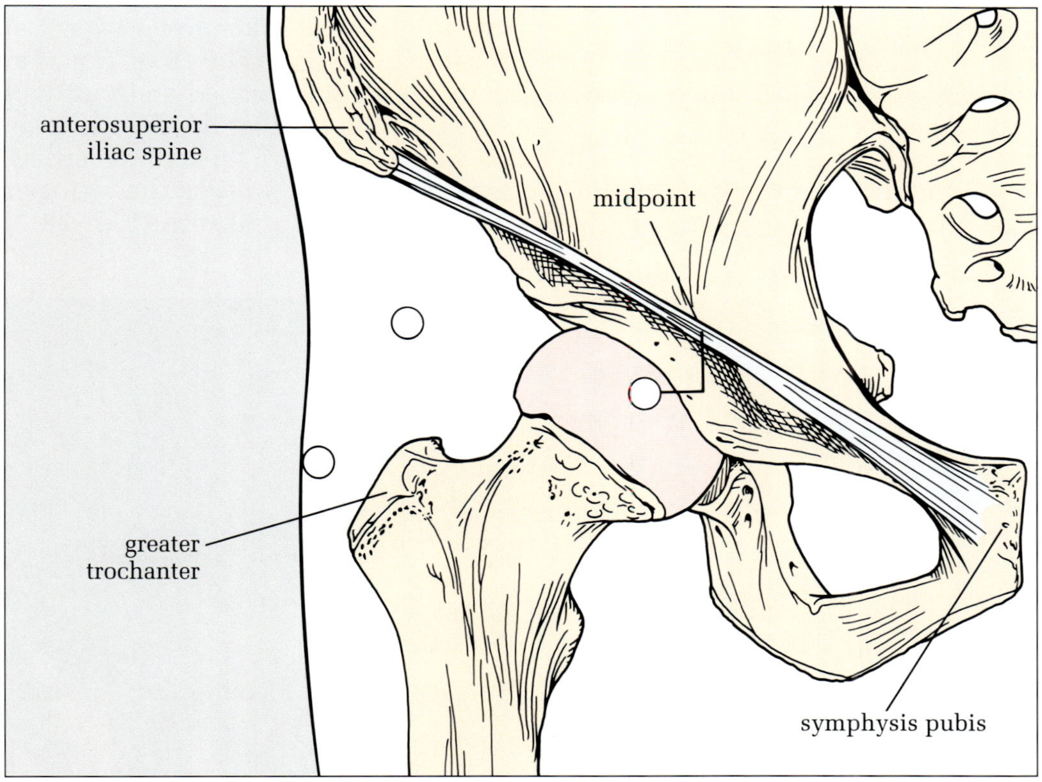

Fig. 23.2 Anatomy of the anterior aspect of the hip joint and portal location.

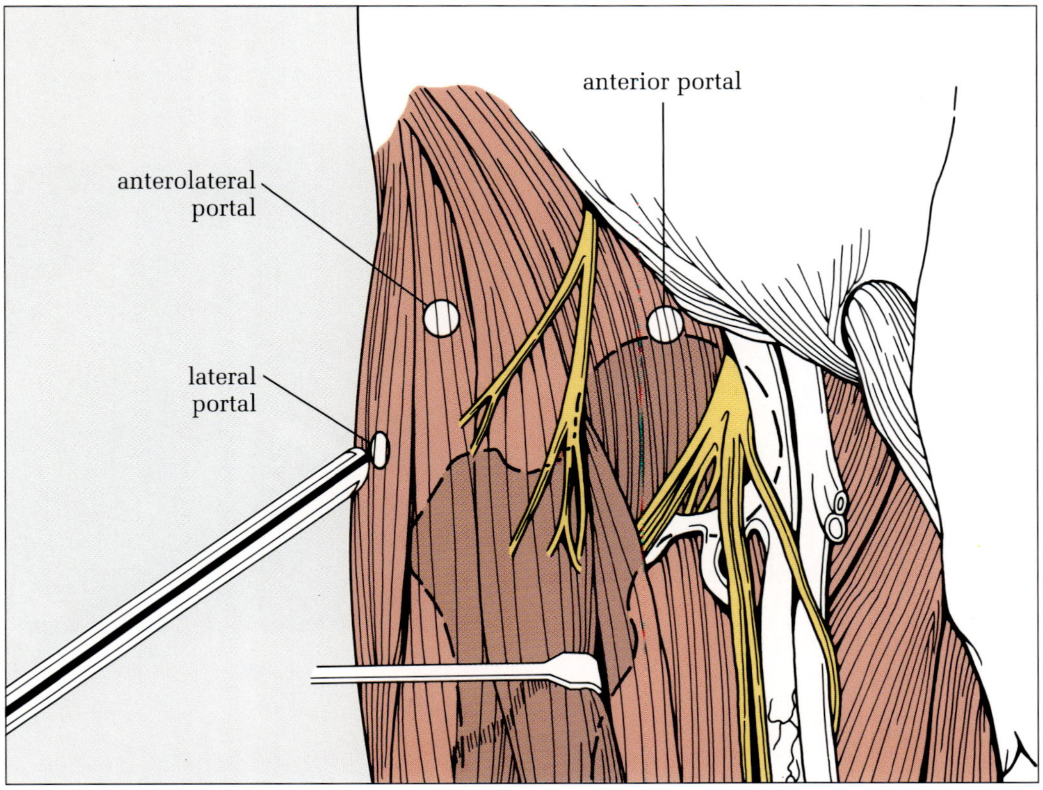

Fig. 23.3 The three portals that can be used for hip arthroscopy in the supine position.

gation, a motorized shaver system and abrader, grasping forceps and basket punch, switching sticks, and a magnetic retriever. An overhead gravity system is used for continuous irrigation.

SURGICAL TECHNIQUE

General or spinal anesthesia can be used. The patient is placed on a fracture table with the leg slightly abducted and in slight flexion (Fig. 23.4). The perineal post in the pubic area should be well padded to minimize excessive pressure against the scrotum and pudendal area. An image intensifier is used. The surgical field is prepped and draped in the usual manner. A sterile plastic bag covers the part of the image intensifier that is placed above the surgical field. An extra long 18- or 22-gauge spinal needle is used laterally above the greater trochanter (Fig. 23.5). The needle is directed towards the femoral head, while some traction is applied to the extremity to distract the hip joint. Normal saline or Ringer's lactate solution, 20 to 30 mL, is used to distend the anterior capsule. Backflow of the solution indicates successful placement into the joint. The needle is replaced by the sharp obturator of a 2.7 mm or 4 mm arthroscope. Further traction is obtained, and before the capsule is penetrated with the sharp obturator the accuracy of the position is confirmed with the image intensifier. A "pop" is felt as the tough capsule is entered. Then the sharp obturator is replaced by the smooth obturator and inserted further into the distracted joint space. The arthroscope (2.7 mm for a child's hip or 4 mm for an adult hip) is then introduced into the joint for the arthroscopic exploration.

The examination begins with the inspection of the femoral head at its lateral aspect. By gently maneuvering the scope it is possible to visualize the anterior aspect of the joint as well as the acetabular area (Fig. 23.6). Rotation of the involved extremity by an unscrubbed assistant will expose the different areas of the femoral head for inspection. It is possible this way to visualize most of the articular cartilage of the femoral head, as well as the articular surface of the acetabulum and the labrum (Fig. 23.7)

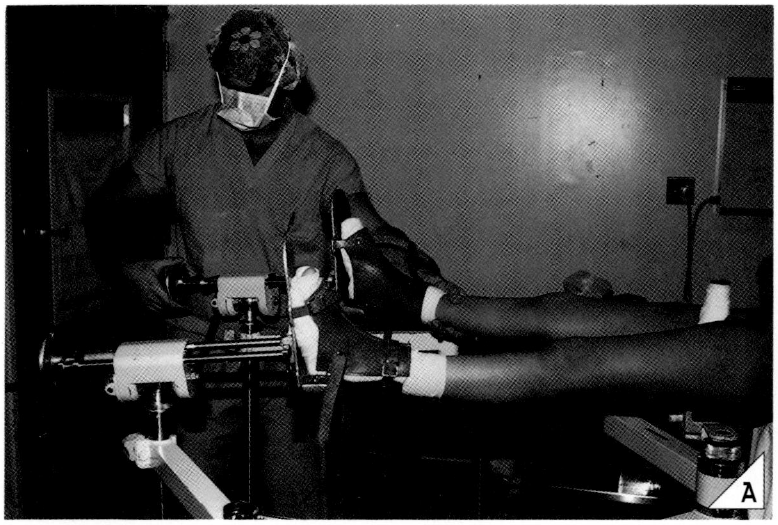

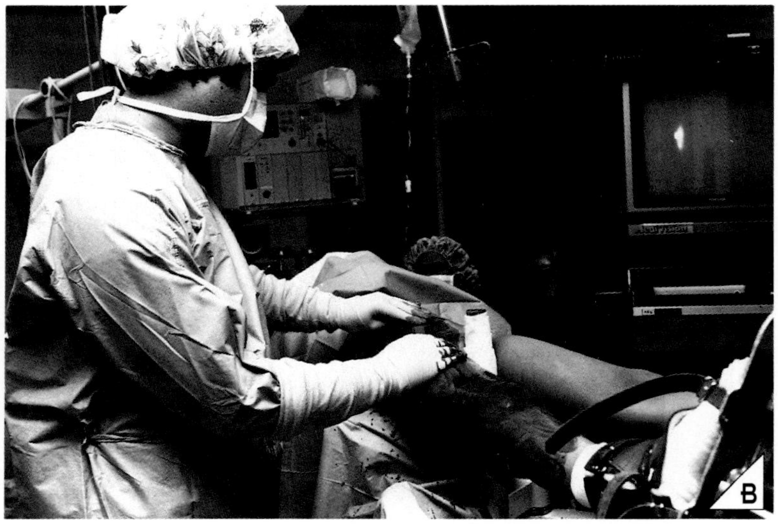

Fig. 23.4
(A, B) The patient is placed on a fracture table for traction with the hip in slight abduction and flexion.

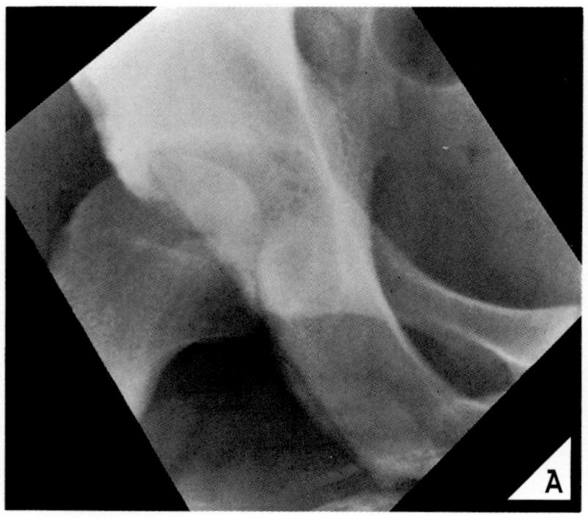

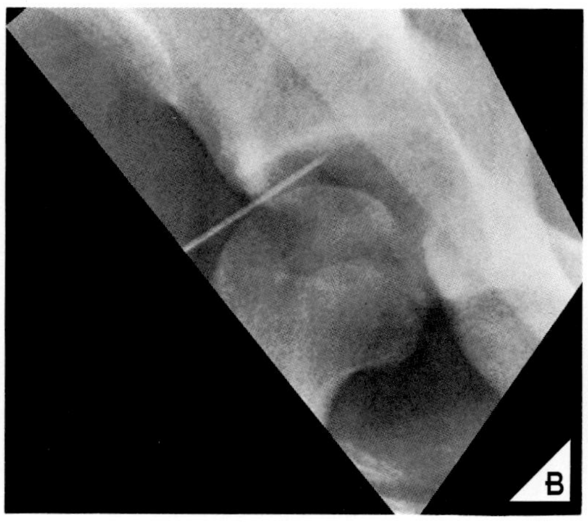

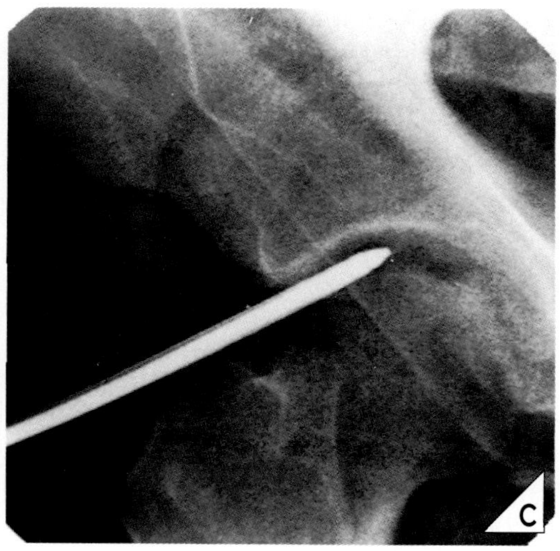

Fig. 23.5
(A, B) The spinal needle position is checked with the image intensifier.

(C) The trocar position is visualized with the image intensifier.

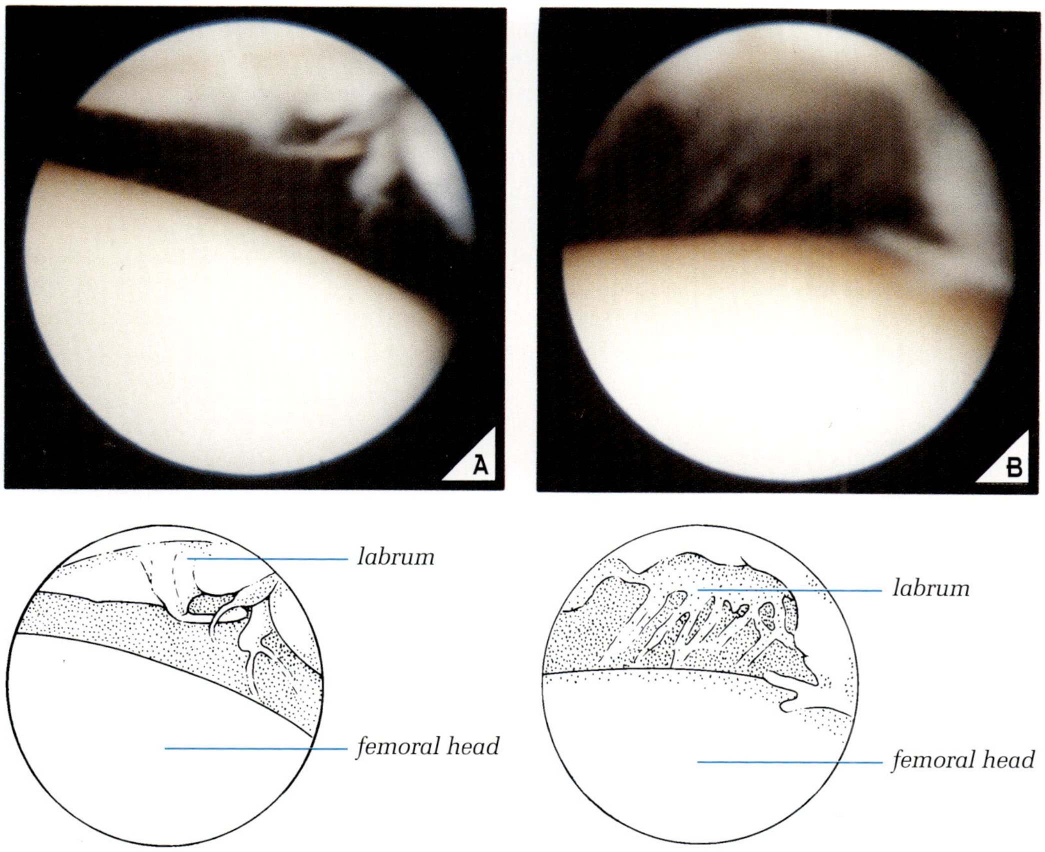

Fig. 23.6
(A, B) Arthroscopic visualization of right hip joint. The femoral head is below and the acetabulum with labrum is on top.

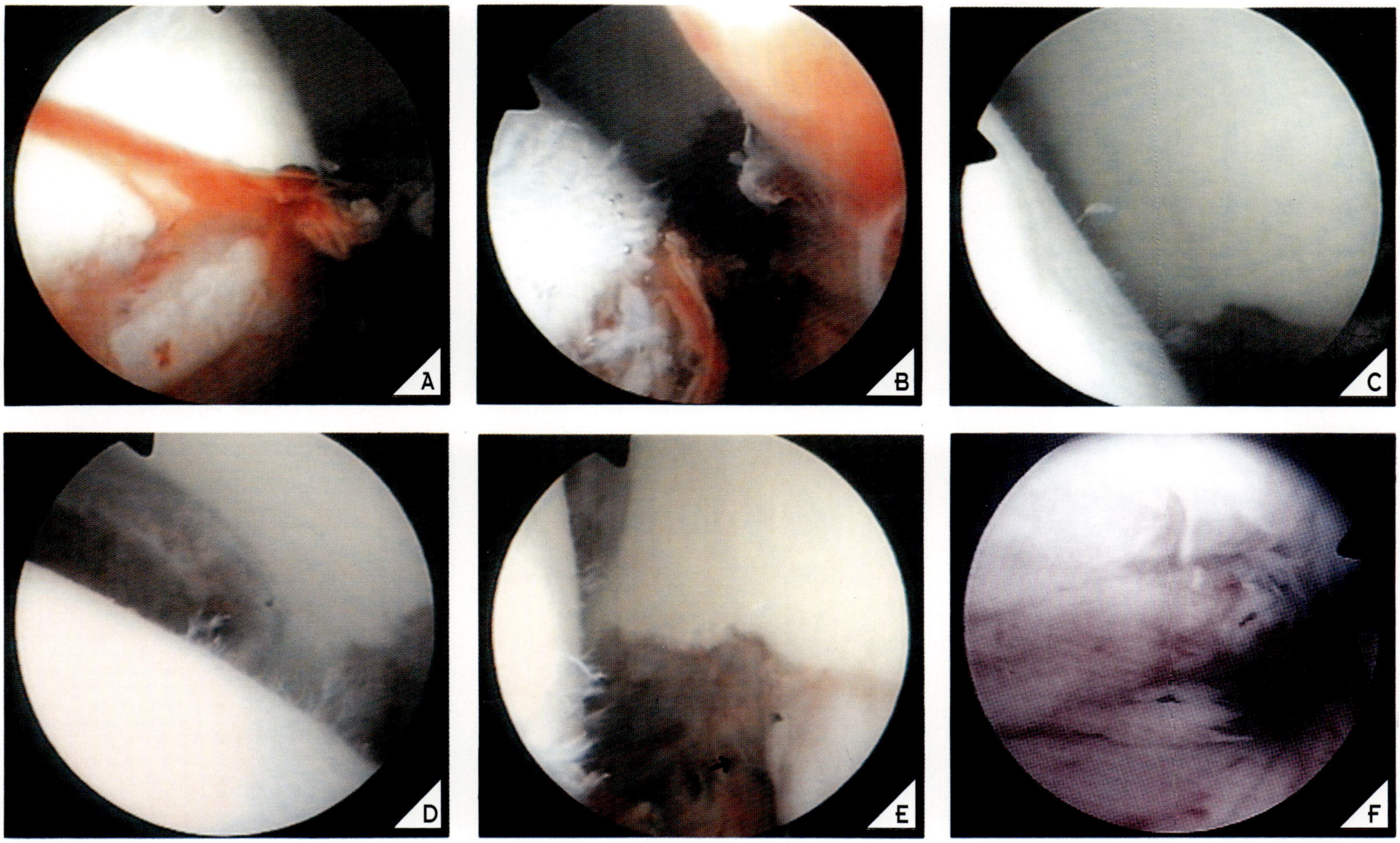

Fig. 23.7
Different areas of the left hip seen with rotation of the femoral head. (A) Lateral aspect of the head with blood clots. (B) Lateral aspect of the labrum. (C) Arthroscope placed inside the confines of the joint. (D) Arthroscope inside the distracted joint. (E) Acetabular notch visualized at the bottom of the picture (arrow=notch). (F) With more internal rotation the posterior aspect of the femoral head is seen with reflexion of the synovium.

Chondromalacic areas of the articular cartilage of the acetabulum and femoral head can be visualized, as can osteochondral defects (Figs. 23.8–23.10). The medial and inferior aspects of the joint can be best visualized from this portal if the 30° scope is replaced by a 70° scope. To improve visualization a second portal is developed, preferably the anterolateral portal. A spinal needle is used midway on the line joining the anterior border of the greater trochanter and the anterosuperior iliac spine. The direction of the needle can be guided with the image intensifier and its accurate placement into the joint cavity is confirmed again by a reflux of fluid from the needle. After the skin incision is made, a mosquito forceps is used to spread the subcutaneous tissue to prevent injury to the lateral femoral cutaneous nerve, which is in proximity to the portal. If the interchangeable cannula system is not available, the cannula for the motorized shaver system is introduced, with its obturator, into the joint. The availability of switching sticks of various sizes will facilitate interchanging the portals. The third (anterior) portal may have to be developed if visualization of the medial aspect of the hip is inadequate or for the purpose of triangulating

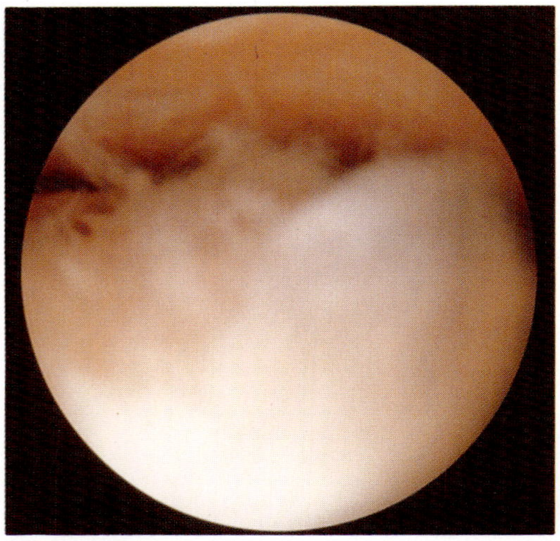

Fig. 23.8
Chondromalacic changes of the femoral head in osteochondritis.

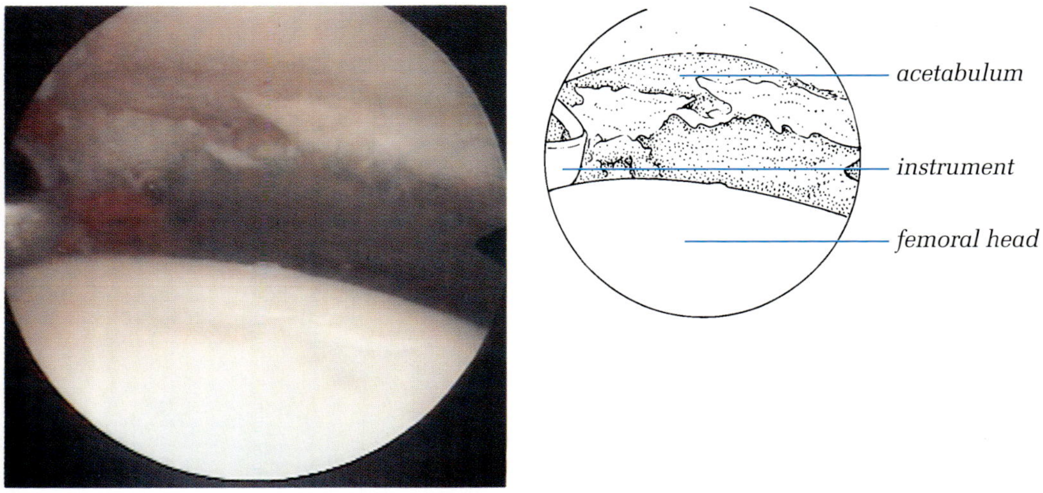

Fig. 23.9
Chondral fracture of the acetabulum of the left hip. The arthroscope is through the lateral portal and the motorized shaver is through the anterolateral portal.

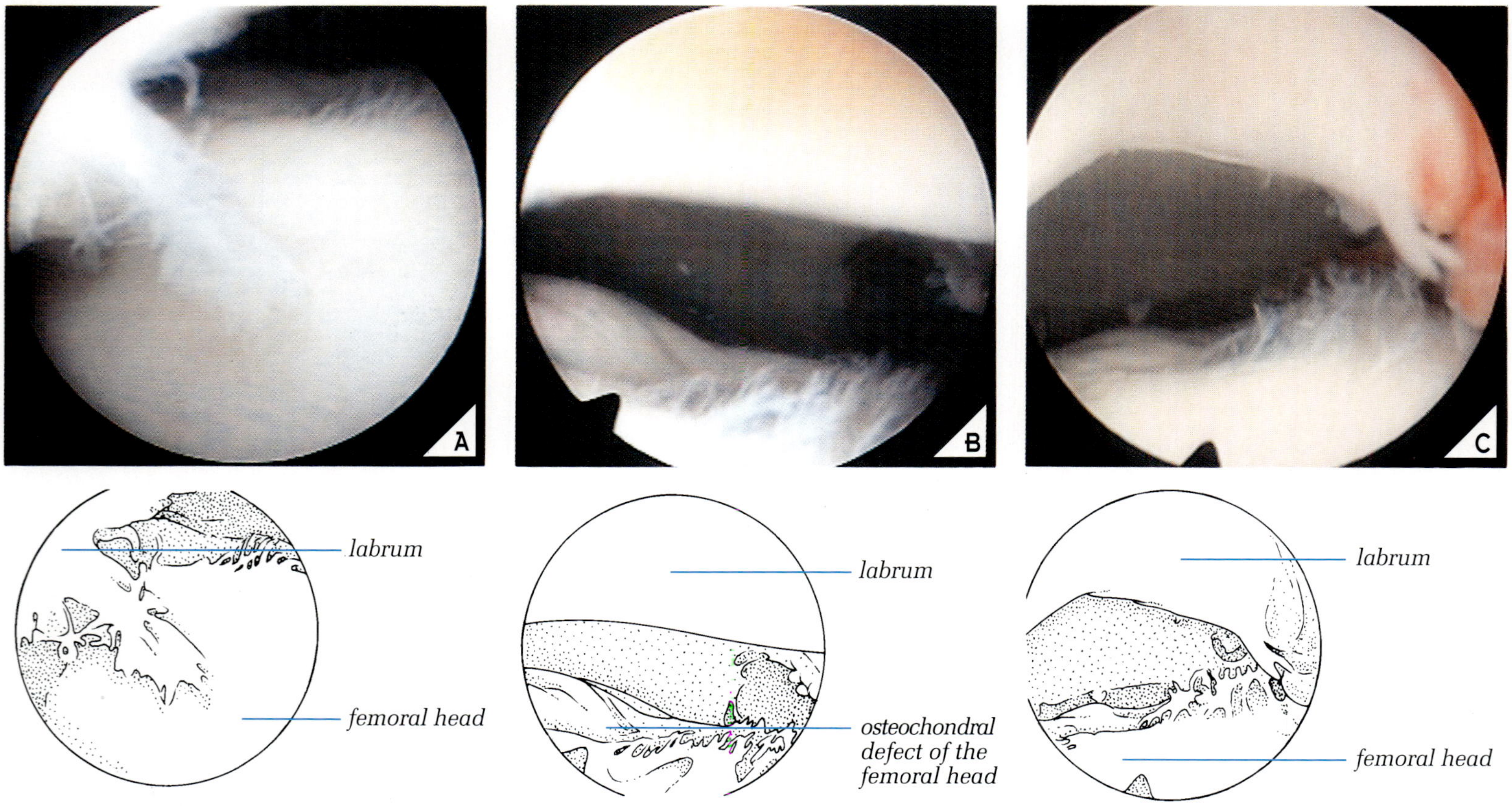

Fig. 23.10
(A–C) Arthroscopic visualization of fracture dislocation of the left hip. An osteochondral defect of the left femoral head is seen in these views.

when surgery is intended. As advocated by Ide et al.,[11] this portal can also be located at an area placed 1 cm lateral and distal to the midpoint of the line between the anterosuperior iliac spine and the symphysis pubis. Surgical procedures such as chondroplasty can be performed (Fig. 23.11). Extraction of large loose bodies from the femoral head or acetabulum can be done with a grasping forceps or motorized instrument using the triangulation technique. Small fragments can be removed by vacuuming (Figs. 23.12–23.14).

Postoperative Management

A light dressing is applied over the hip area. When the procedure is performed on an outpatient basis the patient is discharged the same day. Crutch walking with partial weight-bearing is advisable for a few days, mostly for comfort. With a more extensive procedure (partial synovectomy, debridement for osteochondritis dissecans of the femoral head), a period of non-weight-bearing with crutches is prescribed for 2 to 3 weeks. Active range of motion is encouraged as tolerated by the patient.

Complications and Pitfalls

Positioning of the spinal needle is a very important step in the procedure and is facilitated by the image intensifier. To avoid blockage with soft tissue, it is important to keep the stylet in place when the needle is introduced. Damage to the articular cartilage of the femoral head can be avoided, before using the sharp trocar, by confirming adequate distraction of the joint and proper direction of the instrument with the image intensifier. Using mosquito forceps to spread the skin and subcutaneous tissue will prevent

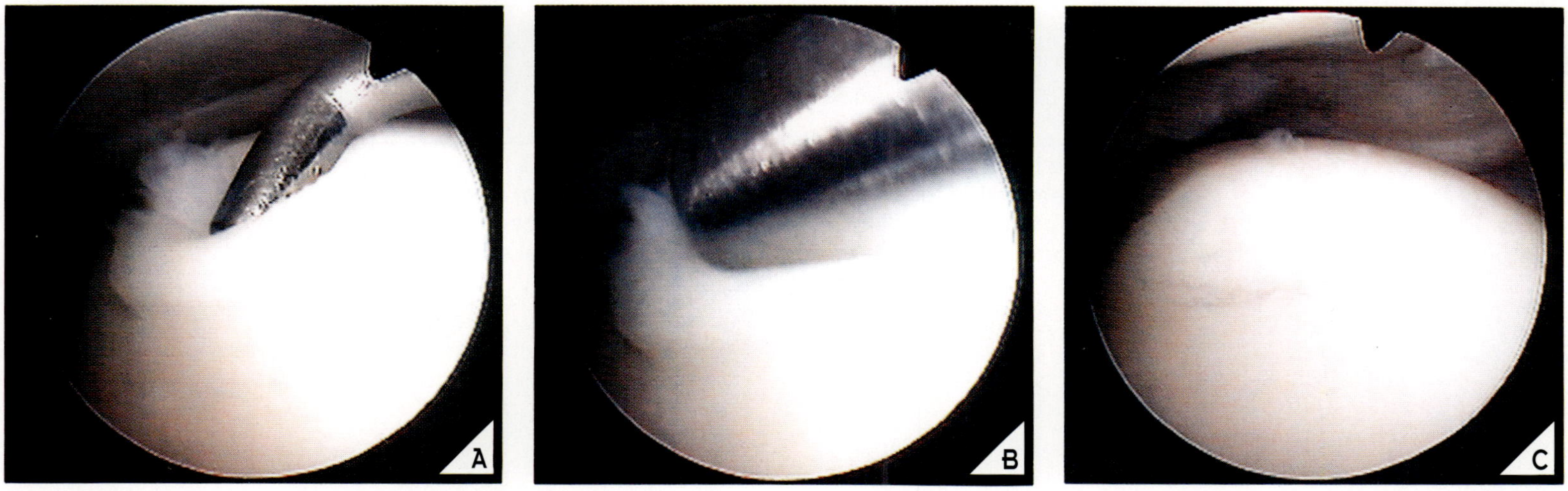

Fig. 23.11
Chondral flap of the medial aspect of the left femoral head. The scope is through the anterior portal. (A) Palpation with probe. (B) Debridement with shaver (C) Status postdebridement.

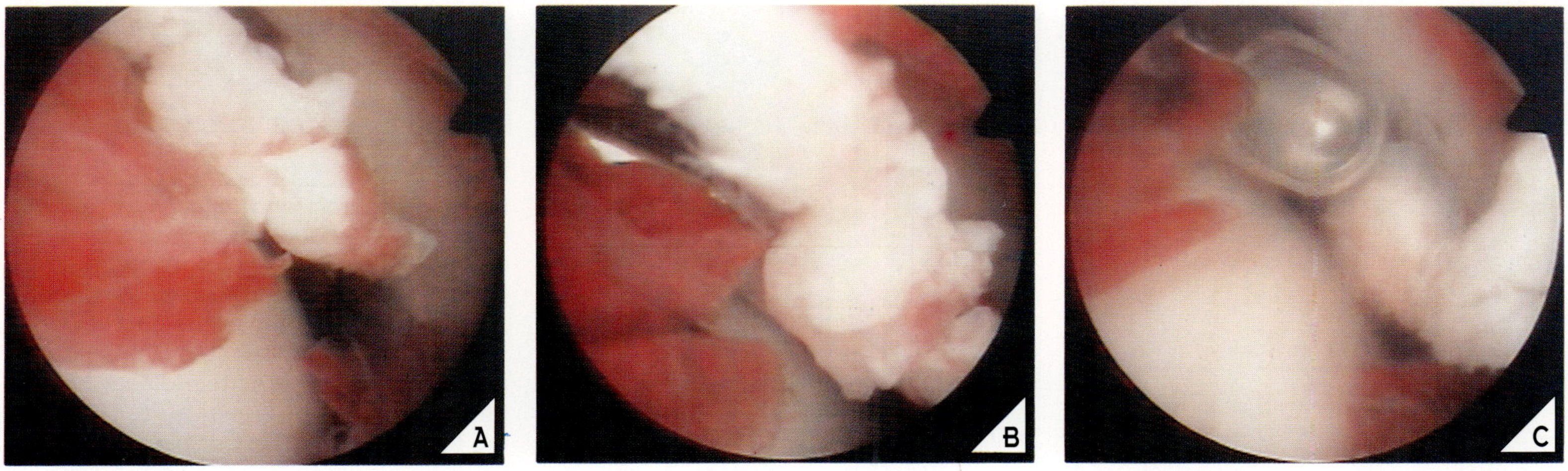

Fig. 23.12
(A–C) Views of loose chondral fracture of the posterior aspect of the femoral head of the left hip with a motorized shaver in the background. The femoral head is on the left.

injury to the lateral femoral cutaneous nerve. The perineal post in the traction table should be carefully padded to avoid abnormal pressure on the scrotum and compression of the branches of the pudendal nerve. Traction on the extremity does not have to be applied constantly. Once the cavity between the femoral head and the acetabulum has been adequately visualized, the traction can be decreased. Continuous traction on the extremity for over 2 hours will probably cause some transient neuropraxia.

Since some pathologic conditions amenable to arthroscopic surgery (synovitis, loose bodies, labral tears) are located in areas that can be visualized without joint distraction, traction may not be mandatory for every arthroscopic hip procedure.

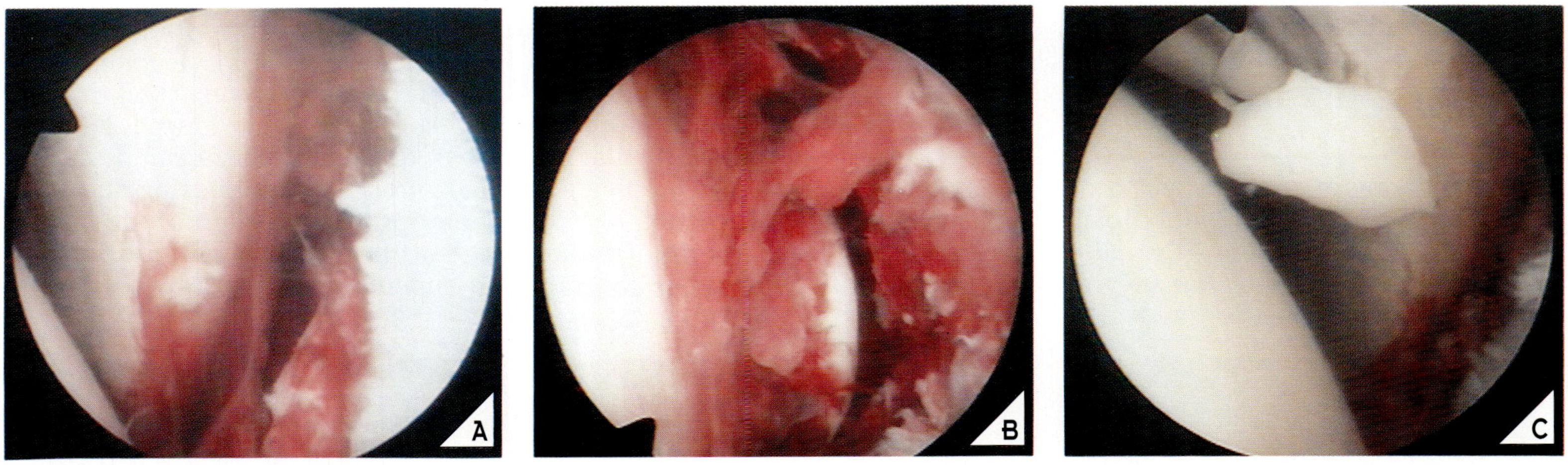

Fig. 23.13
Visualization of an area of fracture located in the posterior aspect of the acetabulum of the left hip. Removal of loose fragments and lavage of joint debris only were performed. Internal fixation was not performed because the fragment was stable and represented less than 10% of the acetabulum. (A) Fracture areas. (B) Close-up of fracture areas. (C) Loose fragment being removed with motorized instrument. The femoral head is on the left and the acetabulum is on the right.

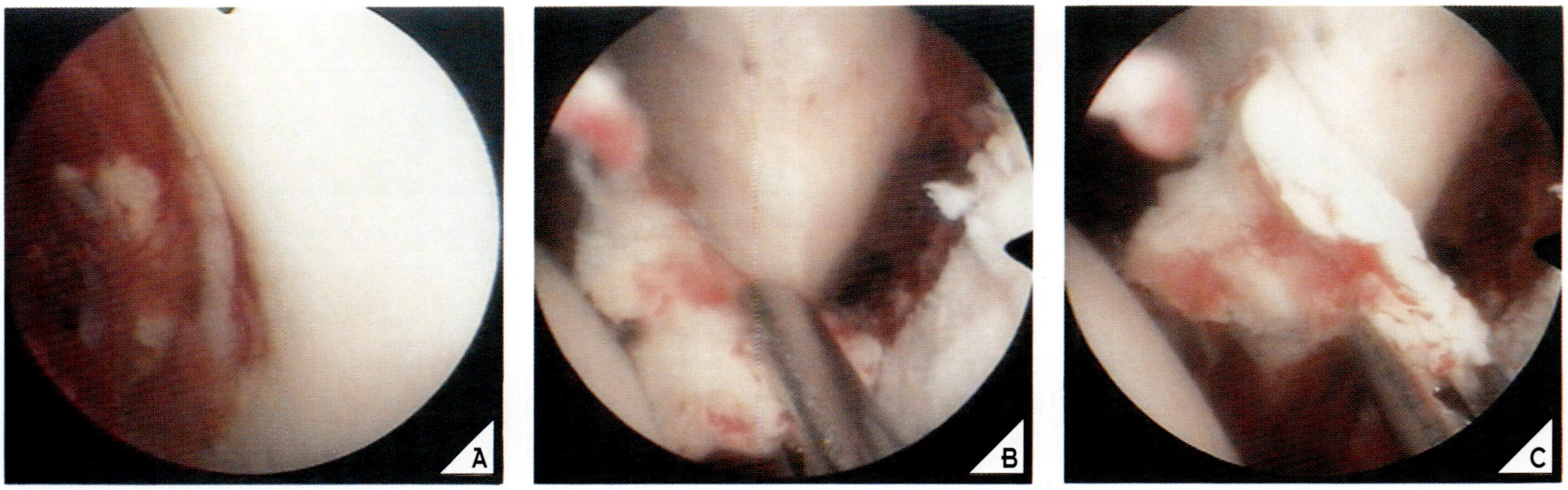

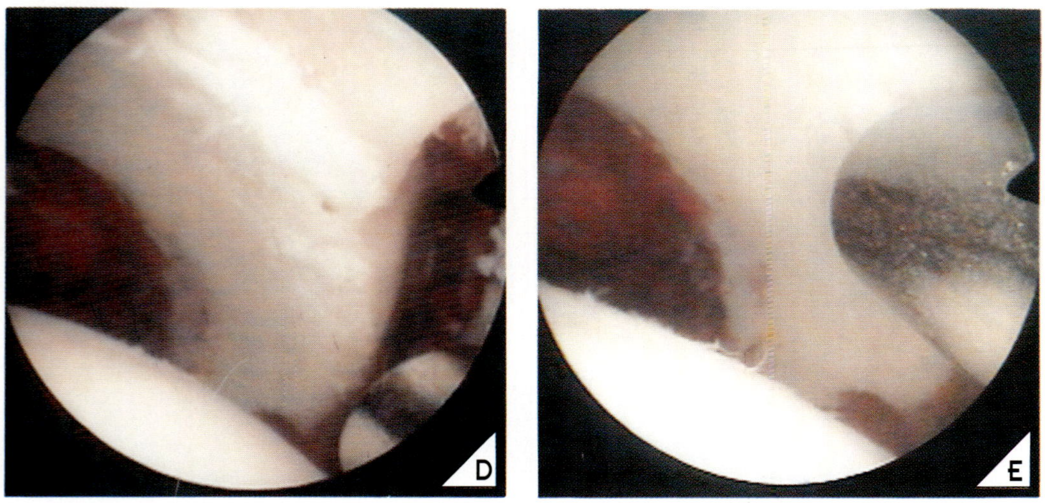

Fig. 23.14
(A) Large osteochondral fragment located deep in the acetabular notch (in the left hip of the preceding photographs). Removal with grasping forceps (B, C) and joint lavage with fluid introduced under pressure through a cannula (D, E). The scope is through the anterolateral portal and the surgical instruments are through the lateral portal. The femoral head is on the left; the acetabulum is on the right.

REFERENCES

1. Altenberg AR. Acetabular labral tears: a cause of hip pain and degenerative arthritis. *South Med J.* 1977;70:174–175.
2. Bowen JR, Kumar VP, Joyce J, Bowen C. Osteochondritis dissecans following Perthes' disease: arthroscopic operative treatment. *Clin Orthop.* 1936;209:49–56.
3. Dorfmann H, Boyer T, Henry P, DeBie B. A simple approach to hip arthroscopy. *Arthroscopy.* 1988;4:141–142.
4. Dorrell JH, Catterall A. The torn acetabular labrum. *J Bone Joint Surg.* 1986;68B:400–403.
5. Dvorak M, Duncan CP, Day B. Arthroscopic anatomy of the hip. *Arthroscopy.* 1990;6:264–273.
6. Eriksson E, Arvidsson I, Arvidsson H. Diagnostic and operative arthroscopy of the hip. *Orthopedics.* 1986;9:169–178.
7. Glick JM, Sampson TG, Gordon RB, et al. Hip arthroscopy by the lateral approach. *Arthroscopy.* 1987;3:4–12.
8. Gross RH. Arthroscopy in hip disorders in children. *Orthop Rev.* 1977;9:43–49.
9. Gross R. Arthroscopy of the hip. In: Grana W, ed. *Update in Arthroscopic Techniques.* Baltimore, Md: University Park Press; 1984:79.
10. Holgersson S, Brattstrom H, Mogensen B, Lidgren L. Arthroscopy of the hip in juvenile chronic arthritis. *J Pediatr Orthop.* 1984;1:273–278.
11. Ide T, Akamatsu N, Nakajima I. Arthroscopic surgery of the hip joint. *Arthroscopy.* 1991;7:204–211.
12. Ikeda T, Awaya G, Susuki S, Yutaka O, Hiroshi T. Torn acetabular labrums in young patients: arthroscopic diagnosis and management. *J Bone Joint Surg.* 1988;70B:13–16.
13. Ikeuchi H. Arthroscopy of the hip joint. In: Watanabe M, ed. *Arthroscopy of Small Joints.* Tokyo: Igaku-Shoin; 1985:97–103.
14. Johnston A, Parisien M. Pathology of reactive (prosthetic) versus septic (revisionary) synovitis. In: Eftekar N, ed. *Infection in Joint Replacement Surgery.* St. Louis, Mo: CV Mosby Co; 1984:97–114.
15. Klapper RC, Silver DM. Hip arthroscopy without traction. *Contemp Orthop.* 1989;18:687–693.
16. Nordt W, Giangarra CE, Levy M, Habermann ET. Arthroscopic removal of entrapped debris following dislocation of a total hip arthroplasty. *Arthroscopy.* 1987;3:196–198.
17. Okada Y, Awaya G, Ikeda T, Tada H, Kamisato S, Futami T. Arthroscopic surgery for synovial chondromatosis of the hip. *J Bone Joint Surg.* 1989;71B:198–199.
18. Parisien JS. Arthroscopy of the hip: present status. *Bull Hosp Jt Dis Orthop Inst.* 1985;45:127.
19. Shifrin LZ, Reis ND. Arthroscopy of a dislocated hip replacement: a case report. *Clin Orthop.* 1980;146:213–214.
20. Ueo T, Suzuki S, Iwasaki R, Yosikawa J. Rupture of the labra acetabularis as a cause of hip pain detected arthroscopically, and partial limbectomy for successful pain relief. *Arthroscopy.* 1990;6:48–51.
21. Vakili F, Salvati EA, Warren RF. Entrapped foreign body within the acetabular cup in total hip replacement. *Clin Orthop.* 1980;150:159.
22. Witwity T, Uhlmann RD, Fischer J. Arthroscopic management of chondromatosis of the hip joint. *Arthroscopy.* 1988;4:55–56.

Section Six

The Wrist, Carpal Tunnel, and Temporomandibular Joint

chapter Twenty Four

Arthroscopic Surgery of the Wrist

Edward S. Bittar

Wrist arthroscopy—described independently by Chen[1] and Watanabe[2]—did not capture popular interest until 1986 when arthroscopic techniques for the wrist were described in detail by Roth[3] and Whipple.[4] Early success with wrist arthroscopy fostered the development of arthroscopic surgical techniques for a variety of surgical procedures that historically required extensive surgical exposure with significant morbidity. Improvements in surgical techniques and the design of small-joint fiberoptic telescopes and accessory arthroscopic equipment have made wrist arthroscopic surgery available for general use.[5] Arthroscopy provides the surgeon with improved visualization and a reduced rate of morbidity and enables the patient to return to activities earlier; thus it has evolved to replace arthrography as the diagnostic "gold standard" of wrist pathology.

INDICATIONS

Wrist arthroscopy has greater diagnostic sensitivity than arthrography. Approximately 40% more wrist pathology can be diagnosed arthroscopically.[6] Additionally, it can often be confirmed arthroscopically that wrist pathology requires treatment via an open procedure prior to committing to an arthrotomy.

As in other joints, a large number of procedures can be performed arthroscopically. Debridement, loose body removal, synovial biopsy or subtotal synovectomy, management of ligament injuries and carpal instability, debridement of a torn articular disc, intraarticular fracture management, management of degenerative disease with radial styloidectomy, or proximal row carpectomy can all be performed with arthroscopic assistance. Procedures requiring extensive debridement, management of intraarticular fractures, and procedures requiring resection of bone are technically demanding and should be attempted only after extensive experience with basic wrist arthroscopy.

PREOPERTATIVE PREPARATION

Anesthesia

Wrist arthroscopy can be performed using general, regional, or local anesthesia. General anesthesia is recommended when experience with wrist arthroscopic techniques is limited or when patients are unusually anxious. Anxious patients managed with regional or local anesthesia tend to move about during the procedure. Even small motions can be disruptive and cause damage to articular surfaces or to the delicate arthroscopic equipment. Arthroscopic

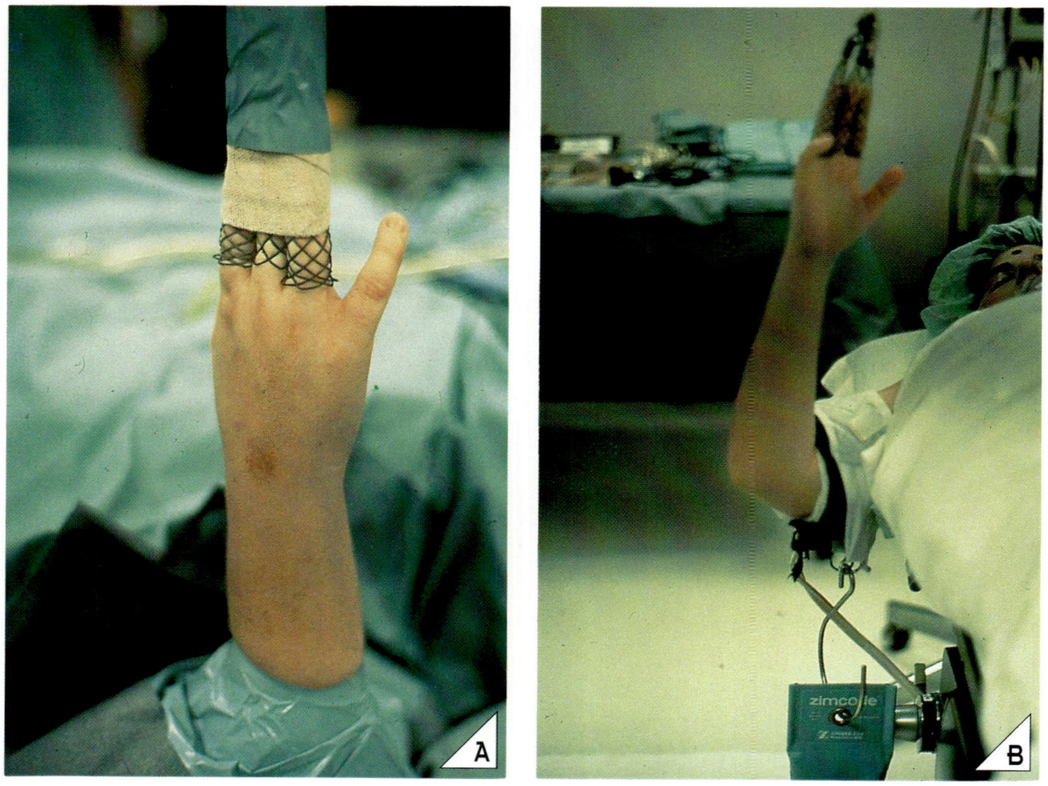

Figure 24.1
(A) Fingertraps on the index, middle, and ring fingers provide adequate distraction of the radiocarpal and midcarpal spaces. (B) Counterweights are suspended by a sling and draped over a pneumatic tourniquet cuff.

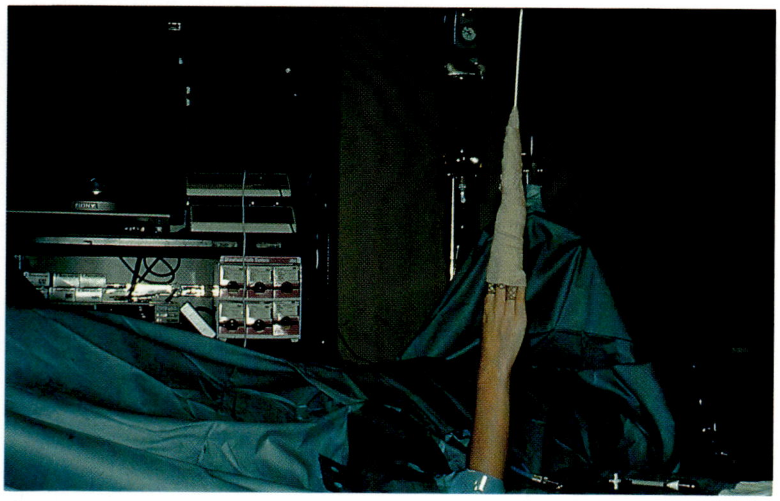

Figure 24.2
Operating room set up. The patient is supine with the head to the left. The right upper extremity is suspended by fingertraps and draped free. Video equipment is on the contralateral side of the operating room table.

procedures performed under a regional or local anesthetic are best accompanied by IV sedation.

Operating Room Set Up

The patient is placed in the supine position with the affected side abducted approximately 45° at the shoulder and with 90° of elbow flexion. The radiocarpal and midcarpal spaces are simultaneously distracted using two or three sterilized fingertraps applied to the index, middle, and ring fingers (Fig. 24.1A). The fingertraps are attached by rope to an overhead bar and pulley system that is fixed to the operating room table. Distraction is usually accomplished with 5 to 10 pounds of weight attached to the rope. A second weight is applied to a sling that is draped over a pneumatic tourniquet wrapped around the upper arm (Fig. 24.1B). The sterilized fingertraps and rope are attached in a sterile fashion to the limb after it has been prepared with a surgical scrub or an antiseptic solution. The limb is draped so that it can be freely manipulated during the procedure (Fig. 24.2).

The surgeon is seated on a rolling stool, facing the dorsum of the wrist and with a clear view of the video equipment placed directly across the patient on the contralateral side of the operating room table (Fig. 24.3A). Hand equipment is placed on a Mayo stand at the volar side of the extremity (Fig. 24.3B). An assistant can be seated at the ulnar side of the extremity (Fig. 24.3C).

Arthroscopic Equipment

A small joint arthroscope approximately 50 mm in length and 2.5 mm in diameter, with a 25° to 30° wide-angle lens, is most versatile for wrist arthroscopy. Arthroscopes that are 1.9 mm in diameter can be useful in the smaller joints of some women and children. The small diameter of the wrist arthroscope lens makes it especially important to transmit high intensity light through the lens to optimize visualization. Quartz light sources with high efficiency fiberoptic light cables improve light transmission and visibility. A high resolution video camera and monitor are equally important in providing an image with adequate detail.

Hand equipment is kept conveniently available on a

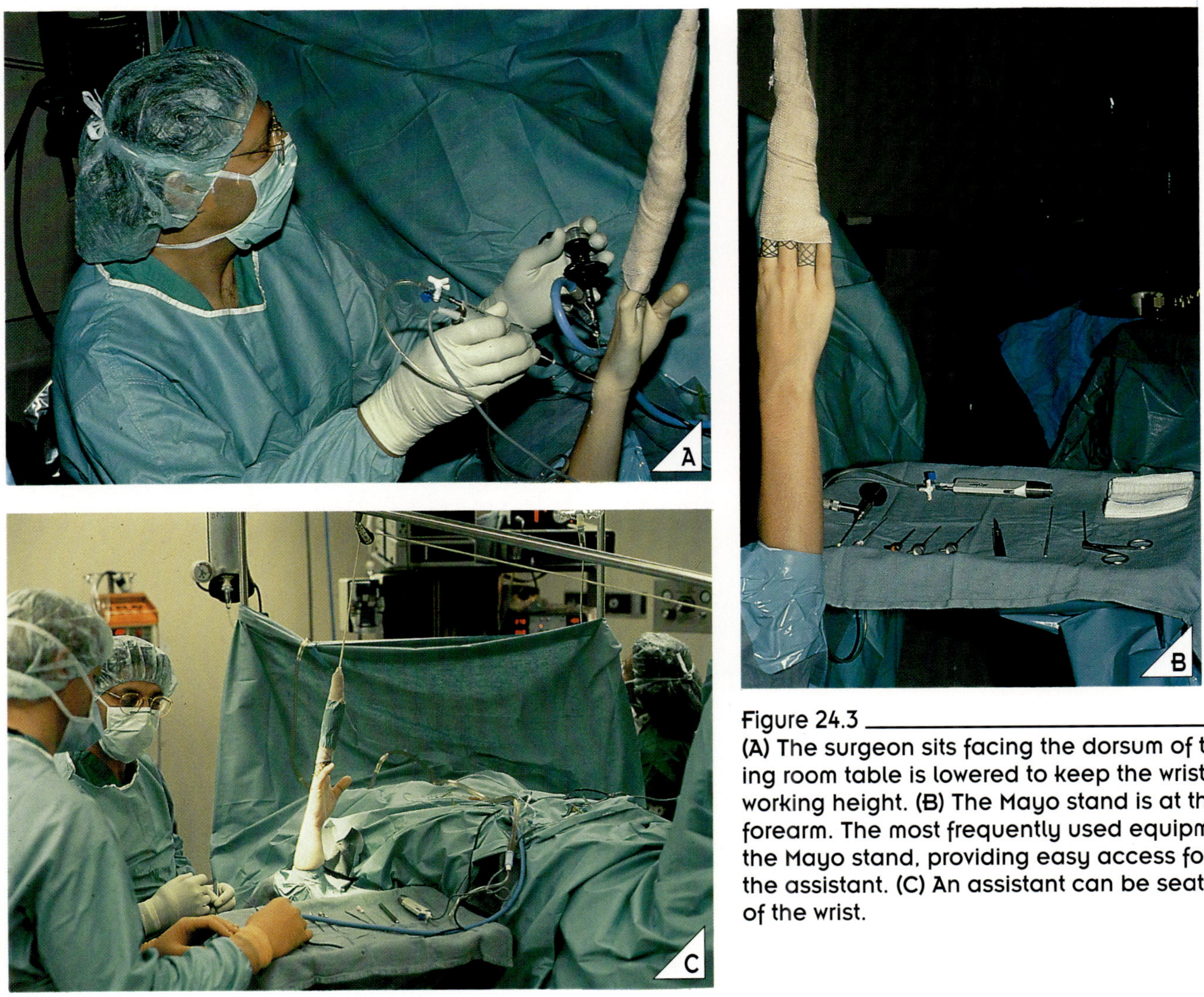

Figure 24.3

(A) The surgeon sits facing the dorsum of the wrist. The operating room table is lowered to keep the wrist at a comfortable working height. (B) The Mayo stand is at the volar side of the forearm. The most frequently used equipment is placed on the Mayo stand, providing easy access for the surgeon and the assistant. (C) An assistant can be seated at the ulnar side of the wrist.

Mayo stand in easy access to the surgeon and assistant (Fig. 24.4). Hand equipment with small, short, or narrow handles is awkward to use and promotes fatigue of intrinsic muscles. One of the most important pieces of hand equipment in wrist arthroscopy is a hook probe, since many lesions cannot be identified by inspection but require probing. The probe should be blunt and less than 2 mm in diameter at the tip. Very sharp, pointed probes have the disadvantage of catching on the subcutaneous tissues, particularly the cutaneous branches of nerves, as the probe is introduced and withdrawn. The short, blunt probes used for large joint arthroscopy are often adequate if their handles are not too large or too heavy.

Conventional arthroscopic grasping forceps and basket forceps 2.7 mm in size are usually small enough for procedures on the ulnar side of the wrist. Occasionally, 2.0 mm hand equipment is necessary at the scapholunate joint or in the midcarpal space where even less space is available. Motorized equipment designed for small joints is preferable. The handles are lightweight and small with shorter rotary blades and burrs to allow the surgeon to operate at a shorter distance from the wrist joint. Two disposable knife blades—the 30° angled "minibanana" blade, and 70° angled "hoe" blade—are effective in performing virtually all cutting tasks at the ulnar side of the wrist. The blade tips are short and rounded with sharp edges on all sides, which minimizes the risk of cutting soft tissue structures, including dorsal ligaments, as the blades are passed through the dorsal portals.

Arthroscopic Technique

Radiocarpal Space

Establishing dorsal wrist arthroscopic portals must be performed with great care and attention to detail. To facilitate portal placement, most arthroscopists advocate distention of the wrist with 5 to 10 mL of saline prior to introducing arthroscopic equipment. Piercing the capsule of the distended joint with an arthroscopic sheath and obturator causes a characteristic popping sensation that indicates entry of the joint. The return of fluid through the sheath also confirms that the distended space has been entered. However, distention of the radiocarpal space in the wrist is not as helpful for protecting articular surfaces and major neurovascular structures from injury as it is in joints like the elbow. Indeed, distention may be counterproductive if not performed with great care. For example, the midcarpal space may be inadvertently distended, and articular surfaces can be damaged by the needle used to inject the fluid.

Additionally, bony landmarks at the wrist disappear once the joint is distended. Anatomic landmarks are especially important in locating the correct interval to introduce the arthroscope sheath and obturator. The first arthroscopic portal is established by locating the interval between the third and fourth extensor compartments at the radiocarpal interval. Locating the radiocarpal interval is facilitated by palmar flexion and palpation of the soft tissue and bony landmarks on the dorsum of the wrist. Palpation of the interval between the dorsal lip of the distal radius just distal to Lister's tubercle and two carpal landmarks, the bony prominence of the dorsal lunate and proximal pole of the scaphoid, will also help to locate the radiocarpal space (Fig. 24.5).

Once the proper interval for the first arthroscopic radiocarpal portal is located, a 2 to 3 mm longitudinal incision is made through the dorsal skin by drawing the skin across a #11 blade. The blade is not plunged into the extracapsular soft tissues—only the skin is incised. Using a fine-tipped hemostat to bluntly dissect subcutaneous tissues to the level of the capsule prevents injury to tendons, tendon sheaths, and cutaneous branches of the radial nerve. An arthroscope sheath with a blunt obturator is then gently introduced into the radiocarpal space with a

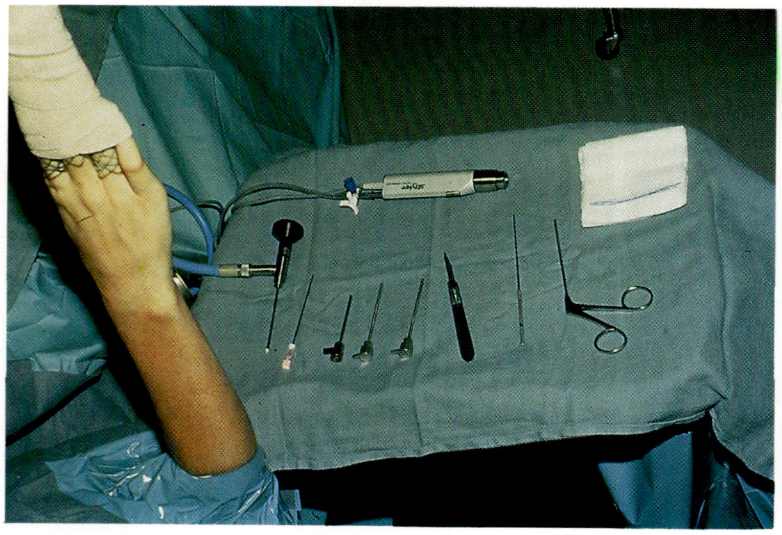

Figure 24.4
Mayo stand showing organization of the small amount of equipment needed for basic wrist arthroscopy.

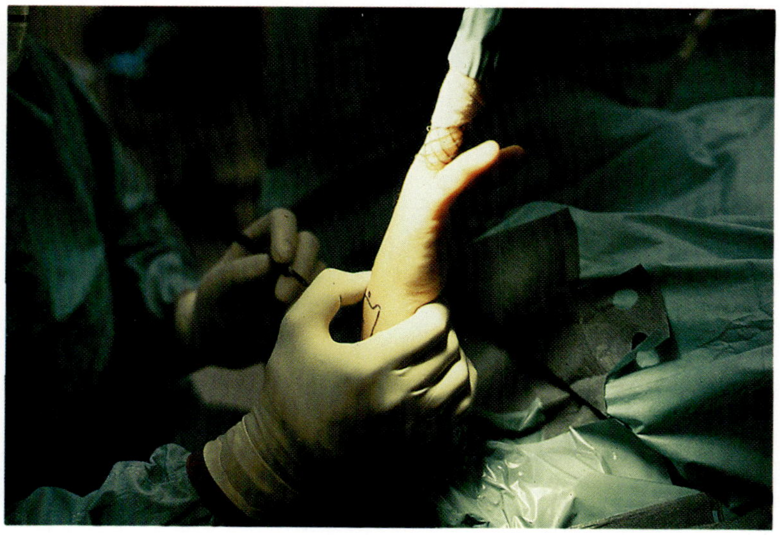

Figure 24.5
Prior to making a dorsal skin incision, the wrist is palmar flexed and dorsal landmarks are identified.

reciprocal twisting motion holding the sheath perpendicular to the skin surface (Fig. 24.6). Minimal force is necessary to push the small diameter sheath and obturator through the capsule. The use of a sharp trocar should be avoided since it can cause injury to articular surfaces and can inadvertently be pushed through the soft cortical and cancellous bone of the metaphysis of the radius or into one of the carpal bones. The use of a blunt obturator and palpation of the dorsum of a palmar flexed nondistended wrist helps prevent incorrect portal placement. Once the sheath has passed through the capsule it is directed toward the ulnar side of the joint. Care should be taken to gently slide the sheath along the dorsal capsular recess to prevent injury, particularly to the articular cartilage surface of the lunate.

Irrigation fluid can be introduced into the radiocarpal space after entry into the space is confirmed arthroscopically. Peristaltic pump irrigation systems have not generally been necessary. Wrapping the IV bag of irrigation fluid in a transfusion pressure cuff, such as that used by anesthesiologists, provides an inexpensive, safe irrigation system that is quickly and easily assembled (Fig. 24.7). The pressure on the cuff-wrapped fluid is manually increased to 150 mm Hg, at which point the fluid is transmitted into the radiocarpal space through IV tubing attached to the inflow portal of the arthroscope sheath. The final pressure transmitted has been measured at 35 to 50 mm Hg using a pressure transducer placed in the radiocarpal space.[7] The transmitted pressure maintains distention of the joint with a constant flow of fluid into the space. The system is very safe since the pressure decreases and cannot increase as fluid is transfused into the joint. Once the joint is irrigated and distended, a routine arthroscopic examination of the radiocarpal space can be performed.

The arthroscopic anatomy of the radiocarpal joint is unclear when seen for the first time. The articular surfaces appear uniform without distinct borders demarcating each of the carpal bones. The intrinsic intercarpal ligaments are smooth sheets that blend into the substance of the articular cartilage of the carpus. The articular surfaces of the radius and the triangular fibrocartilage have poorly defined borders and appear to be continuous and smooth. It is very helpful to review photos or a videotape of arthroscopic wrist anatomy prior to performing an arthroscopic procedure. At the radial limit of the space, the

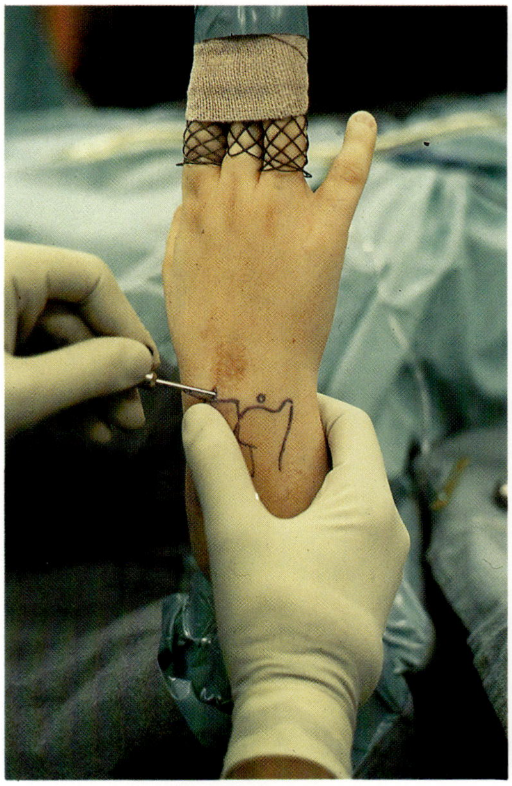

Figure 24.6
The arthroscope sleeve and blunt obturator are introduced with a reciprocal twisting motion and directed ulnarly once they are passed through the capsule.

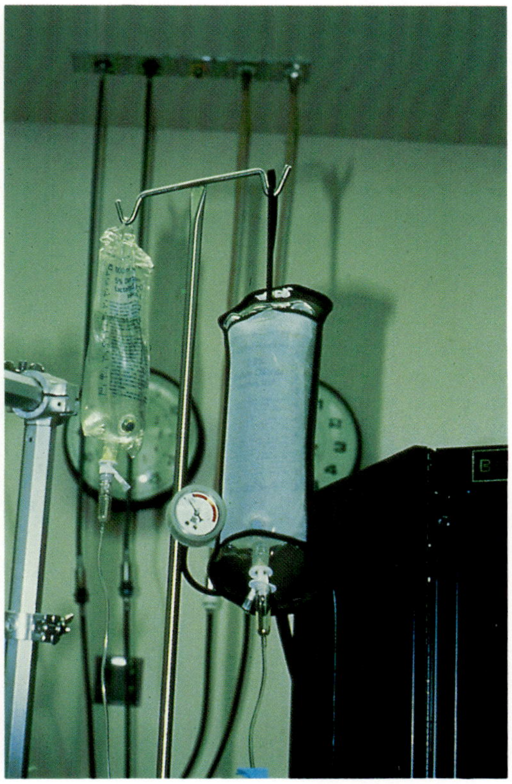

Figure 24.7
A transfusion pressure cuff containing a 1 L bag of sterile fluid is pressurized to 150 mm Hg to pump fluid into the joint at a constant pressure.

radial styloid, the scaphoid fossa of the radius, and the scaphoid are visualized (Figs. 24.8, 24.9A). The scapholunate joint is usually appreciated as only a subtle depression in the articular surface of the proximal row overlying the convexity of the sagittal ridge of the distal radius (Fig. 24.9B). More ulnarly, the lunate and lunate fossa of the radius are visualized (Fig. 24.10).

At the ulnar limit of the radiocarpal space, the lunotriquetral joint is also appreciated as only a modest depression in the convexity of the proximal row (Fig. 24.11). Small tears of the lunotriquetral joint may not be visualized through a radial portal and may require an ulnar portal to be seen (Fig. 24.12A,B). The articular disc of the triangular fibrocartilage complex is seen with both ulnar and radial

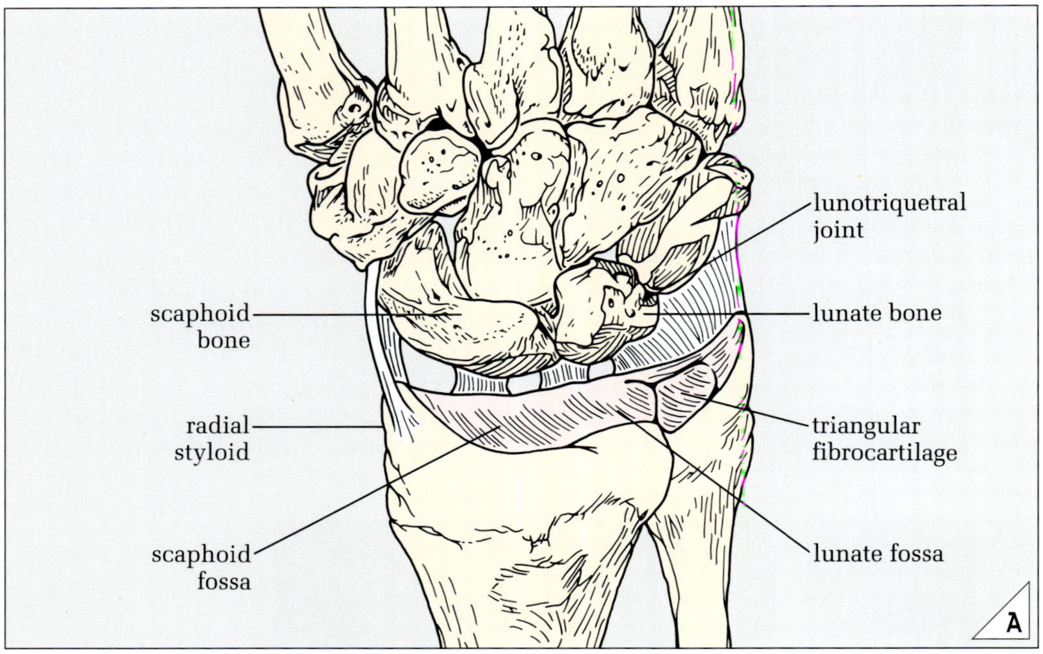

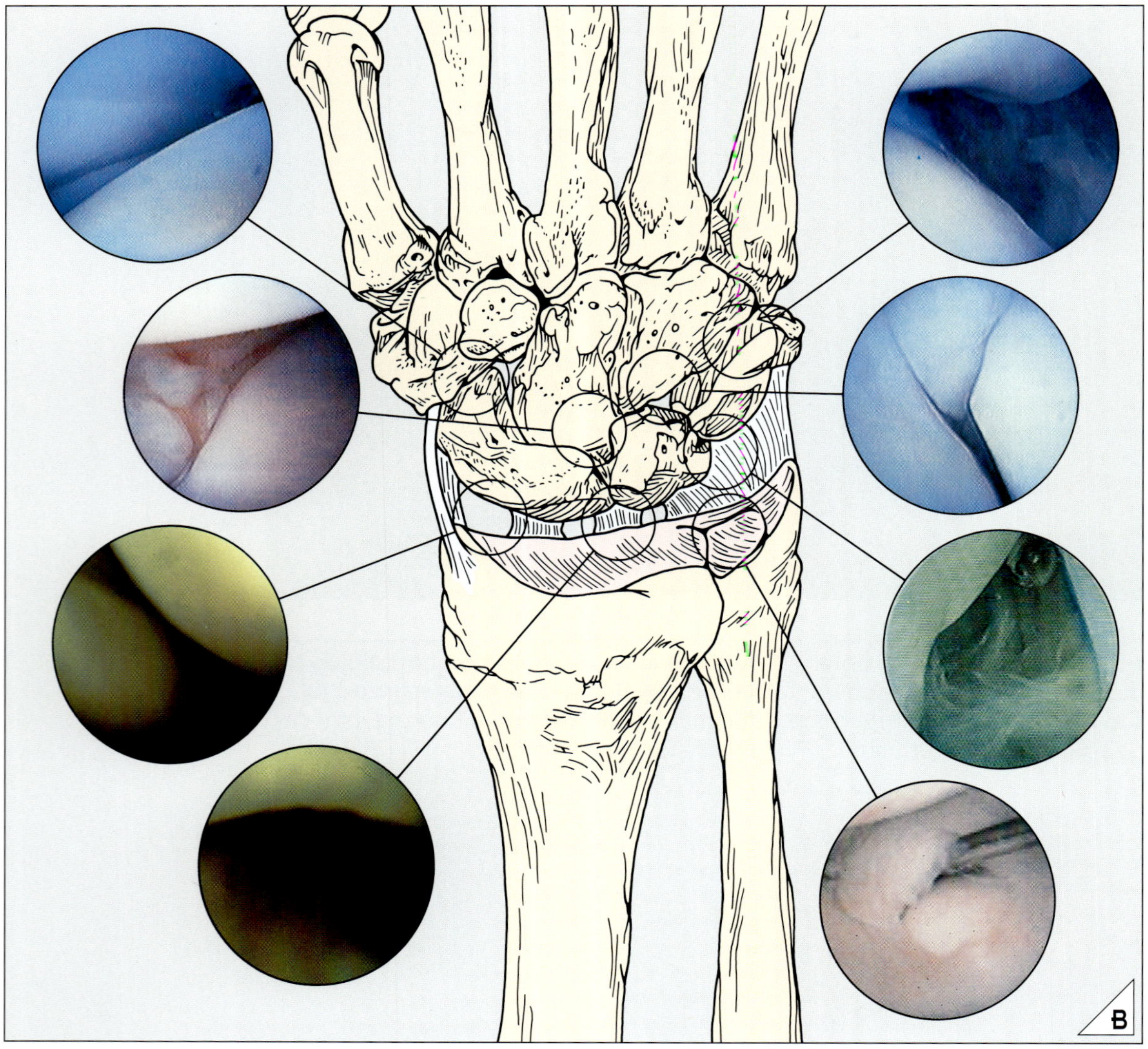

Figure 24.8
(A, B) Radial limit of radiocarpal space, scapholunate joint, lunate and lunate fossa, lunotriquetral joint, and articular disc.

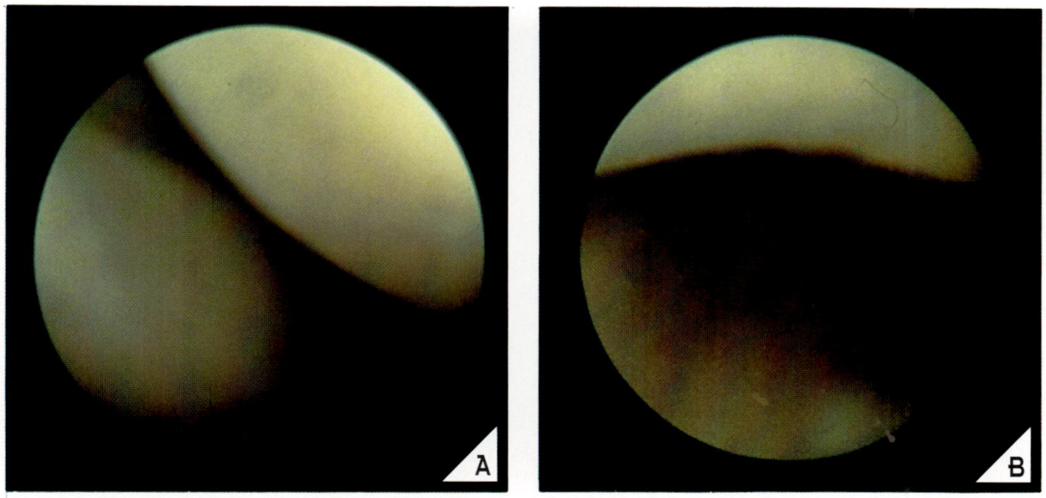

Figure 24.9
(A) Arthroscopic view showing the scaphoid above and the radial styloid and a portion of the scaphoid fossa below. (B) The scapholunate joint is visualized as a subtle depression between the convex articular surfaces of the scaphoid and lunate bones.

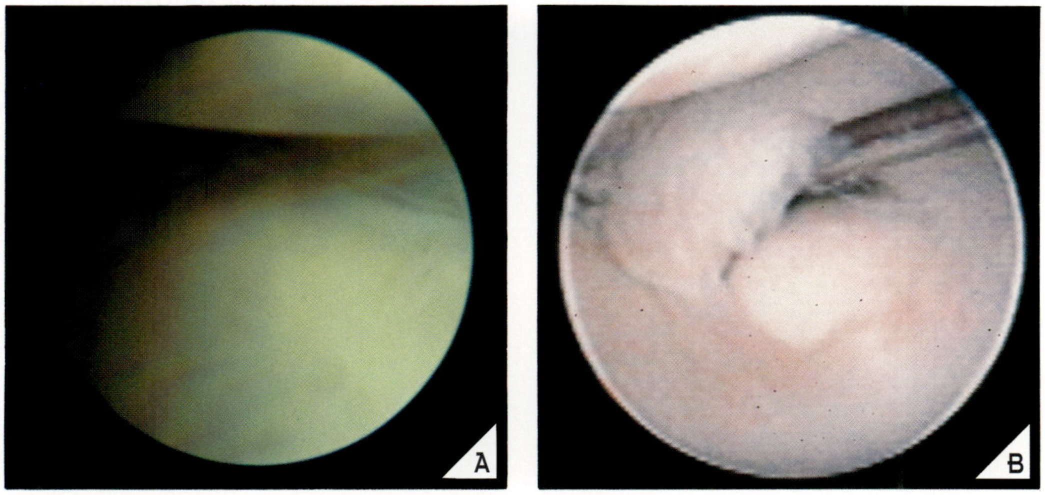

Figure 24.10
(A) The lunate and lunate fossa of the radius. (B) The ulnar limit of the lunate fossa where it merges with the articular disc of the triangular fibrocartilage complex. The disc is torn. The torn flap is being elevated by a hook probe away from the underlying distal ulna.

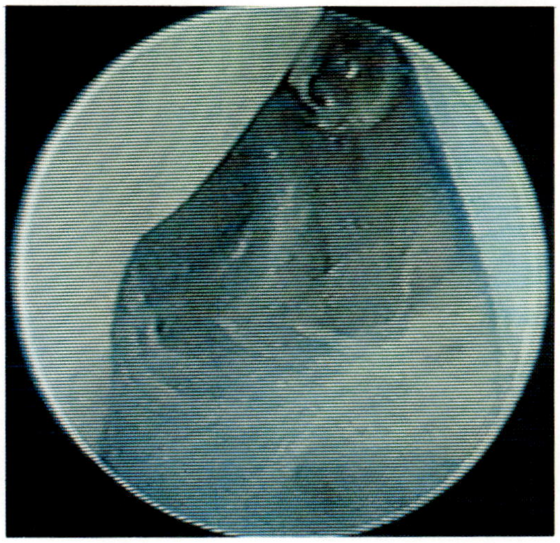

Figure 24.11
A partial-thickness tear of the lunotriquetral ligament seen from a radial portal.

portals (Fig. 24.12C). Tears of the articular disc may not be detected by inspection alone and may require careful probing to be demonstrated (Fig. 24.13; see Fig. 24.10B). It is also helpful to squeeze the distal radioulnar joint to force fluid through a tear of the articular disc. If a tear of the articular disc is present, the transmitted fluid can force open the defect in the articular disc, making the tear more easily recognized. Articular disc tears occur most frequently at the attachment of the disc to the radius.[6]

The extreme ulnar side of the radiocarpal space, the lunotriquetral joint, the dorsal and palmar recesses, and the palmar ligaments are usually best visualized using an ulnar portal and may not be adequately seen through a radial portal (Fig. 24.14). Establishing an ulnar portal is facilitated by arthroscopically viewing the dorsal capsule at the ulnar side of the wrist while palpating the soft tissues between the fourth and fifth or the fifth and sixth extensor compartments. An 18-gauge spinal needle is directed through the dorsal soft tissues into the ulnar side of the joint to confirm optimal portal placement (Fig. 24.15). An ulnar portal is then carefully established by incising only the skin and carefully dissecting subcutaneous tissues with a fine-tipped clamp to avoid injury to cutaneous branches of the ulnar nerve (Fig. 24.16). The arthroscope can then be transferred to the ulnar portal to visualize structures that cannot be seen well from a radial perspective (Fig. 24.17).

Midcarpal Space

It is important to arthroscopically examine the midcarpal space of a patient with wrist pain when pathology is not detected in the radiocarpal joint. An arthroscopic examination of the midcarpal space is also helpful in evaluating carpal instability. Intrinsic carpal ligament insuffi-

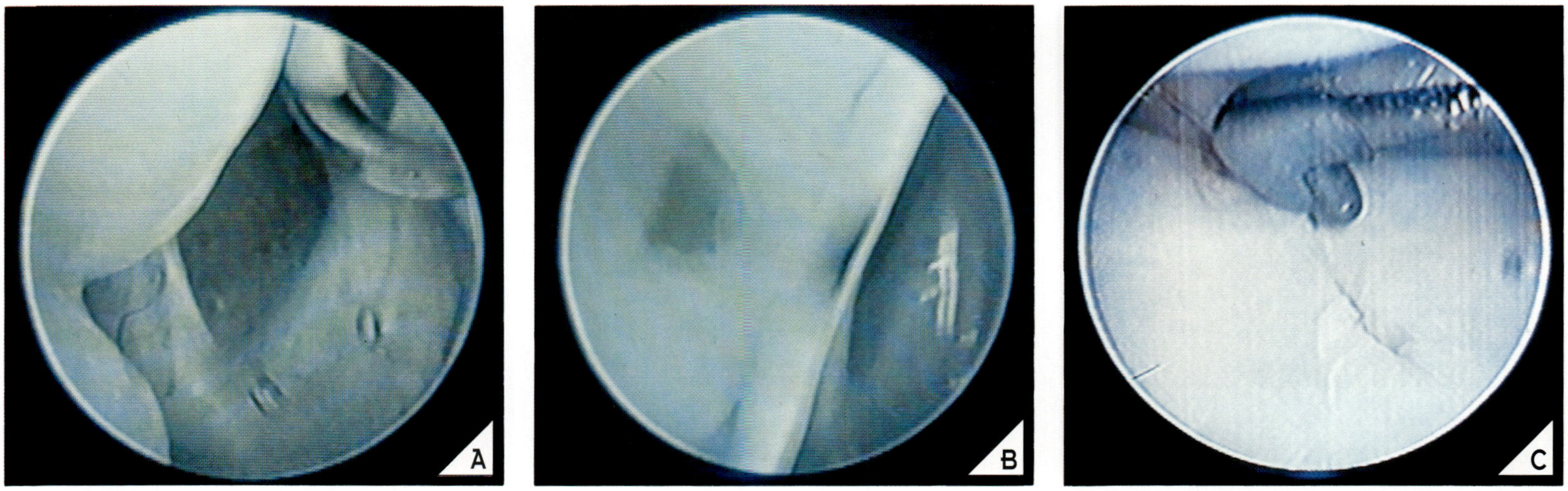

Figure 24.12
(A) A small full-thickness tear of the lunotriquetral ligament in this view cannot be adequately seen arthroscopically from a radial portal. (B) The same lunotriquetral ligament is adequately visualized using an ulnar portal, and the tear is clearly seen to be a small full-thickness defect. (C) A short peripheral tear of the articular disc is located approximately 2 mm from its attachment to the radius. The lunate is above.

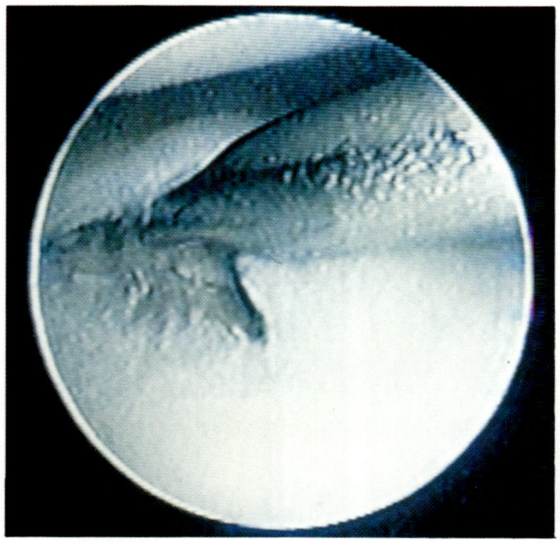

Figure 24.13
Central defect of the articular disc elevated to reveal the apposed, damaged articular surface of the distal ulna.

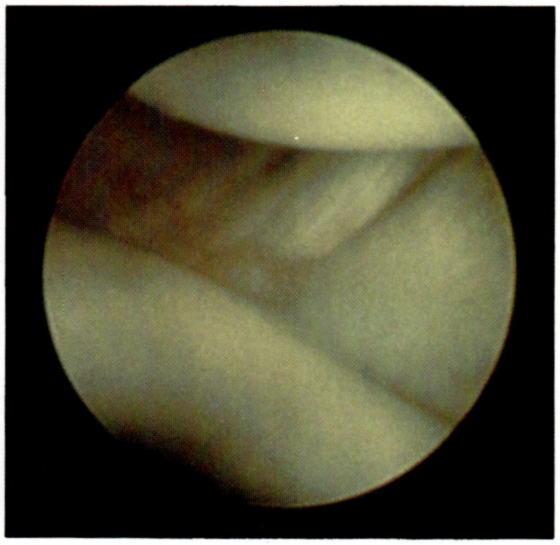

Figure 24.14
The palmar recess of the radiocarpal joint is visualized with an ulnar portal that shows two radiocarpal ligaments.

ciency may not be apparent by inspecting the scapholunate and lunotriquetral ligaments at the radiocarpal space. Midcarpal views of the scapholunate and lunotriquetral joints, however, may show amounts of dissociation when occult tears of the intrinsic carpal ligaments are present (Fig. 24.18).

In general, a radial midcarpal space portal should be established through a separate skin incision made in line with the radiocarpal portal and approximately 1 cm distal to it. The portal is created with the same technique, and care is used to establish other arthroscopic portals. Once the arthroscope has been introduced into the midcarpal space, the midcarpal articular surfaces and the distal scapholunate and lunotriquetral joints can be carefully examined and probed. The arthroscope can be directed radially to demonstrate the articular surfaces of the distal

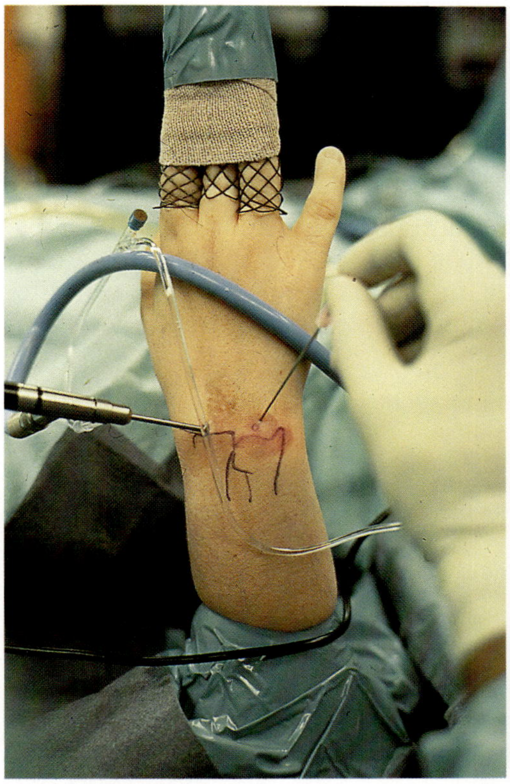

Figure 24.15
Establishing an ulnar portal requires careful selection and testing with an 18-gauge spinal needle prior to making a skin incision.

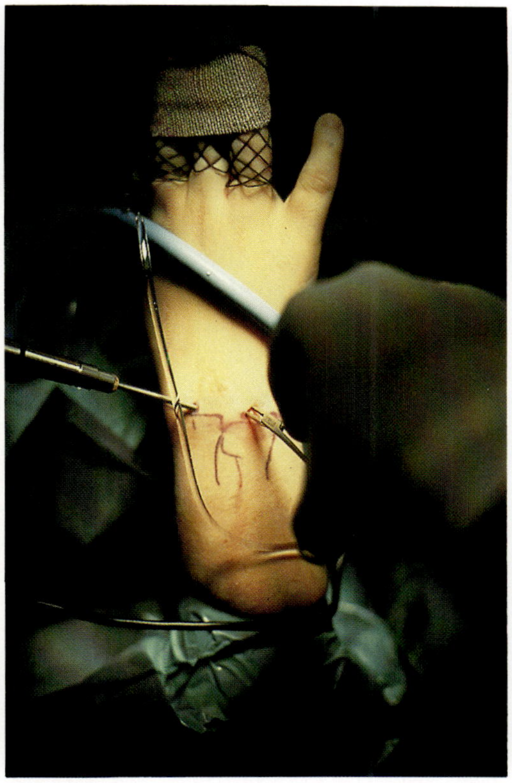

Figure 24.16
Subcutaneous tissues are carefully spread to the level of the capsule to avoid neurovascular injuries.

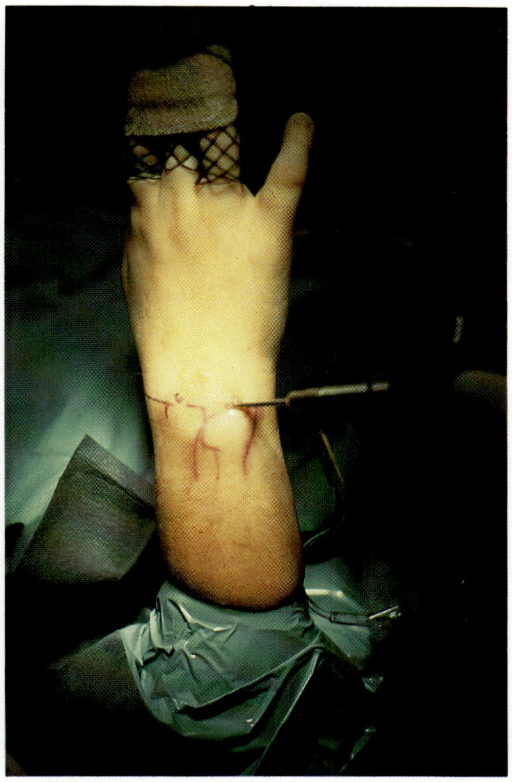

Figure 24.17
The arthroscope is introduced into the radiocarpal joint from an ulnar portal to examine structures that may not be seen adequately from a radial portal.

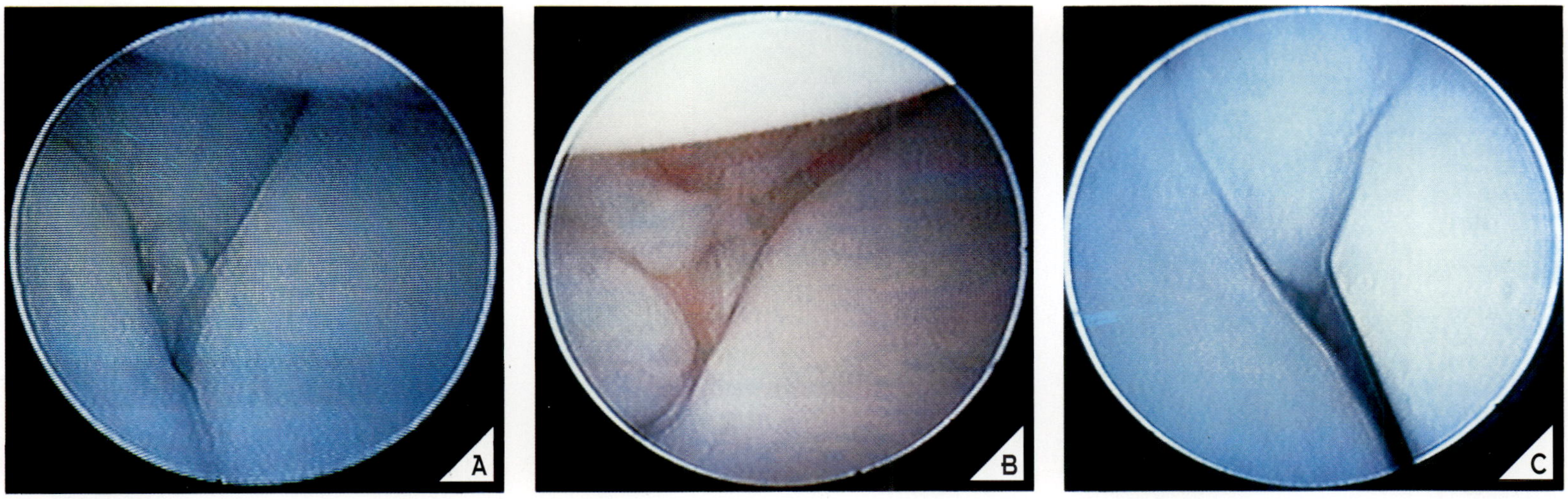

Figure 24.18
(A) Arthroscopic view of the scapholunate joint using a radial midcarpal portal as seen from the midcarpal space. (B) No dissociation of the joint is seen despite a partial-thickness injury to the scapholunate ligament. (C) A tear of the lunotriquetral ligament resulted in the dissociation of the lunotriquetral joint seen in this view of the midcarpal space.

scaphoid and capitate and the scaphocapitate and scaphotrapeziotrapezoid joints (Fig. 24.19). Sweeping the arthroscope ulnarly visualizes the capitohamate (Fig. 24.20A) and triquetrohamate joints (Fig. 24.20B). Small articular defects that are beyond the resolution of arthrography can be demonstrated arthroscopically (Fig. 24.21). Accessory portals in the midcarpal space are necessary for manipulation, probing, and debridement. A midcarpal ulnar portal can be established between the fourth and fifth extensor compartments under direct visualization, using an 18-gauge spinal needle to confirm the placement of the portal prior to making a skin incision. A diagnostic examination for gross pathology of the midcarpal space, however, can usually be adequately performed using a midcarpal radial portal.

Postoperative Management

Patients are generally encouraged to begin motion at home on the morning following an arthroscopic surgical procedure. Patients are wrapped circumferentially with a soft bulky dressing loosely covered with an elastic wrap. Splints are not ordinarily used. Dressings can be removed by the therapist on the second or third postoperative day, when supervised exercises are initiated. Patients can then be examined at 1-week and 3-week intervals by the surgeon.

Surgical Procedures

Excision of the Articular Disc of the Triangular Fibrocartilage Complex

The articular disc, the central component of the triangular fibrocartilage complex, is a triangular fibrocartilage disc that is confluent with the articular surface of the radius and with the dorsal and palmar radioulnar ligaments.

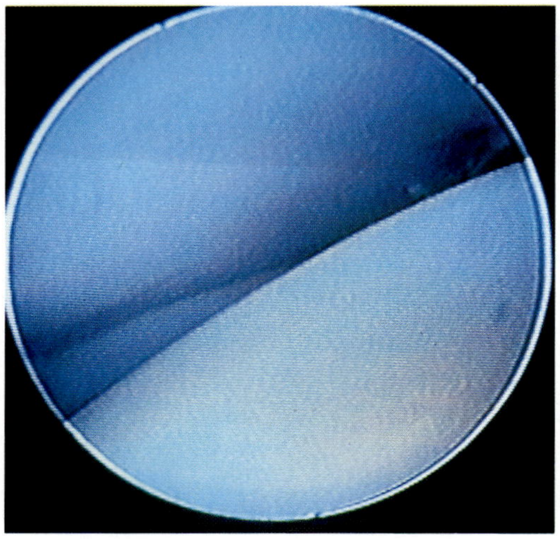

Figure 24.19
Scaphotrapeziotrapezoid joint.

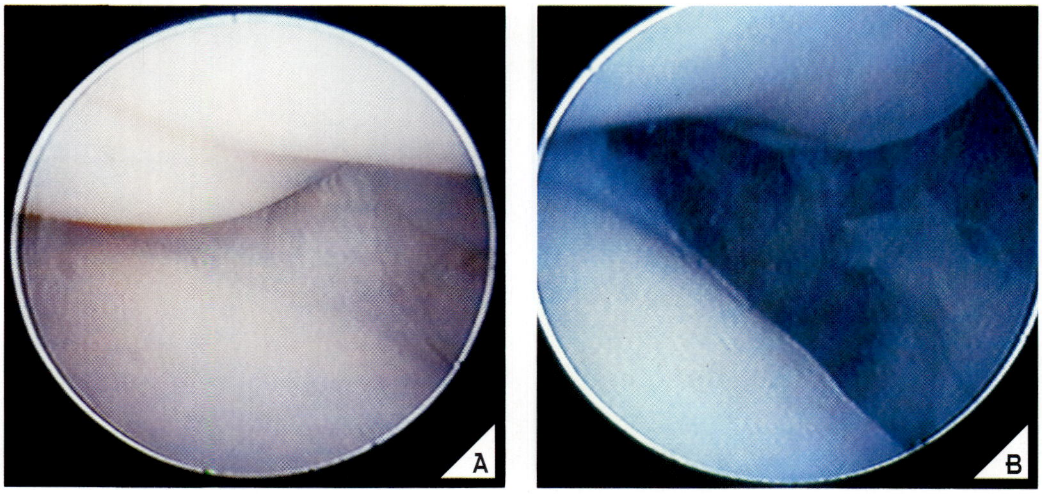

Figure 24.20
(A) The capitohamate joint through the radial midcarpal portal. (B) The triquetrohamate joint is visualized through the radial midcarpal portal.

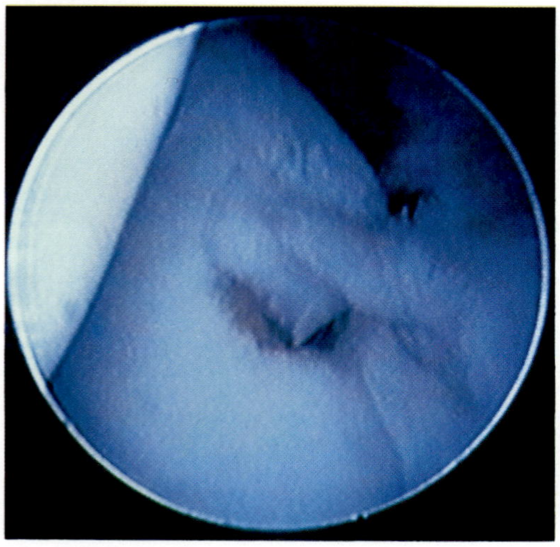

Figure 24.21
Articular defect on the scaphoid. The defect was caused by an arthrography needle introduced into the midcarpal space.

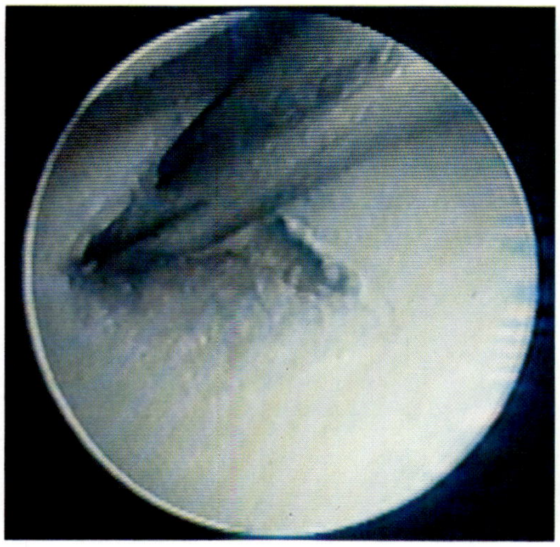

Figure 24.22
A central defect of the articular disc is being probed with arthroscopic guidance prior to excision of the central portion.

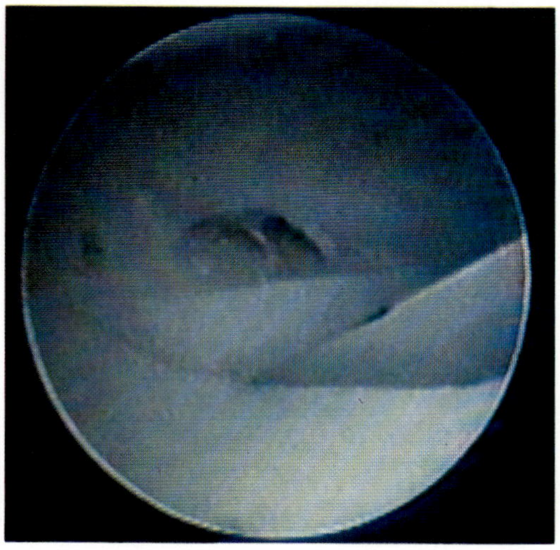

Figure 24.23
A 4 mm "minibanana" blade used arthroscopically to incise the central portion of the articular disc.

Chronic ulnar wrist pain is frequently associated with a tear of the articular disc. Tears of the articular disc usually occur at the peripheral attachments of the disc, or occasionally at its thinner, central portion.

Peripheral tears of the articular disc are more common than central defects. Such tears are generally located approximately 2 mm from the attachment of the articular disc to the articular surface of the radius. Detachment tears are usually short linear tears that parallel the attachment line of the articular disc. Many articular disc tears are not detected by simple inspection, and must be identified by careful probing with a hook probe.[7]

Central defects of the articular disc, less common than peripheral tears, have a high correlation with positive ulnar variance and ulnocarpal impingement. Ulnocarpal abutment may not only cause central articular disc tears, but may also cause tears of the lunotriquetral ligament and chondromalacia of the distal ulna, lunate, and triquetrum. Complete tears of the lunotriquetral ligament may result in diastasis at the lunotriquetral joint that can be demonstrated radiographically. Positive ulnar variance, diastasis of the lunotriquetral joint, or arthrographic evidence of a lunotriquetral ligament tear suggest the presence of a central tear of the articular disc. Central articular disc tears are usually stellate tears with irregular edges and result from compressive loads and chronic wear. Less frequently, central tears can be oblique, partial-thickness tears or full-thickness flap tears. Partial-thickness articular disc tears simply require debridement of the thin superficial fibrocartilage flap.

Most full-thickness tears of the articular disc can be managed with debridement of the central portion of the disc. Excision of the central portion of the articular disc is effective in relieving ulnar wrist pain if neutral or negative ulnar variance is present. The central portion of the torn articular disc can be excised with knives and basket forceps and the resected rim debrided with a rotary motorized shaver (Figs. 24.22–24.24). Care must be taken to excise only the central portion, without injuring the underlying articular surface of the distal ulna or the dorsal and palmar radioulnar ligaments that border the articular disc.

Simple debridement of a torn articular disc will not provide pain relief if the articular disc tear is accompanied by ulnocarpal chondromalacia or a tear of the lunotriquetral ligament, lesions associated with ulnocarpal abutment. Patients will usually remain symptomatic if the torn articular disc is excised and the ulnocarpal abutment is left uncorrected. A tear of the articular disc in a wrist with positive ulnar variance and ulnocarpal abutment can be managed successfully with arthroscopic excision of the central portion of the articular disc and with arthroscopic recession of the distal ulna.

A tear of the articular disc with a tear of the lunotriquetral ligament cannot, in most cases, be managed successfully with only arthroscopic debridement of the torn articular disc structures. The arthroscopic and open management options for treatment of lunotriquetral ligament tears with underlying instability at the lunotriquetral joint remain controversial. The unstable lunotriquetral joint may be surgically treated with either a limited fusion or a proximal row carpectomy. Both procedures can be performed with arthroscopic assistance; they will have essentially the same success as an open procedure but with reduced morbidity.

Distal Ulnar Recession

Central tears of the articular disc are associated with positive ulnar variance. Excising the central portion of the articular disc without shortening the ulna will cause persistent medial wrist pain. Shortening can be accomplished arthroscopically by recessing the distal ulnar articular surface through the defect created in the centrally excised articular disc. A motorized rotary burr is effective in accomplishing the recession. Care must be taken to remove enough bone to recess the distal ulna 2 to 3 mm proximal to the articular surface of the radius. It is also essential to avoid scalloping the soft cancellous bone at the central ulna while leaving the dorsal and palmar cortical bone prominent. Pronation and supination of the wrist while visualizing its ulnar side will help to identify areas of prominence that require further recession. Caution must be used to prevent injury to the dorsal and palmar radioulnar ligaments and to meticulously suction osteochondral debris, which can settle into the distal radioulnar joint and cause persistent pain. Intraoperative x-rays or fluoroscopy in neutral, pronation, and supination are recommended to confirm that an appropriate amount of the distal ulna has been resected. Tears of the articular

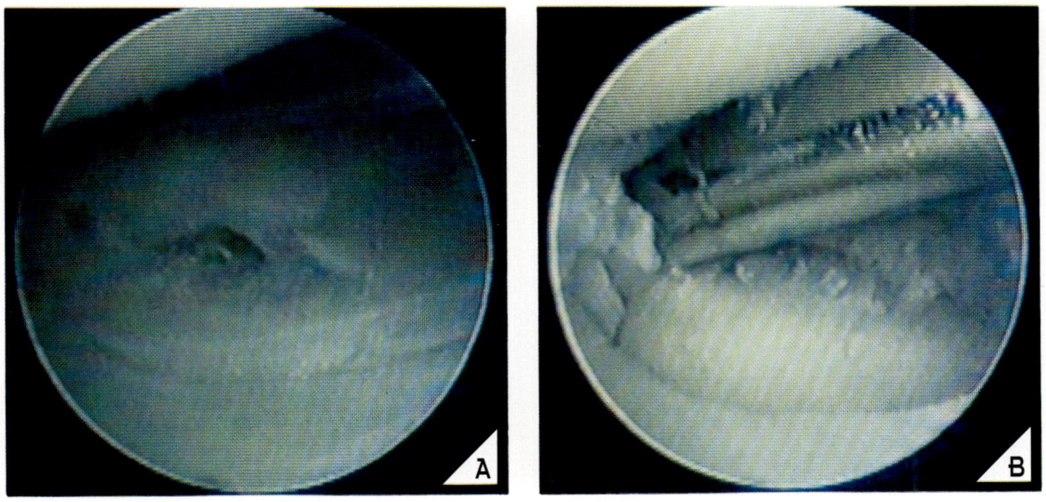

Figure 24.24
(A) The incised articular disc just prior to its removal using a grasping forceps. (B) A rotary motorized shaver is used to "balance" the inner edge of the articular disc.

disc with positive ulnar variance can be adequately treated arthroscopically with articular disc excision and ulnar recession, if intrinsic carpal ligament injuries have not occurred. Debridement and ulnar recession will not relieve pain if a lunotriquetral ligament tear is present and left untreated.

Radial Styloidectomy

In selected cases of advanced osteoarthritis of the radiocarpal space, open radial styloidectomy has traditionally been effective in decompressing the proximal row and eliminating pain. Arthroscopic debridement of the radiocarpal space with a limited synovectomy accompanied by an arthroscopic styloidectomy has reproduced the results obtained with an open styloidectomy (Fig. 24.25). Patients who undergo arthroscopic styloidectomies have less morbidity, and enjoy an earlier return to activities than patients who have undergone open procedures. Arthroscopy offers the additional advantage of simultaneous evaluation and general debridement of the radiocarpal space. Patients with well-localized radioscaphoid pain must be carefully selected to increase the probability of long-lasting success of arthroscopic management.

An arthroscopic styloidectomy is performed using a visualization portal established between the third and fourth extensor compartments. With the arthroscope directed toward the radial side of the wrist, the radiodorsal capsule is palpated through the overlying skin. Soft tissue and bony landmarks between the first and second extensor compartments are also identified by palpation. Then, at the radioscaphoid interval just distal and ulnar to the radial styloid, an 18-gauge spinal needle is introduced to confirm correct portal placement. A small incision is made through the skin only. Caution is necessary to prevent injury to cutaneous branches of the radial nerve. Careful blunt dissection is used to create a soft tissue portal for a motorized rotary burr and its sheath. The radial styloid and one third to one half of the scaphoid fossa are recessed with the burr. Intraoperative x-rays and fluoroscopy are helpful in confirming that an appropriate amount of bone has been resected. A bulky dressing is applied. Postoperative splinting is not necessary. Early range of motion is encouraged.

Arthroscopic Reduction and Internal Fixation of Intraarticular Fractures

The surgical technique for arthroscopic reduction and internal fixation of intraarticular wrist fractures is conceptually the same technique that is used for tibial plateau fractures.[8] From a technical standpoint wrist fractures are less problematic because the upper extremity is smaller

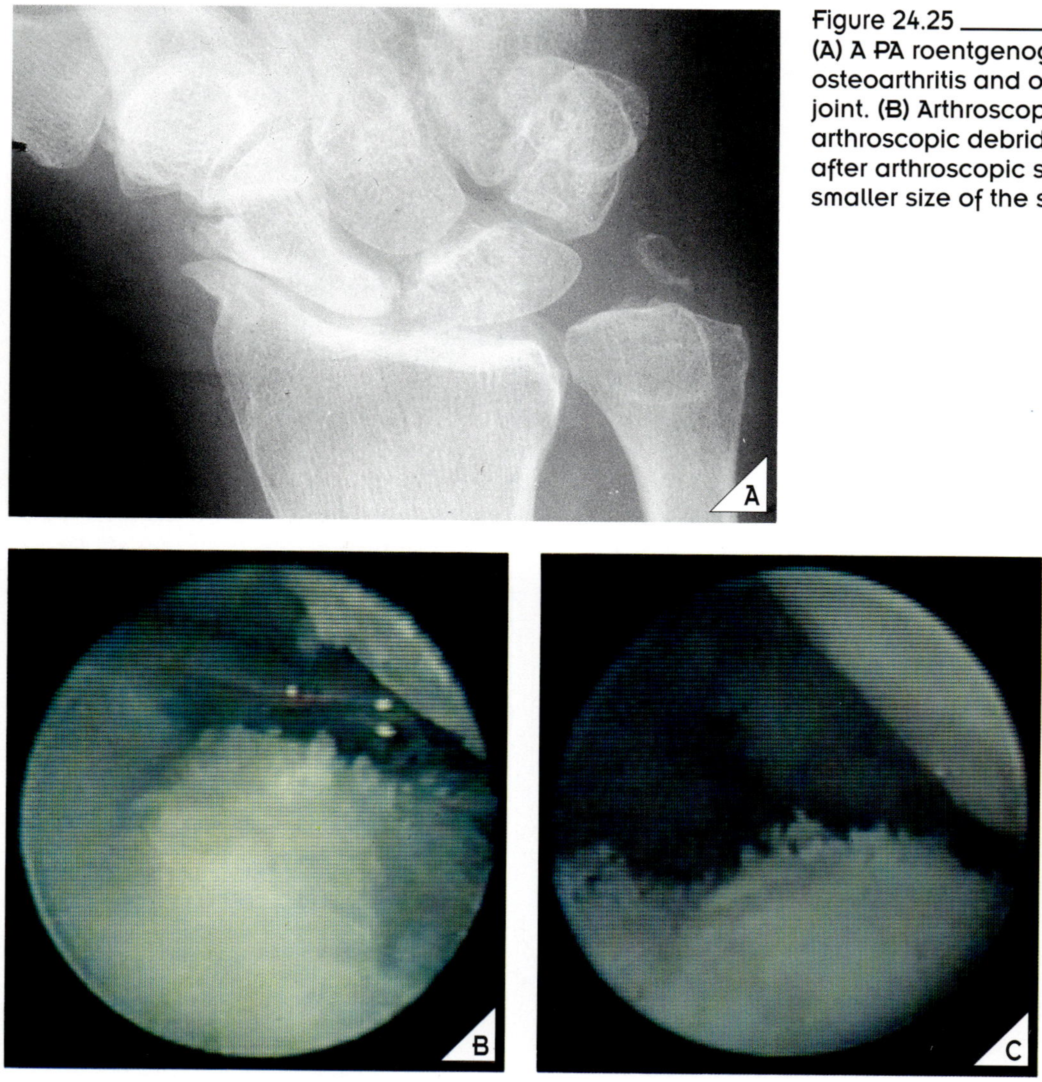

Figure 24.25
(A) A PA roentgenographic view of a wrist confirms advanced osteoarthritis and osteophyte formation at the radioscaphoid joint. (B) Arthroscopic view of the radial styloid seen after arthroscopic debridement. (C) The radial styloid is visualized after arthroscopic styloidectomy was performed. Note the smaller size of the scaphoid fossa.

and more manageable. Distraction of the radiocarpal joint can be easily accomplished using fingertraps. Ligamentotaxis takes advantage of the soft tissue envelope of the wrist to realign the fracture fragments and, in some cases, provide an adequate reduction. Fingertraps are applied to the radial two or three fingers and connected by rope to an overhead bar and pulley system. The fingertrap distraction system has the advantage that it can be easily applied and permits free access to the wrist for x-rays and surgical manipulation. The arm is positioned with the shoulder abducted approximately 30°, the elbow flexed to 90°, and a sling with 10 pounds of weight draped over a pneumatic tourniquet applied to the upper arm. The surgeon is seated facing the dorsum of the wrist. The arthroscopic power equipment and monitor in a video cabinet is directly across from the surgeon on the contralateral side of the operating room table. A C-arm image intensifier is brought into the field. The x-ray beam is parallel to the ground to allow the vertically positioned limb to be monitored in the AP, lateral, and oblique planes using an x-ray monitor, which is adjacent to the video cabinet.

If an anatomic, stable reduction cannot be performed closed, an arthroscopic reduction and internal fixation is considered (Fig. 24.26). The limb is surgically prepared and draped and the image intensifier is draped. The patient and the surgical team are appropriately shielded with lead coverings. Conventional small joint arthroscopy equipment is used. Small rounded periostal elevators, probes, and picks facilitate the reduction of fracture fragments. Cannulated 3.5 and 4.0 mm self-tapping screws are very useful for internal fixation of fracture fragments.

The joint is copiously irrigated with Ringer's lactated solution to remove loose articular debris, fibrinous material and clotted blood. Complete debridement is essential for visualization of the fracture fragments. A small 2.5 mm joint, full radius motorized shaver blade is introduced to debride the radiocarpal space and to separate and carefully debride the fracture fragments (Fig. 24.27). Care must be taken to avoid altering the shapes of the fragments by inadvertent removal of any soft cancellous bone at the edges of the fragments.

After a thorough debridement, a manual reduction of the

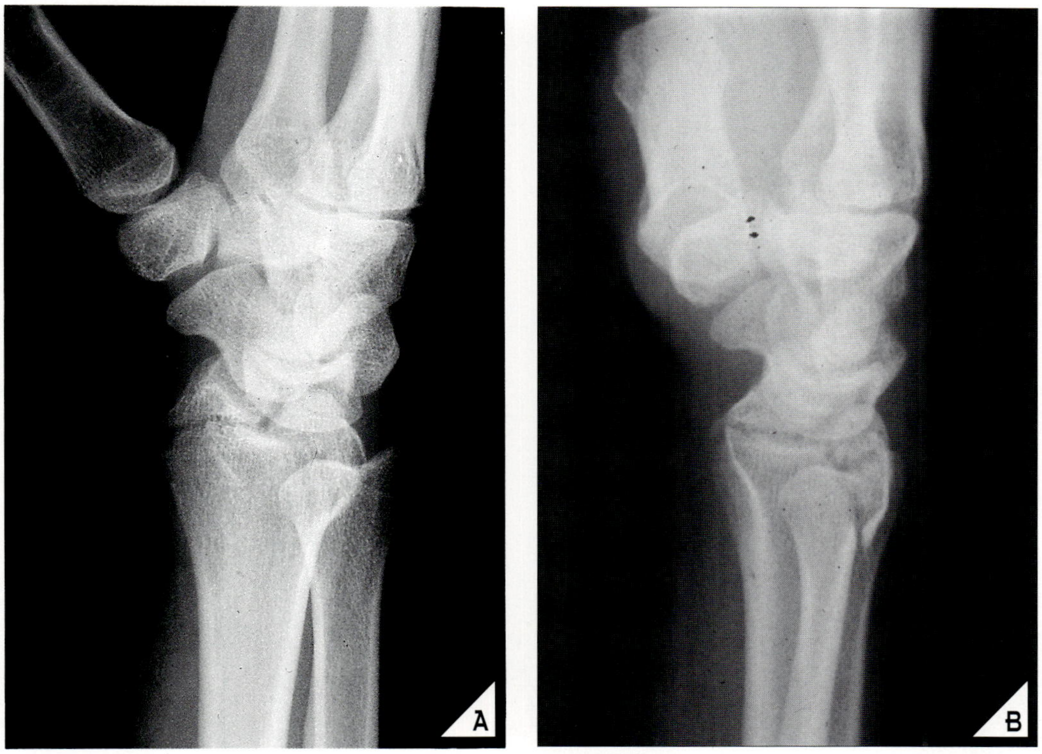

Figure 24.26
Oblique (A) and lateral (B) roentgenographic views of an intraarticular comminuted fracture of the radius seen after an unsuccessful attempt at closed reduction of the fractured fragments.

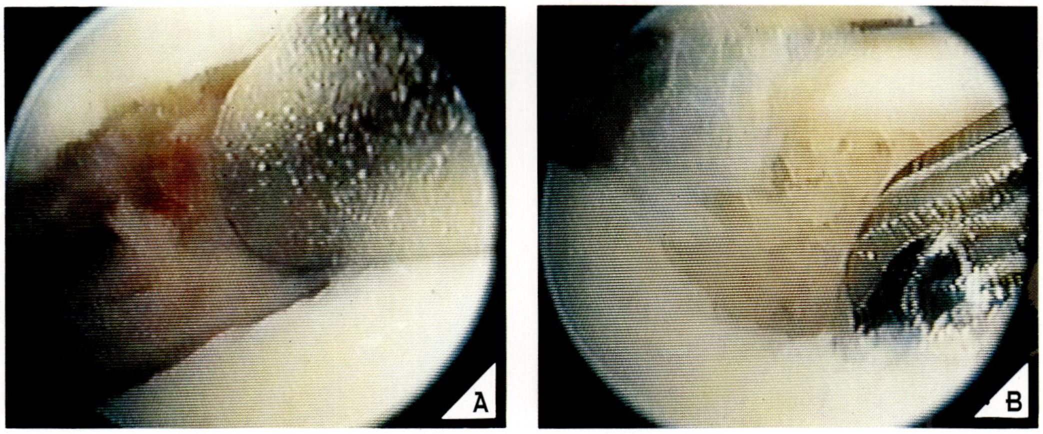

Figure 24.27
(A) Arthroscopic debridement of a fracture using a 2.5 mm full radius motorized blade to debride fibrinous material between fracture fragments. (B) Fracture fragments have been almost completely debrided.

fragments is performed (Fig. 24.28). Fragments can be pinned to each other once they are anatomically reduced. Changing the amount of distraction may assist vith the reduction. The guidewires for cannulated 3.5 and 4.0 mm self-tapping screws are especially useful at this stage. The screws can be passed over the guidewires that are positioned at the center of the bony fragments, thereby avoiding comminution of small fragments. In addition, guidewires can be used to manually reduce the fragments. Once the cannulated screw is firmly seated, the guide-wire can be withdrawn. In some cases, guidewires may be used as the only fixation in fragments too small to accommodate a screw.

Multiple interfragmentary screws accomplish stable fixation, which allows early motion and prevents intraarticular adhesion formation and soft tissue contracture. When introducing pins, guide wires, or screws care must be taken to avoid injury to the cutaneous branches of the radial and ulnar nerves on the dorsum of the wrist. Prior to introducing hardware, soft tissues should be spread bluntly to the level of the capsule. Caution must also be exercised to avoid injury to palmar neurovascular structures when directing metal fixation toward the palmar side of the wrist.

An image intensifier may not provide detail adequate to confirm that fracture reduction is anatomic. Plain x-rays furnish views with higher resolution (Fig. 24.29). The reduction of articular fragments may also be critically assessed intraarticularly under the magnified view seen with an arthroscope. Prior to completing the procedure, a probe is introduced to test the stability of the intraarticular fracture fragments.

Gross motion of the fracture fragments is monitored radiographically by moving the wrist through a full range of motion in the field of the image intensifier. A sugar tong splint is then applied if the fragments are stable. As an alternative, an external fixator may be applied if the fracture fragments can not be adequately stabilized with internal fixation.[9] A short or long arm cast is applied when the splint is removed 1 week after surgery. A wrist-control splint can be applied to provide support and allow daily range of motion exercises 4 to 6 weeks after surgery.

Management of Intrinsic Carpal Ligament Tears

Tears of the intrinsic carpal ligaments can be identified and, in some cases, managed arthroscopically. It is important to remember, however, that the damage detected

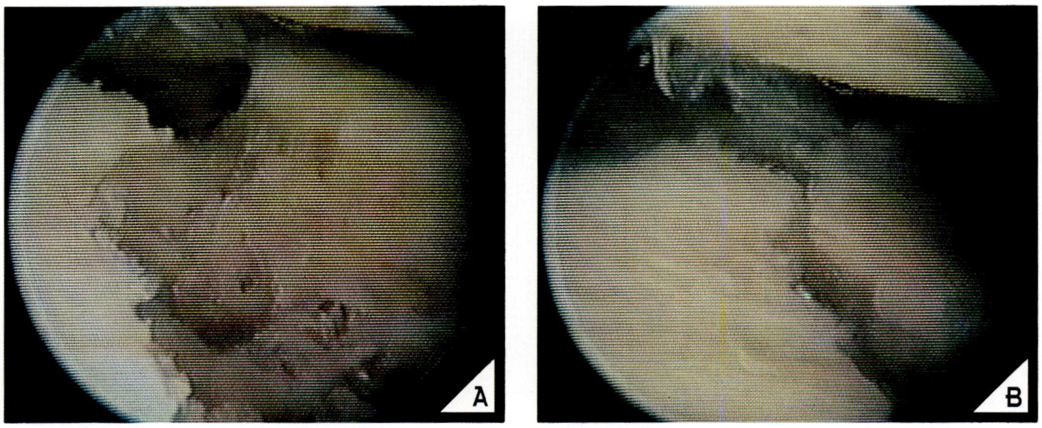

Figure 24.28

(A) Completely debrided fracture fragments are visualized prior to arthroscopic reduction. (B) Fracture fragments reduced manually are visualized arthroscopically prior to internal fixation.

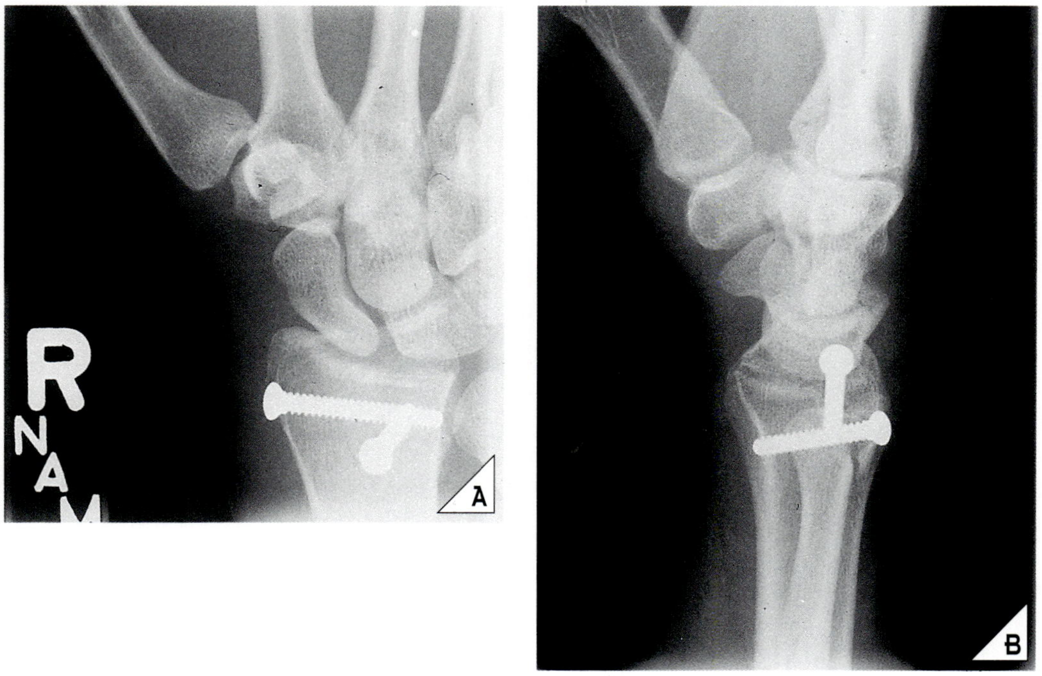

Figure 24.29

A final PA (A) and lateral (B) views is taken of the radius fracture seen in Figures 24.26 to 24.28 after reduction and internal fixation.

arthroscopically may represent only a small part of the global disruption of bone and soft tissues resulting from the original injury.[10–13] Injuries to the scapholunate and lunotriquetral intrinsic carpal ligaments are most common. Nondissociative injuries to the scapholunate and lunotriquetral ligaments may not be radiographically evident. More extensive injuries, with diastasis of the scapholunate or lunotriquetral joint, may be seen with plain x-ray.

X-rays should include PA views in the neutral position and in the radial and ulnar deviations. At least one PA view should be taken with a clenched fist. Lateral x-rays should be taken in the neutral position and in dorsal and palmar flexion. The positional changes required for various roentgenographic views and the concomitant alteration in the transmission of forces across the wrist may demonstrate intercarpal dissociation (Fig. 24.30).

Triple injection arthrography may be helpful when plain x-rays are not diagnostic.[14] For example, the thinner, palmar portion of the scapholunate ligament may fail, leaving the stronger dorsal portion intact. Since the torn palmar portion of the scapholunate ligament cannot be seen arthroscopically, the visible portion of the scapholunate ligament would falsely confirm that it is normal. Arthrography, in some cases, may be the only simple means of detecting small, nondissociative tears of the palmar scapholunate ligament.

The management options for wrist injuries depend on the chronicity of the injury and the extent of tissue damage. Acute, nondissociative tears of the scapholunate ligament or lunotriquetral ligament can be treated with pin fixation using fluoroscopic guidance to select and confirm pin placement. During the pinning procedure, the radiocarpal space can be carefully monitored arthroscopically to prevent inadvertent injury to articular surfaces from the fixation pins. A midcarpal arthroscopic examination can confirm that the anatomic configuration of the scapholunate and lunotriquetral joints has been restored. After pin fixation, the wrist should be immobilized in a long arm cast for 4 to 6 weeks followed by rehabilitation. In essence, a conventional percutaneous pin fixation procedure is performed, but arthroscopy provides the added advantage of directly visualizing the effect of the pinning and can substantially improve the quality of the reduction.

The management of chronic, intercarpal ligament injuries is based primarily on the extent of tissue damage. Nondissociative partial-thickness or small full-thickness tears of the scapholunate ligament may be treated with arthroscopic debridement alone (Fig. 24.31). Arthroscopic debridement of a torn scapholunate ligament is accomplished by alternate use of radial and ulnar portals to gain access to torn ligament fibers. Rehabilitation can begin almost immediately after an arthroscopic debridement procedure.

Complete tears of the scapholunate ligament or of the lunotriquetral ligament with carpal dissociation cannot presently be managed with an arthroscopic repair. Intercarpal fusion, an alternative management option, can be performed with arthroscopic assistance. Arthroscopic debridement of the radiocarpal space can be followed by fusion of the scapholunate or lunotriquetral joint. The arthroscopic fusion is performed by debriding the articular surfaces of the unstable joint with a small joint motorized shaver and a small joint motorized burr. The joint is then reduced and internally fixed with percutaneous pins

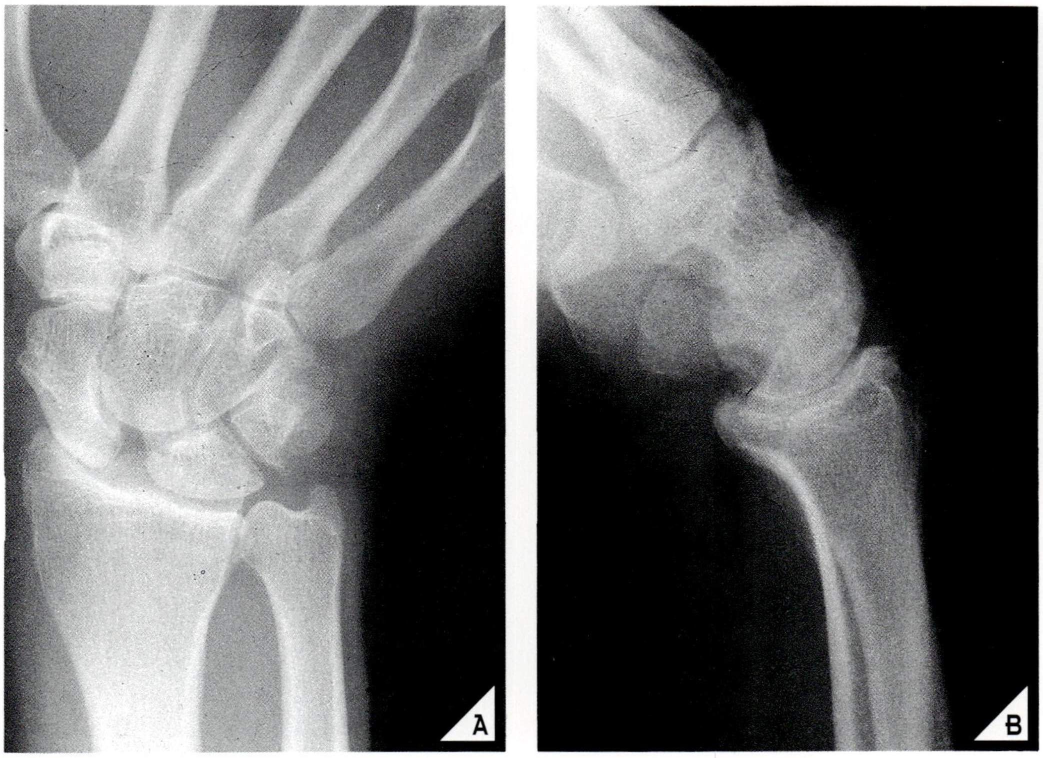

Figure 24.30
(A) Scapholunate ligament disruption with significant joint dissociation is seen with a PA roentgenogram taken in the ulnar deviation. (B) The lateral view shows a widened scapholunate angle.

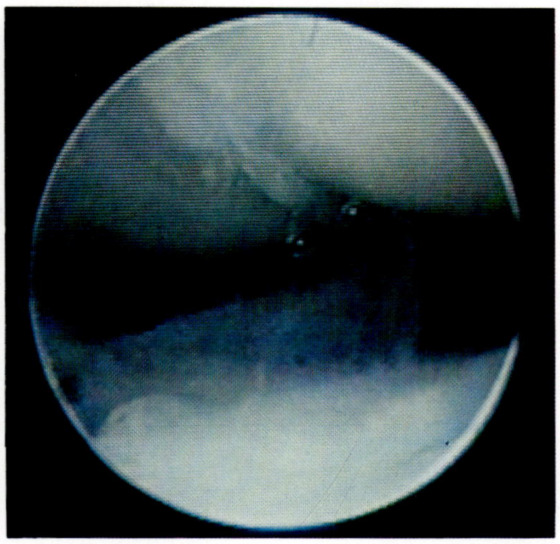

Figure 24.31
A partial-thickness, nondissociative tear of the scapholunate ligament.

or with cannulated screws with the denuded cancellous bony surfaces tightly apposed (Figs. 24.32–24.34). An arthroscopic examination of the midcarpal space confirms that the reduction of the carpus is anatomic.

Open treatment and arthroscopic management of intrinsic carpal ligament injuries with carpal diastasis remains controversial. A significant number of tears of the scapholunate ligament can be managed with simple debridement. Other tears, including full-thickness scapholunate ligament tears and partial-thickness and full-thickness lunotriquetral ligament tears, may require extensive open surgical procedures for management of the associated instability pattern. Arthroscopy can be used to monitor the open surgery if it is selected to treat carpal instability. Choosing the open procedure may be controversial, but soft tissue disruption can be minimized and visualization optimized with arthroscopic assistance.

COMPLICATIONS

Intracapsular debridement is the arthroscopic procedure most commonly performed at the radiocarpal joint. The procedure involves joint distraction and dorsal arthroscopic portals to introduce blunt, sharp, and rotary motorized equipment. Despite the potential for injury, few complications have been reported.

Injury to the soft tissues (including the skin overlying the joints), to the subcutaneous neurovascular structures, and to the dorsal extrinsic ligaments is possible and can be avoided. Short, longitudinal skin incisions made with a sharp #11 blade should extend only through the skin and not into the subcutaneous layer. Meticulous blunt dissection of the subcutaneous tissues must be performed with a fine-tipped clamp to prevent injury to the dorsal

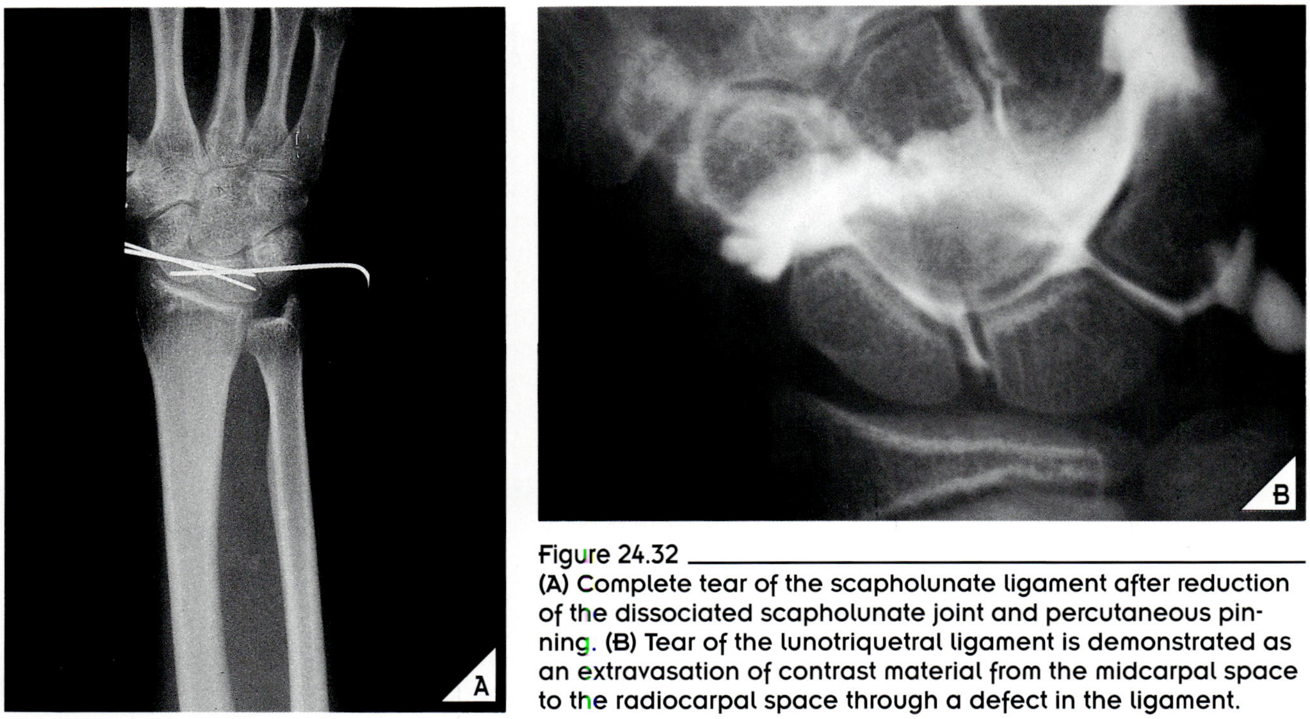

Figure 24.32
(A) Complete tear of the scapholunate ligament after reduction of the dissociated scapholunate joint and percutaneous pinning. (B) Tear of the lunotriquetral ligament is demonstrated as an extravasation of contrast material from the midcarpal space to the radiocarpal space through a defect in the ligament.

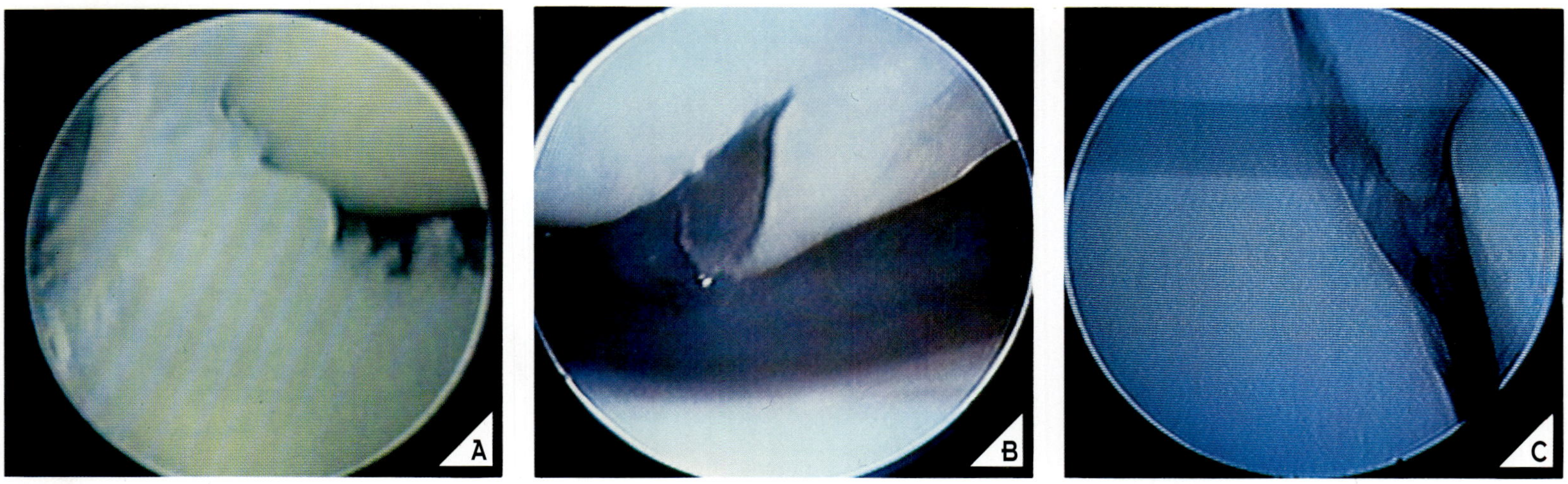

Figure 24.33
(A) Complete dissociative tear of the lunotriquetral ligament, seen arthroscopically, is extensive enough to allow the lunotriquetral joint to be visualized from the radiocarpal space. (B) Large, dissociative flap tear of the lunotriquetral ligament seen from the radiocarpal space. This "trap-door" tear did not allow extravasation of contrast material. (C) A midcarpal view of the lunotriquetral joint seen in B demonstrates that the lunotriquetral ligament tear has caused gross dissociation of the lunotriquetral joint.

cutaneous branches of the radial and ulnar nerves. If possible, avoid portal placement ulnar to the extensor carpi ulnaris and radial to the extensor pollicis longus.

Portals should not be made while the surgeon's finger is applying traction to the dorsal skin. Sliding a superficial soft tissue layer over a deeper layer while a portal is being established causes disruption of the normal topographic anatomy of the tissue layers. After being released, the soft tissues return to their normal anatomic relationship, but the passageway through the tissue planes ceases to be linear. Nonlinear arthroscopic portals are difficult to relocate and make passage of equipment very tedious. In addition, the passage of sharp knives or burrs is impossible to accomplish without causing injury to subcutaneous structures.

Sharp and rotary motorized equipment can injure subcutaneous and intracapsular tissue during excision of the articular disc. The dorsal and palmar radioulnar ligaments can be injured, if articular disc excision is too generous and extends beyond the central portion into the periphery where the ligaments are located. Additionally, care must be exercised to avoid incising the dorsal radioulnar ligament as the blade is passed through an ulnar portal across the ligament and into the ulnar side of the radiocarpal space.

No apparent complications have been related to the traction applied across the joint and no infections have been reported.

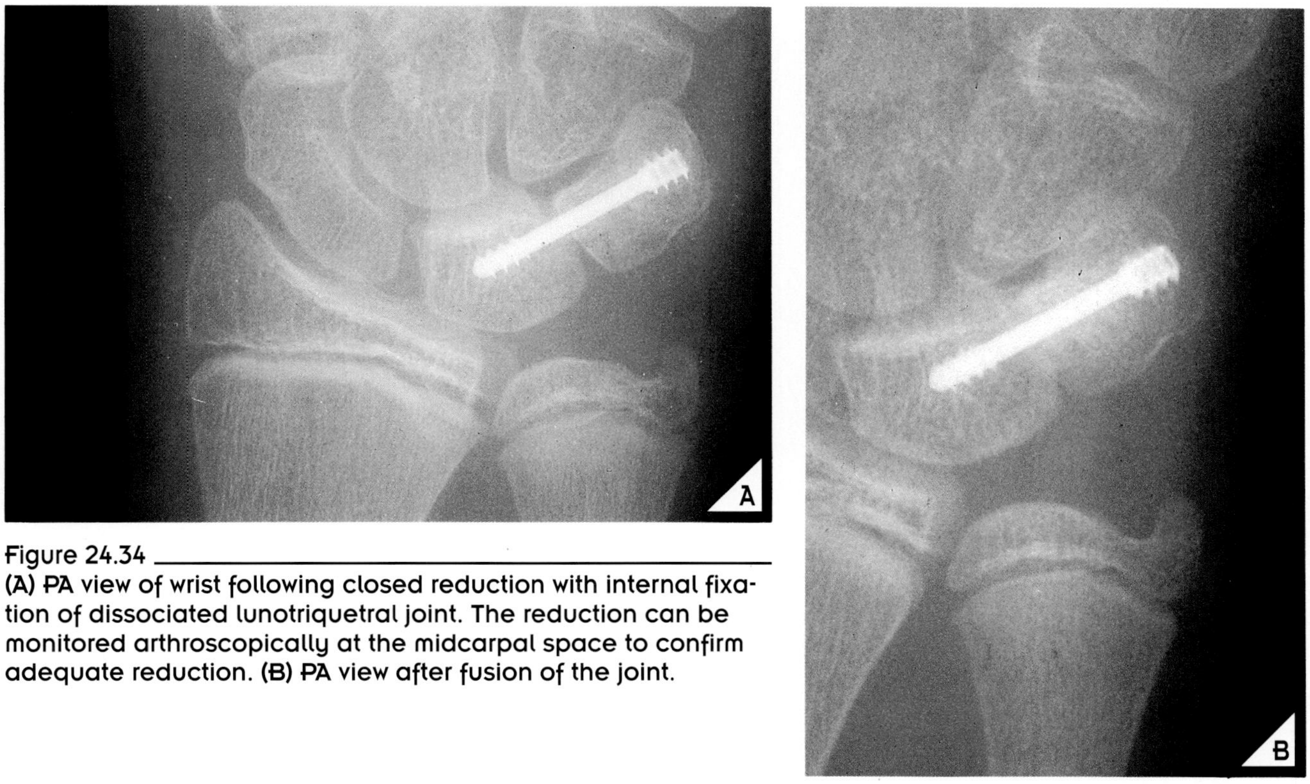

Figure 24.34
(A) PA view of wrist following closed reduction with internal fixation of dissociated lunotriquetral joint. The reduction can be monitored arthroscopically at the midcarpal space to confirm adequate reduction. (B) PA view after fusion of the joint.

REFERENCES

1. Chen YC. Arthroscopy of the wrist and finger joints. *Orthop Clin North Am.* 1979;10:723.
2. Watanabe M. Arthroscopy of the wrist joint. *Arthroscopy of Small Joints.* 1985;85–90.
3. Roth JH, Haddad RG. Radiocarpal arthroscopy and arthrography in the diagnosis of ulnar wrist pain. *J Arthro Rel Surg.* 1986;2:234.
4. Whipple TL, Marotta JJ, Powell JH. Techniques of wrist arthroscopy. *J Arthro Rel Surg.* 1986;2:244.
5. Botte MJ, Cooney WP, Linscheid RL. Arthroscopy of the wrist. Anatomy and technique. *J Hand Surg.* 1989;14A:313.
6. Bittar ES, Dell PC. Comparison of wrist arthrography and arthroscopy in diagnosis wrist pathology. Presented at the 58th annual meeting of the AAOS; March, 1991.
7. Bittar ES. Arthroscopic management of triangular fibrocartilage lesions. Instructional course lecture. Presented at the eighth annual meeting of the AANA; April, 1989.
8. Caspari RB, Patrick MF, Hutton T, Meyers JF. The role of arthroscopy in the management of tibial plateau fractures. *Arthroscopy.* 1985;1:76.
9. Cooney WP. External fixation of distal radius fractures. *Clin Orthop North. Am* 1983;180:44.
10. Mayfield JK, Johnson RP, Kilcoyne RF. Carpal dislocations: pathomechanics and progressive perilunar instability. *J Hand Surg.* 1980;5:226.
11. Mayfield JK. Patterns of injury to carpal ligaments. *Clin Orthop North Am.* 1984;187:36.
12. Linscheid RL, Dobyns JH, Beabont JW. Traumatic instability of the wrist: diagnosis, clarification and pathomechanics. *J Bone Joint Surg.* 1972;56A:1612.
13. North ER, Thomas S. An anatomic guide for arthroscopic visualization of the wrist capsular ligaments. *J Hand Surg.* 13A:815.
14. Belsole RJ, Quinn SF, Greene TL, Beatty ME, Rayhack JM. Digital subtraction arthrography of the wrist: clinical and arthroscopic correlation. *J Bone Joint Surg.* 1991. In press.

chapter Twenty Five

Endoscopic Techniques for Carpal Tunnel Release

James C.Y. Chow

Recent advances in arthroscopic technique and instrumentation permit excellent endoscopic access to and visualization of the carpal ligament. My technique allows complete release of the carpal ligament under direct endoscopic visualization. Clinical results have demonstrated that this technique can be performed safely and offers important advantages. Patients experience a rapid recovery with decreased postoperative pain and scarring and no observable loss of pinch or grip strength.

Preoperative Preparation

Instrumentation

The instrumentation required for the endoscopic carpal tunnel release has been approved by the FDA and is under U.S. patent protection. This system is composed of the following items: a short 4.0 mm and 35 mm videoendoscope; a slotted sheath/conical obturator assembly; a hand-holder and special padding; dissectors; a probe; and a disposable knife set that includes a forward-cutting probe knife, a triangular knife, and a special-design retrograde knife.

Set Up

The patient is placed on the operating table and the skin is prepped and draped in the usual manner. A hand table is used for the involved hand. The surgeon usually sits on the axillary or ulnar side of the patient; the assistant sits facing the surgeon. Two TV monitors are used—one facing the surgeon, the other facing the assistant and patient. The second monitor is usually located on the opposite side of the involved hand. The instrumentation tray is placed at the end of the hand table.

Anesthesia

Local anesthesia plus IV medication are recommended so that the surgeon can communicate with the patient. In addition, an alert patient can inform the surgeon of a variation in the nerve structure. An injection of 1% lidocaine without epinephrine is used at both the entry portal and the exit portal. Versed (1 to 2 mg IV) is given before the surgical incision is made. Sufenta 5 μg IV or Alfenta 100 to 150 μg is given before the insertion of the slotted/conical obturator assembly. This analgesia usually enables the patient to tolerate the procedure quite well.

Tourniquet

An uninflated pneumatic tourniquet is placed on the upper arm and is used only when uncontrollable venous bleeding through the entry portal would obstruct visualization of the underlying structures. This poor visibility could also cause difficulty in dissection and/or insertion of the slotted tube assembly.

It has been our experience in over 95% of cases that endoscopic carpal tunnel release can be performed without the use of a tourniquet. By omission of a pneumatic tourniquet, visualization of the pulsating ulnar artery and identification of the ulnar neurovascular bundle are improved, thereby greatly reducing the risk of damage to these important structures.

Surgical Technique

The basic operative procedure can be divided into two parts: The first is insertion of the slotted sheath/conical obturator assembly into the proper place; the second is the ligament cutting technique. A safety guard added to the cutting technique allows release of the ligament without damage to important structures.

Surgical Landmarks

The surgical landmarks are mapped out with a sterile marker (Fig. 25.1).

The entry portal is approximately 1 cm proximal to the wrist crease between the palmaris longus and the ulnar neurovascular bundle, and the portal should not extend beyond these two points. The proximal pole of the pisiform can be easily palpated and used as the basic landmark, although the landmark can vary depending on the size of the hand. In some hands, the flexor carpi ulnaris tendon can be used to locate that position. A small circle is drawn just to cover the proximal pole of the pisiform. From the center of that circle, a line of approximately 1 cm is drawn radially. From the end of this line another

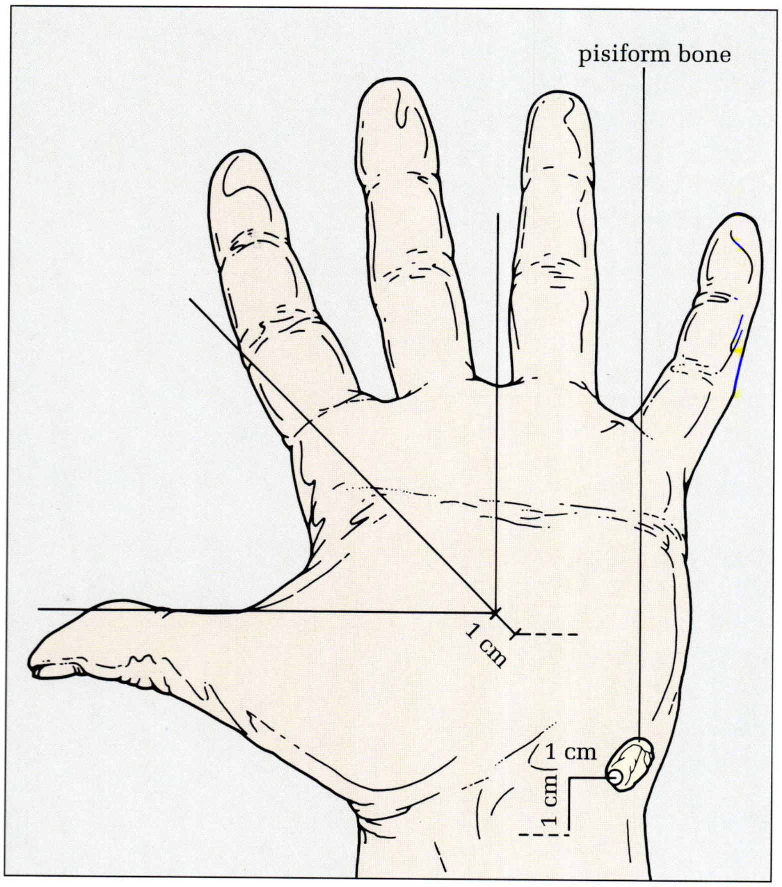

Figure 25.1
The pisiform bone is used as the point to make the incision. Depending on the size of the hand, the incision is made 0.5 to 1 cm proximally and 0.5 to 1 cm radially.

line about 1 cm long is drawn proximally. From the end of this second line, a third line is drawn approximately 1 cm radially. This is the position of the incision for the entry portal (see Fig. 25.1).

With the thumb in full abduction, a line is drawn from the distal border of the thumb across the palm. A second line is drawn from the third web space or between the middle and ring finger. This line usually forms a right angle with the previous line. The exit portal is usually located on the bisect line of this angle, approximately 1 cm proximal to the junction of the angle (see Fig. 25.1). Depending on the size of the hand, it may vary 1 or 2 mm proximally or distally from the mark.

Insertion of Slotted Sheath/Conical Obturator Assembly

The entry portal is created first. The hand is placed on a stack of towels such that the fingers are relaxed. This facilitates retraction of the flexor tendons.

A 1 cm transverse incision is made at the site as previously marked for the entry portal. With the hemostat, the subcutaneous tissue is pushed away with blunt dissection similar to the technique used with wrist arthroscopy. This will push away the superficial vein and possibly some cutaneous nerves to avoid damage to them. The next layer visible is the antebrachial fascia. A longitudinal incision is made through the fascia proximally and distally. Emphasis is placed on making the fascia incision distally as far down as possible under direct vision. This longitudinal distal cut will be picked up endoscopically later, to insure the complete release of the proximal edge of the carpal ligament and also to facilitate endoscopic release of the carpal ligament. If there is no active, uncontrollable bleeding at this time, the pneumatic tourniquet will not be used. A small self-retaining retractor is then placed in the incision, opening towards the proximal and distal side. A small retractor is held towards the ulnar side, allowing the surgeon a good view of the underlying structures.

The next layer seen is the ulnar bursa. A set of dissectors is used. The curved dissector is usually held towards the patient's fingers. The bursa is opened with a blunt dissecting technique. The ulnar neurovascular bundle rests very superficially beneath the fascia, more so than most surgeons realize. Opening the bursa in this manner avoids pulling and thus damaging the ulnar neurovascular bundle. In opening the bursa, care must be taken to start at the radial—not the ulnar—side of the incision. If the dissection begins on the ulnar side the blunt dissector might poke, dissect, and pull directly on the ulnar neurovascular bundle, which would most likely create some uncomfortable complications.

After the bursa is opened the flexor tendon can be viewed, but no entry should be made into the tendon sheath (Fig. 25.2). With the straight dissector, the tendon is identified and retracted gently towards the radial side, grasping with the curved dissector one at a time until the space between the flexor tendon and the ulnar neurovascular bundle is identified. The sheath/conical obturator is guided into the space. When the side of the obturator tip touches the base of the hook of the hamate, the surgeon is assured of being in the carpal canal. Furthermore, by going deep, damage is avoided to the ulnar neurovascular bundle, which usually lies superficially. With this maneuver, the ulnar neurovascular bundle should definitely not be retracted radially along with the flexor tendons. If it is, the obturator will be on the ulnar side of the ulnar neurovascular bundle, lifting the bundle upward, on top of the assembly. This would result in ulnar nerve palsy and potential injury to the ulnar neurovascular bundle.

Following the body of the hook of the hamate, the obturator is rotated upward, palpating the carpal ligament. With the finger and wrist in hyperextension, the obturator

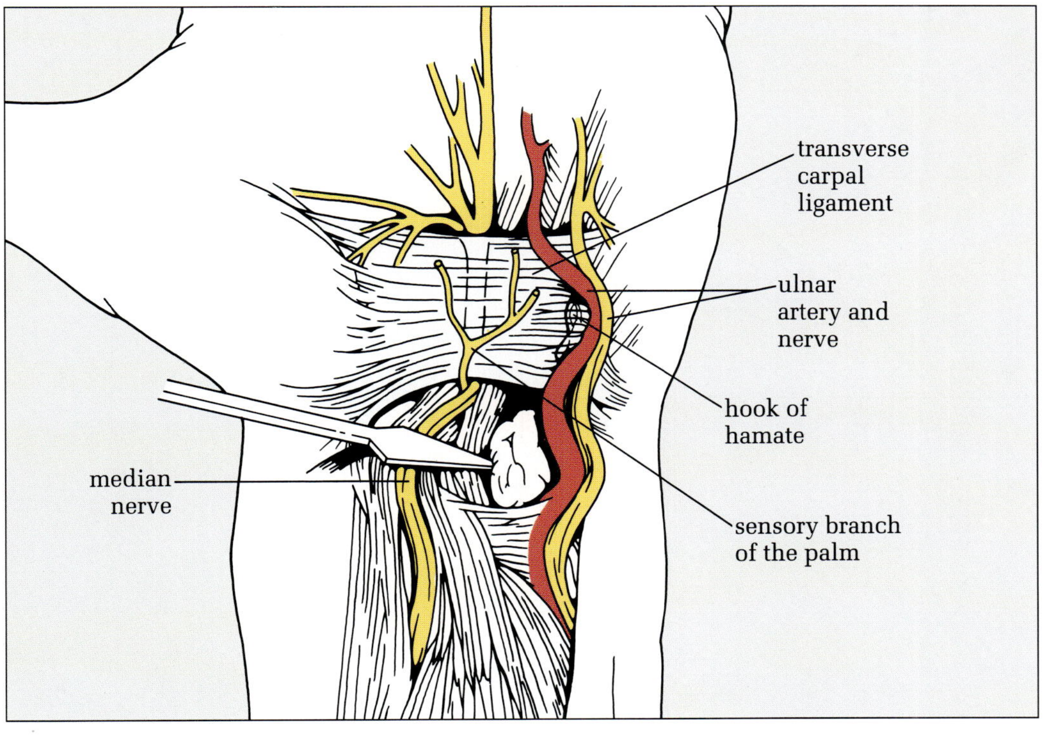

Figure 25.2
The longitudinal incision exposes the flexor tendon. When retracting the tendon, great caution should be taken to avoid the ulnar neurovascular bundle.

assembly is advanced distally (Fig. 25.3). Great caution is taken at this time not to puncture the carpal ligament with the tip of the obturator, which can penetrate through the ligament, later making the release of the carpal ligament incomplete. To avoid puncturing the carpal ligament, the side of the obturator is used to hug the ligaments gently, advancing distally.

The tension created by hyperextending the hand around the geometry of the sheath assembly causes the flexor tendon and other tissues to fall away from the sheath assembly as the obturator is advanced distally. As soon as the obturator passes the distal border of the carpal ligament, its conical tip is felt at the predetermined exit portal, where a second small incision is made. A specially designed catcher is then used to push down the distal part of the palm, actually pushing the superficial palmar arch lower than the obturator. The obturator is gently pushed through the second incision. The hand is then stabilized in a special hand-holder (see Fig. 25.3).

Endoscopic Examination

The videoendoscope is inserted proximally into the sheath. The normal carpal ligament tissue should be visible in the distal half of the tube, through the opening slot (Fig. 25.4). Sometimes a thin bursal membrane covers the opening. Using a blunt hook probe, the membranes are dissected to insure visualization. If there is fogging or obstruction of vision with material, a swab can be used to clear the field of view. The swab should be pressed firmly against the scope and gently rotated radially to clear up the lens. Now the carpal ligaments can be clearly identified. Carpal ligament fibers usually run transversely and can be clearly seen. The light source should be left on manual but dimmed so that there is no strong light reflection through the scope, in order to clearly see the fibers. There is usually some white, swollen-appearing tissue in the proximal opening (Fig. 25.5). Under local anesthesia one can use a probe to poke at the tissue to determine whether it represents an ulnar edge of the median nerve, the bursal tissue, or even the tendon sheath (Fig. 25.6). If this is the median nerve, the patient will usually complain of pain shooting to the middle or index fingers. If the median nerve blocks the opening slot, the slotted tube should be reinserted to avoid damage to the median nerve, aiming about 1 to 2 mm ulnarly to avoid the nerve structure.

Release of Distal Carpal Ligament

With the scope in the proximal sheath, the instrumentation is inserted distally, first using the probe to identify the normal carpal ligament tissue and following through by dissecting and gently palpating distally (Fig. 25.7).

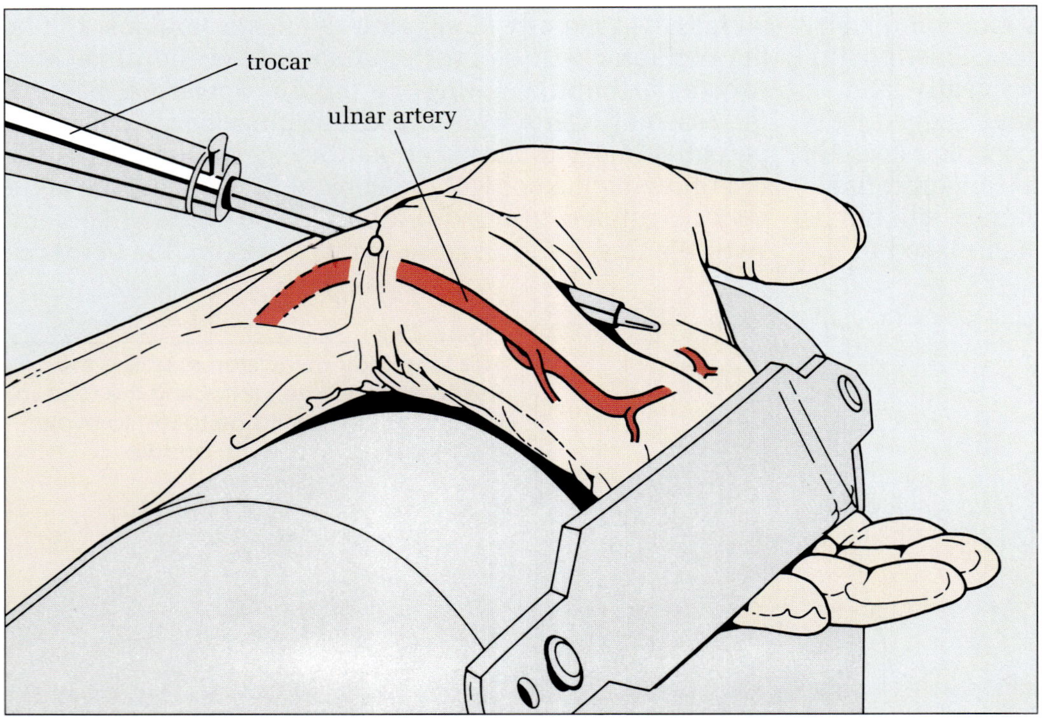

Figure 25.3
The wrist and fingers are hyperextended. The trochar touches the base of the hook of hamate. The trochar is lifted and advanced distally.

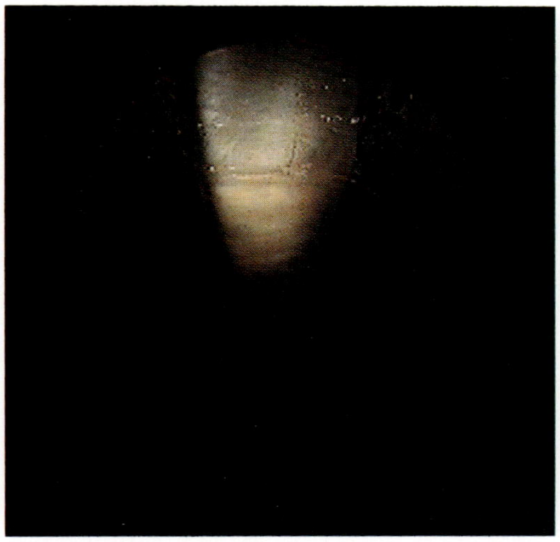

Figure 25.4
Normal carpal ligament tissue.

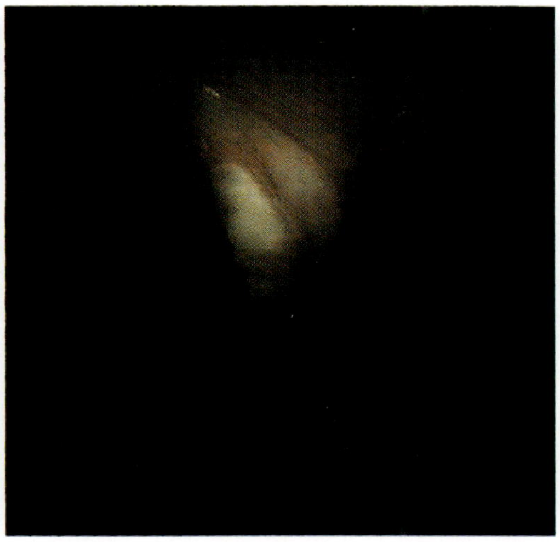

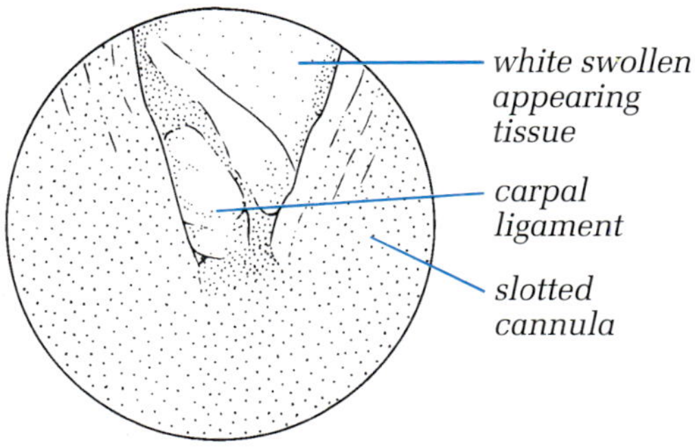

Figure 25.5
Proximal view of the carpal ligament and tissue.

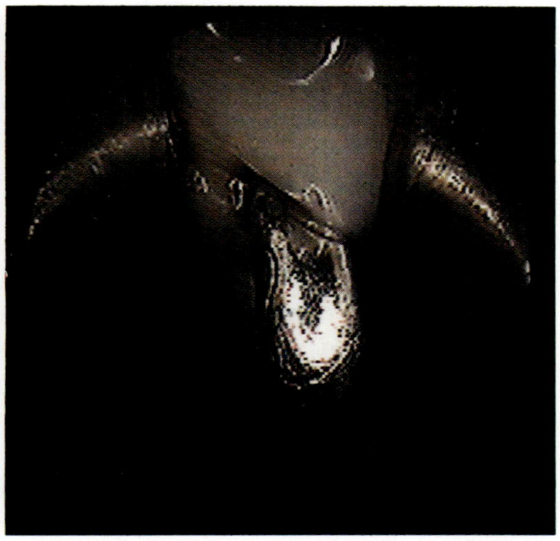

Figure 25.6
The tissue is probed to identify whether it is an ulnar edge of the median nerve, bursal tissue, or tendon sheath.

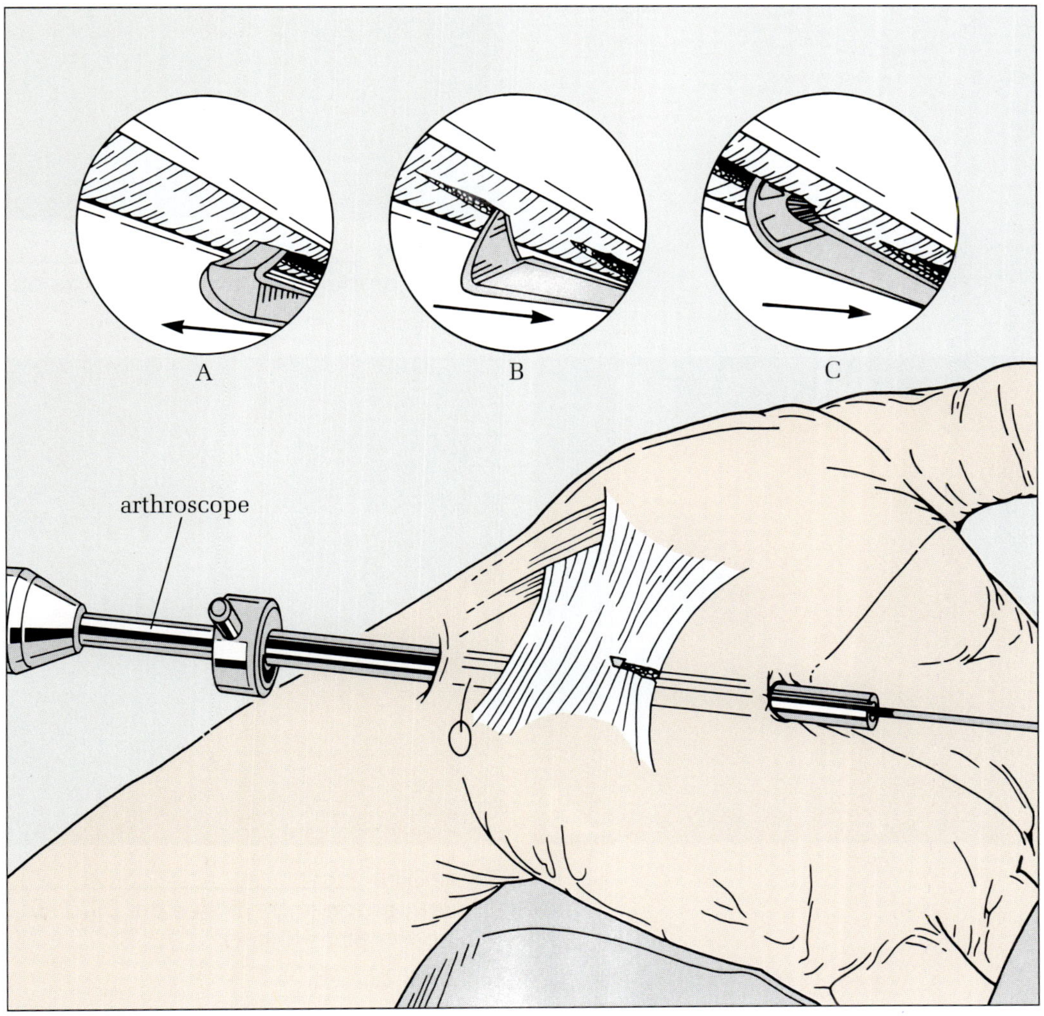

Figure 25.7
With the hand in the hyperextended position in the hand-holder, the videoendoscope is in the proximal portal. (A) The probe knife is inserted through the distal portal. (B) For a controlled upward incision at the midsection of the carpal ligament, use a triangle knife. (C) To complete the release of the distal carpal ligament, the retrograde knife is used to join the previous two incisions.

The distal edge of the carpal ligament is identified (Fig. 25.8). A specially designed probe knife is inserted in the distal opening. The design of the probe knife allows probing of the carpal ligament and permits forward cutting only. Again using the probe, the distal edge of the carpal ligament is identified, cutting from distal to proximal (Fig. 25.9; see Fig. 25.7A). Cutting in this direction keeps the cutting within the safety zone of the ligament. In case the slotted assemblage lifts up some important structures, such as the digital nerves or the superficial palmar arch, this method prevents structural damage. Anatomically, these structures are usually located beyond the distal edge of the carpal ligament.

After the distal edge is released, the scope is retrieved as proximally as possible with clear visualization of the carpal ligament. The triangle knife is inserted, cutting through the midsection of the carpal ligament (Fig. 25.10; see Fig. 25.7B). The design of the triangle blade allows control of the upward cut, which should go through the entire thickness of the carpal ligament. With the triangle knife, a small opening is made, just large enough to allow the retrograde knife to fill in the entire layers of the carpal ligament. (Since the triangle knife has a very sharp blade it should be used with much caution; its extensive use will result in unnecessary bleeding.)

The tip of the specially designed retrograde knife is blunt on the top and on the bottom, with the only cutting edge being axillary or central. Gently insert the retrograde knife through the opening just made with the triangle knife. By looping the entire thickness of the ligament, only the ligament itself is cut, avoiding unnecessary damage to the other tissues. The sharp auxillary cutting edge of the retrograde knife is drawn distally to join the first two cuts, which completely releases the distal aspect of the carpal ligament (Fig. 25.11; see Fig. 25.7C).

When the retrograde knife is unable to cut through the entire thickness of an extremely thick ligament in one motion, to avoid an uncontrolled cut one should not pull strongly and cut the ligament by force. An uncontrolled cut will increase the chance of damage to some important

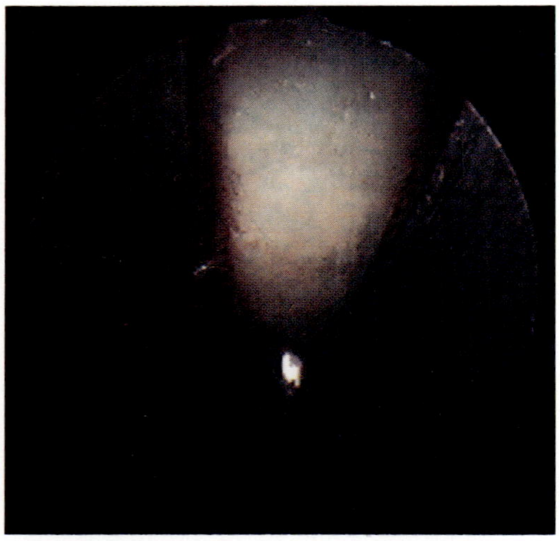

Figure 25.8
The distal border of the carpal ligament is identified.

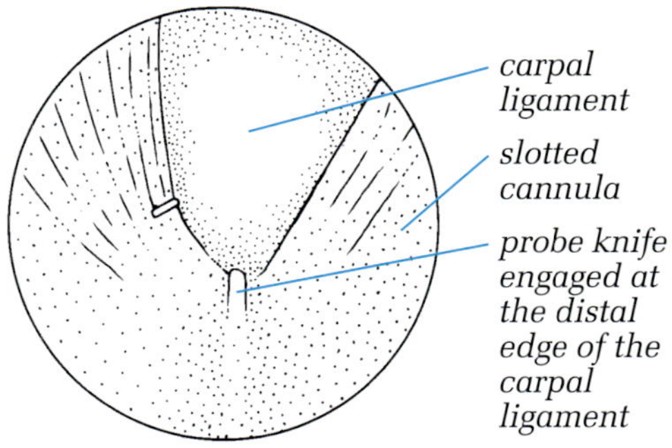

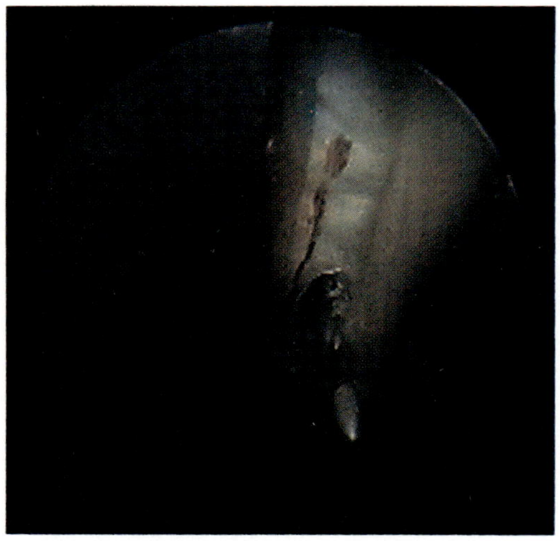

Figure 25.9
With the probe knife, the first cut is made.

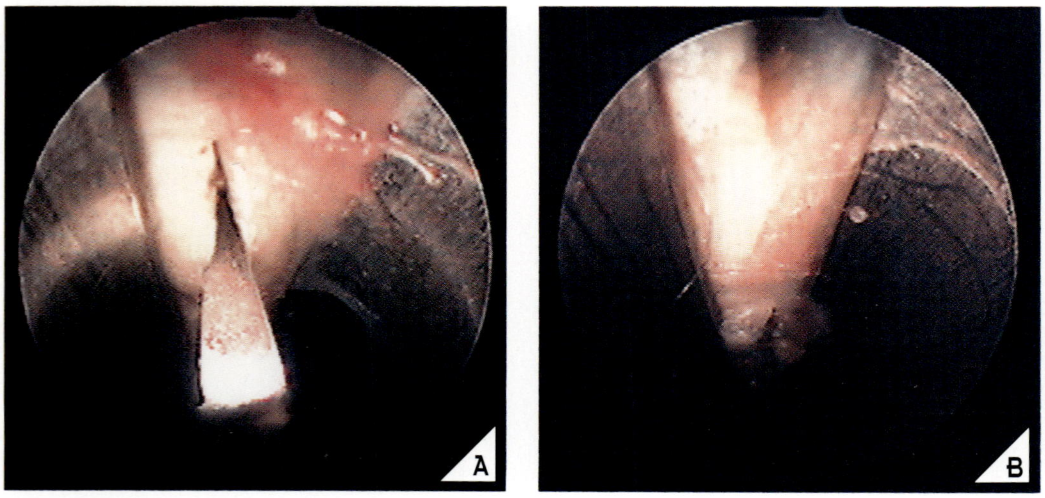

Figure 25.10
(A) The second cut is made with the triangle knife. (B) View of the first and second cut completed.

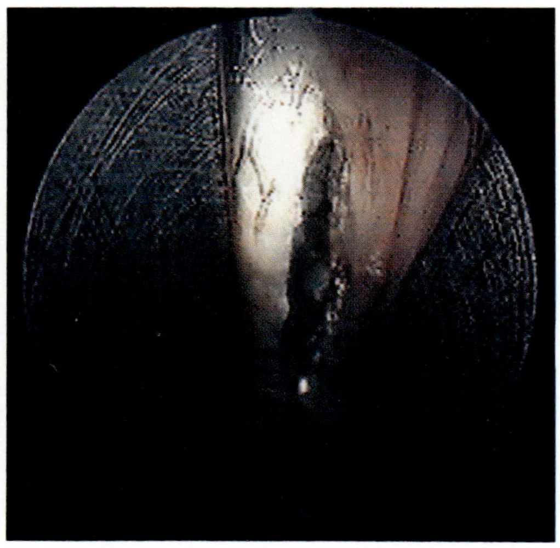

Figure 25.11
The retrograde knife makes the third cut, joining the first two cuts.

distal structures. In this situation a triangle knife is used to cut just halfway to the undersurface of the ligament. The retrograde knife is then used to control the cut of the remaining ligament.

Cutting Proximal Ligament

The endoscope is removed from the proximal opening of the sheath and placed in the distal opening (Fig. 25.12). The previous cut that releases the distal carpal ligament is identified and the uncut ligaments are also identified (Fig. 25.13). With the probe, dissection is begun from the previous cut; identifying the proximal edge of the carpal ligament, the probe knife is used to cut the proximal edge distally (Fig. 25.14; see Fig. 25.12A). Using the probe knife insures that the proximal edge of the ligament is resected and avoids injury to the tissues proximally. The retrograde knife is brought in to release the proximal aspect of the

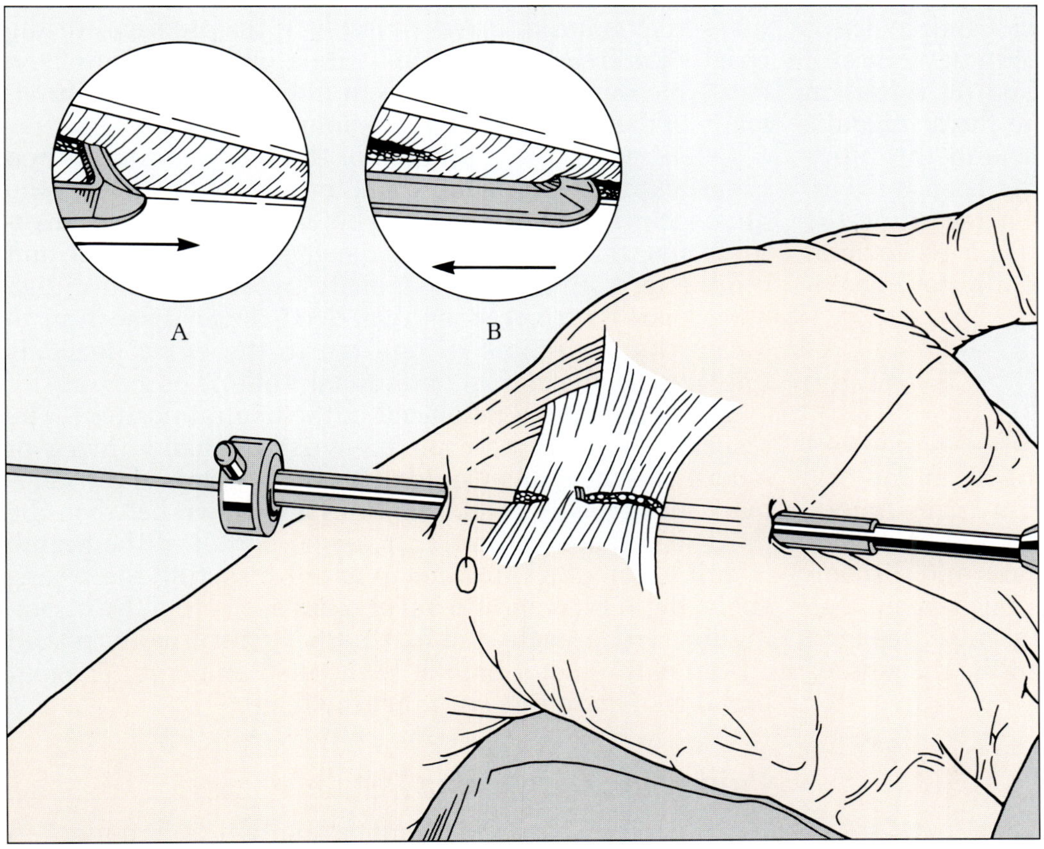

Figure 25.12 The arthroscope is removed from the proximal opening and placed in the distal opening. (A) The probe knife is used to cut the proximal edge distally. (B) The retrograde knife completes the release of the proximal carpal ligament.

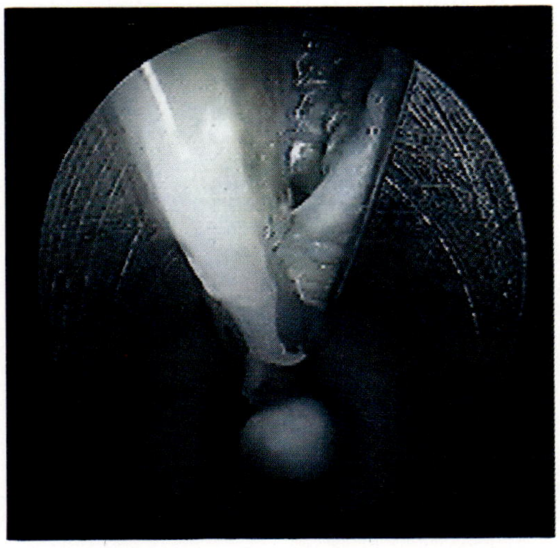

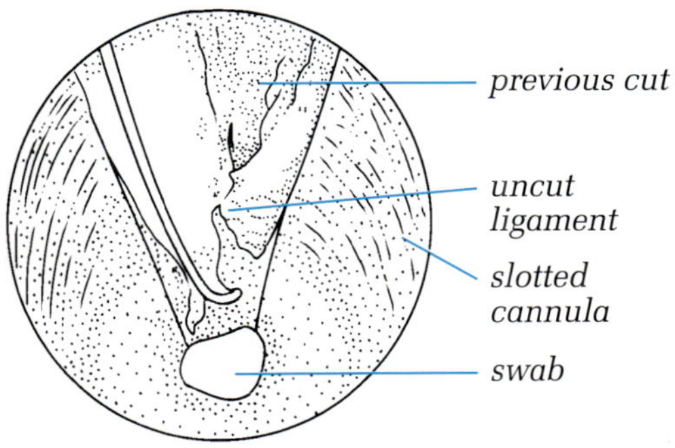

Figure 25.13 The scope is placed distally to identify the previous distal cut.

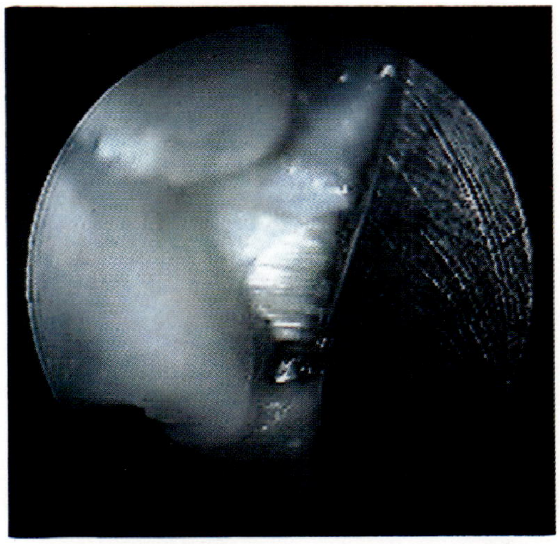

Figure 25.14 The proximal edge of the carpal ligament is identified and the probe knife makes the fourth cut.

ligament (Fig. 25.15; see Fig. 25.12E). The area is meticulously examined endoscopically, both proximally and distally, to insure that the carpal ligament has been fully released. Should further resection be required, the triangle knife can be brought in to cut one fiber at a time until the surgeon is satisfied (Fig. 25.16). Bleeding is rare. If desired, a special probe (an electrocoagulator with a plastic cover up to the tip) can be used to electrocoagulate and stop the bleeding.

The conical obturator is inserted into the sheath and the sheath assembly is removed. Usually only a single suture is required for each portal incision; a simple dressing is applied. Immediately after the procedure, while still on the table, the patient should be checked for sensation in the fingers, circulation, function of the flexor digitalis sublimis and profundus of each finger, and the interosseous muscle functions in case there has been inadvertent surgical injury. If there is a question regarding the surgery, exposure and proper care can be performed immediately while the patient is still under a sterile environment and on the table.

POSTOPERATIVE MANAGEMENT

The patient is advised to keep the dressing clean and dry. Active motion of the fingers should begin immediately. The patient is instructed not to push with the palm region or to lift any heavy objects until the soreness and discomfort in the palm region have completely gone—about 2 to 3 weeks The patient is advised to return to the office for a follow up visit in about 1 week, at which time the sutures are removed.

COMPLICATIONS AND PITFALLS

Failure to Use Proper Anesthesia

Local anesthesia plus IV sedation are recommended for this procedure. By using a local anesthetic the surgeon is more or less assured that he or she has not entered the normal variance. If the surgical instrument enters the normal variance in either the median or ulnar nerve, the patient will have severe discomfort and be unable to tolerate the procedure.

Failure to Mark Proper Landmarks for Entry and Exit Portals

Depending on the size of the patient's hand and wrist, the surgeon should always be aware that the entry portal is located between the palmaris longus and the ulnar neurovascular bundle, *approximately* 1 cm proximal to the wrist skin crease. Since this varies with the size of the hand, measuring precisely 1 cm radially and 1 cm proximally of the pisiform is not recommended.

Often, when the markings of the entry portal are too ulnar, exploration of the incision will be on top of the ulnar neurovascular bundle. This will put the ulnar neurovascular bundle in extreme danger. The ulnar nerve and ulnar artery are located extremely superficial and radial, more than most surgeons realize. Cadaver dissection to locate the structures in relation to the entry portal is important to the correct performance of this procedure.

The hand should be placed in the neutral position. The assistant should not deviate the wrist and hand ulnarly or radially because this would completely displace the landmark for the exit portal. The lines are drawn between the third web space and from the distal border of the thumb in full abduction. In order to avoid bisecting the wrong angle, these lines should never cross each other. By bisecting the wrong angle, the exit portal is incorrectly placed on top of the motor branch of the median nerve. The exit portal is often in line with the ring finger.

Failure to Excise Fascia Distally

When opening the fascia longitudinally it is important to cut the fascia far enough distally. One should learn to use the flexibility of the skin to cut the antebrachial fascia as far distally as possible under direct vision. This can make the endoscopic release of the proximal portion of the carpal ligament much easier. Failure to do so through the entry portal may result in an incomplete release of the entire carpal ligament proximally.

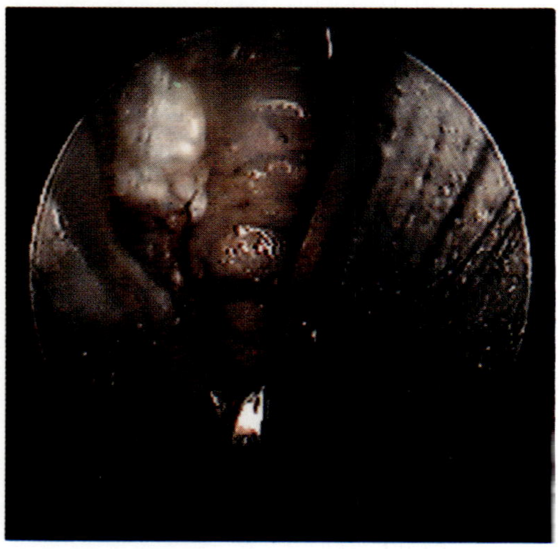

Figure 25.15 The fifth cut with the retrograde knife releases the proximal carpal ligament.

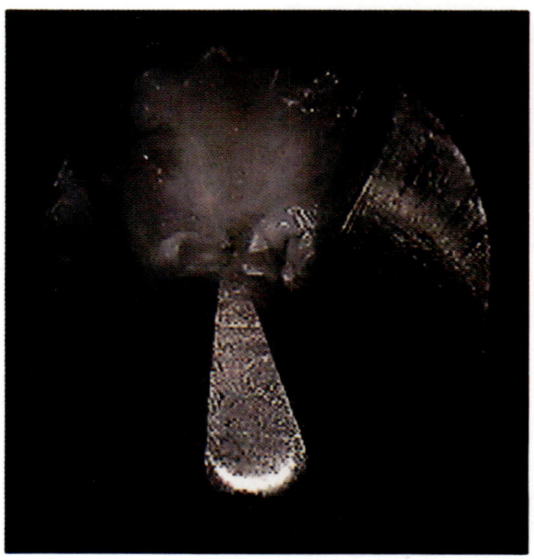

Figure 25.16 The triangle knife releases the remaining fibers if necessary.

Failure to Retract Incision Properly

This can occur after the antebrachial fascia is opened at the entry portal. If the assistant holds the retractor too firmly and pulls the incision ulnarly, the incision will deviate and displace the proper entry portal too ulnarly. If the surgeon is unaware of this danger, dissection will begin on top of the neurovascular bundle and will obviously place the ulnar neurovascular bundle in extreme danger.

Failure to Hold Finger in Relaxed Flexion Position While Dissecting Flexor Tendon

This procedure will be extremely difficult to perform if the assistant fails to relax the patient's fingers in a flexion position during dissection of the flexor tendon to locate the space between that tendon and the ulnar neurovascular bundle. Without this relaxed flexion of the fingers, retraction of the flexor tendon radially will be almost impossible. This struggle may sometimes cause injury to the ulnar neurovascular bundle.

Failure to Place Hand in Complete Supination

The patient's hand should rest on the table in full supination while the dissection is being done. If the hand rotates ulnarly or to a semisupinate position, the surgeon will not be dissecting the flexor tendon straight down but rather with an ulnar deviation. This will also place the ulnar neurovascular bundle in danger.

Failure to Identify Ulnar Neurovascular Bundle

The ulnar neurovascular bundle is extremely superficial and more radial than most surgeons realize. When the flexor tendon is dissected the ulnar bursa should be opened and retracted. Failure to identify the neurovascular bundle and retract it radially will put the slotted tube ulnar to the ulnar neurovascular bundle and cause it to be lifted on top of the slotted tube. This also places the ulnar neurovascular bundle in extreme danger. Local anesthesia without a tourniquet plays an important part in this dissection. It enables the surgeon to see the pulsating ulnar artery during the dissection, and if the ulnar nerve is actually dissected the patient will experience severe discomfort and will not allow the surgeon to continue the procedure.

Failure to Insert Slotted Tube and Cannula Properly

The slotted tube conical obturator assembly should be extremely easy to insert into the carpal canal without resistance. To insure that it is in the carpal canal, the assembly should touch the base of the hook of hamate. Obviously the carpal ligament cannot be resected if the obturator and the slotted cannula slide above the carpal ligament. Of course, if the slotted cannula is inserted into the Gyon's canal it will place the ulnar nerve and ulnar artery in extreme danger.

Failure of Obturator to Hug Carpal Ligament

During insertion of the slotted cannula obturator assembly, the side of the tip of the obturator tip should touch the base of the hook of hamate and gently roll upward so that the obturator hugs the carpal ligament proximally. Failure to do so, or advancing the trochar further down before lifting up, will result in lifting the tendon up on top of the slotted cannula. The finger and wrist should be in full extension so that the tendon can pull away before the trochar is advanced distally. Otherwise, the tendon could loop up on top of the slotted tube and lift some other important structures in the distal part of the hand. If there is doubt that a tendon is looped on top of the slotted tube, the fingers should be taken out of the hand holder and the surgeon should move the fingers and observe the movement of the tendon through the scope to identify the tendon. If the tendon is on top of the slotted tube the surgeon should remove the tube and start the procedure over from the beginning.

Failure to Cut Ligament as Described in Guidelines

Bear in mind that the slotted cannula can loop up some important structures (e.g., the superficial palmar arch, the digital nerve, a tendon) on top of the tube. This is especially true if there is some anatomic variance in the hand. If the superficial palmar arch is located 2 or 3 mm distal to the distal border of the carpal ligament, it can easily loop up on top of the slotted cannula. At this point the proper cutting technique for the carpal ligament becomes extremely important. Failure to use the proper technique may endanger important structures.

Failure to Examine Ligament Thoroughly After Release

Always examine the ligament after the release. The probe should be used to probe proximally to distally. When the ligament is completely released, both edges of the ligament will disappear from the opening slot because the position of the tube in the hand will push the slotted cannula upward toward the skin. A thorough examination will avoid the possibility of incomplete release of the ligament.

Chapter Twenty Six

Arthroscopy of the Temporomandibular Joint

Mohan Thomas

The temporomandibular joint (TMJ) is a unique diarthrodial joint. When compared with other joints in this classification, it shares much of their physiology but differs significantly in anatomy, biomechanics, and purpose. The TMJ is located anterior to the external auditory meatus and caudal to the middle cranial fossa (Fig. 26.1). Normal function of the TMJ allows painless effort in speaking, chewing, and swallowing.

ANATOMY

A good grasp of arthroscopic anatomy and histology[1] is needed in diagnostic arthroscopy in order to recognize the visual fields of each of the puncture sites during the examination. Very careful and systematic diagnostic arthroscopy of the TMJ is necessary for choosing the appropriate operative procedure.

The TMJ is an articulation between the condylar process of the mandible and the glenoid fossa and articular eminence of the temporal bone, with an intervening fibrocartilaginous structure known as the "disc." The joint is enclosed medially and laterally by the capsule (Fig. 26.2). The disc divides the joint space into a superior joint space and an inferior joint space (Fig. 26.3).

Because the joint cavity has no real volume and articular function occurs solely within the synovial fluid, a fluid medium should be injected into the joint cavity under pressure to distend the intra-articular space before arthroscopy is performed.

Distention, although necessary, somewhat distorts the anatomic relations, a point to keep in mind when arthroscopic features are interpreted. The maximum volume of the upper joint cavity is about 2 to 3 mL in the open position of the mandible. The average volume of the lower joint cavity is 1 to 1.5 mL. The upper and lower joint cavities can be subdivided into the intermediate (intraarticular) spaces and synovial pouches (recesses). An avascular articular tissue and synovial membrane lines the inner surface of each joint cavity.

Superior Joint Cavity

The upper joint cavity consists of anterior and posterior synovial pouches and an intermediate space. The osseous landmarks are the highest contour of the mandibular fossa

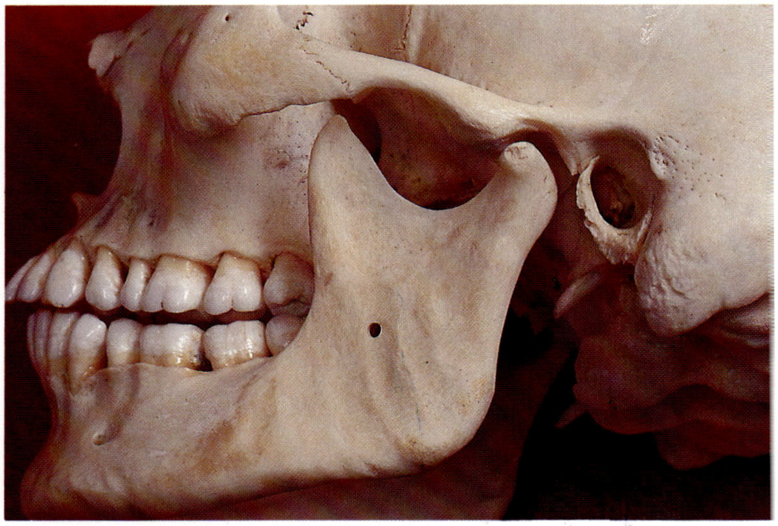

Figure 26.1
Skull showing normal left articulation of the condylar process of the mandible with the glenoid fossa and the articular eminence of the temporal bone.

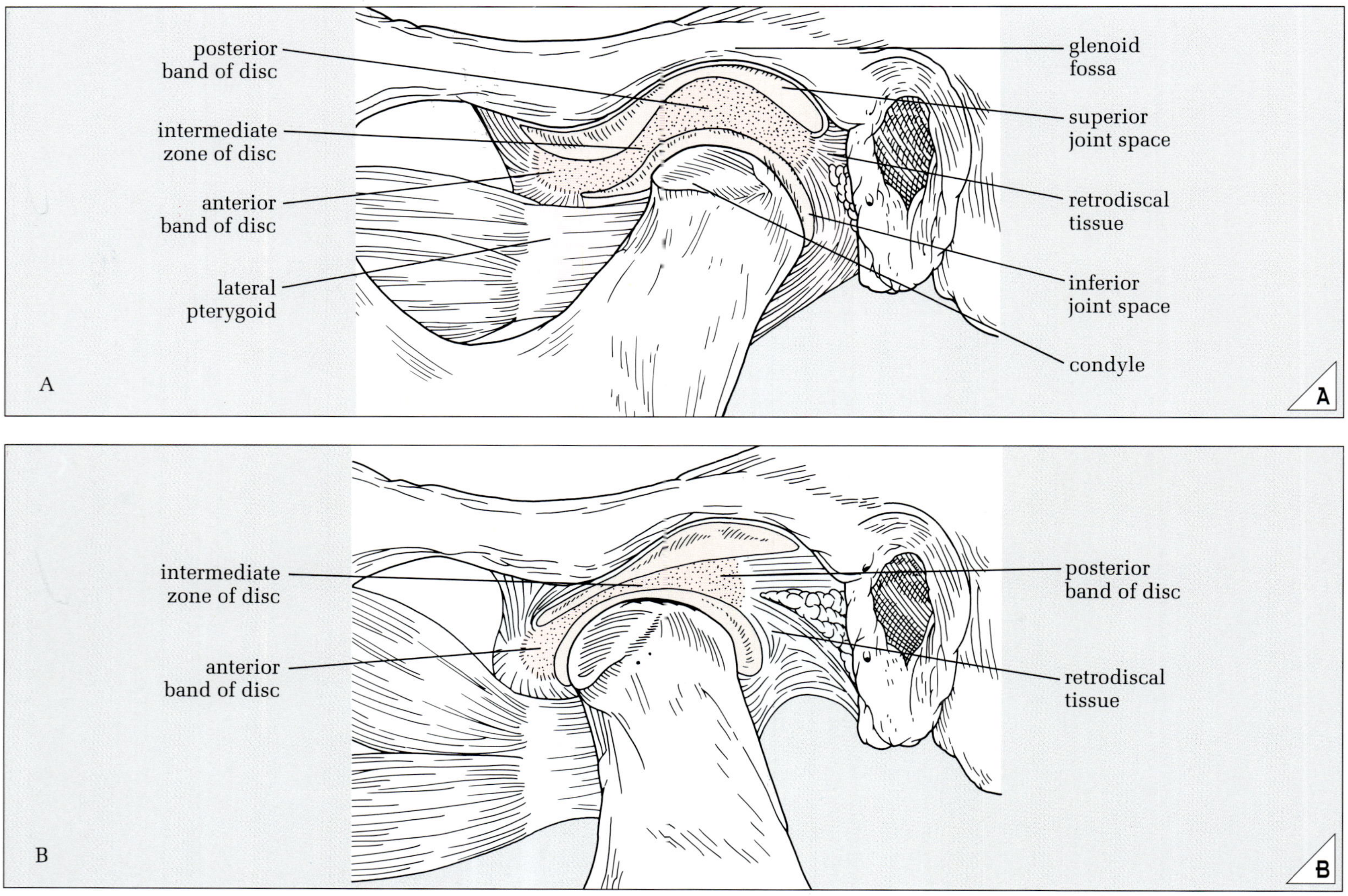

Figure 26.2
Closed mouth (A) and open mouth (B) sagittal views through the left TMJ. (continued on next page)

and the height or the apex of the articular eminence, which are helpful in identifying the compartments of the superior or upper joint cavity (Fig. 26.4). In the most lateral and medial portions of the upper joint cavity, two paradiscal synovial grooves or sulci are formed.

Upper Posterior Synovial Pouch

The synovial membrane in this region is an important anatomic landmark for orientation during arthroscopy of the superior joint space. The synovial membrane appears soft and may have a number of folds on its surface at rest, which often disappear during normal jaw opening. Vascular markings are often seen through the posterior attachment as it runs superiorly and posteriorly to the mandibular fossa, where the attachment blends and joins the articular surface.

Histologically, the synovial membrane consists of a superficial layer composed of a few rows of synovial lining cells, and a deep layer consisting of vascular loose connective tissue containing a great number of short, fine collagen and elastic fibers. A loose vascular connective tissue containing abundant blood vessels lies deep to the two layers of the synovial membrane and blends into the fibrous tissue of the articular disc and into the retrodiscal pad. The synovial membrane covers almost all the posterior pouch except for the articular surfaces and is usually easily distinguishable from the articular surfaces.

Intermediate Space

The intermediate space, located in the central articulating zone, is another important landmark. Viewed through the arthroscope, the articular surface of the posterior slope and the apex of the articular eminence are seen superiorly and the upper surface of the articular disc is seen inferiorly. These structures are relatively close to each other, and their surfaces appear whitish, smooth, shiny, and avascular. When the jaw opens, the articular disc slides along the posterior slope and apex of the articular eminence of the temporal bone. This movement is possible because the articular disc is loosely attached to the capsule but more tightly attached to the underlying mandibular condyle.

Upper Anterior Synovial Pouch

The anatomic landmarks of this recess are superiorly the anterior slope of the articular eminence of the temporal bone and inferiorly the articular disc or the synovium lining the anterior recess. The anterior confine of this recess is the synovial tissue, while medially and laterally it is bounded by the capsule. It is not unusual to see the pterygoid shadow (the texture of the fibers of the lateral pterygoid muscle) through the synovial membrane. In a normal joint this recess enlarges secondary to translation of the disc condyle apparatus anteriorly.

Inflammatory responses such as synovial congestion, hyperemia, and various stages of synovitis may affect this recess. An expanded anterior recess may be observed in

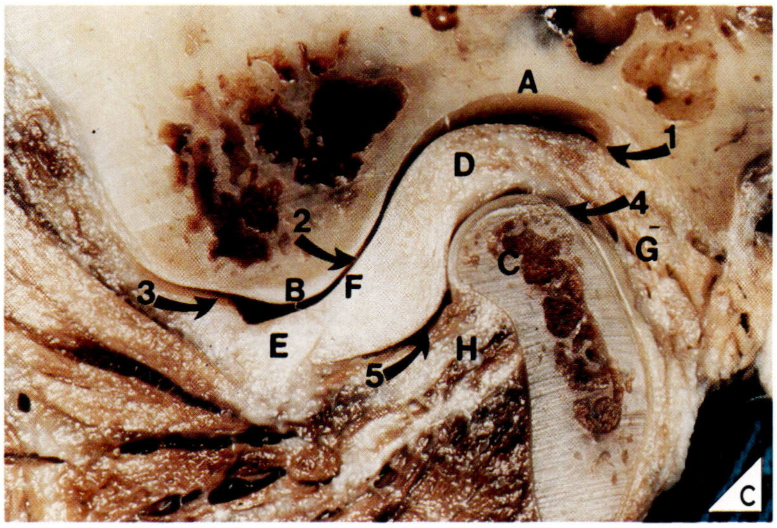

Figure 26.2 (continued)
(C) Sagittal section of the left TMJ. 1=upper posterior synovial pouch; 2=intermediate space; 3=upper anterior synovial recess; 4=lower posterior synovial pouch; 5=lower anterior synovial pouch; A=glenoid fossa; B=articular eminence; C=condylar head; D=posterior band of disc; E=anterior band of disc; F=intermediate portion of disc; G=retrodiscal tissue; H=inferior belly of the lateral pterygoid muscle. (Courtesy of Dr. Ken-Ichiro Murakami)

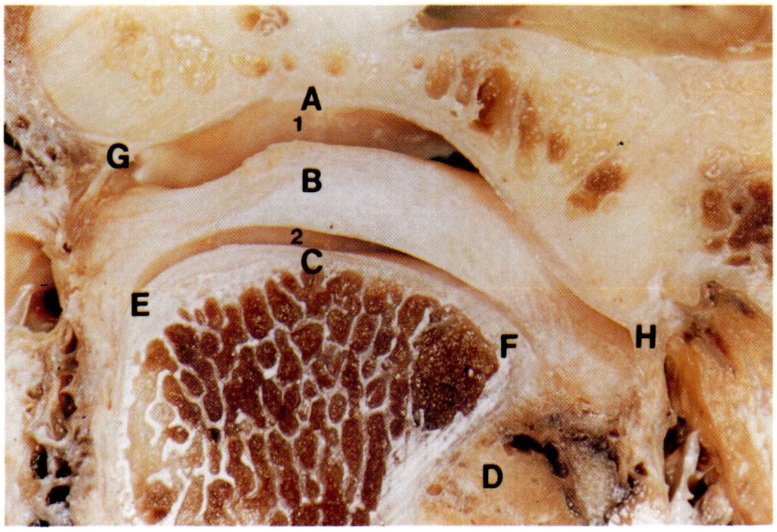

Figure 26.3
Coronal section of the right TMJ. 1=upper joint cavity; 2=lower joint cavity; A=glenoid fossa; B=articular disc; C=condyle; D=lateral pterygoid muscle; E=lateral pole; F=medial pole; G=lateral capsule with synovial lining; H=medial capsule with synovial lining. (Courtesy of Dr. Ken-Ichiro Murakami)

acute anterior disc displacement. Mild to severe fibrous adhesions may be seen in patients with chronically anteriorly displaced discs and arthrosis, in which the volume of this anterior recess is significantly smaller.

Inferior Joint Cavity

The inferior joint cavity has a much smaller volume than the upper joint cavity. Anterior and posterior synovial pouches separated by an intermediate space between the condyle and disc have been described (see Fig. 26.4). Arthroscopic examination of the lower joint cavity is difficult and is not performed routinely by most practitioners. My personal experience has been limited to examination via perforations or at the time of arthrotomy of the TMJ. The arthroscope is moved from the upper joint cavity into the inferior joint cavity through the perforation between the two cavities.

Lower Posterior Synovial Pouch

The lower posterior synovial pouch is bounded superiorly by the disc or retrodiscal tissue and inferiorly by the articular surface of the mandibular condyle, and except for the articular surfaces is lined by synovium. Synovial membrane in this pouch is highly vascularized by the blood vessels in the retrodiscal pad deep to the synovial lining.

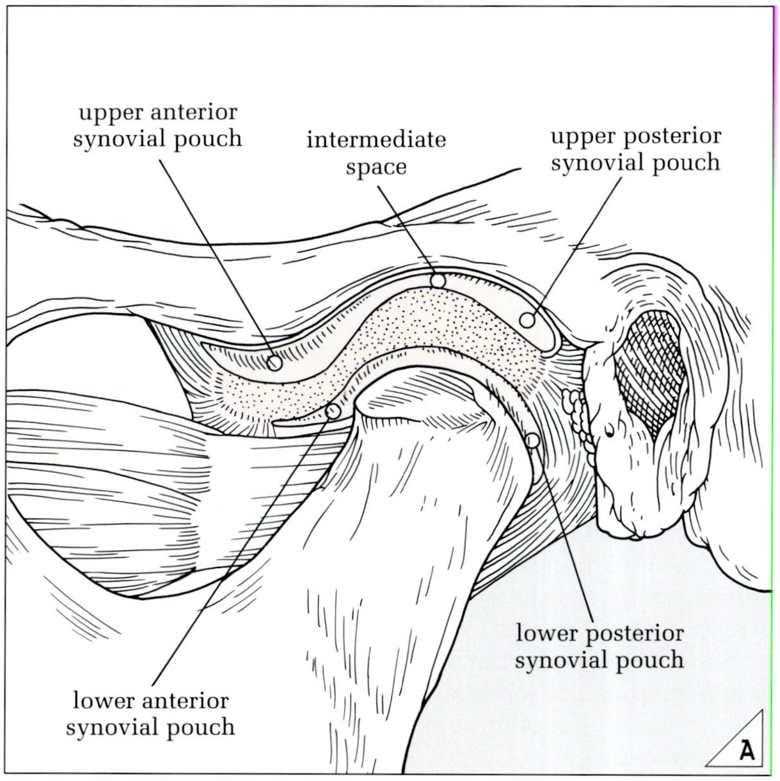

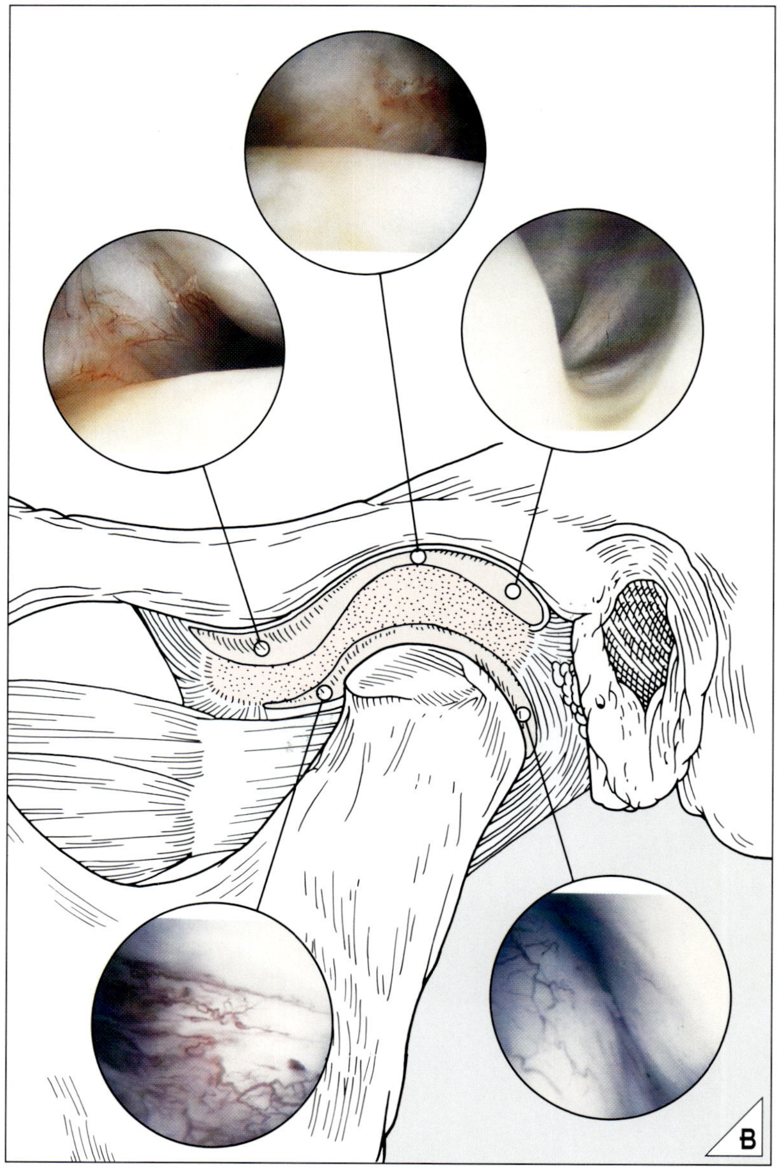

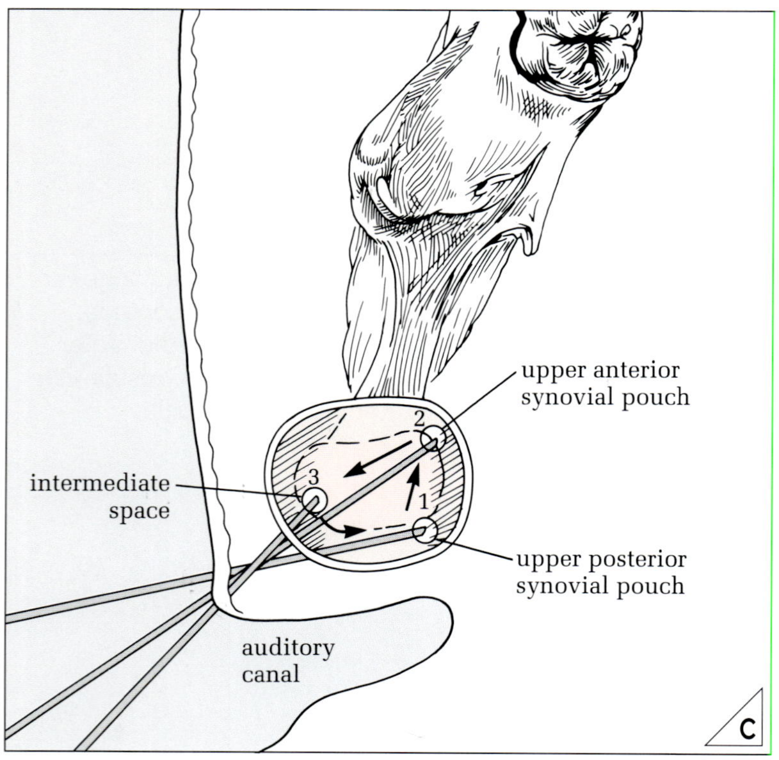

Figure 26.4

(A) Schematic illustration of the arthroscopic anatomy of the left TMJ. (B) Arthroscopic photographs of the subcompartments of the upper and lower joint cavities of the left TMJ. (C) Schematic illustration showing examination of the superior joint space after inferolateral entry when viewed from above.

The retrodiscal pad forms a cushion for the mandibular condyle. Arthroscopically, the undersurface of the retrodiscal pad and the synovial membrane appear to be softer and more cushion-like. Looking anteriorly, one can see the intermediate space between the condyle and the undersurface of the disc. Histologically, the retrodiscal pad consists of loose areolar tissue with connective and adipose components, abundant arteries, and venous plexus.

Lower Anterior Synovial Pouch

This synovial pouch is much smaller than the lower posterior pouch. The undersurface of the articular disc lies superiorly and the articular surface of the mandibular condyle lies inferiorly. The synovial membrane lining this pouch is histologically identical to that of the posterior synovial pouch but is less vascular in the synovial and subsynovial tissues.

Indications

The general indications for diagnostic arthroscopy[2] of the TMJ are unexplained, persistent preauricular or TMJ pain; confirmation of diagnostic findings for surgical treatment decisions as in cases of hypermobility, hypomobility, or painful or noxious clicking; and systemic arthritides or arthropathies involving the TMJ. In addition to these indications, diagnostic arthroscopy may be helpful in disease staging before arthrotomy. Arthroscopy can also be used for synovial or articular surface biopsy to assess joint status and for synovial fluid analysis. Studies of synovial fluid analysis are encouraging and may further elucidate the pathophysiology of TMJ disorders. Indications for operative arthroscopy include internal derangement of the joint or arthropathy that causes functional disability and is not amenable to nonsurgical therapy; synovitis; adhesions; and degenerative joint disease.

The contraindications to arthroscopy include adjacent infection, such as from ear or skin, and the risk of tumor seeding. Relative contraindications include standard medical contraindications and anatomic circumstances unique to the patient such as inability to palpate the preauricular depression or pathologic states such as bony ankylosis.

Instrumentation

Larger-diameter arthroscopes 2.7 mm are recommended for operative procedures (Fig. 26.5A).[3] I prefer the 30° angle, which is most often used for operative arthroscopy. With the more inclined angles orientation is more difficult to obtain, particularly in a small joint such as the TMJ. The 70° angle of inclination is commonly used for posterior viewing via the transcondylar approach.

The instruments used most commonly are probes, spinal needles, switching sticks, knives, ring curettes (Fig. 26.5B), forceps (Fig. 26.5C) and the suction punch

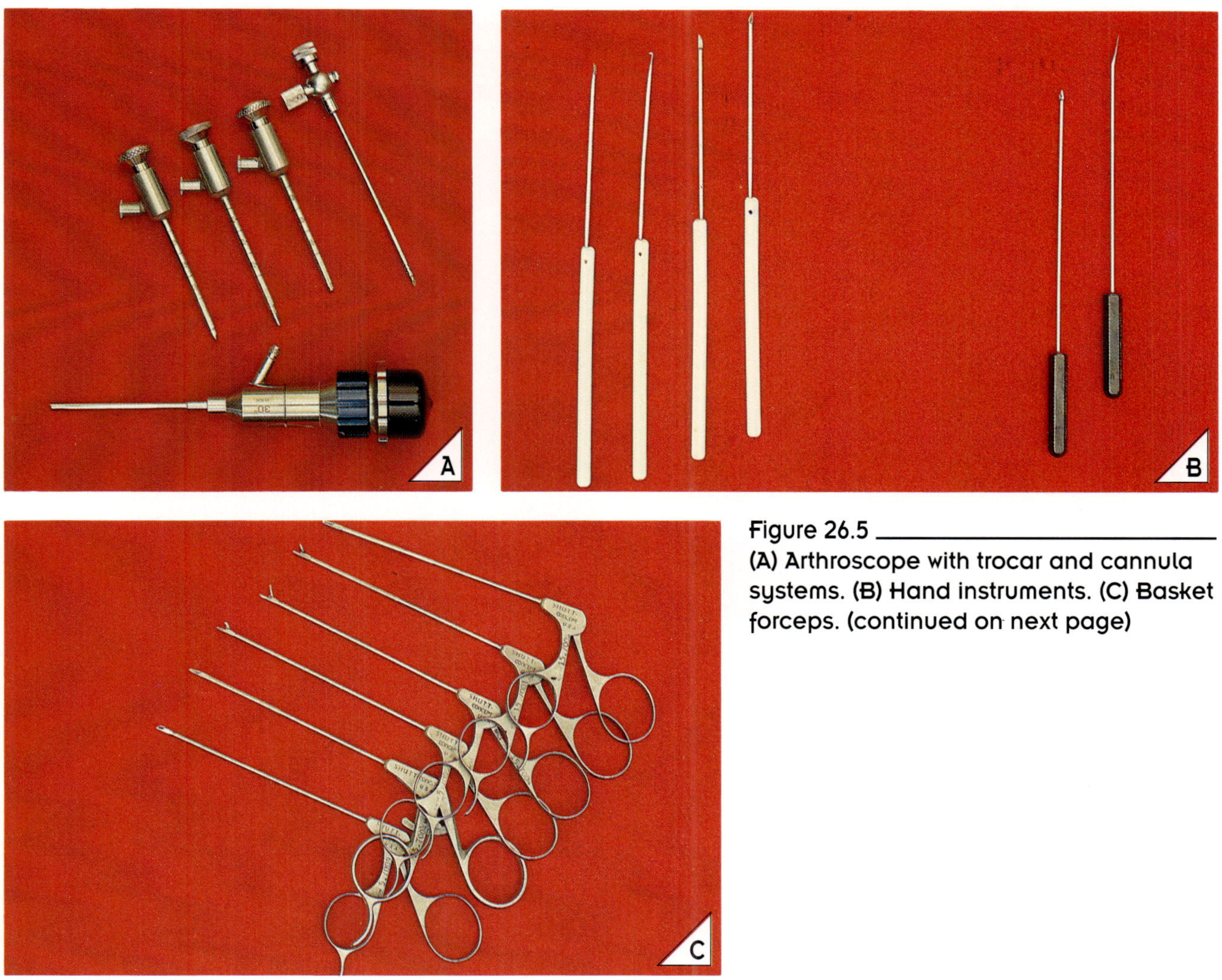

Figure 26.5

(A) Arthroscope with trocar and cannula systems. (B) Hand instruments. (C) Basket forceps. (continued on next page)

(Fig. 26.5D), scissors, bone files, and the "golden retriever." The cartilage shaver (a motorized instrument) (Fig. 26.5E), the mandible manipulator (Leonard Medical), disc suturing devices, or suture sticks (Fig. 26.5F) (Concept), and the meniscus mender (Instrumaker) are used as well. A monitor, VCR, and hard copy printer are recommended for documentation (Fig. 26.5G).

Electrocautery and Fluid Mediums

The use of electrocautery in arthroscopic TMJ surgery evolved after extensive experience with electrocautery in arthroscopic knee surgery. Electrosurgery has become a useful adjunct in a number of procedures, including electrosurgical anterior release, posterior synovial pouch cauterization, electrosurgical synovectomy, and cautery for hemostasis. Both monopolar and bipolar electrosurgical units are used in TMJ arthroscopy.

A nonconductive fluid must be used when electrosurgery is performed. Normal saline has free ions in solution and therefore is usually contraindicated. In theory, Ringer's lactate, a conductive fluid medium, should not be used in electrosurgical applications; however, our experience seems to support its safety in electrosurgery.

The use of viscoelastic solutions such as hyaluronic acid has been reported in TMJ arthroscopy. I was involved in an animal study to determine the deleterious effects of hyaluronic acid, if any, on the intraarticular tissues, and I observed no such effects when sodium hyaluronate was used postsurgically in an animal model. Furthermore, I found an appreciable therapeutic mechanical advantage with this viscoelastic solution, which prompted me to

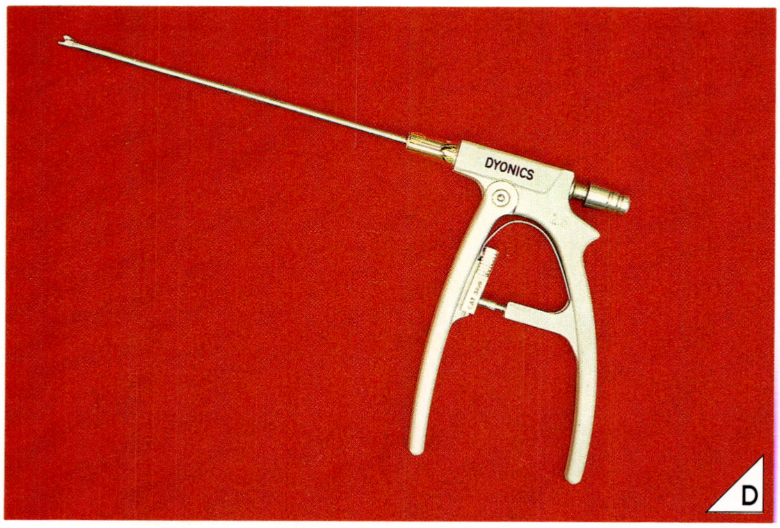

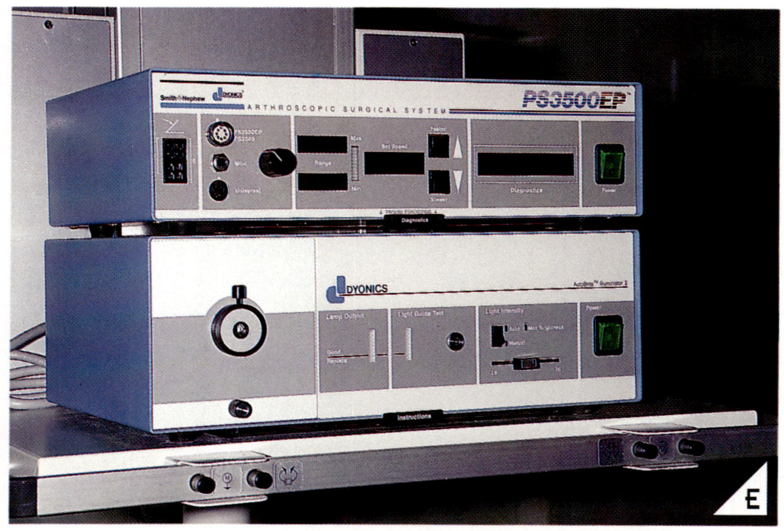

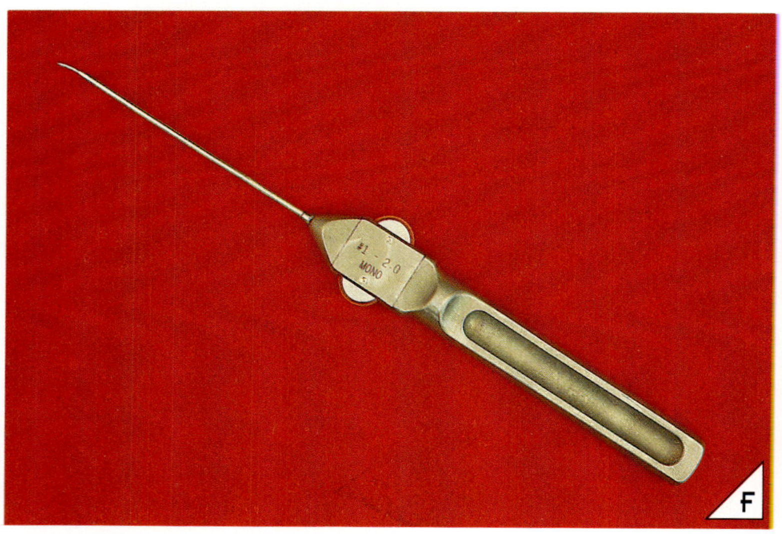

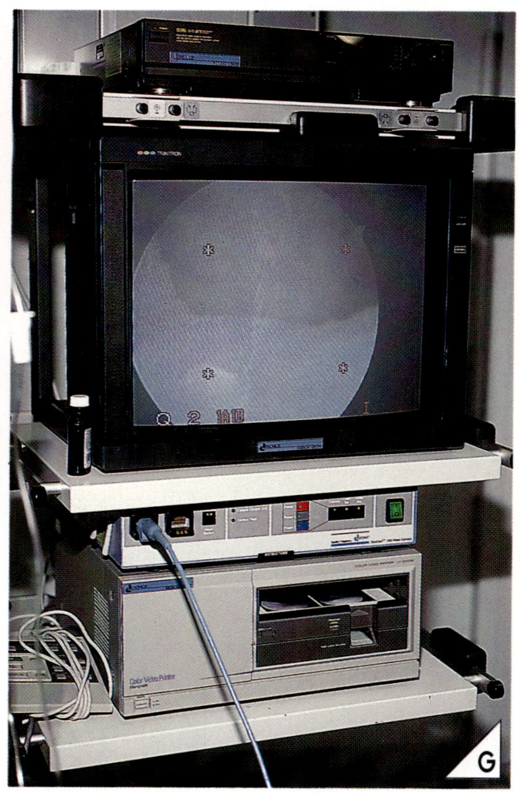

Figure 26.5 (continued)
(D) Suction punch. (E) Motor unit for cartilage shaver and light source for TV camera. (F) Suture stick. (G) Monitor, VCR, and hard-copy printer.

place approximately 0.5 mL of sodium hyaluronate (Healon) into the TMJ after arthroscopy. These patients have reported less pain and greater mobility during the immediate postoperative phase, which in turn led to quicker physical rehabilitation.

Lasers

Electrosurgery has a definite place in TMJ arthoscopy. The neodymium:yttrium–aluminum–garnet (Nd:YAG) and KTP-532 lasers have been used in the TMJ. Pioneer work with the Nd:YAG laser and its effects on cartilage in dogs has been reported by Indresano and Bradrick.[4] One of the newer and safer lasers is the holmium laser, which is called a cold laser because of the reduced amount of heat generated. Lasers seem to have some advantages in operative arthroscopy compared to traditional electrocautery units, but more research is required before they can be fully endorsed.

Surgical Technique

General anesthesia is given, preferably via nasoendotracheal intubation because the mandible must be mobilized often, and the patient is prepped and draped in the sterile manner usual for a TMJ arthrotomy procedure. A special TMJ arthroscopy drape may be employed, which comes with a plastic pouch that is inserted into the patent's mouth so that the assistant surgeon can place a thumb intraorally or employ one of the devices used in the manipulation of the mandible to prevent contamination of the surgical field by the oral cavity (Fig. 26.6).

If an endaural approach or portal is anticipated, the external ear is also prepped to about 2 cm into the external auditory canal with cotton applicators, taking care that the Betadine does not drip onto the tympanic membrane. The external auditory canal is gently packed with a peanut or cotton pledget soaked in mineral oil. The TMJ drape is then applied to the surgical area, and anatomic marks are placed with a marking pen for safe joint entry.

The surgeon can take a position either on the same side or the opposite side of the TMJ to be operated on. The anesthesiologist should be positioned well off to the side of the table so that the surgeon and assistant surgeon have access and can exchange positions during right and left TMJ arthroscopies. The surgeon, assistant surgeon, and scrub nurse should have a direct view of the TV monitor (Fig. 26.7). The arthroscope and camera should be at the head of the table in a sterile, draped basin within the surgeon's easy reach. Placement of the surgical instruments should allow proper positioning of cables, electrical cords, suction tubing, and anesthesia circuit tubing.

A single-portal technique is usually adequate for diagnostic evaluation of the superior joint space. Holmlund and Hellsing[5] reported measured landmarks for joint

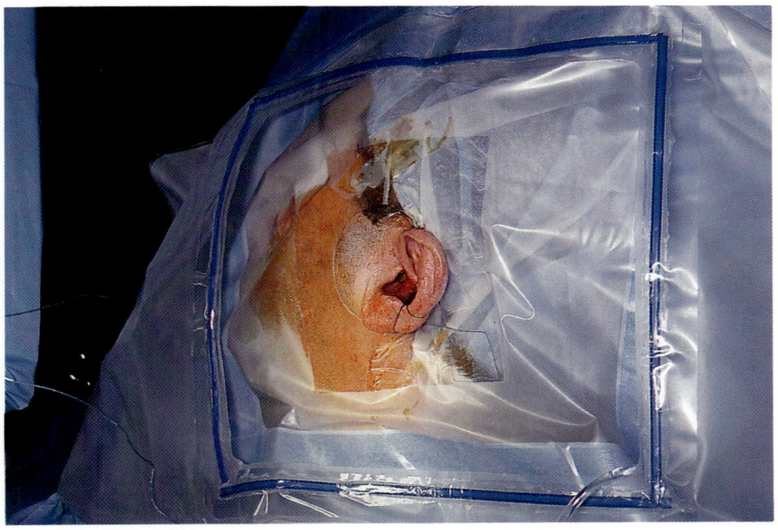

Figure 26.6
TMJ drape.

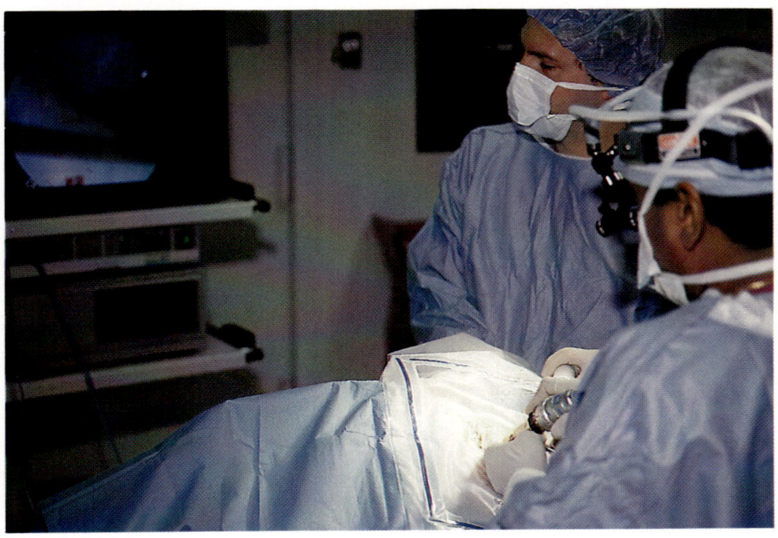

Figure 26.7
Operating room set up with a monitor at the head of the table.

entry after a cadaveric study. They indicated a safe point of entry along a line drawn from the middle of the tragus of the ear to the lateral canthus of the eye, referred to as the "HH line" (Fig. 26.8A). This point for joint entry was found to be 10 mm anterior to the tragus of the ear along the HH line and 2 mm inferior to the line (Fig. 26.8B). This portal corresponds to the inferolateral entry to the TMJ described by Murakami and Ono.[6] Although these landmarks (see Fig. 26.4B) are fairly accurate, one must cross-check against osseous landmarks obtained by palpation of the glenoid fossa and zygomatic arch, which are usually easily palpable except in patients with excessive preauricular bulk. There are several important anatomic structures in the region of joint entry, especially the temporal branch of the facial nerve and the auriculotemporal branch of the trigeminal nerve. In addition, several vascular structures, including the branch of the facial vein, cross the TMJ region. Close attention to detail, particularly the landmarks described, will preclude complications involving these structures (Fig. 26.9).

The surgical assistant usually depresses the mandible in a forward and downward direction so that the surgeon can palpate the glenoid fossa and the posterior margin of the condylar head. I usually place my index finger into the glenoid fossa as the assistant distracts the mandible. A sterile skin marking pen is used to outline the index finger, which provides an outline of the glenoid fossa. This marking, along with the measured landmarks, allows one to enter the superior joint space safely and predictably (see Fig. 26.9C).

Distention of the joint is recommended for easy joint entry, using a 5 mL syringe with a 27-gauge needle about 1.5 inches long (Fig. 26.10). The fluid most often used for joint distention is lactated Ringer's. The surgeon must direct the needle by feel towards the posterior slope of the articular eminence, keeping in mind a three-dimensional picture of the joint anatomy. After the posterior slope of the eminence has been palpated, the tip of the needle is turned slightly medial. Once it is determined that the needle is indeed in the superior joint space, the fluid is slowly injected. The hydraulic effect of a fluid column falling and rising within the syringe when pressure is applied and then released during the distention procedure, along with the assistant sensing the mandible being depressed, confirms the needle's position within the superior joint space. At this point, approximately 2 to 3 mL of lactated Ringer's is injected into the superior joint space. A small amount of local anesthesia (1% lidocaine with 1:100,000

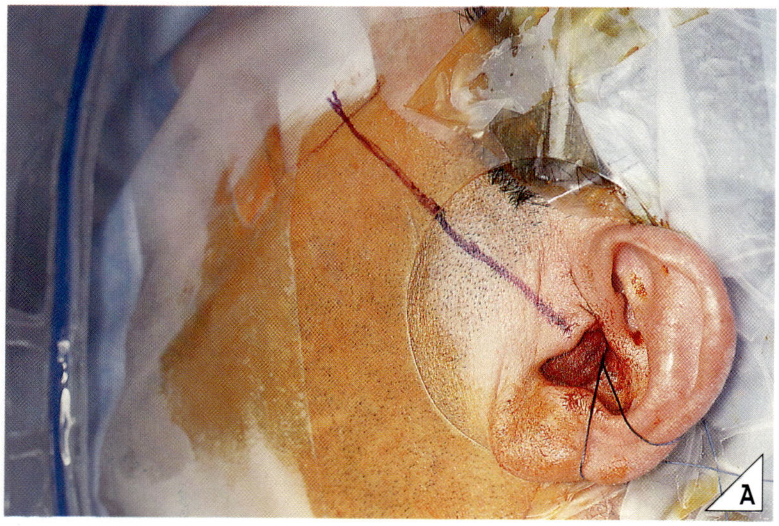

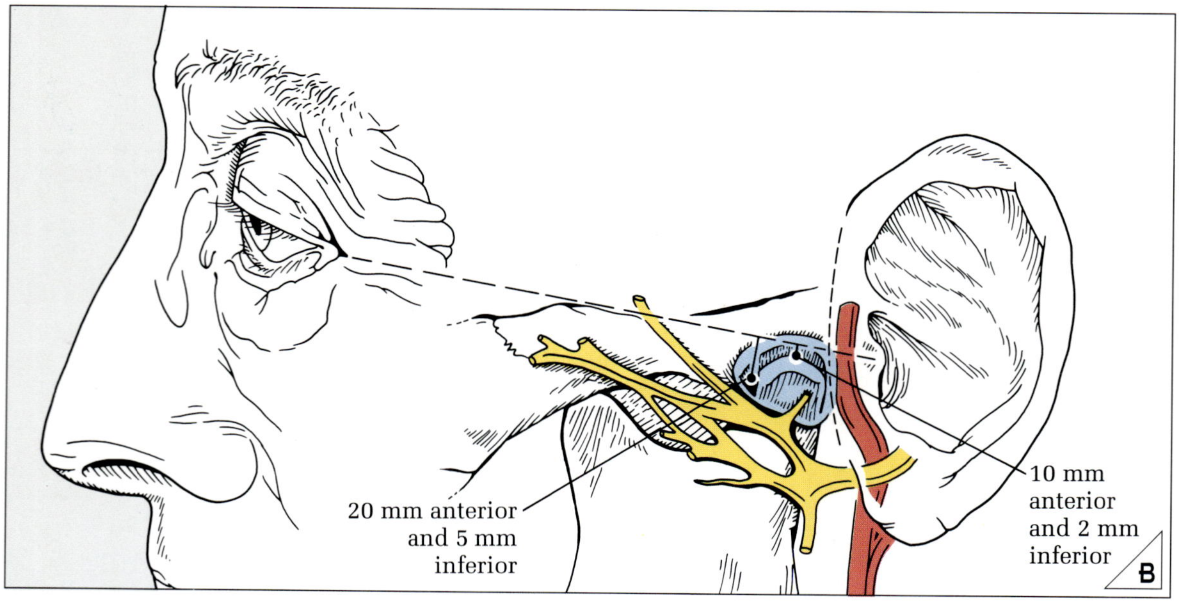

Figure 26.8

(A) The tragus-canthus, or Holmlund-Hellsing (HH), line.
(B) Schematic illustration showing puncture sites with relationship to the HH line, temporal and zygomatic branches of the facial nerve, and superficial temporal artery.

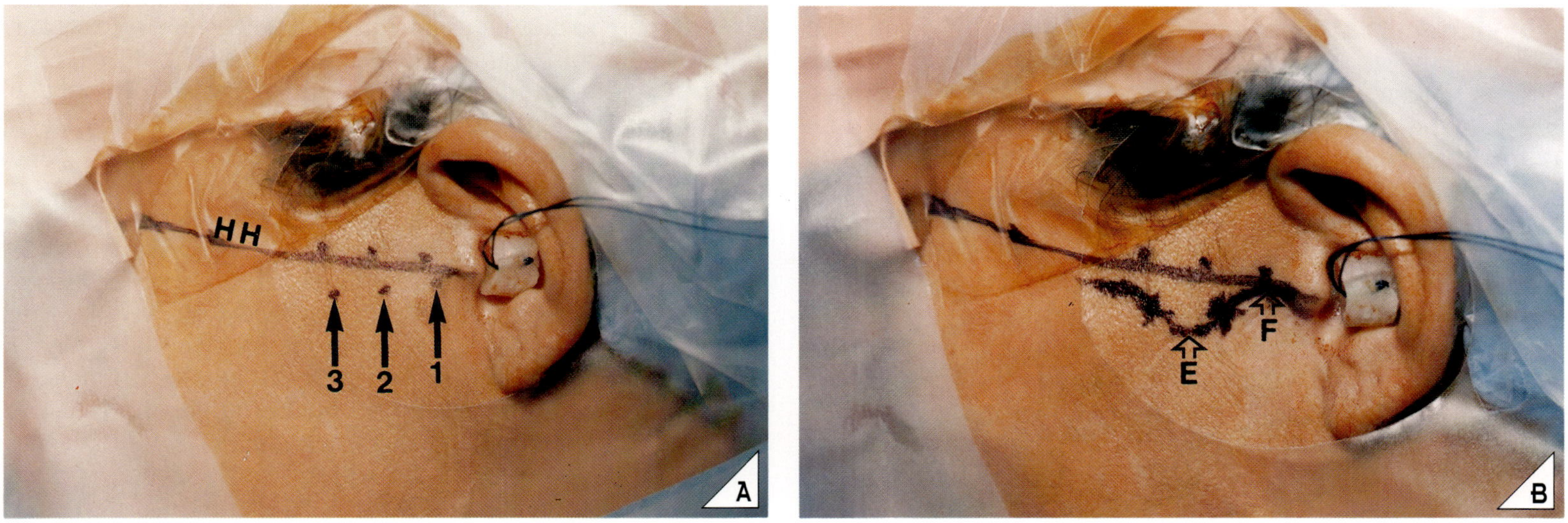

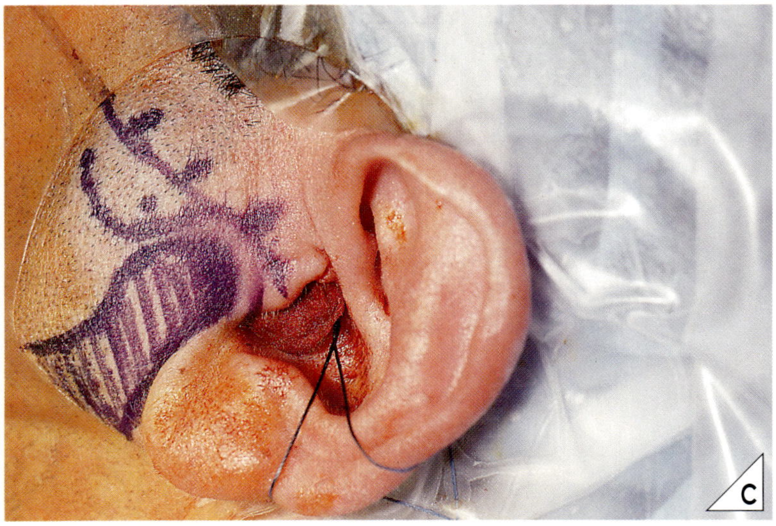

Figure 26.9

(A) The points of safe joint entry with respect to the HH line. 1=10 mm along the HH line and 2 mm inferior to it (fossa puncture); 2=20 mm along the HH line and 5 mm inferior to it; 3=30 mm along the HH line and 10 mm inferior to it. (B) Outline of the fossa after the jaw is distracted downward and forward. E=eminence; F=glenoid fossa. (C) Outline of the left TMJ marked on the skin after palpation and the points for joint entry.

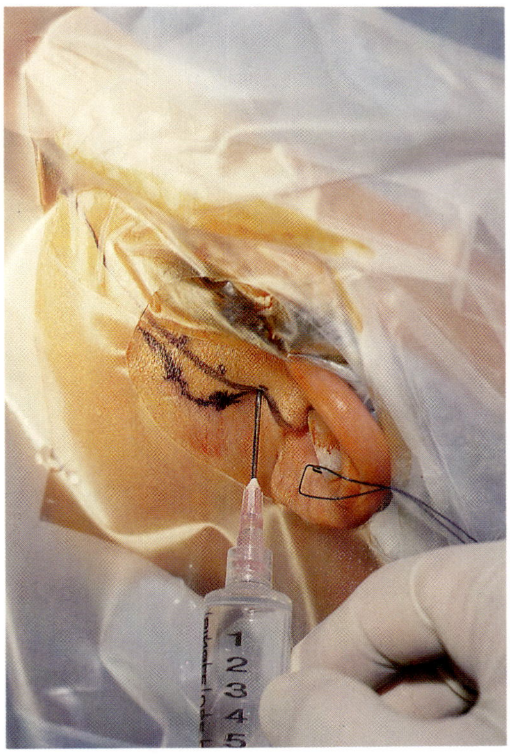

Figure 26.10

Needle inserted inferolaterally to insufflate the left TMJ with irrigating fluid. The goal is to aim the needle towards the posterior slope of the eminence.

epinephrine) can be injected for hemostasis into the skin and preauricular tissues in the region of needle and syringe placement.

A #11 blade is then used to make a vertical stab incision, approximately 3 to 4 mm in length, through the skin. A sharp trocar-and-cannula system (1.9 mm or 2.9 mm in diameter) is inserted through this incision and directed through the preauricular tissues in a swiveling motion towards the posterior slope of the eminence and into the superior joint space (Figs. 26.11, 26.12). The trocar and cannula pierce the capsule and enter the superior joint space with a "snap." The sharp trocar is then exchanged for the blunt trocar, and the trocar-and-cannula system is further advanced into the superior joint space by the same path used for placement of the needle for insufflation. This maneuver achieves clean entry into the joint space without penetrating the retrodiscal tissues (Fig. 26.13).

McCain[7] has described a technique in which the sharp trocar and its sheath are placed through the skin, with or without a small stab incision, at the same site as described above. The trocar is advanced with a rotating motion towards the inferior border of the zygomatic arch approximately 10° horizontally outward from the skin and 10° below the tragus-canthus line. Once the inferior border is contacted, the trocar is further advanced with a swiveling motion along the bony surface to penetrate the lateral capsule. After the capsule is penetrated, the sharp trocar is replaced by the blunt trocar and further advanced into the superior joint space. The surgeon can get a feel for the bony surface anatomy of the upper joint space by gently

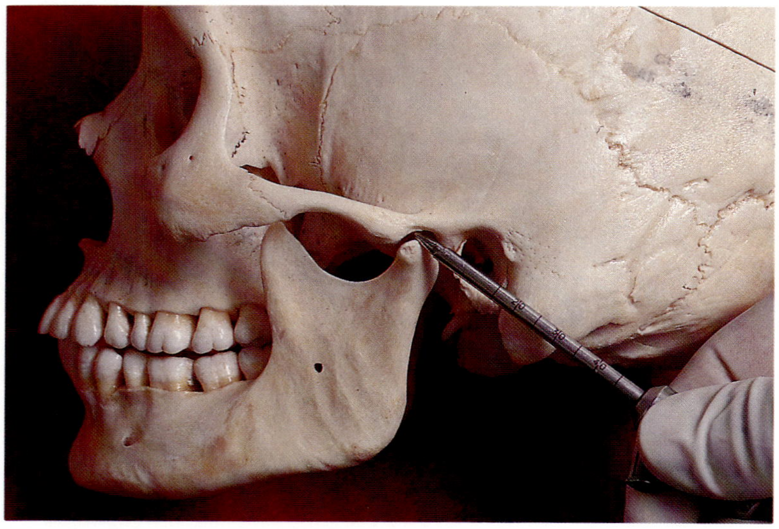

Figure 26.11

Joint entry is depicted on the skull aiming the trocar and cannula towards the posterior slope of the eminence.

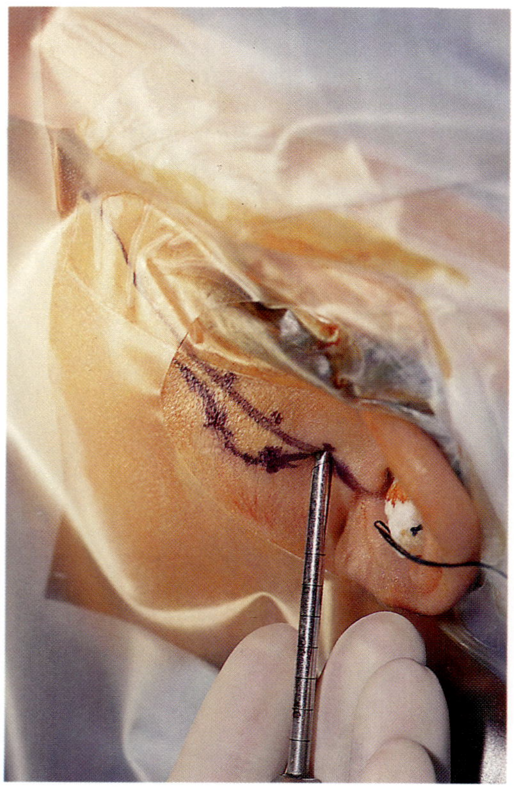

Figure 26.12

The trocar and cannula system is inserted into the superior joint space of the left TMJ through a small vertical stab incision.

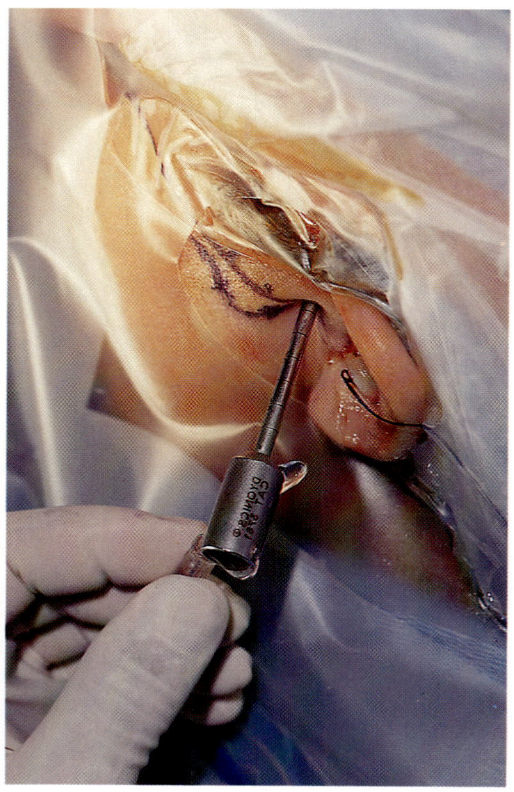

Figure 26.13

The cannula is now placed into the intra-articular space of the superior joint space.

probing with the end of the blunt trocar. Caution must be exercised because the roof of the glenoid fossa is quite thin, averaging about 0.9 mm, and therefore can be easily penetrated. The junction of the bony and cartilaginous auditory canal is another area in which penetration into vital structures may occur.

With the cannula placed in the superior joint space, the arthroscope can be seated in the cannula to confirm successful joint entry. An outflow needle (either an 18-gauge 1.5 inch needle or an 18-gauge spinal needle) can be placed anterior to this cannula to establish through-and-through irrigation (Fig. 26.14). It is assumed that the camera is focused before placement in the superior joint space.

It is essential to develop a systematic method for examining the joint thoroughly, recording the color, texture, surface, and general appearance of all the joint tissues and the position of the disc. The arthroscopist can begin examination at the upper posterior synovial pouch, examining the posterior attachment or retrodiscal tissue as it arises from the pterygotympanic fissure. Although vascular markings are normal in the region of the retrodiscal tissue and synovium, increased vascular markings indicate various stages of synovitis. The upper posterior synovial pouch is best examined when the assistant distracts the mandible forward, displacing the condyle from the glenoid fossa along the slope of the eminence and beyond. The arthroscope is now gently moved from the posterior pouch into the intermediate space. Along the way the tissues lining the roof of the fossa and the slope of the eminence must be evaluated, including the superior surface of the disc, located inferiorly in the visual field. Disc roofing of the condylar head can also be determined at this time. As the operator prepares to advance the scope anteriorly from the intermediate space into the anterior synovial pouch, the scope must be slightly withdrawn and yet still be in the intraarticular space to advance along the lateral trough or lateral paradiscal groove. As the scope is maneuvered into the upper anterior synovial pouch, the assistant should try slowly to reseat the condyle in the glenoid fossa to allow opening and entry to the anterior pouch. An obvious triangular space is formed between the apex of the eminence and the anterior portion of the disc when this movement has been accomplished (see Fig. 26.4).

The color and surface texture of the bone and disc, tissue color of the synovial pouches, fibrillations of the fibrocartilage, vascularity of the synovium, the medial drape of the capsule, and medial and lateral paradiscal grooves are evaluated to establish a diagnosis. The size of the anterior pouch or recess should be assessed and recorded, as it indicates the degree of disc displacement. The results of the preoperative imaging should correlate with the clinical presentation. The disc is further examined for perforations in all directions, particularly lateral-

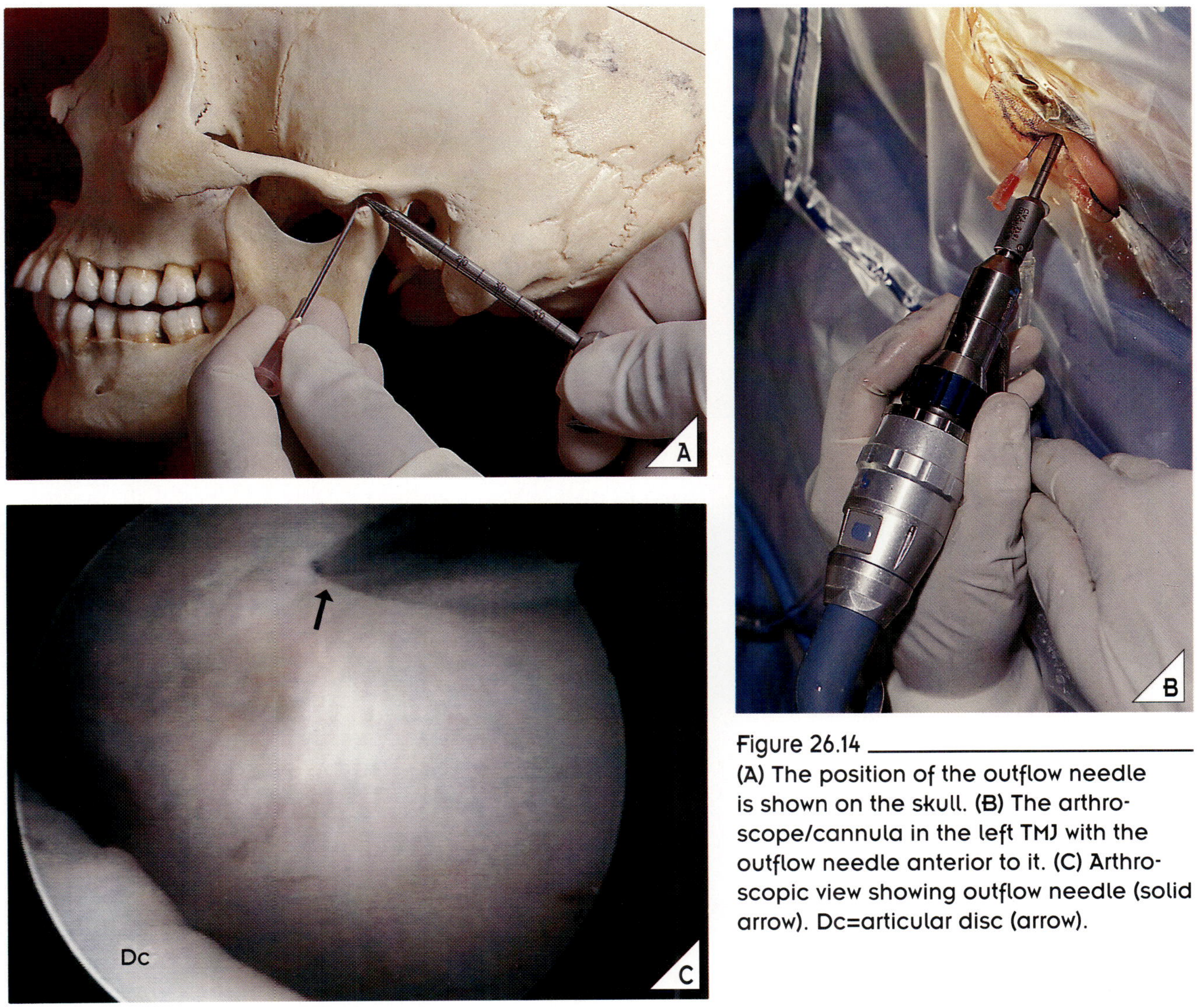

Figure 26.14
(A) The position of the outflow needle is shown on the skull. (B) The arthroscope/cannula in the left TMJ with the outflow needle anterior to it. (C) Arthroscopic view showing outflow needle (solid arrow). Dc=articular disc (arrow).

ly. The condylar head should be examined when perforation is present, and the inferior joint space can be inspected through the perforation.

A double-portal technique requires the placement of a second cannula further anteriorly along the tragus-canthus line so the scope and surgical instruments can be interchanged anteriorly and posteriorly for specific surgical procedures (Fig. 26.15). The double-portal technique is required for triangulation procedures (Fig. 26.16). Triangulation allows direct visualization of the working cannula, and the instruments for the surgical procedures pass through it. An angled lens, such as a 30° arthroscope, makes the triangulation procedure easier, and joint visualization can be achieved by merely rotating the arthroscope, keeping the camera oriented to the 6 o'clock–12 o'clock position so that the joint can be viewed through a full 360°. The instruments must be moved in unison throughout the joint, keeping the working instrument in view as the surgery is performed.

Endaural Approach: Rationale and Technique

The endaural puncture technique was originally described by Ohnishi.[8–10] As described by Dr. Jeffrey Moses, it allows access to the lateral and medial joint. In lateral capsular synovial perforations, capsular herniations, and disc impingement, capsular access is an important diagnostic tool. This approach allows access to the medial and lateral paradiscal grooves for retrieval of loose bodies and broken instruments. To perform this technique, a 30° angled arthroscope is recommended, with the visual access oriented towards the light cord so that the light cord is not forced across the patient's temporal area.

It is best to gain initial entry into the superior joint space via the standard superior posterolateral approach. Once this is accomplished, the arthroscope is rotated and angled superiorly, posteriorly, and laterally so that the light shines through the anterior wall of the external auditory canal, usually about 1 to 1.5 cm medial to the lateral edge of the tragus. The anterior wall of the external auditory canal is perforated with a sharp trocar and cannula while the mandible is distracted forward and downward (Figs. 26.17, 26.18). The direction of the cannula should be anterosuperior and slightly medial, perpendicular to the posterior slope of the eminence. These instruments must enter the joint above the level of the arthroscope to access the superior compartment. Penetration into the joint space through this approach should not be more than 1.5 cm, and visual confirmation can be done with the arthroscope placed in the inferolateral portal.

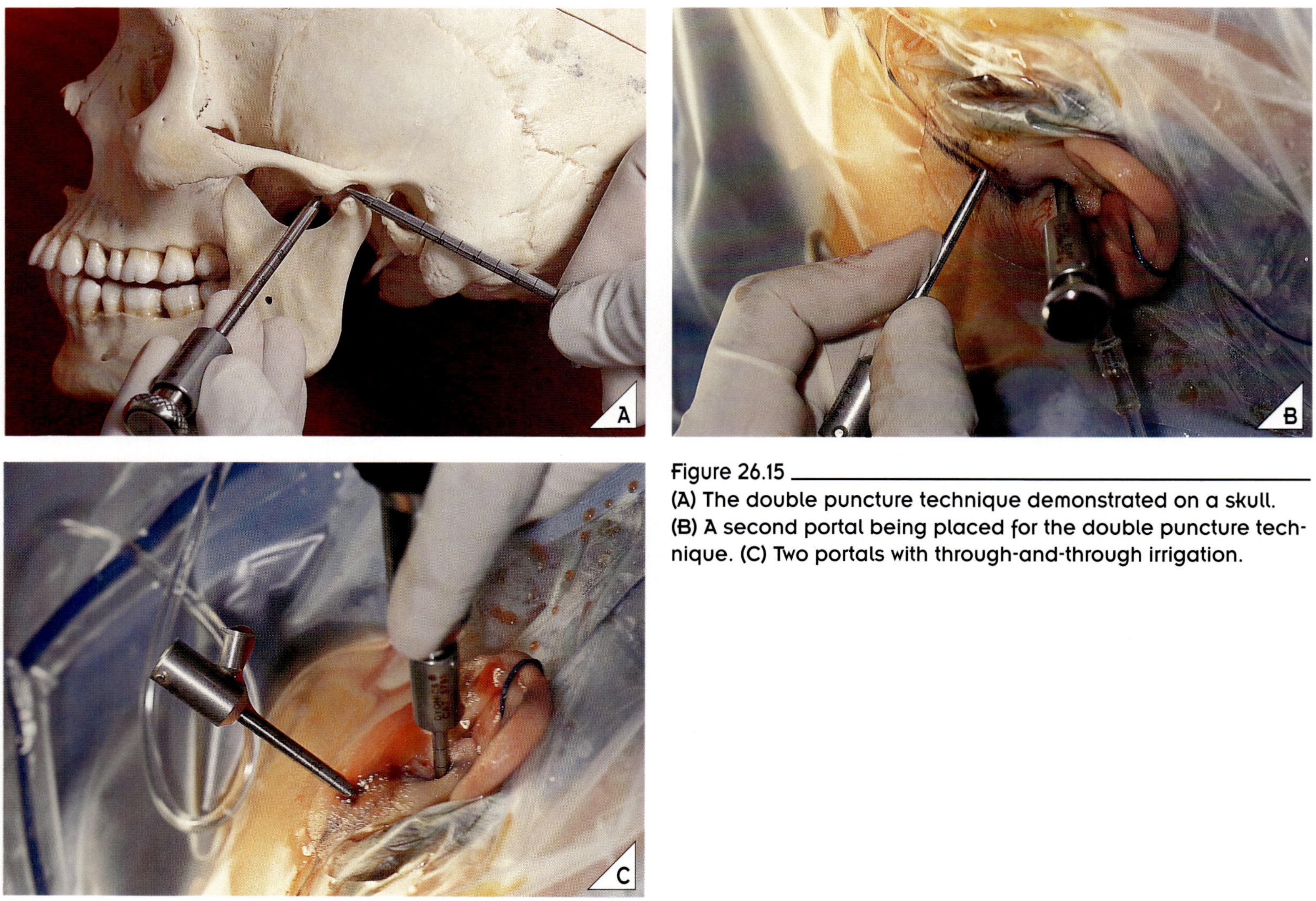

Figure 26.15

(A) The double puncture technique demonstrated on a skull. (B) A second portal being placed for the double puncture technique. (C) Two portals with through-and-through irrigation.

Additional confirmation of the endaural portal can be done by outflow of irrigation from the endaural cannula.

By rotating the arthroscope, the medial, lateral, and superior aspects (superior joint space) of the TMJ can be examined. The anterolateral synovial space can be visualized through this approach, which is difficult to do from any of the other approaches. The skilled operator can achieve direct puncture through the anterior wall of the external auditory canal into the TMJ without the need for superior posterolateral cannulation and transillumination. The cartilaginous elastic membrane of the canal closes the puncture site, which therefore requires no special dressing. Routine otoscopic examination is always performed after arthroscopy to visualize the external auditory meatus and tympanic membrane, particularly when the endaural approach is used, to rule out iatrogenic damage.

Arthroscopic Pathology and Treatment

Soft Tissue Pathology

Intracapsular Fibrosis of the Superior Compartment

This immobility is a common finding in TMJ disease.[11] The disc can be immobilized in many different positions, from within the glenoid fossa to beyond the eminence. These variations in the position of the disc can be found in patients with normal range of motion as well as in those with almost total immobility (e.g., bony ankylosis). Although several factors can contribute to disc immobilization, a major factor is intracapsular fibrosis and fibro-osseous pathosis.

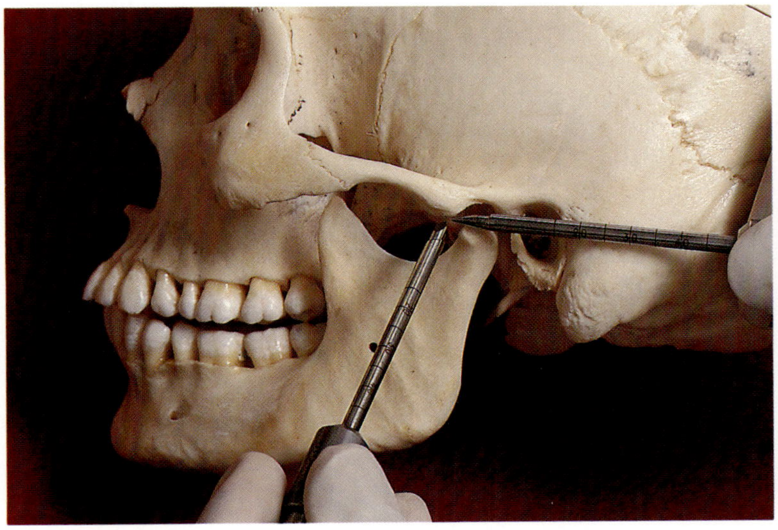

Figure 26.16
The triangulation technique being demonstrated on a skull.

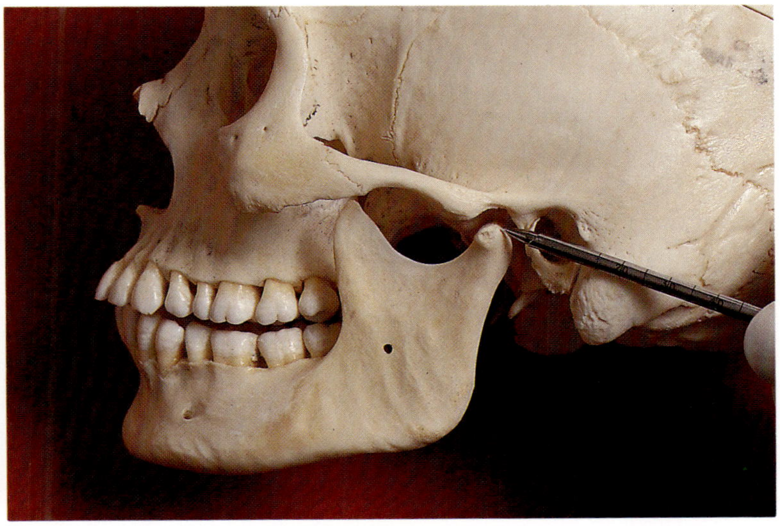

Figure 26.17
The endaural approach demonstrated on a skull.

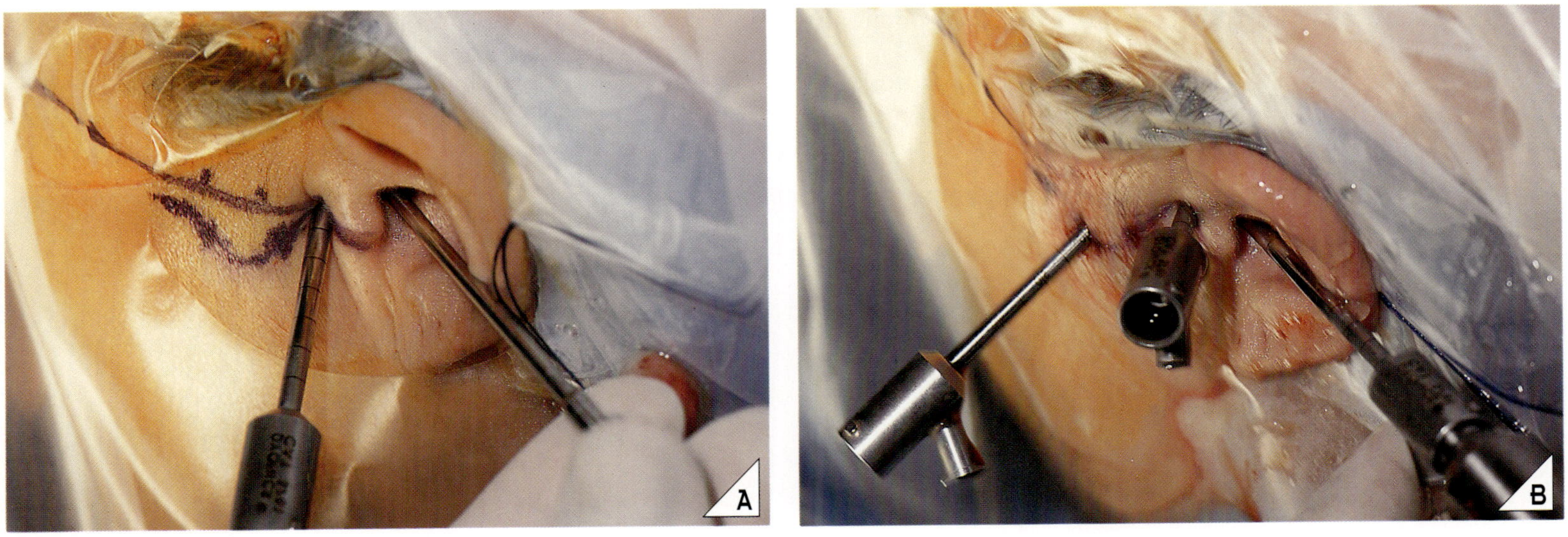

Figure 26.18
(A) Placement of second portal endaurally. (B) Triple puncture including placement of the arthroscope by the endaural approach.

Fibrotic adhesions are the simplest of these fibrous bands, ranging from spider-web-like threads to thick fibrous bands (Fig. 26.19). Histologically, they can range from immature to very mature fibrous tissue. These adhesions usually span the entire joint compartment. Superiorly, they are attached by periosteum of articular cartilage to the bone of the fossa eminence and inferiorly to the retrodiscal tissue, disc, or "pseudodisc" (remodeled or adaptive retrodiscal tissue). In abnormal joint function caused by micro- or macrotrauma, the synovium is easily injured. During the healing phase fibrin forms and becomes a "sticky" surface. In the "suction cup" effect described by Sanders,[12] the surfaces adhere, the fibrin progresses to a fibrous tissue, and intracapsular fibrosis develops. Other causes of intracapsular fibrosis include hematomas, subsynovial hyperemia, and ecchymosis, all of which commonly occur in the TMJ.

Fibrous synovial bands have the same core as the simple fibrous band, except a layer of synovial tissue covers the fibrous tissue. This appears to be a natural progression of the disease process. Histologically, synovial cells at the base of these lesions appears to proliferate and migrate across the fibrous bands. Occasionally there is an area of distinct fibrosis between the eminence and the junction of the bilaminar zone and the disc or pseudodisc.

In capsular fibrosis the normal capsule, both medially and laterally, appears arthroscopically as a homogeneous series of vertical oblique fibers covered by a layer of synovial tissue. In such fibrosis of the lateral capsule, the lateral paradiscal groove along the inferior aspect is usually obliterated.

Discal osseous bands consist of a fibrous band attached to medullary bone, whereas almost all other types of fibrosis attach to the cortical bone via the periosteum. The discal osseous band originates in the medullary bone and penetrates the cortex via an orifice in the layer. This may help to explain one of the factors in intracapsular pain, since there are few pain fibers within the TMJ but many in the bone.

The term "pseudowall" is used to describe fibrous or fibrosynovial "walls" of tissues, partially or completely traversing the joint space from the medial to the lateral capsule. These may arise from the anterior slope, apex, or posterior slope of the eminence, although the majority are found along the anterior slope (Fig. 26.20). Inferiorly, this wall is attached to normal retrodiscal tissue, pseudodisc, or disc. Fibrosynovial pseudowalls completely divide the superior joint space into different compartments. Most of these walls are covered with synovium that exhibits various degrees of inflammation.

Both chronic and severe degenerative joint disease may cause large perforations or loss of large areas of the disc, exposing more than 75% of the articulating surfaces of the condyle to the superior joint space. Interosseous fibrosis usually occurs between the osseous elements of the fossa or eminence and the condyle. Synovial coverings are usually not seen in these cases. Fibroosseous and osseous adhesions are more logically referred to as fibroosseous anklyosis. Occasionally bony ankylosis is indistinguishable from intracapsular fibrosis.

Treatment

In most cases the fibrous tissue is very fragile and soft, so that merely positioning and moving the arthroscope within the superior joint compartment breaks up these tissues spontaneously. Usually a hook probe or a basket forceps can very efficiently take these bands down, opening up the joint space and restoring mobility in the disc. However, if the tissues have matured, resection and surgical release of these bands may be very difficult and time consuming. When the pathologic process has progressed to calcification or ossification, arthrotomy is required. In capsular fibrosis, arthroscopic transection or stretching of these restrictive bands helps improve joint immobility and reduce pain.

Synovial Chondromatosis

Synovial chondromatosis is an uncommon benign condition characterized by formation of multiple cartilaginous nodules in the synovial membrane via metaplasia within the subintimal connective tissue layer of the synovial membrane.[13–15] These nodules may detach from the syn-

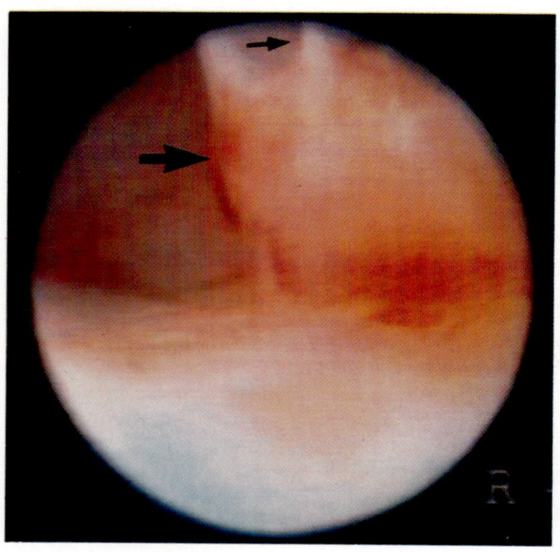

Figure 26.19
Arthroscopic view of the right TMJ showing fibrous adhesions (arrows).

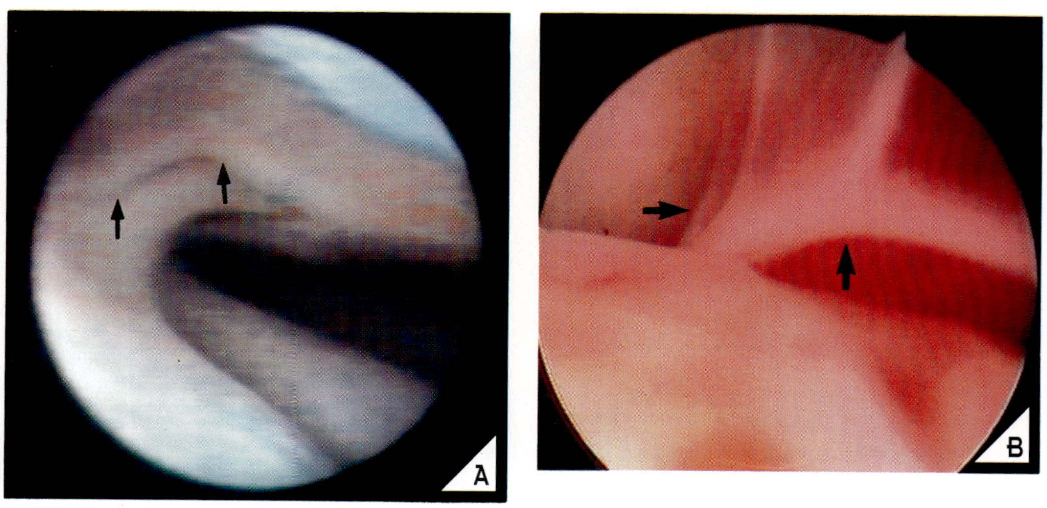

Figure 26.20
(A) Pseudowall (arrows) demonstrated with a probe. (B) Pseudowall formation (arrows) in anterior pouch of the right TMJ.

ovial membrane and move into the joint compartment as free intraarticular loose bodies or "joint mice" (Fig. 26.21). The condition is usually monoarticular and affects the larger joints of the body, especially the knee, hip, ankle, and elbow. The first case of synovial chondromatosis of the TMJ was reported by Axhausen in 1933.[16] Although they are detached in the joint space, the joint mice are nourished by the synovial fluid, and therefore they remain viable and continue to grow. The pathogenesis of synovial chondromatosis remains unsolved, although several proposed etiologic factors affecting the TMJ have been published. These include injury to the joint area (macrotrauma), chronic low-grade trauma (microtrauma), inflammation, malocclusion, and subluxation. Synovial chondromatosis of the larger joints affects men twice as often as women, usually in the fourth and fifth decades. However, when the TMJ is affected the condition shows a great predilection for women, with a 4:1 female-to-male ratio. Most patients are between 18 and 75 years of age, with a mean of 47 years. All reported cases have been monoarticular, the right TMJ being affected more often. TMJ synovial chondromatosis must be considered as a diagnosis for patients who complain of slowly progressive preauricular swelling, pain, crepitus, and limited range of motion in the region of the TMJ. Other signs and symptoms include otologia, malocclusion, stiffness of the joint, popping, deviation of the joint opening, and inability to open the mouth.[13] Confirmation of the diagnosis can be obtained only after a histological examination of the resected specimen.

Treatment

The treatment of synovial chondromatosis described in the literature ranges from conservative surgical removal of the loose bodies and lavage of the joint to removal of the nodules with total synovectomy, meniscectomy, and even condylectomy to gain access to the medial synovial lining.[17–19] The most widely accepted treatment is joint debridement with synovectomy. Most authors advocate a preauricular approach to the joint. After the joint mice have been removed the synovium should be carefully inspected and, if diseased, should be removed as completely as possible to prevent recurrence of the lesion.

Articular Pathology

Discussion of the pathophysiology and progression of disease involving internal derangement of the TMJ is not within the scope of this chapter.

Disc Displacement with Reduction

In displacement of the disc with reduction the disc is in an abnormal position at rest, anteriorly, anteromedially, or anteriorly and laterally (Fig. 26.22). These patients may

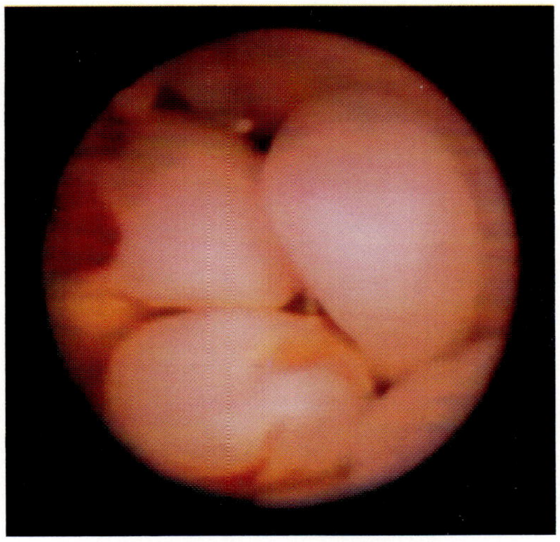

Figure 26.21
A case of synovial chondromatosis. (Courtesy of Dr. Robert Schwartz).

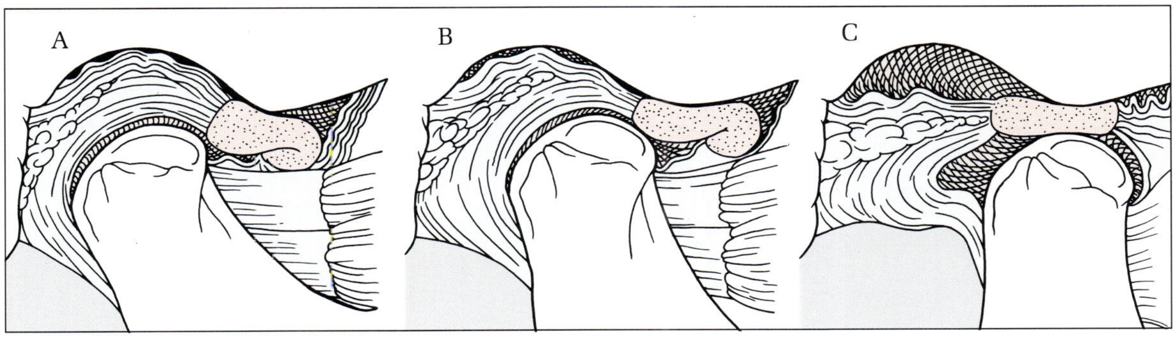

Figure 26.22
(A–C) Sagittal views through the right TMJ showing disc displacement with reduction. C is an open mouth view.

present with clicking on opening and closing of the mouth ("reciprocal clicking") and with lateral and endaural point tenderness of the TMJ region. They may have normal or restricted jaw opening and a compromised range of motion. The degree and direction of the displacement are confirmed by arthrography or MRI (Fig. 26.23).

Treatment

Treatment of the symptomatic patient is usually nonsurgical, with fabrication of an orthotic. Patients who are refractory to nonsurgical therapy become surgical candidates. Such patients can be treated by arthroscopic lysis and lavage of the superior joint space, with possible suturing back of the disc to reduce or eliminate the noxious joint noise.

Disc Displacement Without Reduction

In patients with disc displacement without reduction, the disc is displaced anteriorly, anteromedially, or anteriorly and laterally in the rest position (Fig. 26.24). Clinically, these patients may present in the acute phase with extreme tenderness over the TMJ region, and significantly restricted opening of the mouth and decreased range of motion. In the chronic stage they may continue to exhibit tenderness over the TMJ region, although not quite as exquisite, with some restoration of the range of motion. Restoration to some degree of jaw opening is made possible by the stretching and adaptive remodeling of the retrodiscal tissue. The direction and degree of disc displacement are confirmed by arthrography or MRI (Figs. 26.25, 26.26).

Treatment

Initial treatment consists of fabrication of an orthotic, a restricted nonchewing diet, and nonsteroidal antiinflammatory medication. If the patient's condition continues to be refractory to nonsurgical therapy, arthroscopic surgery becomes an option. This would include lysis and lavage or an anterior release and posterior cauterization, as described by McCain. Lysis and lavage procedures are performed with a blunt or a hooked probe, sweeping the superior joint space from the posterior synovial pouch to the anterior synovial pouch.

The anterior release and posterior cauterization procedure uses a double-puncture technique. The arthroscope is placed into the posterior synovial pouch and then

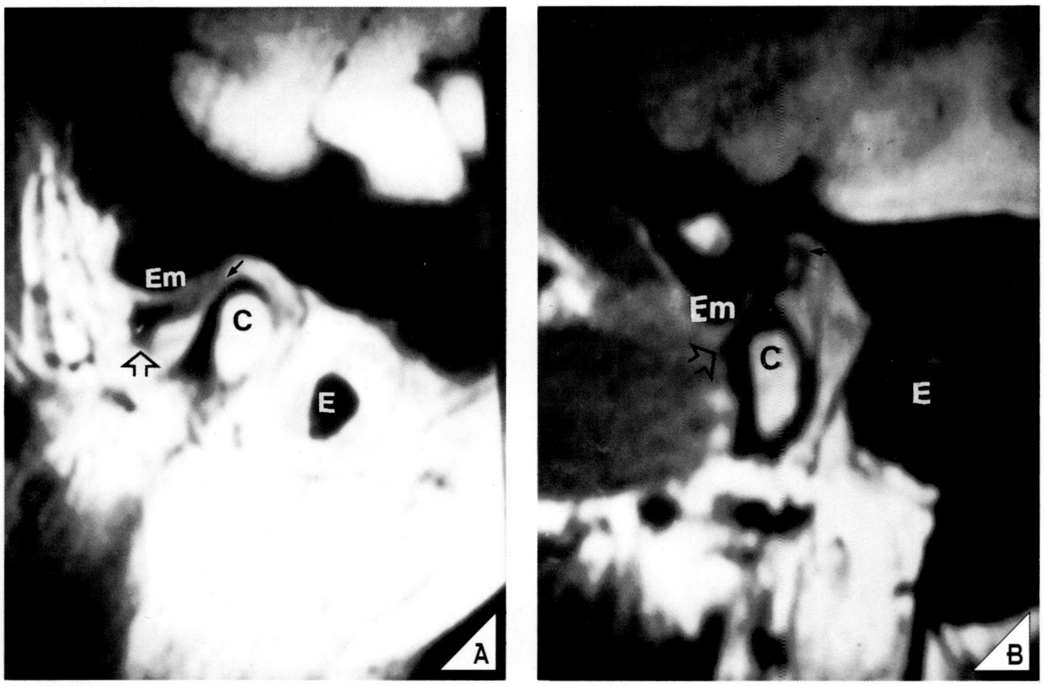

Figure 26.23
MRI of the left TMJ showing displacement with reduction of the disc. (A) Closed mouth view showing displacement of disc (arrows). (B) Open mouth view showing reduction of disc (arrows). C=condyle; E=ear canal; Em=eminence (Courtesy of Dr. Javier Beltran)

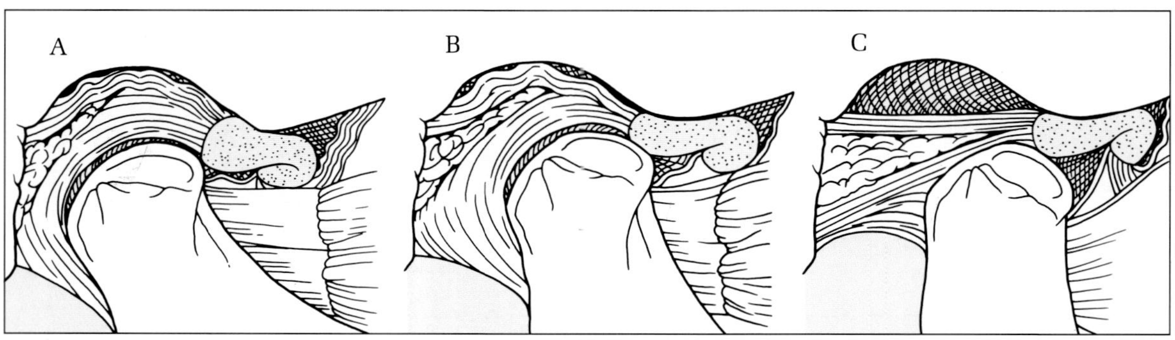

Figure 26.24
(A–C) Sagittal views through the right TMJ showing disc displacement with no reduction. C is an open mouth view.

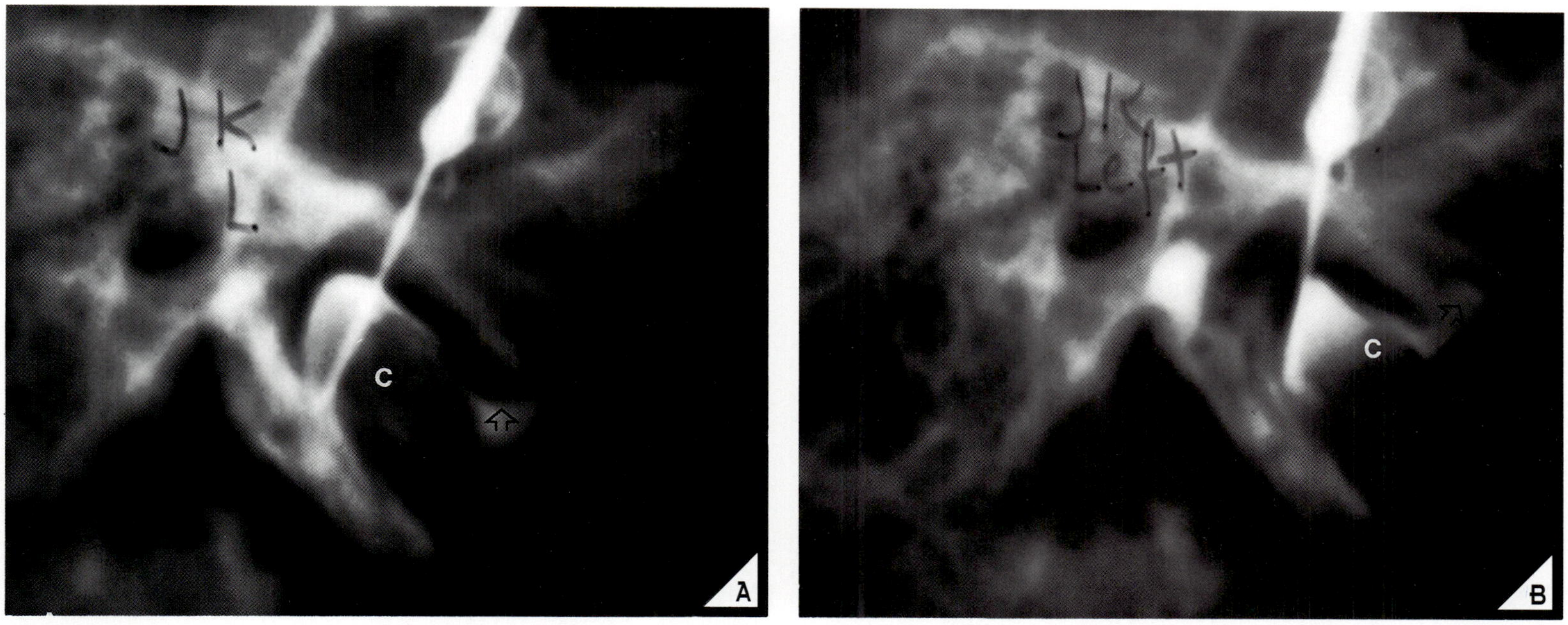

Figure 26.25

(A) Arthrography of the right inferior joint space of the TMJ (closed mouth view) showing displacement of the disc (open arrow). C=condyle. (Courtesy of Dr. Javier Beltran) (B) Open mouth view showing displacement of disc (open arrow). C=condyle. (Courtesy of Dr. Javier Beltran)

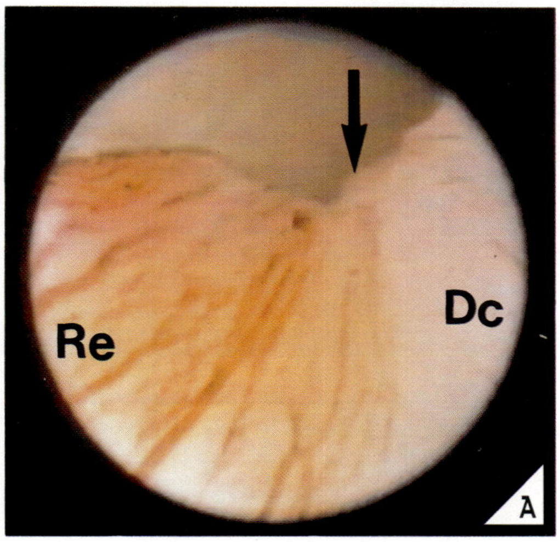

Figure 26.26

(A) Arthroscopic view of anterior displacement with no reduction in the right TMJ. The arrow points towards the junction of retrodiscal tissue and disc. Re=retrodiscal tissue; Dc=disc. (B) MRI of left TMJ showing displacement of disc (arrows), closed mouth, C=condyle; E=ear canal. (C) Open mouth view showing displacement of disc (arrows). C=condyle; E=eminence.

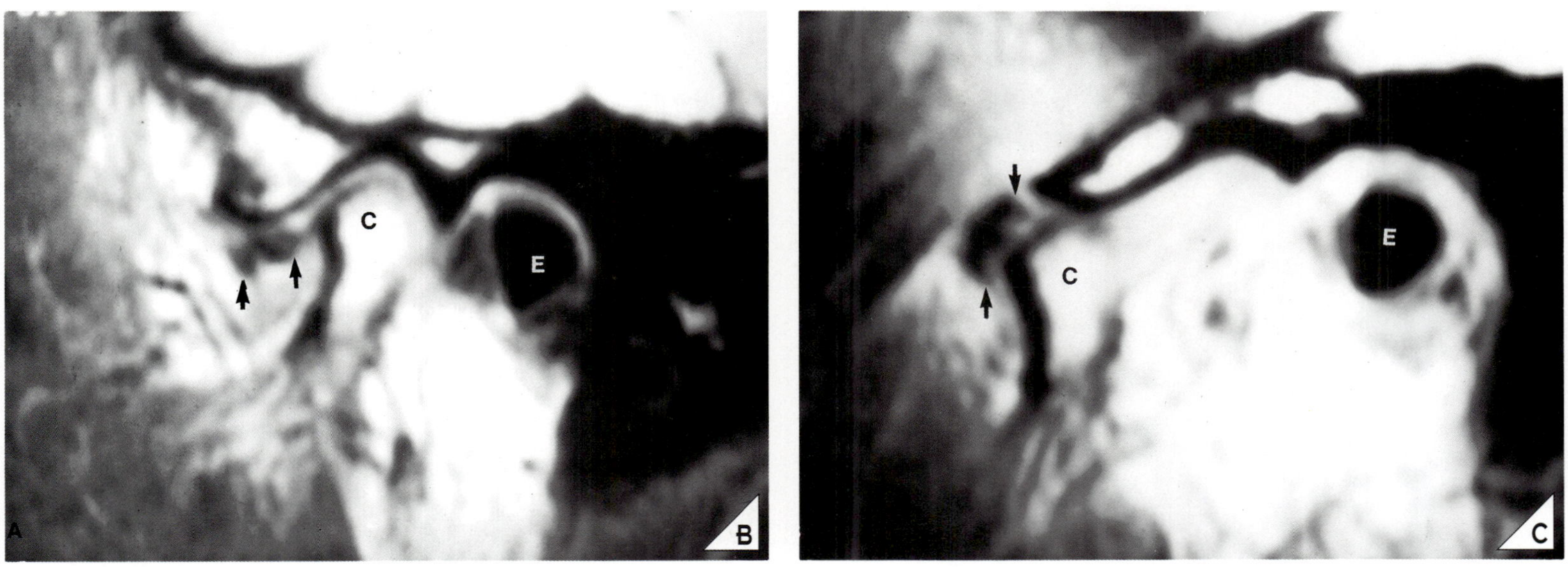

moved into the anterior synovial pouch where, under direct visualization, a working cannula is placed into the anterior synovial pouch. The disc is released anteriorly by an incision in front of the disc through the synovial tissues down to the pterygoid muscle, medial to lateral, with microscissors, electrosurgery, or laser (Fig. 26.27). With blunt hand instruments such as a hook probe, this incision is defined, and the disc is freely moved posteriorly towards the posterior synovial pouch. I prefer to use an electrosurgical unit such as a disposable monopolar cautery (Concept) or a contact laser such as the holmium laser. The arthroscope and the working cannula are next moved from the anterior to the posterior synovial pouch, where attention is directed to the retrodiscal tissue. A blunt probe is inserted through the working cannula and the disc is teased posteriorly to reduce the disc. At this point the cautery tip or the laser contact tip is passed through the working cannula and the retrodiscal tissue is cauterized (Fig. 26.28). The scarification of the retrodiscal tissue achieved by the cautery unit and/or the laser unit should reduce the disc. When the disc has been reduced and is found to maintain its normal position, suturing techniques can be employed either for traction or for suturing the disc back. Suturing of the disc is done with a spinal needle, a suture stick, or a meniscus mender (Fig. 26.29).

Hypermobility Syndrome

Posterior cauterization for hypermobility syndrome was originally described by Ohnishi. Scarification in the retrodiscal tissue achieved by cauterization of this tissue with an electrosurgical unit or a laser unit should restrict

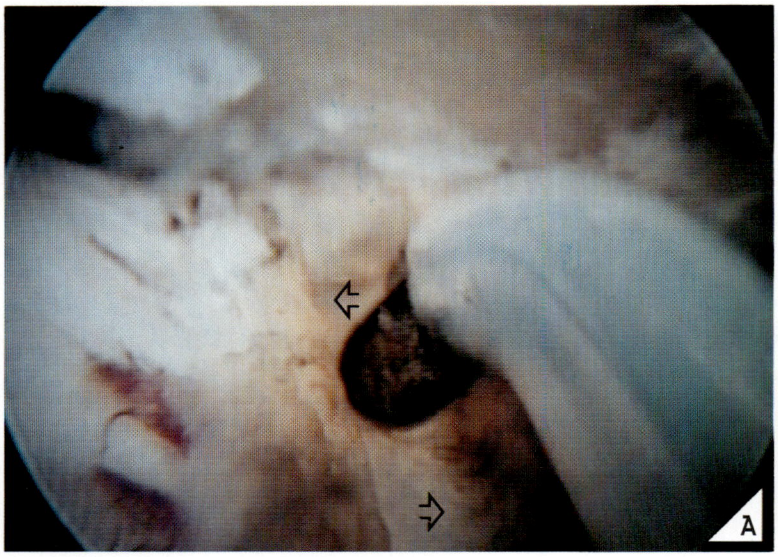

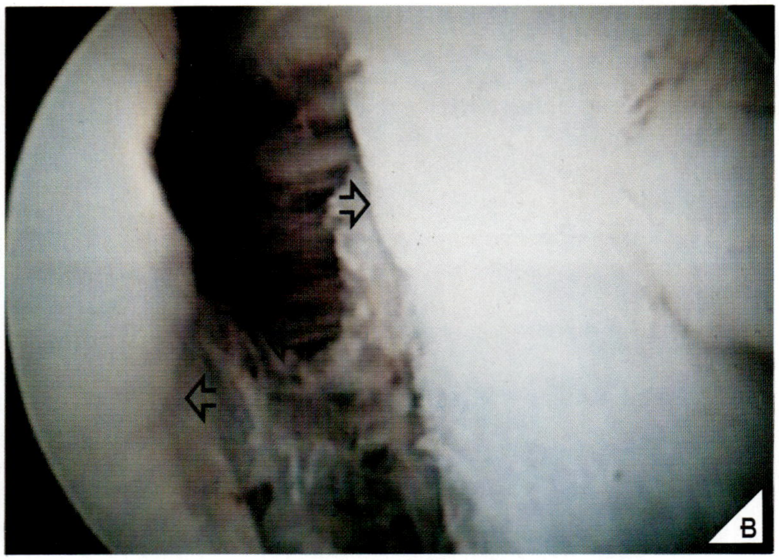

Figure 26.27
(A) Arthroscopic view showing anterior release (arrows) being performed in left TMJ with a monopolar cautery (Concept). (Courtesy of Dr. Allen Tarro) (B) Anterior release completed (arrows). Pterygoid muscle seen in the released area. (Courtesy of Dr. Allen Tarro)

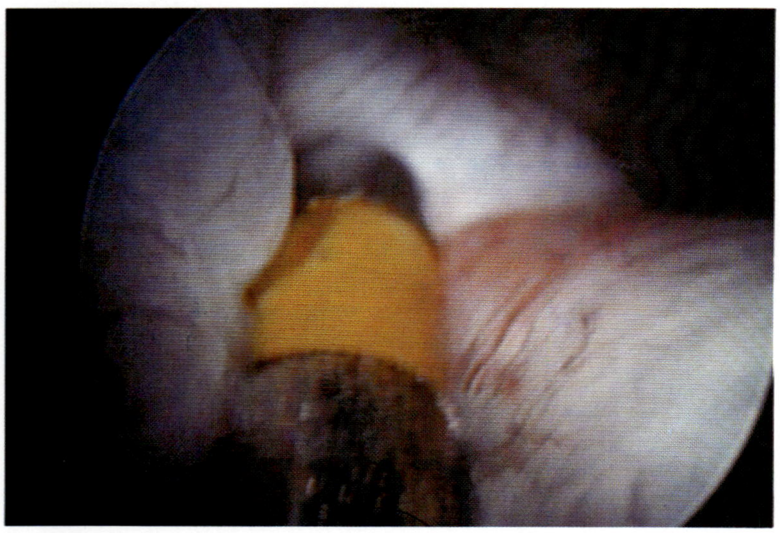

Figure 26.28
Arthroscopic view of the left TMJ showing posterior cauterization (retrodiscal tissue) using a bipolar cautery tip. (Courtesy of Dr. Allen Tarro)

the laxity of the joint (see Fig. 26.28). Merrill advocates injection of 0.25 mL of 1% sodium tetradecyl sulfate (Sotradecol) and 0.5 mL of 0.25% bupivacaine into the oblique protuberance and lateral posterior attachment, to produce the necessary sclerosis and scarring in these structures and to reduce the hypermobility of the joint. Synovial inflammation grades I through IV is addressed by cauterizing these areas or by direct subsynovial injection of betamethasone or dexamethasone into the areas via an 18-gauge spinal needle under arthroscopic control (Fig. 26.30).

Degenerative Joint Disease

Internal derangements over a period of time can progress to degenerative joint disease, in which the patient may or may not present with point tenderness over the TMJ region, with or without functional disability. Auscultation of the joints may reveal a grating sound or crepitus. Radiographic examination is consistent with breakdown of the cortical surface of the condylar head, with or without lipping. There may be corresponding flattening of the apex of the articular eminence. It is not unusual to find large perforations in the disc, secondary to the irregularity

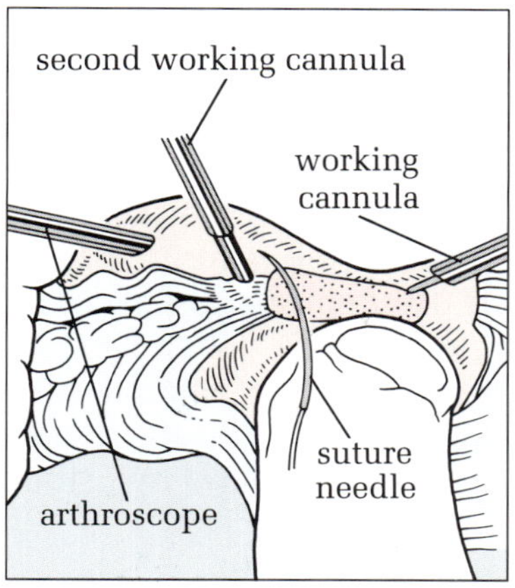

Figure 26.29
Schematic illustration showing a technique for suturing the disc arthroscopically. The arthroscope is placed in the posterior pouch. Two working cannulas and a needle are introduced intraarticularly from inferior to superior, engaging the disc. The suture will be grasped through the second working cannula and tied back to obtain reduction of the displaced disc. (As suggested by Dr. Michael Keslin)

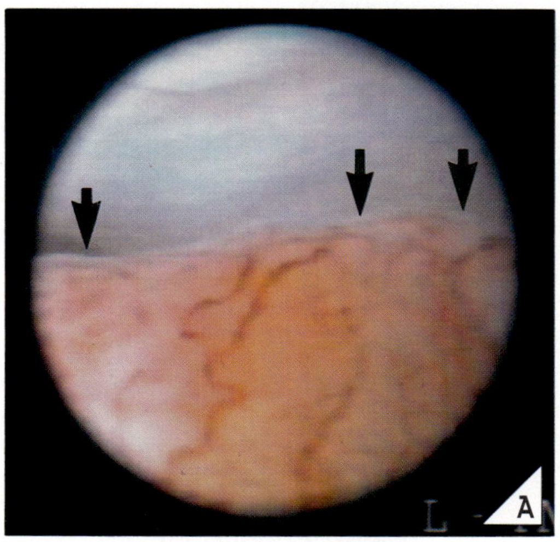

Figure 26.30
(A) Synovitis (grades III and IV) in the left TMJ (arrows). (B) The inflamed tissue is held in place with a straight probe. (C) Holding the inflamed tissue under tension, the spinal needle is placed subsynovially for steroid injection. (Courtesy of Dr. Allen Tarro)

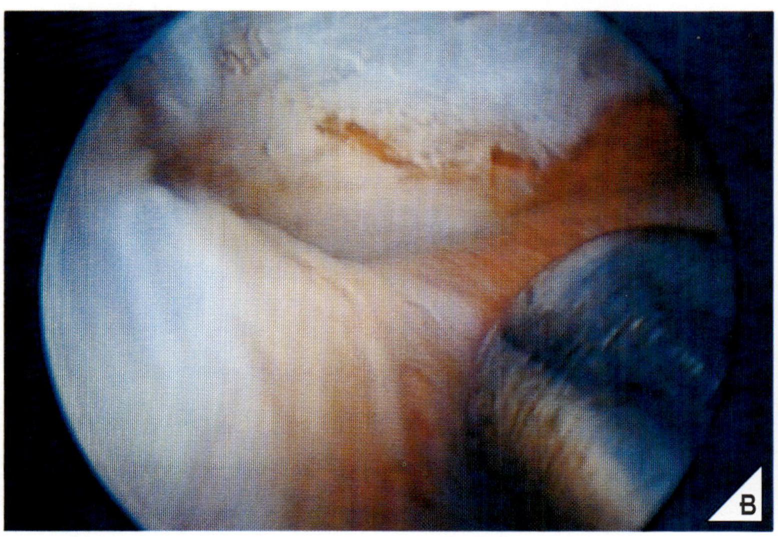

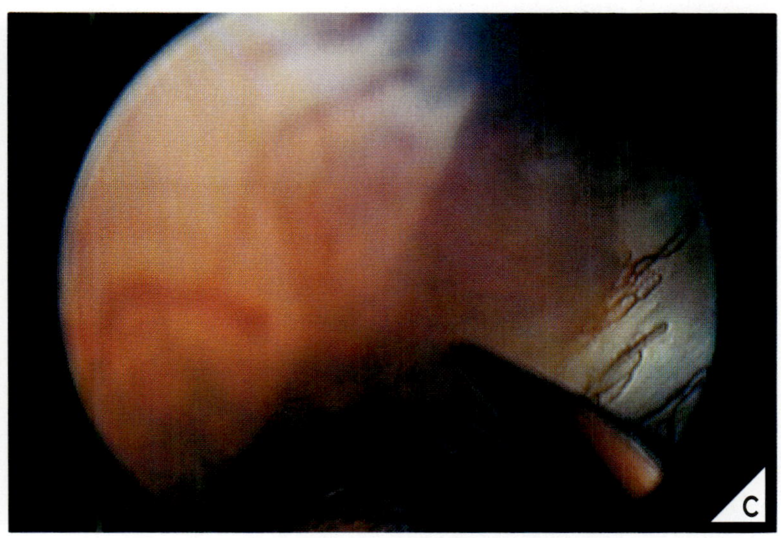

of the underlying condyle (Fig. 26.31). The perforations can be large enough to cause fragmentation of the disc and retrodiscal tissues, anteriorly and posteriorly. Arthrography reveals perforation, evidenced by movement of the dye into the superior joint space from the inferior joint space through the perforation (Fig. 26.32). MRI may reveal fragmentation of the disc and retrodiscal tissue.

Treatment

Arthroscopic treatment in this case consists of partial synovectomy via a cartilage-shaving unit (Fig. 26.33) or a suction punch (Fig. 26.34), followed by taking down and smoothing of the edges of the perforation with motorized and hand instruments. The goal is to restore the translatory movement in the joint.

Disc Displacement and Lateral Impingement Syndrome

The similar symptoms of pain and limitation of motion between the impingement phenomenon of the shoulder and the internal joint derangement of the TMJ led Moses to conclude that an impingement process occurs in the TMJ between the lateral third of the condyle and the eminence. His belief is based on observations with the arthroscopic endaural view, coronal MRI, and anteroposterior protruded-position laminograms in patients who did not respond to conservative treatments for TMJ dysfunction but who did not exhibit classic disc displacement. The pathologic process appears to range from an apparently minor capsulitis with proliferative synovial changes to frank degenerative disease with disc/capsular impingement. The clinical course of this impingement syndrome can range from a reversible condition, to recurrent pain with activity, to progressive disability.

Treatment

In acute capsular synovitis, treatment consists of nonsteroidal antiinflammatory medication, rest, physical therapy, use of an orthotic appliance, intracapsular lysis, and lavage. In chronic adhesive capsulitis, proliferative synovitis, discal displacement or immobility, and synovial plicae the treatment consists of arthroscopic lysis of adhesions, lateral eminence release and capsular stretch, lavage, physical therapy, and use of an orthotic appliance. In discal displacement characterized by immobility, hypoplastic eminence tubercle, and degenerative joint disease, arthroscopic treatment consists of lateral eminence release, capsular stretch, lateral eminence osteoplasty, physical therapy, and an orthotic device.

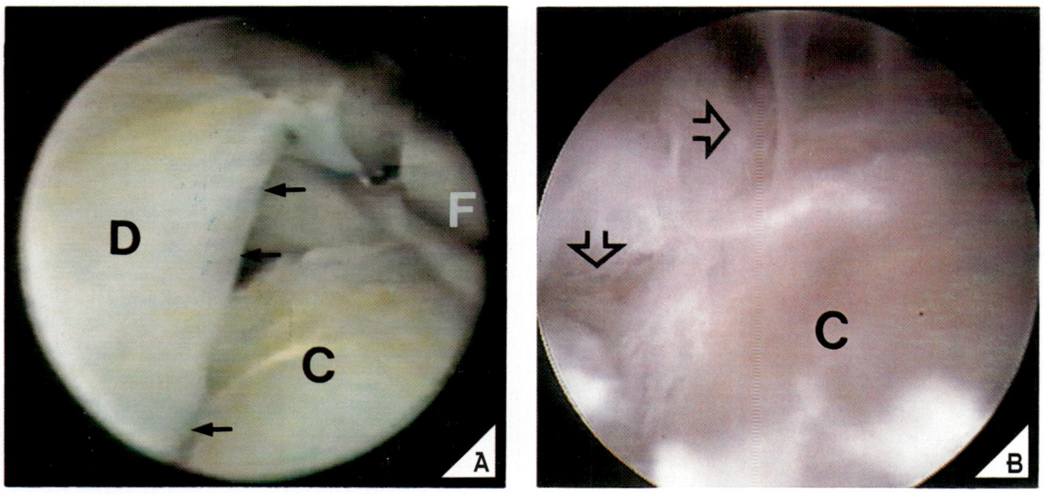

Figure 26.31

(A) Arthroscopic view of perforation (arrows) in the right TMJ. C=condyle; D=disc; F=basket forceps. Basket forceps are holding up the disc through the perforation. (B) Perforation (open arrows) at the junction of the retrodiscal tissue and disc. C=condyle.

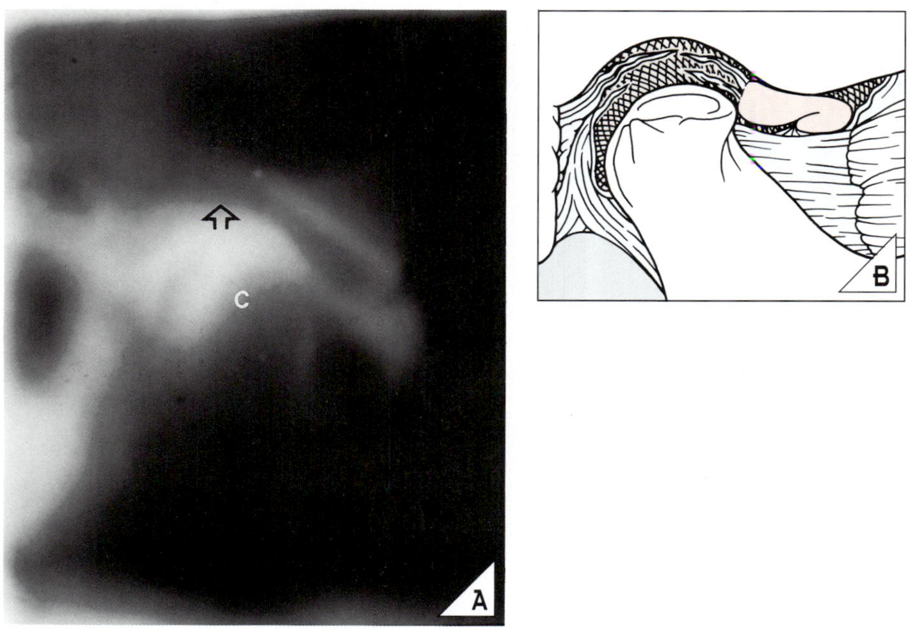

Figure 26.32

(A) Arthrography of the inferior joint space of the right TMJ showing leakage of dye into the superior joint space, suggestive of perforation. (Courtesy of Dr. Javier Beltran) (B) Sagittal view of the right TMJ showing a perforation of the retrodiscal tissue (arrow). C=condyle.

Hard Tissue Pathology

Osteoarthritis

Osteoarthrosis is a noninflammatory disorder that involves the articular cartilage and possibly the synovial membrane and subchondral bone, causing a vicious cycle of cartilage breakdown accompanied by attempts at repair. When the degradative process exceeds the reparative process, the osteoarthritic disorder progresses to a clinically detectable stage.[20,21] Osteoarthrosis of the TMJ is often associated with internal derangement of the joint. The gliding capacity of the articular disc is impaired by the degradative process, which causes disc displacement. Osteoarthrosis is the most common etiology of TMJ disorders, and degenerative changes are easily recognizable during arthroscopy.

Chondromalacia

The term "chondromalacia" was initially used to describe posttraumatic softening of the articular cartilage of the patella in young persons. The anatomic lesions are usually microscopically indistinguishable from those of earlier osteoarthrosis, although several differences have been described. The etiology of chondromalacia is still not well understood. Trauma is considered to be the primary event in the etiology of chondromalacia, and can be divided into two categories: acute trauma and microtrauma. In acute trauma there is a sudden direct injury with high stress loading in a short time frame, leading to loss of a piece of cartilage from the surface of the condyle or death of the chondrocytes over a section of the articular surface. Microtrauma is a repetitive process of damage to the articular surface. Examples of microtrauma affecting the TMJ include clenching and stress bruxism.

According to Quinn,[22] the principal cause of TMJ pain is probably impingement of fragments of degenerative cartilage hanging from the articular eminence between the articular eminence and the disc. Synovitis is one of the earliest signs of degenerative arthritis resulting from microtrauma. Chemical mediators of inflammation and pain, such as bradykinin, prostaglandin E_2, leukotriene B_4, and thromboxane B_2, are believed to be present in the painful dysfunctional TMJ.

The clinical progression chondromalacia of the TMJ is divided into four stages that are observable during

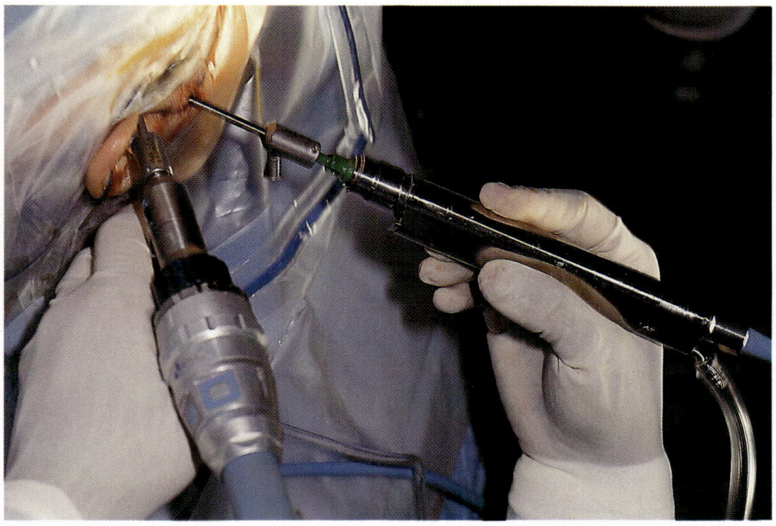

Figure 26.33
The motorized shaver used in the triangulation technique.

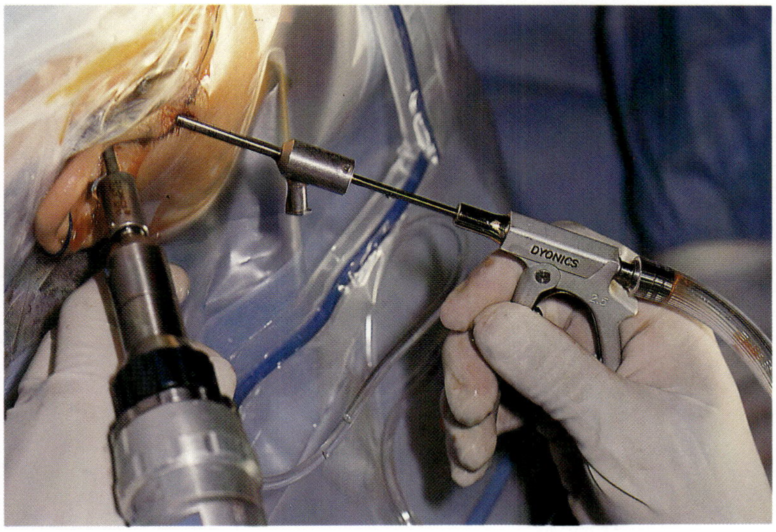

Figure 26.34
The suction punch through the second portal.

arthroscopy. These are stage I softening, stage II furrowing, stage III ulceration and fibrillation, and stage IV crater formation and subchondral bone exposure (Fig. 26.35).

Treatment

Arthroscopy provides a low morbidity approach to the management of chondromalacia. The treatment depends on the stage of degeneration. A motorized shaver is used to carefully remove most of the degenerating hanging strands of fibrillated cartilage in stage III and IV chondromalacia. The cartilaginous loose bodies are removed by suction punch forceps and/or motorized minishavers. In stage IV chondromalacia with exposed bone, abrasion/arthroplasty is performed to remove the surface down to bleeding bone, which encourages granulation tissue to form and possibly cover the bone with fibrocartilage.

The treatment for acute synovitis with moderate to advanced hyperemia is direct injection of betamethasone into the subintimal tissue of the synovial membrane, preferably under arthroscopic control.

Connective Tissue Pathology: Arthritides

Rheumatoid Arthritis

Rheumatoid arthritis (RA) is basically a synovial disease. Although cartilage and bone are frequently involved, this is a consequence of the destructive process in the synovium. The reported incidence of TMJ involvement varies from 2% to 86%, reflecting the lack of definite clinical and radiographic criteria for RA of the TMJ.[23–25] RA of the TMJ largely resembles that of other synovial joints. However, it difficult to differentiate RA from other joint disorders, such as osteoarthrosis, because the clinical signs and symptoms often coincide. When there is symmetric involvement of the TMJ with changes in occlusion that cause a progressive open bite, RA should be suspected. However, the abnormal open bite often occurs late in the disease when destruction of cartilage and subchondral bone has already appeared. Although radiographic examination has been the basis for diagnosis of osteoarthrosis and RA, the radiographic features of TMJ RA are not specific except for erosions, which provide no information on the degree of cartilage destruction.

Arthroscopic Findings

Arthroscopic examination often reveals increased vascularity, capillary hyperemia, granulation formation, villus formation, effusion, and fibrotic synovium. Cartilage exhibits fibrillation, lesions of cartilage and subchondral bone, and bone exposure and eburnation. Other features may be found depending on the severity of the disease. Marked fibrosis or even ankylosis may occur in the joints. In these cases even arthroscopic examination may not be possible. Arthroscopy can be used for obtaining synovial biopsies.

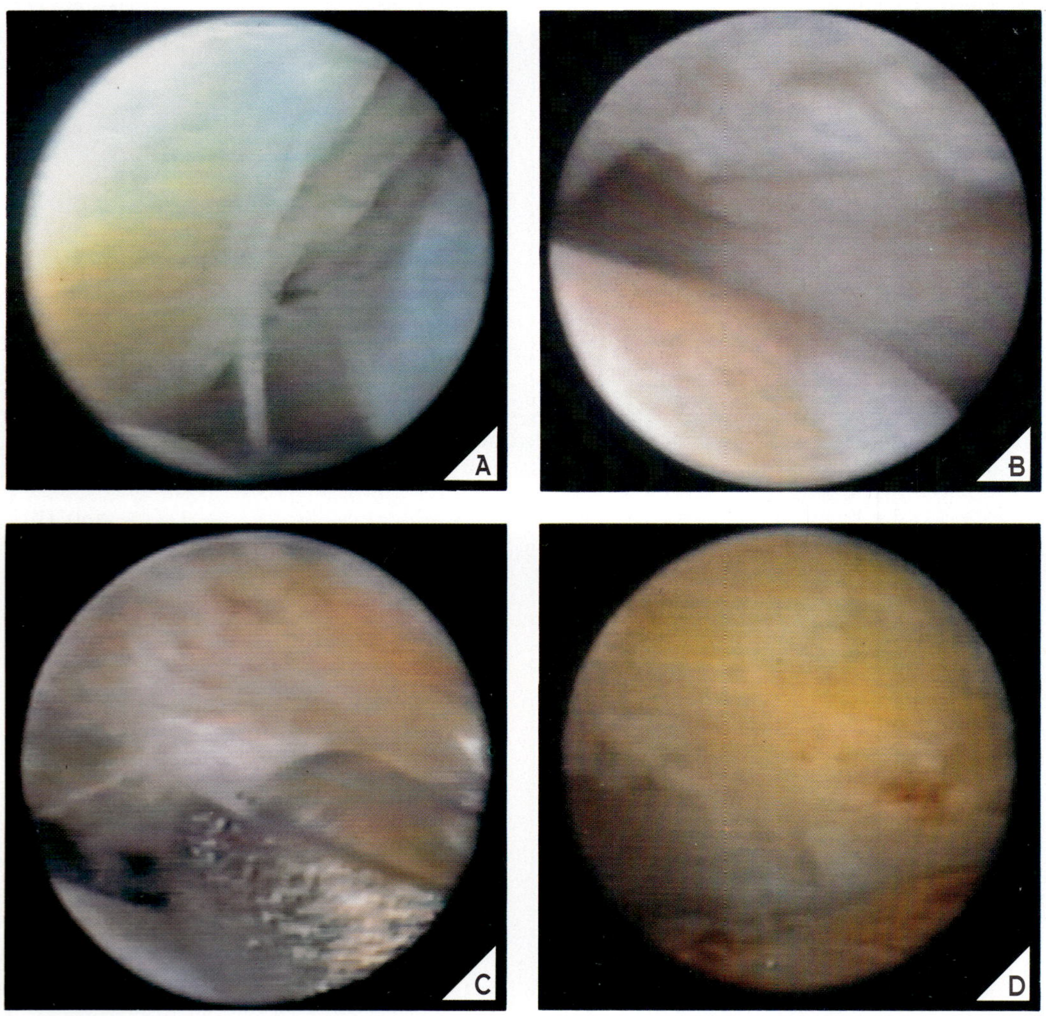

Figure 26.35

(A) Chondromalacia grade I. (B) Chondromalacia grade II. (C) The motorized shaver used in a case of chondromalacia grade III. (D) Chondromalacia grade IV showing subchondral bone exposure. (Courtesy of Dr. Robert Schwartz)

Treatment

Rheumatoid arthritis is a systemic disease and should be treated as such initially. Local treatment of the different joints and physical therapy of the muscle groups involved are often necessary. A team approach involving the various disciplines of medicine and surgery is most appropriate for the management of RA. Nonsurgical management of RA of the TMJ includes fabrication of an orthotic appliance.

Arthroscopic management of RA seems most appropriate (Fig. 26.36). Irrigation of the TMJ with isotonic saline solution has been effective in alleviating symptoms in RA, probably by removing debris and other inflammatory products. Irrigation with diluted sodium hyaluronate seems to be another alternative.[26]

Intraarticular injections of steroids have proven effective, although there is some concern about the local effects on the joint cartilage. No side effects have been reported with the use of sodium hyaluronate, which may therefore be preferable to steroids. Placement of sodium hyaluronate into the TMJ is a relatively simple procedure and can be performed simultaneously with the arthroscopic examination. Subsynovial injections into small areas of inflammation of small quantities of steroids can be done under direct arthroscopic control.

Hypertrophic synovium or redundant tissue is often found in joints with advanced RA, covering the cartilage, isolating it from nutrition, and thereby rendering it nonviable. Synovectomy is best performed with minishavers and should be done under arthroscopic control. Since bleeding often obscures visibility, the procedure is best suited to cases with well-defined lesions.

Fibrosis and adhesions that impair joint mobility are frequently found in RA joints. Hand instruments and motorized shavers can be used to cut or remove these bands under direct arthroscopic observation.

In certain cases involving the TMJ (e.g., marked immobility due to fibrosis or bony ankylosis), arthroscopy may be a poor surgical option. These cases are probably better managed via arthrotomy procedures.

Juvenile Rheumatoid Arthritis

The inflammatory arthritides that begin in childhood are collectively known as juvenile rheumatoid arthritis (JRA) and undoubtedly represent diseases of various etiologies. Patients with JRA become ill before the age of 16. About 25% of patients have involvement of the TMJ.

The classic systemic inflammatory arthritis of childhood is Still's disease, which on rare occasions begins in the third or fourth decade. TMJ involvement is relatively common in children. Inflammation of the joint may lead to ankylosis, and the chronic illness may disturb the growth centers and lead to micrognathia.

One subtype of JRA, primarily affecting very young girls, consists of an oligoarthritis that mainly involves the large joints of the lower extremity. Affected children have chronic, symmetric, erosive polyarthritis that is RF-positive. The disease may progress to a deforming arthritis that is indistinguishable from classic RA in adults. The arthroscopic findings and treatment of JRA with TMJ involvement are identical to those for RA in adults.

Psoriatic Arthritis

Psoriatic arthritis occurs in approximately 5% of patients with psoriasis. Destructive changes in the TMJ may be seen on radiographic studies.[27,28] A confident diagnosis can be made when the patient presents with the typical pattern of joint involvement together with skin lesions of psoriasis or the typical changes of psoriatic nail disease. The arthroscopic findings and surgical treatment are similar to those of RA.

Systemic Lupus Erythematosus

Systemic lupus erythematosus (SLE) is a chronic inflammatory autoimmune disease of unknown etiology. Genetic, hormonal, and environmental factors are all known to play a role. The female-to-male ratio in SLE is 10:1. Musculoskeletal features of SLE include arthralgias, arthritis, and tenosynovitis. Arthropathy findings may mimic those of RA; however, the deformities are easily reducible. Involvement of the TMJ is unusual but has been reported.[29,30]

Classic features of the disease process in the synovium include one or all of the following: synovial proliferation showing increased vascularity and capillary hyperemia, villus formation, effusion, and fibrosis. In cartilage, fibrillation, lesions of cartilage in the subchondral bone, and/or areas of bony exposure with eburnation may be present.

Treatment

SLE is a systemic disease that is managed with systemic therapy (steroids and/or cytotoxic drugs) as well as local treatment. Effective management and treatment when the

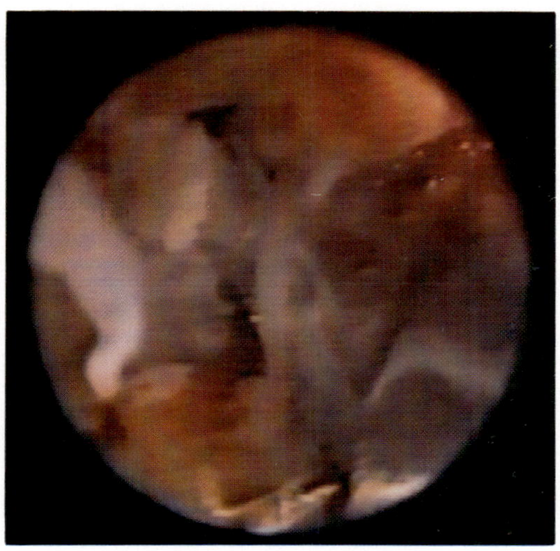

Figure 26.36
Debridement with basket forceps in a case of rheumatoid arthritis.

TMJ is involved uses a combination of nonsurgical and surgical modalities. The former include fabrication and use of an orthotic and physical rehabilitation, along with a change of dietary habits to include nonchewing soft foods. Patients with thrombosis may be treated with anticoagulants, which of course should be discontinued if possible before any surgical procedure. It is very important to have a complete evaluation of the patient (in particular, a hematologic work-up) before surgery.

A patient group treated at the Hospital for Joint Diseases Orthopaedic Institute, New York, has responded fairly well to nonsurgical therapy and alteration of dietary intake. These patients often present with pain specific to the joint area, with a limited interincisal opening registering between 10 and 20 mm.

Arthroscopic treatment includes simple lysis with lavage and/or joint debridement with partial or subtotal synovial resection, using the suction punch or motorized minishavers (Fig. 26.37).

Postoperative Management

Successful arthroscopic outcome is dependent on early mobilization of the joints. Restoration of a normal rotation–translation relationship should be maintained in all phases of opening via joint mobilization of the TMJs bilaterally. The goal is to maintain disc mobility.

The patient is instructed to resume the use of the orthotic postoperatively to unload the joint. Specific instructions for the use of the orthotic will be given by the patient's treating dentist.

A nonchewing diet should be observed for at least 3 months after surgery. Periodic evaluations will determine whether the patient can move up to a normal diet.

Pharmaceutical management after arthroscopy includes a short-term and a long-term postoperative phase. The short-term postoperative phase begins with the hospital discharge and continues for approximately 6 to 8 weeks. The considerations during this period include control of postoperative pain so that physical therapy can be initiated and reduction of swelling or stiffness and inflammation of the joints, for which nonsteroidal antiinflammatory agents are useful. The long-term postoperative phase begins 6 weeks after surgery. If pain persists beyond this period, the preoperative diagnosis should be reconsidered to rule out coexisting disease and search for a nonarticular origin. Semisynthetic narcotic combinations and nonsteroidal antiinflammatory agents are useful during this period, and mood elevators and antianxiety drugs have also been shown to be effective.

Complications and Pitfalls

When arthroscopy of the TMJ was billed as a less invasive procedure with a higher therapeutic success rate than traditional arthrotomy, there was a stampede towards clinical application of this new technology. Although our initial experiences were with diagnosis, lysis, and lavage, few isolated complications were reported in the literature. Intraoperative bleeding and transient peripheral facial nerve weakness were reported by Goss and Bosanquet[31] and Holmlund and colleagues.[32] However, these complications were similar to those reported for traditional arthrotomy procedures. Several serious surgical misadventures started to appear in the literature as more complex operative arthroscopic procedures were undertaken. In 1987, Carter and Testa[33] performed the first multicenter retrospective study. The large patient sample underwent diagnostic procedures, lysis, and lavage, with a global complication rate of 10%. Small's prospective study reported an overall complication rate of 1.86% for arthroscopy of the knee and other joints. Review of the complications revealed, first, that most were perioperative and transient and, second, that some of the more serious complications had not been previously seen with TMJ arthrotomy.

Upper airway obstruction has been reported secondary to puncture of the medial capsule of the TMJ by an improperly placed outflow cannula or extravasation of irrigant into the lateral pharyngeal space. White[34] described two such cases that required prolonged intubation in the recovery room. A sound knowledge of the joint anatomy and strict attention to puncture techniques, including the depth of insertion of the trocar and cannula into the intraarticular space, can reduce the risk of complications. The airway should be checked before extubation.

Some practitioners use local anesthetics to distend the joint and promote hemostasis during the diagnostic

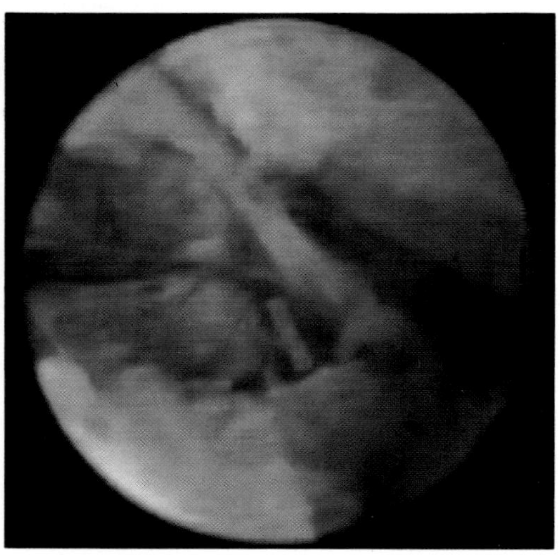

Figure 26.37
A case of SLE being debrided with a suction punch.

phase. Too rapid absorption of the anesthetic can cause cardiac arrhythmias. Jones and Horn reported a case in which a patient developed premature ventricular contractions with bigeminy. Inadvertent massage of the carotid body during forced manipulation of the mandible may cause bradycardia.

The overall rate of infection in TMJ arthroscopy was less than 1%, as reported by Carter and Testa.[33] Although arthroscopic procedures may be contraindicated in the presence of an infection, Murakami and colleagues[35] reported the successful use of arthroscopy to diagnose suppurative arthritis in the TMJ. Sanders[36] reported one case of otitis media secondary to TMJ arthroscopy. Greene and Van Sickels[37] reported a case of external otitis after lysis and lavage. Although Small[38] implicated both staphylococcal and streptococcal organisms in postoperative infection, no causative organism was named in the reported cases of infection after TMJ arthroscopy. Surgeons, including myself, have approached this problem empirically; an example is the prophylactic use of 1 g cephalexin preoperatively followed by oral cephalexin 500 mg every 6 hours for 5 days.

Neurologic injuries are the most common complications reported in the larger retrospective studies by Greene and Van Sickels[37] and by Carter and Testa.[33] As noted earlier, the roof of the glenoid fossa is a thin bony lamina that is at risk for perforation by an arthroscope or trocar. McCain[7] reported puncture of the fossa and dura resulting in a cerebrospinal fluid leak. A neurosurgeon was consulted and the planned procedure was carried out, with an uneventful postoperative course. Schellhas and colleagues reported destruction of the roof of the fossa by enlarging granulomas in patients who had received a Teflon–Proplast implant. Arthroscopy in these patients may be contraindicated because of the increased risk of perforation into the middle cranial fossa.

The proximity of the cranial nerves V and VII to the capsule of the TMJ renders them more vulnerable to injury. Injuries to these nerves are usually secondary to extravasation of fluid during arthroscopic procedures. There is a greater risk of injury to the branch of the facial nerve compared with those of the trigeminal nerve, although this is usually transient. These risks are important because of the cosmetic and ophthalmologic considerations (Fig. 26.38).

The infraorbital nerve, lingual nerve, and inferior alveolar nerve—all branches of the trigeminal nerve—may be involved by fluid extravasation during arthroscopy. The resulting hypoesthesia is often transient. Inadvertent puncture of the medial capsule causes medial extravasation of fluid into the pterygomandibular space and exerts hydrostatic pressure on the lingual and inferior alveolar nerves. Mechanical injury to the inferior alveolar nerve has been reported by Heffez and Blaustein.[39] It is speculated that the jaws of the towel clamp placed at the angle of the mandible to distract it for interarticular procedures

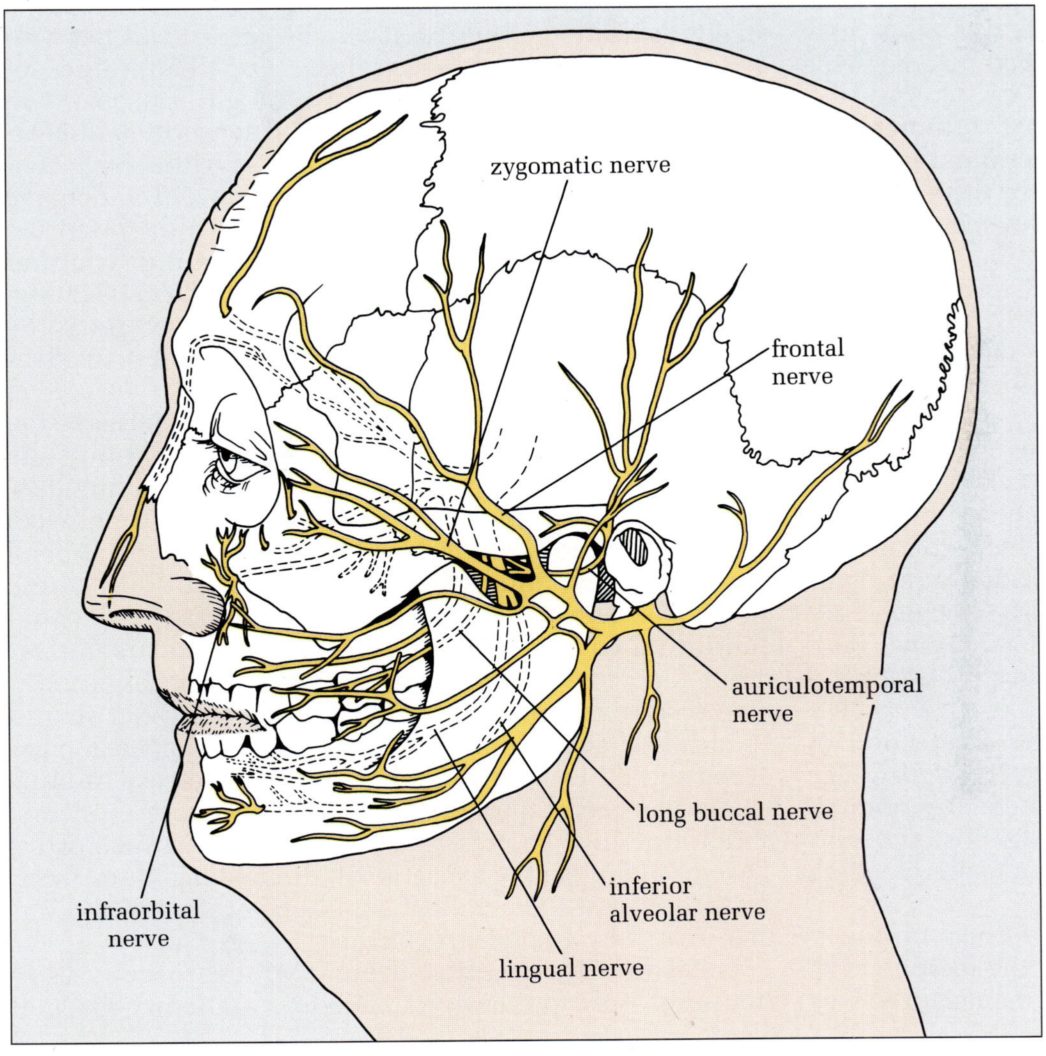

Figure 26.38
Neuroanatomy surrounding the TMJ.

perforated the lateral cortex of the mandible, resulting in compression injury. Postoperative hypoesthesia of the auriculotemporal nerve is frequently encountered in TMJ arthroscopy because of its proximity to the lateral capsule of the joint. The most common injuries include severance, contusion, hydrostatic pressure, and local hematoma secondary to rupture of the adjacent posterior capsular veins. Operative time may be prolonged and fluid extravasation is most likely to occur when surgeons are first becoming acquainted with arthroscopy or when they are performing advanced operative techniques. My practical advice is to limit operative time to approximately 1 hour per joint.

The most common VII nerve injury reported is to the temporozygomatic branch of the facial nerve. Joint entry as described by Murakami and Ono[40] was designed to reduce the risk of injury to this nerve. Although various techniques to reduce the risk have been described by others, reports of injury to this nerve remain frequent. The incidence was reported as 4% in the review by Carter and Testa and as 0.56% by Greene and Van Sickels. All of these injuries were transient except for one documented case of complete facial nerve paralysis reported by Appelbaum and colleagues. The patient in this case had previously undergone open joint surgery and may therefore have represented a higher risk for arthroscopy.

Management of a persistent temporozygomatic injury is directed towards prevention of corneal desiccation and abrasion. Taping of the eyelid at night and use of artificial tears are beneficial. Oculoplastic consultation for a lateral tarsorrhaphy is mandated for the unusual case of total paralysis. The potential risk for injury to this nerve may increase as more advanced operative procedures requiring greater access are developed.

The vascular structures that are most vulnerable to injury during TMJ arthroscopy are the terminal branches of the external carotid and the branches of the superficial temporal vein (Fig. 26.39). Operative arthroscopy requires multiple portals and multiple punctures. Palpation of the superficial temporal artery before joint distention will help to avoid penetration of the vessel. Injury to the superficial temporal artery will result in rapid high-pressure bleeding, which can usually be controlled by direct digital pressure. A hematoma may result, and the arthroscopic procedure should be aborted if the anatomic landmarks are obscured. Greene and Van Sickels[37] reported a case that required ligation. Moses and Topper[41] reported a postoperative arteriovenous fistula after TMJ arthroscopy. A secondary surgical procedure was performed to ligate the fistula. Preisler and associates[42] reported a case of AV fistula that was treated initially with interventional radiology. Successful embolization was followed by surgical resection of the lesion.

Carter and Testa[33] reported that the likelihood of venous injury was much greater than arterial injury. The two posterior capsular veins, which are usually nonpalpable, and the possible engorgement of the posterior portion of the deep temporal vein represent a major bleeding hazard.

Advanced operative techniques and the use of power shavers for synovectomy have increased the likelihood of intraarticular bleeding. Small reported hemarthrosis as the most frequent complication of orthopedic arthroscopy, although to date there have been no reported cases of postoperative hemarthrosis of the TMJ. Hypotensive anesthesia, local vasoconstrictors, and good visualization during the use of power instrumentation will help to prevent or control intraarticular bleeding.

For the most part, instrument failure in TMJ arthroscopy has occurred as a result of metal defects. Most of the newer instruments for TMJ arthroscopy are merely scaled-down versions of existing orthopedic instruments, and are therefore more delicate and fragile. Instrument retrieval is often performed by either grasping forceps or a magnetic probe. The "golden retriever" is helpful in retrieving metal fragments. In two reported cases the use of an angiocatheter as an evacuation cannula resulted in fragmentation of the distal tip, which became a loose body within the joint. In one case the tip was retrieved by grasping forceps; the other required an arthrotomy procedure. The use of nonmetallic instruments is strongly discouraged.

Most of the otologic injuries resulting from TMJ arthroscopy have been transient. However, a few patients have sustained permanent deficits. The close proximity of the temporomandibular joint to the ear canal is responsible for most of these complications.

Sanders reported the first case of otitis media with a slight hearing impairment as the only complication in a large series of cases. Van Sickels and colleagues[43] reported a case in which a blunt trocar accidentally slid posteromedially through the ear canal and entered the inner ear, causing perforation of the tympanic membrane and a slight dislocation of the malleus. The patient was left with a residual 15 dB conductive loss. Appelbaum and coworkers reported three cases of otologic injuries. Two patients developed severe to profound sensorineural hearing loss, and the third had a hearing loss with a large conductive component. Two of these patients had undergone previous open joint surgery that may have distorted the anatomic structures and landmarks. The authors further postulated that the sensorineural loss may have been secondary to damage to the oval or round window caused by increased pressure of the irrigation solution that accidentally entered the middle ear.

There have been several reports of minor injuries to the external auditory canal resulting from contusion of the anterior wall. Several patients had transient hearing loss. Reported perforations of the external auditory canal were usually between the junction of the tragus and the bony portion of the canal. Bleeding from such lacerations should be controlled with cautery, and the ear canal should be treated with antibiotics/hydrocortisone ear drops for 1 to 2 weeks. In external otitis probably caused by moisture remaining in the ear canal, the canal should be cleansed and antibiotic/hydrocortisone suspension ear drops should be placed. Although only one case of otitis media has been reported after TMJ arthroscopy, systemic antibiotics must be prescribed immediately in such cases. The antibiotic of choice is amoxicillin 500 mg, three times daily for 7 days. The patient should be evaluated and further treated by an otolaryngologist.

Local injuries resulting from TMJ arthroscopy have included postoperative capsulitis, cutaneous thermal injury, and atrophy of the subcutaneous fat in the preauricular area. Postoperative capsulitis occurs quite often, due to violation of the skin and capsular structures by the arthroscopic instruments. It is usually transient and the pain is managed with nonsteroidal antiinflammatory medications.

Cutaneous injury resulting from the cautery is rare. The surgeon should be aware of the position of the electrode tip relative to the cannula, since contact between the active electrode and the cannula can result in a circumferential cutaneous injury.

Goldberg and colleagues[44] reported a case of subcutaneous fat atrophy after TMJ arthroscopy with the use of 10% triamcinolone acetonide. This phenomenon is most often observed in premenopausal women. The resultant postoperative preauricular depression was presumed to be secondary to fat atrophy. The authors state that this complication appeared after 6 months, and have suggested limiting the site of insoluble steroids to deep in injections, using the lowest effective concentration, and avoiding drug escape from deeper to superficial planes to minimize problems of fat atrophy.

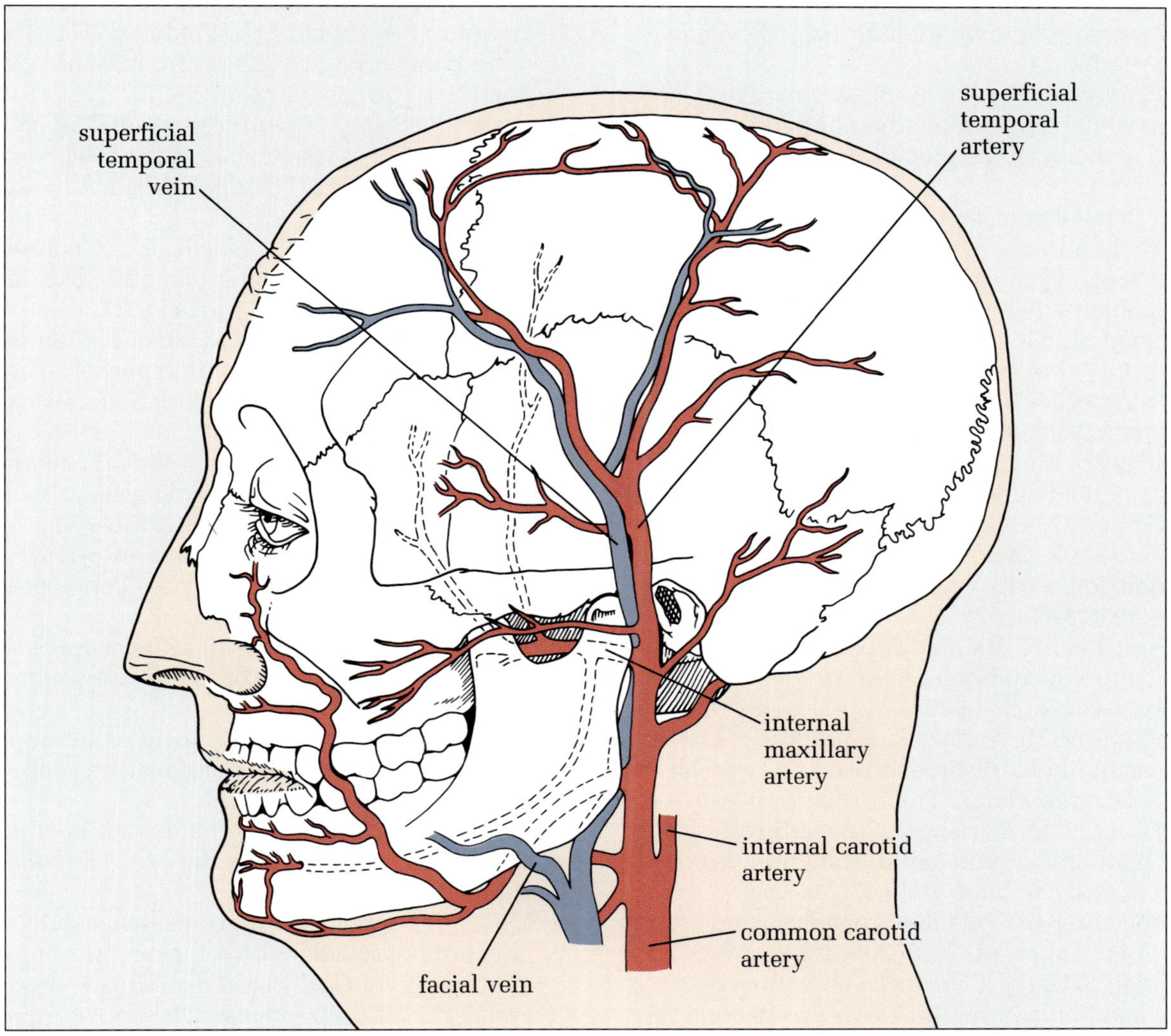

Figure 26.39
Arterial and venous blood supply around the TMJ.

REFERENCES

1. Murakami K-I. Arthroscopic anatomy, histology and visual fields in the temporomandibular joint. In: Thomas M, Bronstein SL, eds. *Arthroscopy of the Temporomandibular Joint.* Philadelphia, Pa: WB Saunders Co; 1991:140–153.
2. Thomas M. Diagnostic and operative arthroscopy of the temporomandibular joint. In: Thomas M, Bronstein SL, eds. *Arthroscopy of the Temporomandibular Joint.* Philadelphia, Pa: WB Saunders Co; 1991:154–164.
3. Bronstein SL. Surgical procedures and techniques. In: Thomas M, Bronstein SL, eds. *Arthroscopy of the Temporomandibular Joint.* Philadelphia, Pa: WB Saunders Co; 1991:166–186.
4. Bradrick JP, Eckhauser ML, Indresano AT. Morphologic and histologic changes in canine temporomandibular joint tissues following arthroscopic guided neodymium: YAG laser exposure. *J Oral Maxillofac Surg.* 1989;47:1177
5. Holmlund A, Hellsing G. Arthroscopy of the temporomandibular joint. *Int J Oral Surg.* 1985;14:169–175.
6. Murakami K-I, Ono T: Temporomandibular joint arthroscopy by infero-lateral approach. *J Oral Maxillofac Surg.* 1986;15:410–417.

7. McCain JP. Arthroscopy of the human temporomandibular joint. *J Oral Maxillofac Surg.* 1988;46:648–655.
8. Ohnishi M. Kokubyu Gakkai, Zasshi J. *Japan Stomatol Soc.* 1982;31:487–512.
9. Ohnishi M. *Arthroscopy.* 1984;9:43–48.
10. Ohnishi M. Proceedings of the Symposium on TMJ Arthroscopy. Southern California OMFS Foundation; 1986.
11. Kaminishi RM, Davis CL. Intra-capsular fibrosis of the superior compartment of the temporomandibular joint. In: Thomas M, Bronstein SL, eds. *Arthroscopy of the Temporomandibular Joint.* Philadelphia, Pa: WB Saunders Co; 1991:235–243.
12. Sanders B, Buoncristiani R. Diagnostic and surgical arthroscopy of the TMJ: clinical experience with 137 patients over 2 years. *Craniomandibular Disorder Facial Oral Pain.* 1987;1:202–213.
13. Blankestijn J, Panders A, Vermey A, Scherpbier AJ. Synovial chondromatosis of the temporomandibular joint: report of three cases and a review of the literature. *Cancer.* 1985; 55:479–485.
14. Casselman JW, Demeulemeister L, Bossuyt M, et al. CT findings in synovial chondromatosis of the temporomandibular joint. *J Comput Assist Tomogr.* 1987;11:898–900.
15. Forsell K, Happonen R, Forsell H. Synovial chondromatosis of the temporomandibular joint: report of a case and review of the literature. *Int J Oral Maxillofac Surg.* 1988;17:237–241.
16. Axhausen G. Pathologie und Therapie des Kiefergelenkes. *Fortschr Zahnheilk.* 1933;9:171–186.
17. Silver CM, Simon SD, Litchman HM, Dyckman J. Synovial chondromatosis of the temporomandibular joint. *J Bone Joint Surg.* 1971;53A:777–780.
18. Sun S, Helmy E, Bays R. Synovial chondromatosis with intracranial extension: a case report. *Oral Surg Oral Med Oral Pathol.* 1990;70:5–9.
19. Von Arx DP, Simpson MT, Batman P. Synovial chondromatosis of the temporomandibular joint. *Br J Oral Maxillofac Surg.* 1988;26:297–305.
20. Stegenga B, de Bont LGM, Boering G. A proposed classification of temporomandibular disorders based on synovial joint pathology. *J Craniomandib Pract.* 1989;7:107–118.
21. Stegenga B, de Bont LGM, Boering G. Osteoarthrosis as the cause of craniomandibular pain and dysfunction: a unifying concept. *J Oral Maxillofac Surg.* 1989;47:249–256.
22. Quinn JH. Pathogenesis of TMJ chondromalacia and arthralgia. *Oral Maxillofac Surg Clin North Am.* 1989;1:47–57.
23. Carlsson GE, Kopp S, Oberg T. Arthritis and allied diseases of the temporomandibular joint. In: Zarb GA, Carlsson GE, eds. *Temporomandibular Joint Function and Dysfunction.* St. Louis, Mo: CV Mosby Co: 1979:293–320.
24. Ogus H. Rheumatoid arthritis of the temporomandibular joint. *Br J Oral Surg.* 1975;12:275–284.
25. Tegelberg A, Kopp S. Clinical findings in the stomatognathic system for individuals with rheumatoid arthritis and osteoarthritis. *Acta Odontol Scand.* 1987;45:65–75.
26. Weiss C. Basic structures of di-arthrodial joints. In: Parisien JS, ed. *Arthroscopic Surgery.* New York, NY: McGraw-Hill; 1988:3–18.
27. Kononen M. Clinical signs of craniomandibular disorders in patients with psoriatic arthritis. *Scand J Dent Res.* 1987; 95:340–346.
28. Kudryk WH, Baker GL, Percy JS. Ankylosis of the temporomandibular joint from psoriatic arthritis. *J Otolaryngol.* 1985;14:336.
29. Liebling MR Gold RH. Erosions of the temporomandibular joint in systemic lupus erythematosus. *Arthritis Rheum.* 1981;24:948.
30. Gerbracht D, Shapiro L. Temporomandibular joint erosions in systemic lupus erythematosus. *Arthritis Rheum.* 1982;25:597. Letter.
31. Goss AN, Bosanquet AG. Temporomandibular joint arthroscopy. *J Oral Maxillofac Surg.* 1986;44:614–617.
32. Holmlund A, Hellsing G, Wredmark T. Arthroscopy of the temporomandibular joint: a clinical study. *Int J Oral Maxillofac Surg.* 1986;15:715–721.
33. Carter JB, Testa L. Complications of TMJ arthroscopy: a reviews 2,225 cases. Review of the 1988 Annual Scientific Sessions Abstracts. *J Oral Maxillofacial Surg.* 1988;46: M14–M15.
34. White RD. Retrospective analysis 100 consecutive surgical arthroscopies of the temporomandibular joint. *J Oral Maxillofac Surg.* 1989;47:1014–1021.
35. Murakami K, Matsumoto K, Izuka T. Suppurative arthritis of the temporomandibular joint: report of a case with special reference to arthroscopy observations. *J Maxillofac Surg.* 1984;112:41–45.
36. Sanders B. Arthroscopic surgery of the temporomandibular joint: treatment of internal derangement with persistent closed lock. *Oral Surg.* 1986;62:361–372.
37. Greene MW, Van Sickels JE. Survey of TMJ arthroscopy in oral and maxillofacial surgery residency programs. *J Oral Maxillofac Surg.* 47:574–576.
38. Small NC. Complications in arthroscopic surgery performed by experienced arthroscopists. *J Arthroscopic Rel Surg.* 1988;4:215–221.
39. Heffez L, Blaustein D. Diagnostic arthroscopy of the temporomandibular joint, I: normal arthroscopy findings. *Oral Surg.* 1987;64:653–670.
40. Murakami K, Ono T. Temporomandibular joint arthroscopy by infero-lateral approach. *Int J Oral Maxillofac Surg.* 1986;15:410–417.
41. Moses JJ, Topper DL. Arteriovenous fistula: an unusual complication associated with arthroscopic temporomandibular joint surgery. *J Oral Maxillofac Surg.* 1990;48:1220–1222.
42. Preisler SA, Koorbusch GF, Olson RAJ. An acquired arteriovenous fistula secondary to temporomandibular joint arthroscopy: report of a case. *J Oral Maxillofac Surg.* 1991;49:187–190.
43. Van Sickels JE, Nishioka GJ, Hegewald MD, et al. Middle ear injury resulting from temporomandibular joint arthroscopy. *J Oral Maxillofacial Surg.* 1987;45:962–965.
44 Goldberg JS, Julian JB, Dachille R. Local subcutaneous atrophy following arthroscopy of the TMJ. *J Oral Maxillofac Surg.* 1989;47:986–987.

Index